Marilyn Barrett, PhD
Editor

The Handbook
of Clinically Tested
Herbal Remedies
Volume 1

More pre-publication
REVIEWS, COMMENTARIES, EVALUATIONS . . .

"This book includes profiles on thirty-two individual herbal medicines and ten combination formulas. These profiles include descriptions of most of the major published clinical studies, which have been analyzed by a panel of authoritative reviewers. It is obvious that great care was taken to ensure completeness and accuracy of information, and the reviewers' comments regarding study quality are especially informative and helpful.

Clinicians searching for detailed and accurate information on herbal clinical trials will find much in this text that is useful. It is a significant achievement in the field of evidence-based analyses of herbal medicine. It should be of most help to clinicians or researchers who want specific details on herbal clinical studies that are not readily available, or who are interested in clinical-trial-quality assessments by authoritative reviewers."

Michael Rotblatt, MD, PharmD
Associate Clinical Professor of Medicine, UCLA; Co-author,
Evidence-Based Herbal Medicine

❧

"The purpose of this book is to provide both consumers and health care providers with concise, evidence-based information on the most widely used herbs and herbal formulas tested in clinical trials. The focus is on what preparations have been studied in clin-ical trials and how good the evidence is as assessed by preset criteria applied by botanical experts.

The book is broken down into three parts. The first section is very informative and sets the stage nicely for a discussion of individual herbs. The second part describes the process of evidence gathering, sorting, grading, and peer review. Those readers familiar with the Natural Standard database of natural products will recognize the editor's use of 'levels of evidence' criteria as a useful tool to distill the information available from clinical trials. In the third part, the authors provide monographs on the various herbals listed alphabetically. These are concise and cover basic questions of whether the trial was randomized and whether the methods were clearly described. One unique feature is a detailed description of specific products used in clinical trials. These are very helpful to both clinicians interested in recommending specific products and to patients interested in finding these same products at their local health food stores.

This book provides valuable information to providers and patients looking to sort out which commonly used herbs are evidence-based and particularly which specific products they should be looking for."

Philippe O. Szapary, MD
Assistant Professor of Medicine, Division of General Internal Medicine, University of Pennsylvania School of Medicine

The Handbook
of Clinically Tested
Herbal Remedies
Volume 1

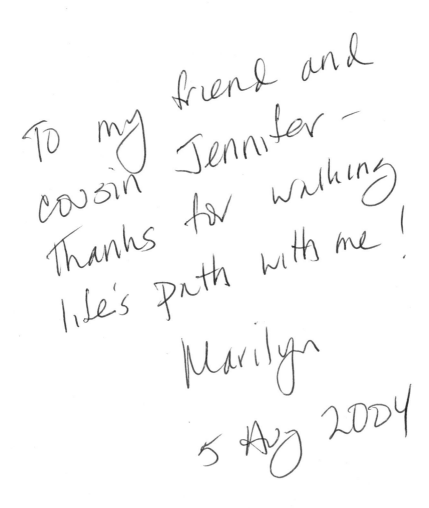

To my friend and
cousin Jennifer —
Thanks for walking
life's path with me!

Marilyn

5 Aug 2004

Haworth Series in Evidence-Based Phytotherapy
Marilyn Barrett, PhD
Editor

The Handbook of Clinically Tested Herbal Remedies edited by Marilyn Barrett

Other titles of related interest:

Herbal Medicine: Chaos in the Marketplace by Rowena K. Richter

Botanical Medicines: The Desk Reference for Major Herbal Supplements, Second Edition by Dennis J. McKenna, Kenneth Jones, and Kerry Hughes

Tyler's Tips: The Shopper's Guide for Herbal Remedies by George H. Constantine

Handbook of Psychotropic Herbs: A Scientific Analysis of Herbal Remedies for Psychiatric Conditions by Ethan B. Russo

Tyler's Honest Herbal: A Sensible Guide to the Use of Herbs and Related Remedies, Fourth Edition by Steven Foster and Varro E. Tyler

Tyler's Herbs of Choice: The Therapeutic Use of Phytomedicinals, Second Edition by James E. Robbers and Varro E. Tyler

The Handbook
of Clinically Tested
Herbal Remedies
Volume 1

Part I: Fundamentals of Herbal Medicine
Part II: Methods
Part III: Botanical Profiles—
Product and Clinical Trial Information
(Artichoke–Ginseng)

Marilyn Barrett, PhD
Editor

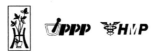

The Haworth Herbal Press®
Pharmaceutical Products Press®
The Haworth Medical Press®
Imprints of The Haworth Press, Inc.
New York • London • Oxford

Published by

The Haworth Herbal Press®, Pharmaceutical Products Press®, and The Haworth Medical Press®, imprints of The Haworth Press, Inc., 10 Alice Street, Binghamton, NY 13904-1580.

PUBLISHER'S NOTE
This book has been published solely for educational purposes and is not intended to substitute for the medical advice of a treating physician. Medicine is an ever-changing science. As new research and clinical experience broaden our knowledge, changes in treatment may be required. While many potential treatment options are made herein, some or all of the options may not be applicable to a particular individual. Therefore, the author, editor and publisher do not accept responsibility in the event of negative consequences incurred as a result of the information presented in this book. We do not claim that this information is necessarily accurate by the rigid scientific and regulatory standards applied for medical treatment. **No Warranty, Expressed or Implied, is furnished with respect to the material contained in this book. The reader is urged to consult with his/her personal physician with respect to the treatment of any medical condition.**

Cover design by Marylouise E. Doyle.

Photography by Linda Nikaya.

Library of Congress Cataloging-in-Publication Data

The handbook of clinically tested herbal remedies, volumes 1 and 2 / Marilyn Barrett, editor.
    p. ; cm.
  Includes bibliographical references and index.
  ISBN 0-7890-1068-2 Volumes 1 and 2 (hard : alk. paper)
  ISBN 0-7890-2723-2 Volume 1 (hard : alk. paper)
  ISBN 0-7890-2724-0 Volume 2 (hard : alk. paper)
  1. Herbs—Therapeutic use—Handbooks, manuals, etc. [DNLM: 1. Plant Preparations—Handbooks. QV 39 H2362 2004] I. Barrett, Marilyn.
RM666.H33H363 2004
615'.321—dc22
                                         2003025270

To Dr. Varro (Tip) Tyler, who believed in my abilities and sold the idea of this book to the publisher of The Haworth Press

To my parents, Geoffrey and Elizabeth Barrett, whose faith and confidence in me has enabled me to embark on this book, and many other adventures

CONTENTS

VOLUME 1

ABOUT THE EDITOR

Marilyn Barrett, PhD, is founder and principal of Pharmacognosy Consulting, whose mission is to provide a scientific foundation for botanical medicine. She was awarded a PhD in pharmacognosy from the School of Pharmacy, University of London, UK, in 1985 and a BA in botany from the University of California, Berkeley, CA, in 1977.

Since 1994, Dr. Barrett has provided scientific information and technical expertise to manufacturers, associations, and government concerning medicinal plant products through her consulting business. She is a member of the United States Pharmacopeia Committee of Experts for Dietary Supplements Information, an external advisory board member for the University of California at Los Angeles Center for Dietary Supplements (an NIH-funded center) and a consultant to the Office of Dietary Supplements in preparation of their botanical fact sheets. Dr. Barrett served on a working group for the Institute of Medicine of the National Academy of Sciences Committee developing a Framework for Evaluating the Safety of Dietary Supplements. She is a member of the American Botanical Council Advisory Board, the American Herbal Pharmacopoeia and Therapeutic Compendium Technical Advisory Board, and the American Herbal Products Association's Scientific Advisory Board.

Dr. Barrett has published over 30 publications in peer-reviewed journals and a booklet titled *Reference on Evaluating Botanicals* for the Council for Responsible Nutrition, in 1998. More information is available on her Web site at <www.pharmacognosy.com>.

CONTRIBUTORS

Authors of Chapters in Part I

Anthony L. Almada, MSc, has worked within the dietary supplement industry since 1975. He has a BSc in physiology with a nutritional biochemistry minor from California State University, Long Beach, and an MSc from Berkeley (with a research thesis in antioxidant-exercise biochemistry). He is the cofounder/past president of Experimental and Applied Sciences (EAS) and is the founder/CSO of IMAGINutrition, Inc., a nutritional technology creation, clinical research, and intellectual property-driven think tank/incubator. He has been a coinvestigator on over 65 university and research institute clinical trials, ranging from AIDS/HIV to osteoarthritis.

Ezra Béjar, PhD, is a phytopharmacologist with more than 15 years of experience in the concept development, testing, and launching of botanical supplements. He is the principal of Plant Bioassay, a consulting company that serves the dietary supplement industry, government, and academia. Dr. Béjar also acts as adjunct professor in the College of Sciences at San Diego State University. He is the author of two books, several chapters, and numerous scientific articles. Dr. Béjar currently serves as a book review editor for the journal *Phytomedicine* and as a member of the advisory board of the journal *Phytotherapy Research*.

Joseph M. Betz, PhD, is Director of the Dietary Supplements Methods and Reference Materials Program at the National Institutes of Health (NIH) Office of Dietary Supplements. Prior to this, he spent 12 years as a research chemist at the Food and Drug Administration (FDA) Center for Food Safety and Applied Nutrition. He has been a principal investigator in the National Cancer Institute's (NCI) "Designer Foods" program as well as project manager for FDA's "Plant Toxins" and "Chemical, Biological, and Toxicological Characterization of Food Plants" research programs. Dr. Betz has a PhD in pharmacognosy and over 30 publications in the areas of plant toxins and botanical dietary supplements.

Anton Biber, PhD, studied food chemistry at the University of Karlsruhe. He received his PhD at the University of Würzburg in 1984 and subsequently joined a research group at the University of Munich. Since 1987 he has been head of the Bioanalytical Department of Dr. Willmar Schwabe GmbH & Co., Karlsruhe, Germany. His interest is pharmacokinetics of herbal medicinal products.

Joerg Gruenwald, PhD, is an international expert in the field of botanicals and natural ingredients and the author of the *Physicians' Desk Reference (PDR) for Herbal Medicines.* He is a member of the Ad Hoc Advisory Committee of the Office of Dietary Supplements of the NIH and chairman of the International Committee of the American Herbal Products Association. Dr. Gruenwald is president of Analyze & Realize, Inc. with its subsidiaries Phytopharm Consulting and Phytopharm Research in Berlin. The companies' activities range from market analysis, product development, and clinical trials to regulatory affairs for the natural and functional food industry.

Loren D. Israelsen, JD, is president of the LDI Group in Salt Lake City, Utah, a consulting firm specializing in the regulatory and commercial development of herbs, dietary supplements, and other natural products. Mr. Israelsen has previously served as president of Nature's Way Products, Inc., and as an advisor to the National Institutes of Health, the Food and Drug Administration, and foreign governments on dietary supplement policy.

Uwe Koetter, PhD, is Director of New Product Development with GlaxoSmithKline Consumer Healthcare, where he has been for the past ten years. He is responsible for development and research of over-the-counter (OTC) drugs and dietary supplements. Dr. Koetter is the author of 22 publications. He completed his PhD in pharmaceutical biology under the supervision of Professor Heinz Schilcher, president of the German Commission E. He is a fully accredited pharmacist, licensed in Germany.

Friedrich Lang, PhD, studied chemistry at the University of Heidelberg and received his PhD in 1980. He is head of the Analytical Development Department of Dr. Willmar Schwabe GmbH & Co., Karlsruhe, Germany. His special interest is stability testing and biopharmaceutical characterization of herbal medicinal products.

Tieraona Low Dog, MD, currently serves as chair of the U.S. Pharmacopeia Dietary Supplements/Botanicals Expert Panel and was a member of the White House Commission on Complementary and Alternative Medicine. A former president of the American Herbalists Guild, she has researched, practiced, and taught about herbs for more than twenty years. Dr. Low Dog is in private practice and serves on the executive advisory board for the National Institutes of Health National Center for Complementary and Alternative Medicine (NCCAM).

Stefan Spiess, RPh, is a pharmacist and food scientist. He is president of Grunwalder GmbH, a company that sells drugs and supplements of mainly natural origin in Europe, is active in the development of new products, and provides consulting advice. Prior to this, he held senior positions in quality control, research and development, regulatory, and business development for HEXAL AG. Mr. Spiess is a member of the Gesellschaft deutscher Chemiker Food Chemistry section, the Arbeitskreis pharmazeutische Verfahrenstechnik, and the Panel for Medical/Pharmaceutical Affairs of the Bundesverband der Arzneimittelhersteller.

Vijayaraghavan (Srini) Srinivasan, PhD, currently serves as Vice President of the Dietary Supplement Verification Program of the U.S. Pharmacopeia. Prior to this, Dr. Srinivasan was Director of the OTC Drugs and Dietary Supplements Division of the Information and Standards Development Department in the USP. Dr. Srinivasan has numerous publications covering various aspects of nutritional supplements such as bioavailability, in vitro dissolution of oral solid dosage forms, botanicals, aerosols, and synthetic organic chemistry. His current interest is the establishment of public standards for in vitro dissolution for botanical dietary supplements.

Varro E. Tyler, PhD, was Editor in Chief of The Haworth Herbal Press and Distinguished Professor Emeritus of Pharmacognosy in the School of Pharmacy and Pharmacal Sciences at Purdue University before his recent passing in 2001. A recognized authority on plant drugs (herbs) and their uses, he was a co-author of *Pharmacognosy and Pharmacobiotechnology,* the standard U.S. textbook in the field. Dr. Tyler authored over 300 scientific and educational publications, including more than two dozen books. He served as Purdue University's Executive Vice President for Academic Affairs for five years, and for 20 years as dean of its School of Pharmacy and Pharmacal Sciences.

Roy Upton, RH, is the executive director and editor of the American Herbal Pharmacopoeia, an organization dedicated to the development of quality control standards for botanical medicines. Mr. Upton is also vice president of the American Herbalists Guild, serves on the board of directors of the Botanical Medicine Academy, is general manager of the herbal company Planetary Formulas, and is a member of the Standards Committee of the American Herbal Products Association. Mr. Upton has also authored several books, including *St. John's Wort* and *Echinacea,* in the Good Herb series of Keats Publishing and the *Botanical Safety Handbook* published by CRC Press.

Reviewers of Clinical Trials in Part III

Karriem Ali, MD, obtained his medical degree with honors in research from Stanford University School of Medicine, along with his residency in anesthesia, intensive care, and pain management. He has extensive experience in ethnobotanical field work and is a recognized consultant and lecturer in the fields of ethnobiology and rational development of herbal products. Dr. Ali reviewed trials on dragon's blood, ginger, milk thistle, and the formulas Gastrim and Iberogast in conjunction with Dr. Aranda.

Richard Aranda, MD, obtained his degree from Stanford University School of Medicine and is board certified in internal medicine and gastroenterology. He also obtained advanced training in immunology at UCLA where he was on the faculty in the Division of Digestive Diseases. Currently, he holds the position of Associate Director, Clinical Design and Evaluation, Immunology, Bristol-Myers Squibb Co., Princeton, New Jersey. Dr. Aranda reviewed trials on dragon's blood, ginger, milk thistle, and the formulas Gastrim and Iberogast in conjunction with Dr. Ali.

Elliot Fagelman, MD, is an attending urologist at Good Samaritan Hospital, Suffern, New York, and Nyack Hospital, Nyack, New York. Dr. Fagelman reviewed trials on cranberry, pygeum, saw palmetto, grass pollen, and the formulas Cystone and Prostane in conjunction with Dr. Lowe.

Deborah A. Goebert, PhD, is assistant professor and associate director of research at the Department of Psychiatry, John A. Burns School of Medicine, University of Hawaii. She has conducted research on St. John's wort, melatonin, and kava as well as traditional healing and acupuncture. Dr. Goebert reviewed trials on St. John's wort in conjunction with Dr. Kim.

Mary Hardy, MD, a board-certified internist, is the medical director of the Cedars-Sinai Medical Center program in Integrative Medicine. Her research projects include clinical trials for herbal remedies as well as participating in an NCCAM-funded project to study barriers to integration of a hospital center of integrative medicine. Most recently, Dr. Hardy has been appointed Associate Director for the Center for Dietary Supplement Research in Botanicals at UCLA. Dr. Hardy obtained her medical degree from Louisiana State University School of Medicine in New Orleans and completed her residency in internal medicine at Tufts-New England Medical Center in Boston. Dr. Hardy reviewed trials on grape seed, hawthorn, and horse chestnut, as well as the formulas 2nd Wind and Padma.

David Heber, MD, PhD, FACP, FACN, is Director of the Center for Human Nutrition, Professor of Medicine and Public Health, Founding Chief of the Division of Clinical Nutrition in the Department of Medicine, and Founding Director of the Center for Human Nutrition, all at the University of California, Los Angeles. Dr. Heber directs the NIH Center for Dietary Supplement Research in Botanicals, the NCI-funded Clinical Nutrition Research Unit, and the NIH Nutrition and Obesity Training grants. He is a director of the American Board of Nutrition and past chair of the Education Committee of the American Society for Clinical Nutrition. Dr. Heber reviewed trials on artichoke, bilberry, cordyceps, garlic, green tea, and red yeast rice.

John Trimmer Hicks, MD, FACP, FACR, is president of Greenwood Regional Rheumatology Center, South Carolina, is on the editorial board of the journal *Phytomedicine,* and is a visiting professor at the College of Pharmacy, University of Illinois at Chicago. Dr. Hicks has over 20 years of experience in treating patients with various rheumatologic and arthritic conditions. He orchestrated worldwide clinical trials with Smith Kline (now GlaxoSmithKline) and spearheaded trials as director of the Arthritis Institute in Arlington, Virginia. He has been a member of the clinical teaching faculties of Georgetown University, West Virginia University, and Temple University. Dr. Hicks reviewed trials on cat's claw, devil's claw, evening primrose oil, and the formula Phytodolor.

Hannah L. Kim, MD, is board certified in both child/adolescent psychiatry and adult psychiatry and is in private practice in Honolulu.

She is also clinical assistant professor at the Department of Psychiatry, John A. Burns School of Medicine, University of Hawaii. She and colleagues previously published a review of St. John's wort clinical studies. For this book, Dr. Kim reviewed trials on St. John's wort in conjunction with Dr. Goebert.

Tieraona Low Dog, MD, currently serves as chair of the U.S. Pharmacopeia Dietary Supplements/Botanicals Expert Panel and was a member of the White House Commission on Complementary and Alternative Medicine. A former president of the American Herbalists Guild, she has researched, practiced, and taught about herbs for more than 20 years. Dr. Low Dog is in private practice and serves on the Executive Advisory Board for the National Institutes of Health National Center for Complementary and Alternative Medicine. Dr. Low Dog reviewed trials on black cohosh, chaste tree, red clover, and the formula Geriforte.

Franklin C. Lowe, MD, MPH, is Associate Professor of Clinical Urology at Columbia University, College of Physicians and Surgeons, Associate Director of Urology at St. Luke's-Roosevelt Hospital, chairperson of the American Urological Association Committee on Complementary and Alternative Medicine, and a member of the American Urological Association Benign Prostatic Hyperplasia Guidelines Committee. He has published extensively on phytotherapy for benign prostatic hyperplasia. Dr. Lowe reviewed trials on cranberry, pygeum, saw palmetto, grass pollen, and the formulas Cystone and Prostane in conjunction with Dr. Fagelman.

Richard D. O'Connor, MD, is Director of the Department of Clinical Research, Director of the Department of Quality Management, and chief of division and staff physician in the Division of Asthma, Allergy, and Clinical Immunology, all at Sharp Rees-Stealy Medical Group in San Diego, California. He is also Clinical Professor of Pediatrics at the School of Medicine at the University of California, San Diego. Dr. O'Connor has more than 90 publications and has participated as an investigator in over 135 phase II and phase III clinical trials. In addition, he was chairperson of the Institutional Review Board for Sharp HealthCare for six years and supervised more than 250 clinical trials annually. Dr. O'Connor reviewed trials on boxwood, butterbur, echinacea, elderberry lemon balm, and the formulas Resistex and Sinupret.

Barry S. Oken, MD, has been a member of the faculty at Oregon Health and Science University (OHSU) since 1985, where he is currently Professor in the Departments of Neurology and Behavioral Neuroscience and Director of the Oregon Center for Complementary and Alternative Medicine (CAM) in Neurological Disorders (www. ohsu.edu/orccamind) whose mission is to facilitate research and education on the effectiveness and mechanisms of action of CAM therapies in the treatment of neurological disorders. Dr. Oken reviewed trials on kava and valerian in conjunction with Dr. Shinto.

Lynn Shinto, ND, received a degree in naturopathic medicine from Bastyr University, Kenmore, Washington. She is currently a research assistant professor in the Department of Neurology at Oregon Health and Science University and a clinical research professor at the National College of Naturopathic Medicine, Portland, Oregon. Dr. Shinto reviewed trials on kava and valerian in conjunction with Dr. Oken.

Keith Wesnes, PhD, founded Cognitive Drug Research in 1986, which has since grown to be the world's leading provider of automated cognitive function testing facilities for clinical trials. The company was honored to receive the Queen's Award for Enterprise for International Trade in 2002, and the Queen's Award in Innovation in 2003. Professor Wesnes has published over 100 peer-reviewed research articles and chapters and holds several university appointments, including a visiting professorship at the Human Cognitive Neuroscience Unit, University of Northumbria. He is a member of numerous advisory boards and frequently speaks at national and international meetings. Dr. Wesnes reviewed trials on ginkgo and ginseng.

Assistants

Eva Boyd, AB, worked with me in the summer of 2000. She searched scientific literature databases for clinical trials, retrieved those studies, and entered the information into the database.

Julie Dennis, BA, worked with me at the beginning of this project, from June 1999 to January 2000. She made the initial contact with U.S. manufacturers and gathered product information from them. She was also instrumental in establishing the electronic database that was used to collect the trial and product information included in this book.

Eva Dusek, BS, worked with me in 2001. She also collected and summarized information from clinical studies and entered it into the database.

Clea Lopez, BA, worked with me during the last year and a half on this project, from January 2002 through June 2003. She conducted scientific literature searches, reviewed and extracted information from clinical trials, and obtained product information from manufacturers. Clea compiled the pharmacopoeial therapeutic information in the summary sections in Part III of the book. She also assisted in editing the chapters in Part I, Part II, and the summary sections in Part III.

Preface

I believe that if herbal medicine is to play a significant role in future health care, the therapeutic effects of the individual herbs must be carefully evaluated by well-designed, randomized, double-blind, placebo-controlled studies involving a significant number of human subjects.

Varro E. Tyler (1999)
"Phytomedicines: Back to the Future"
In *Journal of Natural Products*

Background of the Project

The genesis of the idea for this book came from a conversation with my childhood physician, Larry Posner, MD, at a party in September 1998. He told me of his interest in botanicals due to the number of patients he had taking dietary supplements and of the limited knowledge he had of those products. He knew of my work with medicinal herbs and asked me to speak to him in his language regarding the evidence for these herbs. I inquired what language that might be and he replied, "double-blind, controlled, randomized clinical trials." My response was that quite a few studies have been conducted on herbal remedies, probably more than he realized. Thus, the idea of this book was born.

Purpose and Scope of the Book

This book provides consumers and health professionals with a means to distinguish those herbal products that have the backing of clinical evidence to substantiate claims of efficacy. It includes product descriptions provided largely from label information. In addition, this book describes in detail the trials associated with those products and provides an assessment of the quality of those trials.

Only products that have undergone controlled clinical trials are included, as this research design is considered the most persuasive and is generally given the most weight by researchers and practitioners. Many herbal preparations commonly sold on the market are not included in this text, as they have not been subjected to controlled clinical trials.

The book lists products, made with 32 herbs and ten formulas, that have been studied in a total of 369 clinical trials. Attempts were made to be systematic and inclusive in gathering products and trials; however, due to the magnitude of the effort and the amount of time required to complete the project, I acknowledge that it is essentially a snapshot—a sampling of the existing products and their clinical trials at the time when we were doing research for the book.

It is my hope that this snapshot will assist in the evaluation of the clinical science behind botanical medicine and will help with the evaluation of the evidence for herbal product efficacy. I also hope that this book will help to bridge the gap between herbal medicine and standard Western therapies by using the language of the latter to describe the former. Ultimately it is my desire that this book will assist in establishing an appropriate place for botanical medicine alongside standard Western therapies in the medicine cabinet.

The chapters in *Part I: Fundamentals of Herbal Medicine* provide background as well as context for the product and trial summaries that follow. These chapters provide information on the regulatory status of botanicals in the United States, the characterization and standardization of products, as well as the means to establish bioavailability, efficacy, and safety. Also included is a discussion on the "borrowing" of science from one product to support claims of efficacy for another. In addition, there is a discourse on the motives for conducting trials in the United States and in Europe, particularly in Germany. Finally, a chapter on pharmacopoeial monographs describes what they are and what information they provide.

Part II: Methods describes the methods used to gather information on products and clinical studies. It includes the criteria for entry into the book and the means used to evaluate the efficacy of the individual trials.

Part III: Botanical Profiles contains information on products and clinical trials. Products are grouped according to the principal botanical ingredient. If the products are multi-ingredient formulas, without a primary ingredient, then they are listed separately. Each botanical section is headed by a summary review of the products and trials. This summary section contains an at-a-glance table listing the products included in that section, the indications addressed by the clinical studies, and the number and quality of those studies. The summary section also includes information from therapeutic monographs with use information for that herb. The summary section is followed by details on the products, which is in turn followed by a detailed account of the clinical trials for each product.

Indexes allow for easy access to the product and trial information through the botanical common and scientific names, as well as by product and manufacturer names and therapeutic indication.

Acknowledgments

This book was a long time in the making, and like many large projects, it has gone through several stages. Many people have given me advice and/or assistance over that time and to mention all of them would be prohibitive. I will therefore mention a few and hope that those whose names do not appear will forgive me.

When I embarked on this book, I had only a vague sort of notion as to what it would entail. Initial encouragement from Joerg Gruenwald regarding the idea of this book resulted in a joint attempt to contact U.S. manufacturers. We asked manufacturers if they had products whose efficacy was supported by clinical studies. The scant response revealed to us that it would not necessarily be easy to obtain this product information and the project was abandoned.

However, Dr. Varro (Tip) Tyler approached me regarding a contract with The Haworth Herbal Press in June 1999, starting the process anew. With the assistance of Julie Dennis, we expanded our mailing list and contacted approximately 200 manufacturers, initially asking only for a sign of interest. This time, with the publisher's name clearly on the letterhead, we got better results. We set out to collect not only those products which had been tested in clinical studies, but also those which had similar specifications. Julie tirelessly collected information on 300 products, designed and established a database for that information, and entered the information into the database. Her enthusiasm and positive attitude were a boon throughout this stage of the project.

In the meantime, conversations with Loren Israelsen, Ulrich Mathes, and others revealed to me the complexity of evaluating product equivalency and the issues behind "borrowing" the science for one product to support the efficacy of another. I soon realized that I could include only products that had themselves been tested in clinical trials. However, now I was seven months into the project, had spent most of the generous grant from The Haworth Press, and, in some ways, was starting over. I began to concentrate on the clinical trials themselves: retrieving studies from scientific databases and then specifically contacting manufacturers who made those products. Both Eva Boyd and Eva Dusek helped tremendously with the massive job of identifying and collecting clinical trials as well as entering them into the database.

Conversations with Marie Mulligan, MD, and others helped me with ideas regarding the evaluation of the quality of clinical studies. Paramount in these conversations were those methodological qualities required by the medical community for a trial to be considered credible. Thankfully, Tieraona Low Dog, MD, stepped in and designed the checklist used to evaluate the trials. Her guidance was also instrumental in the overall concept and design of the book.

With the trials gathered and the checklist in place, I began to send those trials out to MDs for review. I am deeply indebted to all those who reviewed trials, for this is not a quick process. Concurrent with the gathering and evaluation of trials was the writing of Part I of the book, encompassing the fundamentals of herbal medicine. I am indebted to the authors of those chapters for their contributions. In addition, I am grateful to Mitch Bakos for his computer advice and assistance with the database. Also, the advice of Cathirose Petrone, who taught me how to juggle many tasks at the same time with a minimum of stress, was a blessing.

Thinking that I had only a few months left before finishing the book, I asked Clea Lopez to assist me. Those several months turned into a year and a half. Clea assisted with just about every aspect of the book during that time. With her help, we again conducted literature searches, looking for trials that had been published since our initial search. Her editing skills were a very pleasant surprise to me, with a wonderful ability to spot where the text needed to be clearer or where I needed to provide additional information. Her excellent editorial advice and attention to detail has made this book a much better one than it would have been without her.

EDITOR'S NOTE

The purpose of this book is informational. It is not intended as a guide to self-medication or as a substitute for the advice of a health practitioner.

The production of this book was partially supported by a grant from The Haworth Press. No monetary assistance was provided by any manufacturer whose product is, or is not, included in the book.

This book is not meant to promote any product(s) in particular. The purpose of the book is to examine the scientific data supporting the efficacy of herbal preparations. As therapeutic equivalence of these products has not been proven, examining the clinical evidence cannot be done without profiling individual products.

Manufacturers who wish to submit their product(s) for inclusion in future editions of this book should contact the editor via e-mail at <marilyn@pharmacognosy.com> or via the Internet at <http://www.pharmacognosy.com>.

PART I:
FUNDAMENTALS
OF HERBAL MEDICINE

Chapter 1

History and Regulation of Botanicals in the United States

Loren D. Israelsen
Marilyn Barrett

INTRODUCTION

At least four regulatory classifications are now possible for botanicals in the United States: (1) food, (2) dietary supplement, (3) over-the-counter (OTC) drug, and (4) prescription (Rx) drug. However, most botanical products are regulated as dietary supplements according to provisions in the Dietary Supplement Health and Education Act (DSHEA) of 1994. This chapter gives a brief description of how botanicals were historically regulated in the United States, the subsequent genesis of DSHEA, and the means that DSHEA provides to regulate herbs and other botanicals. It also briefly covers the regulations regarding botanicals as drugs, either sold without a doctor's prescription over-the-counter or requiring a doctor's prescription.

HISTORY

Plants have, at one time, supplied virtually all cultures with food, clothing, shelter, and medicines. It is estimated that approximately 10 to 15 percent of the roughly 300,000 species of higher plants have a history of use in traditional medicine. By contrast, only 1 percent of plant species have a history of food use (McChesney, 1995).

One hundred years ago, herbs were well established as medicines in the United States. They were widely listed in the *United States*

Pharmacopeia (USP) and prescribed by physicians. Herbal tinctures, extracts, salves, and so forth, were the materia medica of the day.

Regulation of medicines in this country began when the authority to set and enforce drug safety standards was given to the Food and Drug Administration (FDA) in 1938. The passage of the Food, Drug, and Cosmetic Act gave the FDA the responsibility to prosecute the adulteration or misbranding of foods, drugs, and cosmetics.

Herbal preparations soon gave way to single-entity chemical drugs. World War II created a demand for more powerful drugs of all kinds, particularly antibiotics and trauma treatment agents. The federal government urged drug companies, then largely botanical crude-drug houses, such as Merck, Lily, and Parke-Davis, to invest in new synthetic chemistry-based research. Single-entity chemicals were more consistent, easier to measure, and judged more specific in their therapeutic focus than botanical preparations.

In 1951, Congress passed the Durham-Humphrey Act which defined a prescription drug as any drug that because of its toxicity or other potential for harmful effect or method of use is not safe for use except under the supervision of a practitioner licensed by law to administer such a drug (Young, 1995). Manufacturers at that time had to position their drugs as either Rx or OTC.

In 1962, the Food, Drug, and Cosmetic Act was expanded to require all drugs marketed at that time to be proven *both* safe and effective. The FDA then issued guidelines for safety and efficacy testing requirements for new drugs. As a result, new drugs now required the FDA's approval before marketing. Old drugs were permitted to remain on the market as long as their ingredients and labeling remained unchanged.

In 1972, the FDA began a comprehensive review of all OTC drug products to assess their safety and efficacy. Drug ingredients found to be generally recognized as safe and effective (GRASE) were placed into Category I and approved for marketing. Those determined to be unsafe or ineffective were placed in Category II and banned from use in any OTC drug. If safety and efficacy could not be determined due to a lack of information, then the ingredient went into Category III. With few commercial sponsors to conduct safety and efficacy studies, many botanicals, listed as possible or known ingredients in OTC products, were relegated to Category II status and some were placed in Category III. With few herbs retaining drug status after the OTC review, the botanical industry had no other regulatory option but to offer their products as foods.

In the late 1970s, the FDA began to apply the food additive provisions of the Food, Drug, and Cosmetic Act to botanicals. Under provisions added to the Federal Food, Drug, and Cosmetic Act of 1958, food additives already on the market in 1958 were accepted without FDA review. However, substances added to the food supply after this date were required to gain FDA approval prior to marketing, unless they were considered GRAS (generally recognized as safe). A fair number of herbs were included on a list of GRAS food additives that had been prepared by the Flavor and Extract Manufacturers Association as flavorings for alcoholic beverages. However, the FDA viewed commonly used herbs as unapproved food additives and therefore subject to FDA approval prior to marketing. This interpretation led to a series of bitterly fought court cases and several herbs being taken off the market.

Congress passed the Nutrition Labeling Education Act of 1990 (NLEA) to reform food labeling and to allow, for the first time, a new class of health claims based on disease-nutrient relationships. For the most part, this legislation did not apply to botanicals because of the way it was written and the way it was interpreted by the FDA.

With lawsuits between herbal manufacturers and the FDA commonplace, a group of leading herb companies met with Senator Orrin G. Hatch (R-Utah) and Congressman Bill Richardson (D-New Mexico) who drafted legislation that became the Dietary Supplement Health and Education Act of 1994. This law was passed by Congress and signed into law by President Clinton on October 25, 1994. This was the first time a U.S. law defined the terms *herb* or *botanical*.

DSHEA EXPLAINED

As with most federal laws, the legislative language of DSHEA is arcane, if not mystifying. The core provisions of the act, however, are straightforward and create an expansive framework for all dietary supplements. The following summary of DSHEA is an "herbs-only" interpretation which provides a useful tool for those wishing to see how DSHEA creates a new architecture for the manufacture, sale, and promotion of herbs.

Definition

DSHEA defines the term *dietary supplement* as an herb or other botanical or concentrate, constituent, extract, or combination of any botanical that is intended for ingestion as a tablet, capsule, or liquid, is not represented for use as a conventional food or as a sole item of a meal or the diet, and is labeled as a dietary supplement. This includes new drugs that were marketed as botanicals prior to such approval; it does not include a botanical approved as a new drug, or authorized for investigation as a new drug, and not previously marketed as a dietary supplement. Botanicals are not classified as food additives.

Safety

Dietary supplement products are allowed to contain botanicals that have been present in the food supply and in a form in which the food (botanical) has not been chemically altered. Dietary supplement ingredients marketed in the Unites States before October 15, 1994, are regarded as safe because of their long history of use. Those ingredients not marketed before then are "new" ingredients. At least 75 days before introduction into commerce, manufacturers must provide the FDA with information that shows the new botanical can reasonably be expected to be safe under conditions of use or labeling.

DSHEA states that a botanical is considered unsafe under one of two conditions: (1) it presents a significant or unreasonable risk of illness or injury under conditions of use recommended or suggested in labeling, or (2) it is a new botanical for which inadequate information exists to provide reasonable assurance that it does not present a significant or unreasonable risk of illness or injury. In any case, the FDA shall have the burden of proof to show that a botanical is unsafe.

Good Manufacturing Practices

A botanical is also considered unsafe if it is prepared, packed, or held under conditions that do not meet current good manufacturing practice regulations (GMPs). For the moment, the preparation and packaging of dietary supplements is covered by the same GMPs that apply to conventional foods. However, DSHEA authorizes the FDA to establish separate GMPs for dietary supplements, and rule making by the FDA is imminent.

Labeling

The label must identify the product by the term *dietary supplement*. Botanical dietary supplement labels must list the name of each ingredient, the quantity of such ingredients, or, if a proprietary blend, the total quantity of all ingredients. The label must also identify any part of the plant from which the ingredient is derived.

Botanical dietary supplements are misbranded if they are represented as conforming to such official compendium as *USP* and fail to do so, fail to have the identity and strength which they represent to have, or fail to meet the quality, purity, or compositional specifications, based on validated assays or other appropriate methods, which they are represented to meet.

Literature, including an article, a chapter in a book, or an official abstract of a peer-reviewed scientific publication which appears in an article shall not be defined as labeling when used in connection with the sale of botanicals to consumers provided that it is not false or misleading, does not promote a particular manufacturer or brand of botanical, is displayed or presented with other items on the same subject matter so as to present a balanced view of the available scientific information on a botanical, and, if displayed in an establishment, is physically separate from the botanical and does not have appended to it a sticker or other method that associates it with the product.

Claims of Benefit or "Statements of Nutritional Support" Allowed in Labeling

Under DSHEA, a statement for a botanical dietary supplement may be made if the statement describes how a botanical is intended to affect the structure or function of humans, characterizes the documented mechanism by which a botanical acts to maintain such structure or function, or describes general well-being from consumption of a botanical. The statement must contain, prominently displayed and in bold-faced type, the following: "This statement has not been evaluated by the Food and Drug Administration. This product is not intended to diagnose, treat, cure or prevent any disease."

The FDA published a final rule in the Federal Register on February 7, 2000 (docket No. 98N-0044), which describes how the agency will distinguish disease claims from structure/function claims. The rule permits health maintenance claims ("maintains a healthy circulatory system"), other nondisease claims ("for muscle enhancement," "helps you relax"), and claims for common, minor symptoms associated with life stages ("for common symptoms of PMS," "for hot flashes"). It does not allow for claims regarding diseases ("prevents osteoporosis") or implied disease claims ("prevents bone fragility in postmenopausal women") (FDA, 2000).

As with all food labeling, statements must be truthful and not misleading. Statements of nutritional support may be made without prior FDA review, but the manufacturer must notify the FDA within 30 days of marketing a product with a new claim and must have substantiation for the claim. Criteria for substantiating a claim are not yet defined by the FDA. However, advertising guidelines for benefit statements for dietary supplements have been published by the Federal Trade Commission (1998) and can be found on their Web site (www.ftc.gov).

DSHEA establishes that a botanical is not a drug solely because its label or labeling contains a statement of nutritional support. Also, a botanical shall not be deemed misbranded if its label or labeling contains directions or conditions of use or warnings.

Commission on Dietary Supplement Labels

DSHEA established a presidential commission to study and provide recommendations for the regulation of label claims and statements for botanicals, including the use of literature in connection with the sale of botanicals, and procedures for evaluation of such claims. The seven members of the Commission on Dietary Supplement Labels were appointed by the president to evaluate how best to provide truthful and scientifically valid information about dietary supplements to consumers. The commission's final report, which was submitted to the president and Congress in November 1997, included guidance regarding statements of nutritional support and the substantiation of such claims. The commission recognized that under DSHEA, botanical products should continue to be marketed as dietary supplements, when properly labeled. However, they recommended that a review panel be established to review claims for OTC drug uses (Commission on Dietary Supplement Labels, 1997).

Office of Dietary Supplements

DSHEA also established an Office of Dietary Supplements (ODS) within the National Institutes of Health (NIH). The purposes of the office are to explore the potential ability of botanicals to improve health care and to promote scientific study of the benefits of botanicals in maintaining health and preventing chronic disease.

The director of the ODS is to conduct and coordinate scientific research relating to botanicals that can limit or reduce the risk of diseases such as heart disease, cancer, birth defects, osteoporosis, cataracts, or prostatism, collect results of scientific research related to botanicals and compile a database, and serve as a principal advisor to the NIH, the Centers for Disease Control and Prevention (CDCP), and the commissioner of the FDA on issues relating to botanicals and scientific issues arising in connection with the labeling and composition of botanicals.

Currently the ODS, in collaboration with the National Center for Complementary and Alternative Medicine (NCCAM), sponsors six botanical research centers. The ODS Web site hosts two databases: one containing information regarding federally funded research on dietary supplements (CARDS, "Computer Access to Research on Dietary Supplements") and the other containing scientific literature regarding dietary supplement ingredients (IBIDS, "International Bibliographic Information on Dietary Supplements") (http://dietary-supplements.info. nih.gov). The ODS is also conducting systematic reviews of the literature in order to determine areas needing research and to assist in the development of clinical guidelines. Fact sheets with information on the most commonly used botanicals are in preparation. The ODS, again in conjunction with NCCAM, has sponsored clinical trials on St. John's wort and ginkgo. Several dozen other trials on botanicals are currently listed on the NCCAM Web site (nccam. nih.gov). The ODS is also currently supporting the development of validated analytical methods, standards, and reference materials for the most commonly used botanicals.

DRUGS: OTC AND Rx

Before a botanical product is marketed as a drug with a claim to diagnose, treat, cure, or prevent a disease, it must first be approved by the FDA. The revision of the Food, Drug, and Cosmetic Act in 1962 required all drugs marketed after that time to be proven both safe and effective. This revision presented the FDA with the challenge of updating its approval of hundreds of drugs already on the market that had not been proven effective. The FDA set up panels of experts to review the active ingredients of these drugs, many of which were sold over-the-counter. However, many herbal products were found to be either unsafe, ineffective, or simply lacking sufficient evidence to evaluate (Tyler, 1993).

In order to obtain drug status for a new botanical product, or for one that failed a previous evaluation, manufacturers must submit a New Drug Application (NDA) to the FDA. This requirement holds whether the new drug is to be sold as an OTC or Rx drug. The NDA must contain evidence of the product's safety and efficacy. This evidence is usually in the form of pharmacological studies, ranging in scope from in vitro assays and small animal studies to randomized, double-blinded clinical trials in humans, with an emphasis on the clinical studies. The benefit to pharmaceutical firms which manufacture synthetic chemical drugs is that their research is rewarded by patent protection for a substantial period of time. However, as most herbs have previously been marketed in a traditional form, and thus are not new or unique, they are not eligible for patent protection. There are some exceptions when a botanical is prepared in a unique form (for example, the ginkgo extract EGb 761) or for a previously unknown use. Without patent protection, most manufacturers are unwilling to spend the money necessary to conduct the research required for a new drug application. In addition, manufacturers may find it easier to forego scientific studies as they can easily sell their products as dietary supplements.

The Commission on Dietary Supplement Labels (1997) recommended that the FDA establish a "review panel for OTC claims for botanical products that are proposed by manufacturers for drug uses" (p. 57). However, in April 1998 the FDA published a notice responding to the commission report, indicating that the agency considers such a review to be "premature" at this time. The FDA did not give an explanation for their decision (FDA Notice, 1998).

Petitions formally requesting that valerian and ginger be recognized as old OTC drug ingredients were filed with the FDA in 1994. Nearly six years later, the agency issued a response provisionally accepting the supporting data, which was largely European, but only under very stringent conditions. Valerian and ginger have yet to become OTC drugs.

Numerous experts agree that a select number of botanicals are proper candidates for OTC drug status. Although this would mean that some plant extracts would be available both as dietary supplements and OTC drugs, it is likely that many American consumers who currently would not use a certain herb as a dietary supplement would accept and use that same herb if it were offered as a drug that has received FDA (government) approval. Likewise, physicians, pharmacists, and other health care providers would be far more inclined to recommend, or at least not discourage, the use of an herbal OTC drug. The reasons being that OTC drugs are manufactured under stricter good manufacturing practices, and OTC products have mandatory labeling which includes dosage recommendations, cautions, and warnings. Although manufacturers of botanical products are welcome to submit their products for review under the new drug approval process, it does not appear that the FDA is prepared to actively welcome OTC applications for botanicals as old drug ingredients. That is, for a botanical to achieve OTC status, it must have all the scientific research required for a new drug. It is unlikely to be "grandfathered in" as an old drug without that documentation.

PROSPECTUS

Canada has created a natural health products category, which is intermediate between the formal OTC drug review process and the less formal dietary supplement regime in the United States. Many in the herbal industry now feel that such a category would be beneficial for the United States as well. However, this would require a new regulatory category to be created.

In the meantime, it is entirely possible for a botanical to be marketed and sold as a food, a dietary supplement, and a drug at the same time, depending on its label claim. For example, ginger root can be sold as a food ingredient, as a dietary supplement "to maintain a calm stomach," or (if approved by the FDA) as an OTC drug "to prevent and treat nausea or motion sickness."

REFERENCES

Commission on Dietary Supplement Labels (1997). Commission on Dietary Supplement Labels Report to the President, the Congress and the Secretary of the Department of Health and Human Services. Final Report, November 24.

Dietary Supplement Health and Education Act (DSHEA) (1994). Public Law 103-417, October 25.

Food and Drug Administration (FDA) (2000). Regulations on Statements Made for Dietary Supplements Concerning the Effect of the Product on the Structure or Function of the Body. *Federal Register* 65 (4): 1000-1050.

Food and Drug Administration (FDA) Notice (1998). Dietary supplements: Comments on report of the Commission on Dietary Supplement Labels. *Federal Register* 63: 23633-23637 (April 29).

Federal Trade Commission (1998). *Dietary Supplements: An Advertising Guide for Industry.* Federal Trade Commission, Bureau of Consumer Protection (www.ftc.gov).

McChesney (1995). Botanicals, Historical Role. Presented at the Drug Information Association (DIA) Alternative Medicine Workshop on Botanicals, March 30-31.

Office of Dietary Supplements (ODS) Web site: <http://dietary-supplements.info.nih.gov>.

Tyler VE (1993). *The Honest Herbal, A Sensible Guide to the Use of Herbs and Related Remedies,* Third Edition. Binghamton, NY: Pharmaceutical Products Press.

Young JH (1995). Federal Drug and Narcotic Legislation. *Pharmacy in History* 37 (2): 59-67; citation of amendments to sections 303(c) and 503(b) of the Federal Food, Drug, and Cosmetic Act, 82nd Congress, First Session, October 26, 1951, 65 *U.S. Statutes* 648.

Chapter 2

Product Definition Deficiencies in Clinical Studies of Herbal Medicines

Varro E. Tyler

Clinical studies and case reports of herbal medicines have recently begun to appear in major medical journals of the United States. The clinicians responsible for these publications are apparently unaware that no standards of quality exist for herbal products in this and many other countries. Accustomed to working with drugs that must conform to official specifications, these authors often fail to define adequately the botanicals employed, and their failure to do so raises more questions than are answered. The following examples, some of them selected from the special November 11, 1998, alternative medicine issue of the *Journal of the American Medical Association*, will illustrate this problem.

One of the major clinical trials published in that issue was a study conducted in Australia by Bensoussan et al. (1998), involving the treatment of irritable bowel syndrome with a multi-ingredient Chinese herbal formula. None of the 20 botanicals employed was identified by its correct Latin binomial (genus, species; followed by author citation) nor was any assurance provided that the identification given only as a Latin drug title was confirmed in any way (botanical or chemical characterization).

The quantities of the herbs were provided only as a percentage basis (presumably by weight), and the amount administered was stated only as five capsules (size not specified) three times daily. On the basis of the data provided, the study could never be replicated or its pur-

Chapter 2 originates from *The Scientific Review of Alternative Medicine,* by Varro E. Tyler, "Product Definition Deficiencies in Clinical Studies of Herbal Medicines," Vol. 4, No. 2 (Fall/Winter 2000), pp. 17-21. Reprinted by permission of the publisher.

13

ported results verified. Further, no follow-up was conducted to determine which of the herbs contributed to the reported positive effects and which were merely adjuvants, correctives, or flavors.

A letter to the editor by Grush et al. (1998) in the same issue warns against the use of St. John's wort during pregnancy as a result of observations on two gravid women. Both of them were said to be consuming 900 mg/day of the herb. Because the dose of St. John's wort ranges from 2 to 4 g, what is probably being referred to here is 900 mg of a St. John's wort concentrated extract standardized to contain 0.3 percent hypericin. There is a considerable difference between this and the crude herb. Further, no botanical or chemical studies verifying that the herbal product labeled St. John's wort was indeed *Hypericum perforatum* L. were apparently conducted.

Garges, Varia, and Doraiswamy (1998) attribute a case of cardiac complications and delirium to the withdrawal of valerian root extract, even though the patient was consuming seven other medications plus minerals and vitamins. Although the designation valerian root is commonly misused to described both the rhizome (underground stem) and roots of the plant, no data were presented to assure readers that the extract was prepared from *Valeriana officinalis* L. as specified. Several species of valerian are commonly employed as central nervous system depressants.

Further, the preparation involved is defined only as an "extract," without specifying the solvents used to prepare it or the degree of concentration. It was apparently consumed in substantial quantities, ranging from 30 mg to 2 g per dose five times daily. The authors conclude that in view of the multiple factors involved (e.g., numerous other drugs, surgery) "we cannot causally link valerian root to his symptoms." This statement contradicts an earlier one, which reported "a case of serious cardiac complications and delirium associated with the withdrawal of valerian roots." It also renders inaccurate the similarly worded title of the publication. In actuality, information provided in the paper is inadequate to allow any firm conclusion as to what herbal product was being consumed.

A letter from Lawson (1998) in the same issue of *JAMA* commented on the negative results achieved with a steam-distilled garlic oil (*Allium sativum* L.) preparation tableted in combination with beta-cyclodextrin. The author pointed out that the prepared garlic oil has little hypocholesterolemic activity in the first place and that only about 25-40 percent of it was ever released from the binder. Some of the tablets were compressed so compactly that they passed through the intestinal tract of human intact or in large pieces.

Although the authors of the original paper replied that the binding of the oil to the beta-cyclodextrin was intentional, thus providing a slow release of activity, they failed to address the more difficult problem of whether therapeutic levels of allyl sulfides were ever attained (Berthold, Sudhop, and von Bergmann, 1998). In their minds, this was considered unnecessary because "convincing evidence of lipid-lowering effects of any garlic preparation is still lacking." No reference in support of this assertion is provided. The 17 positive of 20 total studies cited by Lawson are dismissed as lacking rigorous design, but the defects are not specified. They do concede that "conclusions of our study apply only to the preparation we used. . . ." Unfortunately, that was not the way it was reported in the popular press, which labeled all garlic preparations ineffective for blood lipid reduction.

Berthold and colleagues (1998) could have precluded much of the concern about their original study simply by including in it a better definition of the product utilized. Characterization of the proven activity (or lack thereof) of allyl sulfides, quantitative figures regarding the slow release of these principles from the beta-cyclodextrin binder with estimates of predictable blood levels, and data on tablet disintegration time under controlled conditions should certainly have been presented. This study is an excellent example of the pronounced effect dosage form design can have on the purported activity of an herbal product.

In the report of their clinical trial on *Garcinia cambogia* Desr. for weight loss, Heymsfield et al. (1998) made more than the usual effort to define the product utilized. However, something went awry. The authors indicate that caplets containing the plant extract (50 percent hydroxycitric acid) plus added hydroxycitric acid were administered in daily doses totaling 3000 mg of extract and 1500 mg of hydroxycitric acid. The problem here is that hydroxycitric acid (HCA) does not exist in that form in nature. Instead, it occurs as a lactone which lacks the ability to inhibit ATP-citrate lyase (Clauatre and Rosenbaum, 1994). That enzyme is responsible for the formation of acetyl-CoA, the metabolite necessary for fatty acid and cholesterol biosynthesis. Lacking this inhibiting activity, the plant extract could not be expected to have any antiobesity activity and, of course, none was found.

However, the authors state that the extract used was found to contain 50 percent hydroxycitric acid by analysis. This is almost certainly inaccurate because HCA is an unstable hygroscopic compound that reverts to the inactive lactone over time. Probably the HCA was present in the extract as a more stable salt of some type. This raises concerns about the absorbability and ultimate activity of the undefined salt. Presumably the HCA administered with the plant extract was also in the form of a salt rather than the free acid.

Once again, failure to define precisely the nature of the herbal extract utilized has resulted in confusion. Replication of the study on the basis of the published data would be impossible.

Confusion in the medical literature due to inadequate herbal product definition is certainly not confined to one journal, nor is it of recent origin. In 1989, MacGregor et al. published a report in the *British Medical Journal* of four women who suffered hepatotoxic effects after consuming two different proprietary herbal remedies. Both of these remedies presumably contained scullcap (*Scutellaria lateriflora* L.) and valerian *(Valeriana officinalis),* and the authors concluded that the deleterious effects noted probably resulted from the consumption of these two herbs. This assumption was based in part on the reported toxicity of valepotriates in valerian. No analysis of the products was conducted to determine if they actually contained the two herbs in question.

Since that time, it has been determined that the unstable iridoid compounds known as valepotriates are not found in significant amounts in commercial valerian preparations. Further, in Britain the known hepatotoxic herb germander *(Teucrium chamaedrys* L.) is often substituted for scullcap, and this substitution was, in all likelihood, the cause of the observed effects (Tyler, 1993). Once again, failure to characterize an herbal product properly resulted in a false report of potential toxicity of two herbs.

Probably more confusion has been produced in the herbal literature by so-called Siberian ginseng, better designated eleuthero, than any other herb. Eleuthero is not a true ginseng, a designation properly reserved for species of *Panax*. Botanically, it is *Eleutherococcus senticosus* (Rupr. and Maxim.) Maxim., and although it belongs to the same family as ginseng, the *Araliaceae,* its constituents are very different. Family relationships of botanicals do not necessarily reflect similar constituents or activities. Potatoes (*Solanum tuberosum* L.) and the deadly nightshade (*Atropa belladonna* L.) are both members of the Solanaceae.

Eleuthero is seldom obtainable in this country in the form of pieces sufficiently large to allow identification by means of organoleptic evaluation. Instead, it is usually seen either as a powder, which is more difficult to identify, or as an extract. In China, where much of the herb originates, it is known as *wujia,* a name also applied to entirely different plants, especially Chinese silk vine (*Periploca sepium* Bunge) (Keville, 1992). Eleuthero is utilized in various herbal mixtures touted to enhance athletic performance, so it is also subject to adulteration with stimulants.

In 1990, Koren et al. published a report of a mother whose newborn infant suffered from neonatal androgenization. They attributed the effect to the mother's consumption of "pure ginseng" and discussed the literature on ginseng's (*Panax ginseng* C.A. Mey.) effect on hormones. In fact, the product consumed was labeled Siberian ginseng, but the authors failed to recognize the difference between it and ginseng.

Unfortunately, the product actually consumed was no longer available for analysis, but additional samples of the same lot from the original supplier were subsequently shown to be Chinese silk vine (Awang, 1991). Additional analyses of various specimens revealed one that was actually eleuthero, but it contained caffeine, which is not a normal constituent of that herb (Tyler, 1994). Moreover, none of the natural constituents of either species is known to induce androgenization. The hairy baby case has thus become an infamous example of poor herbal quality. One herb, eleuthero, was mistaken for another, ginseng, but eleuthero was replaced by Chinese silk vine, which in turn was almost certainly adulterated with an androgen. This entire muddle could have been avoided if the dosage form initially utilized had been properly analyzed and defined prior to publication.

Eleuthero substituted with Chinese silk vine has also been implicated in a case involving elevated digoxin levels in a cardiac patient. McRae, the attending physician, reported that eleutherosides in Siberian ginseng may have been converted to digoxin in vivo, thus causing the increased serum levels (McRae, 1996).

No eleutheroside is known to be related chemically to digoxin or to have cardiotonic properties, but Chinese silk vine has related compounds with such properties. Therefore, as Awang has surmised, the apparent rise in serum digoxin levels was probably due to the substitution of *P. sepium* for *E. senticosus* (Awang, 1996). The erroneous attribution of digitalis-like effects to constituents of eleuthero could have been avoided if the dosage form utilized had been tested for the presence of eleutherosides, thus assuring its identity before publication.

A particularly egregious case of inadequate product definition appeared in a 1998 article by DiPaola et al. in the *New England Journal of Medicine*. An eight-herb formula designated PC-SPES, promoted for the treatment of prostate cancer, was defined as consisting in part of five plants designated by common names only. These included chrysanthemum, licorice, scutellaria (scullcap), isitis, and saw palmetto. Of these, the first three may be obtained from at least two different species, so the composition of the formula is unclear. The remaining three botanicals in the formula were designated by Latin binomials but without author citations.

The formula was said to have been purchased from a commercial source in four different batches, each of which was analyzed. Exactly what the products were analyzed for, how they were analyzed, and the results of the analyses are not stated in the paper. The concentration of each of the eight herbs in the total formula is likewise not mentioned. Stock solutions of the formula and other herbs studied were prepared by exposing them to alcohol for 24 hours. Nowhere is the method of "exposure" explained.

Rather than continuing to describe examples of inadequate herbal product characterization in the medical literature, it seems more profitable to review exactly what is necessary to provide adequate herbal product definition. First of all, the botanical should be identified by its Latin binomial, followed on the first citation by the name of the author who assigned that designation. This latter specification, often overlooked by those unfamiliar with botanical nomenclature, is nevertheless important because it increases the clarity and accuracy of the designation (Laurence, 1995).

Plants often have more than one scientific name, each assigned by a different author. The long-used medicinal herb chamomile has at least 12 scientific names, each more or less accurate depending on one's interpretation of its characteristics. *Matricaria recutita* L. (the L. is an abbreviation of Linnaeus) is now considered the most appropriate binomial, but other authors have assigned it to different genera and utilized different specific epithets. The genera include *Chamomilla, Chrysanthemum, Leucanthemum,* and *Athemis,* in addition to *Matricaria* (List and Hörhammer, 1976). Unless the author's name is cited, it is impossible for a reader to know that *Matricaria recutita* L. and *Chamomilla vulgaris* K. Koch, for example, refer to the same plant, specifically, chamomile. Chamomile, which is also commonly referred to as German chamomile, Hungarian chamomile, or genuine chamomile, is distinct from Roman or English chamomile, an altogether different plant. Common names also cause serious problems because the same one may be applied to several different plants.

Correctly written, a Latin binomial includes a genus name that is capitalized and a species epithet in lower case; both words are italicized. Such scientific names should not be confused with the seldom-used (in the United States) Latin drug names, which in the case of chamomile is Matricariae flos (Matricaria flowers).

Following the proper name of the herb, the part used should be specified (root, rhizome, bark, leaves, flowers, seeds, etc.) and the method of identification (botanical, chemical) specified. Next, a profile or fingerprint of the principal constituents, particularly if an extract is employed, obtained by HPLC, CG-MS, or some appropriate analytical methodology, should be reported. If the product tested is a mixture of herbs, the above information should be specified for each.

The appropriate data concerning the identity of the herbs and their composition are available from any quality producer of botanical products. It is essential, however, that they be reported in a clinical study on a particular dosage form because they vary greatly from product to product. Further, the composition of a particular product may change from time to time without notice.

Herbal mixtures, particularly the complex formulas utilized in Asiatic traditional medical systems, require special consideration. Clinicians need to remember that determination of the activity of the entire formula is not an end point but simply the beginning of the study. The Old Woman of Shropshire's dropsy formula is a good example. The astute physician William Withering was able to narrow down her secret remedy of some 20 plants to a single effective herb, foxglove (digitalis) (Mann, 1992). In almost all such cases, the significant activity of such remedies can ultimately be attributed to a single herb and the remaining botanicals, whether called adjuvants, correctives, or flavors, are found to be more or less window dressing. Clinical studies of complex mixtures must eventually determine what is active and what is not, in order to be truly useful.

Finally, the composition of the dosage form and the method of administration must be specified. Diluents used in capsules and tablets may have a decided influence on the availability of the active constituents. Likewise, appropriate data concerning such important factors as the dissolution time of compressed tablets, the properties of tablet or capsule coatings, and the like need to be specified.

Inclusion of the above information may at first seem superfluous to clinicians accustomed to working with drugs for which standards covering such matters are in place. However, no such standards exist for herbal products, and it is necessary to include sufficient information to allow the study to be reproduced. Many of the problem studies reviewed in the initial section of this paper could never be replicated because the necessary data are not provided in the original publication.

Authors and editors also have the responsibility to assure that titles of papers accurately describe the specific nature of the study and the conclusions reached. A paper dealing with the activity or inactivity of a particular herbal dosage form should not be titled so broadly as to allow the inference, especially by the popular media, that all dosage forms of that herb have the same properties.

While applicable to all clinical trials, this caveat is most important for herbal studies, which in the past have often utilized ill-defined dosage forms, and the results of which are of extreme interest to the popular press. Just because a particular dosage form of garlic oil did not show antihypercholesterolemic activity does not in any way invalidate the utility of other garlic preparations. Similarly, data indicating that a specific preparation of echinacea did not prevent colds following prophylactic administration does not necessarily invalidate the results of studies indicating that some echinacea preparations ameliorated the symptoms of colds following remedial use.

Most clinical studies involve participation of a relatively large number of investigators with different areas of expertise. It seems obvious that any future studies will find it necessary to involve individuals with experience in the broad field of phytotherapy ranging from botanical nomenclature to analytics to dosage form design, if the investigation is to be conducted in such a way as to produce meaningful, reproducible results. Editors of clinically oriented journals have an important responsibility to utilize referees capable of judging whether herbal dosage forms have been adequately defined in submitted manuscripts.

REFERENCES

Awang DVC (1991). Maternal use of ginseng and neonatal androgenization [comment]. *Journal of the American Medical Association* 266 (3): 363.

Awang DVC (1996). Siberian ginseng toxicity may be case of mistaken identity. *Canadian Medical Association Journal* 155 (9): 293-295.

Bensoussan A, Talley NJ, Hing M, Menzies R, Guo A, Ngu M (1998). Treatment of irritable bowel syndrome with Chinese herbal medicine. *Journal of the American Medical Association* 280 (18): 1585-1589.

Berthold HK, Sudhop T, von Bergmann K (1998). In reply. *Journal of the American Medical Association* 280 (18): 1568.

Clauatre D, Rosenbaum M (1994). *The Diet and Health Benefits of HCA (Hydroxycitric Acid)*. New Canaan, CT: Keats Publishing.

DiPaola RS, Zhang H, Lambert GH, Meeker R, Licitra E, Rafi MM, Zhu BT, Spaulding H, Goodin S, Toledano MB, et al. (1998). Clinical and biologic activity of an estrogenic herbal combination (PC-SPES) in prostate cancer. *New England Journal of Medicine* 339 (12): 785-791.

Garges HP, Varia I, Doraiswamy PM (1998). Cardiac complications and delirium associated with valerian root withdrawal. *Journal of the American Medical Association* 280 (18): 1566-1567.

Grush LR, Nierenberg A, Keefe B, Cohen LS (1998). St. John's wort during pregnancy. *Journal of the American Medical Association* 280 (18): 1566.

Heymsfield SB, Allison DB, Vasselli JR, Pietrobelli A, Greenfield D, Nunez C (1998). *Garcinia cambogia* (hydroxycitric acid) as a potential antiobesity agent—A randomized clinical trial. *Journal of the American Medical Association* 280 (18): 1596-1600.

Keville K (1992). Siberian ginseng—False accusation. *American Herbalists Association Quarterly* 4 (2): 9.

Koren G, Randor S, Martin S, Dannerman D (1990). Maternal ginseng use associated with neonatal androgenization. *Journal of the American Medical Association* 264 (22): 2866.

Laurence GHM (1995). *An Introduction to Plant Taxonomy.* New York, NY: Macmillan.

Lawson LD (1998). Effect of garlic on serum lipids. *Journal of the American Medical Association* 280 (18): 1568.

List PH, Hörhammer L, eds. (1976). *Hagers Handbuch der Pharmazeutischen Praxis,* Fourth Edition, Volume 5. Berlin: Springer Verlag.

MacGregor FB, Abernethy VE, Dahabra S, Cobden I, Hayes PC (1989). Hepatotoxicity of herbal remedies. *British Medical Journal* 299 (6708): 1156-1157.

Mann J (1992). *Murder, Magic, and Medicine.* Oxford, UK: Oxford University Press.

McRae S (1996). Elevated serum digoxin levels in a patient taking digoxin and Siberian ginseng. *Canadian Medical Association Journal* 155 (3): 293-295.

Tyler VE (1993). *The Honest Herbal,* Third Edition. Binghamton, NY: Pharmaceutical Products Press.

Tyler VE (1994). *Herbs of Choice.* Binghamton, NY: Pharmaceutical Products Press.

Chapter 3

Identifying and Characterizing Botanical Products

Marilyn Barrett

When referring to a botanical product in a scientific report, details such as the scientific name of the plant, plant part, preparation, formulation, and dose must be included as the basis of any discussion of therapeutics. Without a full description of the test material, there can be no assurance of a reproducible effect.

In Chapter 2, Dr. Varro Tyler addresses the lack of proper characterization of botanical materials in clinical study publications. The omissions he describes are still more common than not, even in the most prestigious medical journals. The need for guidelines in the characterization of botanicals has been acknowledged by the National Center for Complementary and Alternative Medicine of the U.S. National Institutes of Health (NCCAM). NCCAM recently added a description of characterization parameters expected of botanical products to the grant application guidelines on their Web site (http://nccam.nih.gov).

An unfortunate recent example of an inadequately described product was a report of a trial studying the effectiveness of echinacea for the prevention of experimental rhinovirus colds. The authors acknowledge in their report that three species of echinacea are used medicinally and that different echinacea preparations differ in their chemical composition. They therefore present chemical analysis of the test sample as 0.16 percent cichoric acid with almost no echinacoside or alkamides (Turner, Riker, and Gangemi, 2000). However, the paper does not state whether the echinacea preparation was powdered plant material or an extract. Further, we are not told the species or the plant part (the flowering tops and/or roots of echinacea are both commonly used). When I contacted the lead author, Dr. Turner, it was apparent that he was not informed of the taxonomic identity of the material that he tested, although he did tell me it was powdered plant material. Further inquiries by Dr. Tyler of the supplier led to the information that the material was 85 percent *Echinacea purpurea* root and herb with 15 percent *E. angustifolia* root extract powder. However, Dr. Tyler and I were still puzzled, as the results of the chemical analysis did not fit the suggested identification. The combination of *E. purpurea* root and herb with *E. angustifolia* root would be expected to contain both alkamides and echinacoside, as alkamides are present in both species and echinacoside is present in *E. angustifolia* roots.

Lack of adequate identification can lead not only to scientific confusion, but also to substitutions that can have toxic consequences. In one incident the similar-looking leaves of a species of digitalis (*Digitalis lanata* Ehrhart) were accidentally substituted for plantain (*Plantago lanceolata* L.), thereby causing heart arrhythmia (Slifman et al., 1998). In several other incidents confusion over traditional Chinese names led to the substitution of guang fang-ji root, also known as fang-chi (*Aristolochia fangchi* Y.C. Wu ex L.D.), for han fang-ji (*Stephania tetrandra* S. Moore) root. Unfortunately, the use of the *Aristolochia* species caused liver failure and death in several individuals (Vanhaelen et al., 1994).

In the hope that this sort of confusion may be prevented in the future, this chapter describes the means for assuring the identity of plant material, common forms of botanical preparations, and the influence of the dosage form on the dose and bioavailability of the product.

IDENTIFYING PLANTS BY NAME

Purple coneflower, black samson, red sunflower, comb flower, cock-up-hat, Indian head, and Missouri snakeroot are all common names for the same plant as defined by its Latin binomial, *Echinacea purpurea* (L.) Moench (Hobbs, 1994). Another plant, also known locally in the U.S. Midwest as snakeroot, has a completely different Latin name: *Parthenium integrifolium* L. Confusion over the similar common names is thought to be the cause of exportation of *Parthenium* root as *Echinacea purpurea* root to Europe. The substitution of *Parthenium* for *Echinacea* has raised doubt over which plant material was used in clinical trials conducted in Germany before 1986 (Awang and Kindack, 1991).

Common names are not definitive, as demonstrated in the previous example. Different plants may have the same common name, or the same plant may have different common names. Common names are given in the local language and often vary depending upon the region. In contrast, the scientific name, or Latin binomial, is a definitive name, and if used properly should eliminate confusion. The name is composed of the taxonomic categories of genus and species followed by the name of the scientific authority, or authorities, who officially described the plant. Thus in the binomial for garlic, *Allium sativum* L., the "L." at the end is an abbreviation for Linnaeus, the famous botanist of the 1700s.

Scientific names are based on guidelines laid down by the International Code of Botanical Nomenclature (ICBN). These rules were originally established in 1930 and are periodically revised (Greuter et al., 2000). According to the ICBN, the Latin binomial is accompanied by a published description and a "type" specimen upon which that description is based.

Although Latin names are definitive, they can be revised. All taxonomic revisions are conducted according to a detailed set of guidelines established by the ICBN. An old name can be replaced by a new one, or the definition of a name can be altered. When the definition is altered, but the name remains the same, both authorities are listed after the binomial, with the previous authority listed in parentheses. As an example, we have the name for milk thistle, *Silybum marianum* (L.) Gaertn.

Latin names are commonly listed with the taxonomic family to which they belong. Milk thistle is in the sunflower family, or Asteraceae. Thus, the complete name for milk thistle is *Silybum marianum* (L.) Gaertn., Asteraceae.

The American Herbal Products Association (AHPA) has attempted to solve the confusion over common names by establishing definitive common names to be used in trade. In a publication titled *Herbs of Commerce,* AHPA has defined common trade names by pairing them with their Latin binomials (McGuffin et al., 2000). The FDA, in its dietary supplement labeling regulations, has recognized the common names listed in *Herbs of Commerce* as official trade names (CFR 21 Part 101.36, 1997).

MEANS OF ASSURING PLANT IDENTITY

The primary way to identify plant material is through physical examination of the features of the entire plant, especially the flowers. Those features are compared to descriptions in plant taxonomy books and/or to specimens whose identity has already been established by a botanist. When a specimen is identified by a botanist, it is said to be authenticated.

Sensory information, referred to as organoleptic features (color, texture, smell, taste), can also yield information on the identity of whole, chopped, or milled plant material. Further information on identity of milled or powdered plant material is provided by microscopic examination that allows for viewing of tissue structures, organization, cell types, and cell contents.

Chemical constituents are also important in identification. Plants contain thousands of chemical components, including basic proteins and sugars necessary for metabolism and structure. They also contain secondary compounds that were originally thought not to be essential to the life of the plant, but have important medicinal qualities for mammals. The best known of these secondary components are the alkaloids, a group which includes nicotine, caffeine, morphine, and cocaine. Other classes of secondary compounds include phenolics, terpenoids, and steroids (Trease and Evans, 1978). Chemical analysis can be useful in identification even when physical examination of plant structures is not possible, such as with fine powders and extracts.

For any material studied scientifically, or sold in retail, a sample should be retained for a period of time. This sample could be examined in the future, should any questions arise regarding identity or quality. In the case of fresh plant material, this can be a voucher specimen that is pressed and dried. If the test material is milled or powdered, or even in final product form, a retained sample, in that form, may still be used to answer any possible inquiries that might arise regarding identity or quality.

Voucher Specimens

Voucher specimens include the whole plant, or representative parts of the plant (ideally including flowers and seeds), pressed, dried, and fastened to an 11.5" by 16.5" card. Included along with the plant material is information as to the location and environment from which the plant was collected. Prepared in this way, the taxonomic identity of the specimen can be determined by a botanist. The specimen also serves as a lasting record.

Millions of plant specimens have been collected and stored in herbaria, to serve as reference collections of the world's flora. Most universities and many private organizations that work with plants house herbaria. The largest herbarium in the United States is the National Herbarium in Washington, DC, which houses 4.5 million specimens and contains collections from the exploration of North America in the 1800s (http://www.nmnh.si.edu/botany/colls.htm). The world's largest herbarium is the Royal Botanical Gardens in Kew, England, with over seven million specimens from all over the world, including 250,000 type specimens (specimens that define taxonomic species) (http://www.rbgkew.org.uk).

Voucher specimens are the most appropriate form of identification for primary suppliers of botanicals, i.e., farms, collectors, and those who have access to the entire plant.

Organoleptic Identification

Sensory, or organoleptic, information is very useful to those experienced with plant materials in establishing identity. Sight, touch, smell, taste, and sound can also assist in assessment of the quality of the material.

Organoleptic features are included in the following characterization of cinnamon bark (*Cinnamomum verum* J. Presl.):

> The matt pieces of bark, 0.2 to 0.7 mm thick, in the form of single or double compounds quills, light brown on the outside and somewhat darker on the inside; the surface longitudinally striated and the fracture is short and splintery. The odor is characteristic and pleasantly aromatic. The taste is pungently spicy, somewhat sweet and mucilaginous and only slightly sharp. (Wichtl, 1994, 148)

Microscopic Identification

Characteristic tissue structures, tissue organization, cell types, and cell contents can be viewed under magnification. For example, the glandular (rounded, multicellular) hairs common to mint leaves are quite distinct from the stellate (star-shaped) hairs of witch hazel leaves when viewed under a microscope. The addition of chemical reagents to the microscope slide can verify the presence and location, or absence, of starch grains, calcium carbonate, and/or oxalate crystals, as well as lignin (a plant cell wall component). Starch grains will appear purple following the addition of iodine, and their size and pattern are indicative of certain plants. Lignin will appear red with the addition of acidic phloroglucinol solution and is present in the cell walls of woody plants. The appearance of uncharacteristic components is an indication of adulteration or substitution.

Chemical Identification

Simple chemical tests can be performed on milled or powdered plant material by adding a few drops of a particular chemical reagent to the plant material. These tests usually indicate the presence or absence of a characteristic class of chemical constituent, for example, steroids or alkaloids. The presence of alkaloids, for example, can be determined by a purple (reddish-brown) color reaction following addition of Dragendorff's reagent (a solution of potassium bismuth iodide).

Extracts of plant material can be analyzed in more detail for characteristic compounds using spectroscopic analysis and chromatographic techniques. Spectroscopic analyses employ light absorption techniques to analyze classes of compounds. They include ultraviolet (UV), infrared (IR), and Fourier-transfom infrared (FTIR) spectroscopy.

Chromatographic techniques allow for the isolation and quantification of individual compounds. Components of the mixture are separated through chemical affinity to either the mobile phase (liquid or gas) or the stationary phase (solid substance such as silica over which the mobile phase runs). These techniques include thin layer chromatography (TLC), high performance thin layer chromatography (HPTLC), gas chromatography (GC), capillary electrophoresis (CE), and high performance liquid chromatography (HPLC).

Plant extracts examined using either spectroscopic or chromatographic techniques will display a characteristic profile, or "fingerprint," which is useful in identification. Even without chemical identification of all the individual components, a particular pattern accompanied with the identification of a few components can be an assurance of identity.

Chemical analysis is often offered as proof of identity of plant material, but it is not necessarily enough by itself. To prove this point, Dr. Alvin B. Segelman (1995) demonstrated that belladonna alkaloids added to sterilized cow dung could pass the *U.S. Pharmacopeia* chemical identification test. However, when the material was examined microscopically it was clear that it was neither belladonna leaves nor roots. Conversely, if plant material has been depleted chemically, through extraction, it may pass microscopic examination due to the remaining cell structure, but not chemical analysis. Therefore, both physical characterization (microscopic examination) and chemical analyses are needed for optimal identification.

When the results of chemical analysis are given as descriptors of a product, some indication of the test method must be provided. For example, extracts of St. John's wort (*Hypericum perforatum* L.) are often described as standardized to 0.3 percent hypericins. Hypericin is one of a group of biologically active dianthrones (phenolic compounds) in the herb that includes hypericin, pseudohypericin, protohypericin, and protopseudohypericin. The dianthrones in the extract can be measured using either UV spectroscopy or HPLC. UV spectroscopy will provide information as to absorption of light by compounds at a specific wavelength. Thus UV spectroscopy will indicate the total quantity of the dianthrones in the extract (as well as other compounds that absorb light at the tested frequency), and the results can be described as total hypericins. In contrast, HPLC analysis allows for the separation and quantification of the individual compounds. HPLC allows the quantities of hypericin, pseudohypericin, and other dianthrones to be determined individually. Therefore, the quantity of total hypericins as determined by UV will be different from the amount of the individual hypericin as quantified by HPLC.

As another example, the *U.S. Pharmacopeia* (2004) method of measuring the alkaloids in belladonna extract via HPLC will give a slightly different number from the European Pharmacopoeial (Ph Eur) method which measures total alkaloid content via titration (Ph Eur, 2002). Thus in describing the amount of any constituent in a botanical, the method of analysis must be indicated.

PREPARATIONS AND FORMULATIONS

Herbs are sold in many forms, as fresh plant material in the produce department of a grocery store, and as dried plant material in bulk, tea bags, capsules, or tablets. Fresh or dried plant material can be prepared as extracts, either sold in liquid form, or dried and formulated into tablets or capsules, both hard and soft. Some basic botanical preparations and formulations are described in the appendix to this chapter.

The diversity in plant preparations is illustrated by those available for commercially supplied Asian ginseng roots, which are graded according to their source, age, part of the root, and method of preparation (Bahrke and Morgan, 1994). The root can be used fresh, or prepared as "white" ginseng (peeled and dried) or "red" ginseng (steamed and dried). The fresh root is often thinly sliced and taken with or without honey, or it can be boiled in soup. White or red ginseng can be powdered, extracted, or made into a tea (Yun and Choi, 1998). The different ginseng root preparations differ in their chemical composition. As an example, we know that the heating process in the production of red ginseng converts the malonylginsenosides to their ginsenoside counterparts and also results in other chemical transformations (Chuang et al., 1995).

DOSE

The preparations described are, by definition, of different strengths and composition. Thus the type of preparation will have an influence on the recommended dose. Teas prepared with hot water are usually quite dilute in contrast with extracts that are more concentrated. So it follows that the type of preparation must be taken into account in determining the dose. For example, peppermint tea may be drunk by the cupful, while peppermint oil is administered in doses of five hundredths of a milliliter (Wren, 1988).

BIOAVAILABILITY

The type of preparation, and formulation of the preparation, will have an influence on the ability of the chemical components of the herb to be assimilated into the body. This is especially a concern with tablets and capsules whose contents must first dissolve before being absorbed. Coatings on the surface of tablet or capsules may be designed to either accelerate or delay dissolution (release of chemical constituents) in the gastrointestinal tract.

As an example, garlic products often have enteric coatings to delay dissolution until the garlic preparation reaches the intestine. The reason for this is that garlic powder contains the enzyme allinase, which is necessary to produce the active constituent allicin, and that enzyme is destroyed by the acidic pH of the stomach. Studies on the effectiveness of Kwai garlic to reduce elevated serum cholesterol levels have been inconsistent. A review found a highly significant difference in effectiveness between studies conducted before 1993 and those conducted in 1993 and later. The authors found that the amount of allicin released under simulated gastrointestinal conditions correlated well with the success or failure of the tablets to lower serum cholesterol values. The sharp decline in the effectiveness of the tablets is paralleled by sharp declines in both the acid resistance and the allicin release from the tablets, apparently caused by a change in the coating of the tablet (Lawson, Wang, and Papadimitriou, 2001).

GUIDELINES

As demonstrated in this chapter, therapeutic effect is a result of the following variables: botanical identity, chemical profile, formulation, bioavailability, and dose. Therefore, characterization of botanical products, in publications and scientific studies, needs to include all of that information. An adequate description of botanical products is needed in order to ensure a consistent therapeutic effect. It is also needed to be able to compare products and to conduct statistical analyses on the results of multiple trials.

Editors of scientific, particularly medical, literature need to be cognizant of the breadth of information required. The *Journal of Natural Products,* published by the American Chemical Society and the American Society of Pharmacognosy, provides guidance to its authors in the characterization of botanical substances. It requires that experimental biological material be authenticated as to its identity and that the herbarium which holds the voucher specimen be given along with the voucher number. It further requires that the scientific name (genus, species, authority citation, and family) be given. It also requires authors who purchase dried "herbal remedies" or other materials from companies to deposit a specimen in an herbarium, for future access. It requires that the extraction procedure be specified when studying a commercially available extract and that the identification of the extract be supported by an HPLC trace of known secondary metabolite constituents (*Journal of Natural Products*, 2003).

NCCAM, in its guidelines for clinical trial grant applications, suggests that when plant material is used in a trial, it be accompanied by a botanical description, extraction procedure, the quantity of any known active constituent(s), as well as identity and stability tests. When a product is used, information about the manufacturing process, analysis for impurities, and quality controls for manufacturing must be included. In addition, disintegration/dissolution rates are required to estimate bioavailability (NCCAM, 2003).

APPENDIX: PREPARATIONS AND FORMULATIONS

Preparations

Teas and Decoctions

A tea, or infusion, is made by pouring boiling water over finely chopped plant material (usually leaves and flowers). The mixture is allowed to stand for a period of time before straining. The usual ratio is 500 ml (1 pint) of water to 30 g (1 oz) plant material. A decoction is made by adding cold water to the plant material and then heating it to a boil. The mixture is allowed to simmer before cooling and straining. Decoctions are often made of roots, bark, and berries, which may require more forceful treatment than more fragile plant parts such as leaves and flowers. The same proportions of water to plant material apply, but it is best to start with 800 ml (1½ pints) to allow for evaporation. Teas and decoctions may be consumed either hot or cold.

Plant Juices

Freshly harvested plant parts can be pressed to release their juices. The shelf life of the expressed juice is usually extended by pasteurization or by rapid, ultra-high-temperature treatment. In addition, alcohol may be added as a preservative.

Tinctures

A tincture is made by soaking the plant material in a solution of alcohol and water for a period of time followed by filtering. Tinctures are sold in liquid form and are useful for both concentrating and preserving an herb. They are made in different strengths that are expressed as ratios. Traditionally, a ratio of 1 part herb to 5 or 10 parts liquid (1:5 or 1:10) has been used. These ratios represent 100 g (3½ oz) plant material in 500 ml (1 pint) of solvent, or 100 g plant material in 1000 ml (2 pints) solvent.

Extracts

Extracts are concentrated preparations that can be in liquid, viscous, or powdered form. They are prepared from fresh or dried plant material by distillation, maceration (soaking then filtering), or percolation. The extraction liquid or solvent is chosen for its chemical properties, as it will selectively extract components in the plant that match those chemical properties. Typical solvents include water-alcohol mixtures, glycerin (a colorless, odorless, syrupy, sweet liquid), oils, supercritical gases (carbon dioxide can be liquefied at certain temperatures and pressures), hexane, methylene chloride, acetone, and ethyl acetate. Some or all of the liquid solvent can then be evaporated to make a dry extract, which can be easily placed into capsules or made into tablets. This is often accomplished by evaporating the liquid in the presence of a carrier such as cellulose, lactose, maltodextrose, or even dried plant material.

Again, ratios are used to describe the strength of the extract. Most crude plant materials have a content of roughly 20 percent extractable substances which corresponds to an herb to extract ratio of 5:1. If the extract is further purified, even greater ratios can be obtained. However, this means that some components of the plant have been selected over other components. For example, the standardized ginkgo extracts, which are made in a multistep purification process, are highly purified extracts with an average ratio of 50:1. This ratio means that 50 parts of plant material went into producing one part extract. Essentially the extract is a concentration of certain flavonoids and terpenes present in ginkgo leaves.

Syrups

Medicinal syrups are viscous liquids that contain a minimum of 50 percent sugar, more typically 65 percent, added to a plant extract. This high concentration of sugar acts as a preservative.

Oils

Oils can be produced by pressing or extracting plant materials such as seeds and fruits. Crude oils can be refined by distillation. Alternatively, medicinal oils can contain plant substances dissolved in oil. These oil-based extracts are typically used as salves or in other topical applications.

Formulations

Tablets

Tablets are made by compressing powdered or granulated material. Besides the active ingredients, tablets may contain diluents, binders, lubricants, coloring, and flavoring agents. They also contain disintegrators that help the compressed tablet to dissolve when it comes in contact with water. Tablets can be coated with sugar, dyes, fat, wax, or film-forming polymers. The function of the coating may be to extend the life of the tablet by protecting the active ingredients. It also may be to control or delay the release of the active ingredient. Coated tablets may mask any unpleasant taste of the active ingredient and may make the tablet easier to swallow.

Capsules

Hard gelatin capsules consist of a two-part cylindrical shell. They usually enclose plant material or dried extracts. Soft gelatin capsules are spherical, oval, oblong, or teardrop shaped and consist of a gelatin shell enclosing semisolid or liquid contents. The composition of the capsule can be designed to control the release of the contents. For example, an enteric coating, which resists the acid in the stomach, will dissolve in the intestine when the pH rises above 7.

Lozenges

Lozenges have a tabletlike appearance but differ in that they are not made by compression. They are molded or cut from a gummy mass. Lozenges are designed to release the active ingredient slowly in the mouth while being sucked or chewed. They are often made with sugar, gums, gelatin, and water.

REFERENCES

Awang DVC, Kindack DG (1991). Echinacea. *Canadian Pharmaceutical Journal* 124 (11): 512-516.

Bahrke MS, Morgan WP (1994). Evaluation of the ergogenic properties of ginseng. *Sports Medicine* 18 (4): 229-248.

Chuang WC, Wu HK, Sheu SJ, Chiou SH, Chang HC, Chen YP (1995). A comparative study on commercial samples of ginseng radix. *Planta Medica* 61: 459-465.

European Pharmacopoeia (Ph Eur) (2002). Belladonna Leaf Dry Extract standardized. *European Pharmacopoeia,* Fourth Edition. Strasbourg Cedex, France: Council of Europe, p. 700.

Greuter W, McNeill J, Barrie FR, Burdet HM, Demoulin V, Filgueiras RS, Nicholson DH, Silva PC, Skog JE, Trehane P, et al. (2000). *International Code of Botanical Nomenclature (St Louis Code). Regnum Vegetable 131.* Königstein, Germany: Koeltz Scientific Books.

Hobbs C (1994). Echinacea, a literature review. *HerbalGram* 30: 33-47.

Journal of Natural Products (2003). Preparation of manuscripts. *Journal of Natural Products* 66 (1): 10A.

Lawson LD, Wang ZJ, Papadimitriou D (2001). Allicin release under simulated gastrointestinal conditions from garlic powder tablets employed in clinical trials on serum cholesterol. *Planta Medica* 67 (1): 13-18.

McGuffin M, Kartesz JT, Leung AY, Tucker AO (2000). *The American Herbal Products Association's Herbs of Commerce,* Second Edition. Silver Spring, MD: American Herbal Products Association.

National Center for Complementary and Alternative Medicine (NCCAM) (2003). Considerations for NCCAM Clinical Trial Grant Applications (nccam.nih.gov).

Segelman AB (1995). Quality control in the herb industry. American Chemical Society Middle Atlantic Regional Meeting, American University, Washington DC, May 25. Abstract 224.

Slifman NR, Obermeyer WR, Aloi BK, Musser SM, Correll WA, Cichowicz SM, Betz JM, Love LA (1998). Contamination of botanical dietary supplements by *Digitalis lanata. New England Journal of Medicine* 339 (12): 806-811.

Trease GE, Evans WC (1978). *Pharmacognosy,* Eleventh Edition. London: Bailliere Tindall.

Turner RB, Riker DK, Gangemi JD (2000). Ineffectiveness of echinacea for prevention of experimental rhinovirus colds. *Antimicrobial Agents and Chemotherapy* 44 (6): 1708-1709.

U.S. Pharmacopeia (USP) (2004). Belladonna Extract. *US Pharmacopeia and National Formulary,* USP 27, NF 22: 211. Rockville, MD: U.S. Pharmacopeial Convention.

Vanhaelen M, Vanhaelen-Fastre R, But P, Vanherweghem L (1994). Identification of aristolochic acid in Chinese herbs. *The Lancet* 343 (8890): 174.

Wichtl M (1994). *Herbal Drugs and Phytopharmaceuticals, a Handbook for Practice on a Scientific Basis.* Trans. NG Bisset. Stuttgart: Medpharm Scientific Publishers, and Boca Raton, FL: CRC Press.

Wren RC (1988). *Potter's New Cyclopaedia of Botanical Drugs and Preparations.* Revised by EM Williamson, FJ Evans. Saffron Walden, England: The CW Daniel Company Ltd.

Yun TK, Choi SY (1998). Non-organ specific cancer prevention of ginseng: A prospective study in Korea. *International Journal of Epidemiology* 27 (3): 359-364.

Chapter 4

Standardization of Botanical Preparations: What It Does and Does Not Tell Us

Uwe Koetter
Marilyn Barrett

INTRODUCTION

Standardization is probably one of the most controversial terms used to describe herbal supplements. Most would agree that the goal of standardizing herbal products is to provide product consistency and thus a reliable health benefit. However, the term has been defined in several different ways. Standardization can mean the establishment of a consistent biological effect, a consistent chemical profile, or simply a quality assurance program for production and manufacturing.

How the process of standardization is applied depends, in part, on whether the active constituents in the botanical are well established. For that reason, the European Union has defined three categories of botanical products: (1) those containing constituents (single compounds or families of compounds) with known and acknowledged therapeutic activity that are deemed solely responsible for the clinical efficacy; (2) those containing chemically defined constituents possessing relevant pharmacological properties which are likely to contribute to the clinical efficacy; and (3) those in which no constituents have been identified as being responsible for the therapeutic activity (Lang and Stumpf, 1999).

This chapter will discuss how the extent of knowledge regarding the active constituents in the botanical relates to standardizing botanical products either to a consistent biological effect, a consistent chemical profile, or as part of a quality assurance program. The most important point is that there is no one definition of standardization and that this term has been applied differently to different products in the marketplace. In addition, no legal or regulatory definition of standardization for herbal products has been established in the United States.

STANDARDIZATION OF THERAPEUTIC ACTIVITY

The standardization of active ingredients in botanical preparations is a well-established procedure that has been used for over a century. Before sophisticated chemical analytical methods were available, and when the active principles were unknown, preparations were standardized to biological activity. This was accomplished with the help of bioassays: measurements of activity in animals or animal tissues. Bioassays were especially important tools for normalizing the activity of powerful drugs, such as digitalis, in which small variances in the glycoside content could lead to sufficient differences in the cardiac stimulating effect that could be dangerous. Still today, the potency of digitalis preparations is determined using a pigeon assay, which compares the activity of the new preparation to that of a standard preparation (U.S. Pharmacopeia [USP], 2004b).

In those instances in which the chemical constituents deemed responsible for the clinical efficacy (active ingredients or active components) are known and easily measured, chemical analysis can indirectly determine biological activity. With the advent of more sophisticated chemical analytical techniques, it became more efficient to replace bioassays with the measurement of chemical constituents.

Standardization of a botanical product with established active components is achieved by adjusting the preparation to contain a defined level of active substance or group of substances in the dosage form. This can be achieved by adjusting the final amount of raw material (i.e., extract or powdered herb) in the dosage form so as to include a consistent amount of active constituent. It can also be achieved by including a consistent amount of raw material that contains a consistent amount of active ingredient. In the latter case, the consistency of the raw material is achieved by blending different lots of material. As an example, milk thistle preparations contain silymarin, which is accepted as the active component of the botanical. So, the amount of product in the dosage form could be either a fixed amount of silymarin in a variable amount of total extract, or a fixed amount of extract that has been adjusted to contain a fixed amount of silymarin.

Guidelines for the standardization of specific botanical preparations can be found in pharmacopoeial monographs. These guidelines include the methods used to determine the levels of active ingredients. As an example, the *United States Pharmacopeia* defines belladonna extract as containing not less than 1.15 g, and not more than 1.35 g, of alkaloids (measured as atropine [*dl*-hyoscyamine] and scopolamine via high performance liquid chromatography [HPLC]) in 100 g extract (USP, 2004a). The *European Pharmacopoeia* defines standardized belladonna leaf dry extract as containing not less than 0.95 percent, and not more than 1.05 percent, total alkaloids calculated as hyoscyamine measured via titration (European Pharmacopoeia [Ph Eur], 2002a).

An important distinction can be made between single chemical compounds that are *active ingredients* and *active components* of a mixture. For example, hyoscyamine as an isolated compound may be an active ingredient in a pharmaceutical formula. However, as a component of belladonna extract, and one of several alkaloids in the extract with activity, it is an active component of the extract.

Standardization to active constituents can ensure consistency between lots produced by the same manufacturer. However, it is just one step toward comparing a proprietary preparation that has been tested in clinical studies with another proprietary preparation of the same botanical. Even if the claimed level of constituents is accurate, the inherent variability in the undefined portion of the extract must be considered. In addition, different formulations or routes of administration may affect the bioavailability (levels of active components present at the site of action in the body).

STANDARDIZATION TO MEET A CHEMICAL NORM

Botanical products can be standardized to a norm that may or may not relate to the expected biological activity of the product. Usually this norm is a level of a constituent chemical or group of chemicals called marker compounds. The concept of determining levels of marker compounds was developed because it is not feasible to test for all compounds in an extract and final formula for content and consistency. *Markers* are chemically defined constituents of an herbal drug, ideally specific to that herb, which are of interest for quality control purposes independent of whether they have any therapeutic activity (European Agency for the Evaluation of Medicinal Products [EMEA], 2000).

By providing product characterization, marker compounds can be used to facilitate botanical identification and detection of adulteration. They can also be used as indicators of consistency throughout manufacturing, handling, and storage. When marker levels are determined in the starting materials they can be used to calculate the quantity of herbal drug or preparation in the finished product. Setting minimum limits for marker compounds can be a useful indicator of quality in preparations in which there is little, or contradictory, knowledge regarding the active constituents.

As there is no established active ingredient in this class of botanicals, the whole preparation is considered to be the active principle. Standardization is achieved by including a consistent amount of raw material (i.e., extract or powdered herb) in the dosage form. Preparations that contain powdered herb are filled with a set amount of powder. The amount of marker compound in the powdered herb can be controlled through blending different lots of powder. Preparations that contain extracts can be made consistent by controlling the ratio of plant material to extract and including either a fixed amount of plant material or a fixed amount of extract.

For consistency, determinations regarding levels of markers in finished products should be made with validated methods for specific formulations. For some botanicals, detailed analytical procedures are provided by pharmacopoeial monographs. However, adherence to pharmacopoeial guidelines may be regional or voluntary, and compliance may not be apparent from product labels.

Analytical methods can be used to measure either classes of compounds or individual constituents. Thus the measurement can be general in nature or highly specific. Ultraviolet/visible light spectroscopy (UV/VIS) results in detection and quantification of a general class of compounds, compared to high performance liquid chromatography (HPLC), which allows for analysis of individual compounds. Thin layer chromatography (TLC) presents a general profile of the plant and can detect whether the product contains a full spectrum extract or a few isolated compounds.

As an example, some echinacea products are standardized to contain 4 percent phenolics. This measurement will mean something quite different if the determination is made using the Folin-Ciocalteu spectrophotometric (UV) method detecting phenolics as a class of compounds, than if it is made using an HPLC method detecting specific phenolics, i.e., cichoric acid, 2-caffeoyl tartaric acid, and echinacoside. In addition, two HPLC analyses can yield different results if different test parameters are used and/or if different phenolic constituents are measured.

In addition, the purity of chemical reference standards, as well as sampling methods, sample preparation, sample matrix (excipients used in formulation of the sample), solvents, and the equipment used, all contribute to the results achieved in chemical analysis.

Thus, it is important to realize that no global consensus has yet been made regarding standards or test methods for herbal products, although attempts are being made in this direction.

STANDARDIZATION AS A REFLECTION OF QUALITY ASSURANCE PROGRAMS

Standardization is also understood to be, and perhaps better described as, a quality assurance program. This type of standardization is the result of following guidelines that cover all aspects of production from seed selection, cultivation, collection, extraction, and formulation to production of the final product. Throughout this process, the measurement of a particular chemical or chemicals can be used to indicate the consistency of one lot throughout production and the consistency of numerous lots to one another.

The quality assurance process starts with the cultivation and/or harvesting of the plant material. The chemical profile of plant material can vary due to genetics, environmental factors, seasonal and/or diurnal variation, the age of the plant, selection of the plant part, the time of harvest, postharvest treatment (drying and storage conditions), and processing.

For example, there are 72 cultivars of the same species of kava growing in Vanuatu (South Pacific) with kavalactone contents ranging from 3 to 20 percent (Dentali, 1997). In another example, St. John's wort growing conditions are important for consistent chemical profiling. Studies have shown that the phenolic content increases in dry climates and when the ambient temperature is above 57°F (Upton et al., 1997). Harvest time is important for ginseng roots. The content in American ginseng varies from 3 percent in the first year to 8 percent in the fourth year (Court, Reynolds, and Hendel, 1996).

Awareness of the possible variation of a particular botanical can be used to guide the control of each step of the process. Under controlled conditions, a plant variety can be bred for consistency, the growing environment can be carefully selected, and watering and the use or avoidance of pesticides, herbicides, and fertilizers can be directed and monitored. In addition, the plant can be harvested at the optimal time, and processing after harvest can take place in a controlled environment. Careful management of postharvest processing can prevent or control enzymatic processes and preserve the content of volatile oils.

As part of the standardization process, manufacturing protocols must be in place to guarantee consistency in the extraction process. Extraction of plant materials is a process of using a liquid or *solvent* to remove substances from the crude plant material. This is a process many of us use daily to make tea or coffee. As everyone knows from experience, the consistent quality of the raw material accounts only partly for the quality of the end product. Both the water temperature and the amount of water used will also influence the quality of the drink. In addition, there is consideration with coffee as to whether the beans are boiled in water, percolated with boiling water, or steamed under pressure. So, too, with commercial botanical extraction procedures, the quality of the extracts will vary depending upon the conditions of the extraction process, including solvent type, temperature, method of extraction, and the ratio of plant material to solvent.

The ratio of plant material (by weight) to solvent (by volume) is referred to as the *strength* of the extract. This ratio is sometimes listed on the product label as a description of the extract. For example, an extract made with 100 g of plant material in 1000 ml solvent would be described as having a ratio of 1 to 10 and might appear on a label as 1:10. The ratio can also appear as a range. For example, the German Commission E monograph for hawthorn leaf and flower extract allows for the ratio of plant material to extract to be from 4 to 7:1, with a defined flavonoid or procyanidin content calculated according to the *German Pharmacopoeia* (Blumenthal et al., 1998).

GUIDANCE

The lack of uniform understanding of the term *standardization* is reflected in a guidance note drafted by the European Agency for the Evaluation of Medicinal Products. Standardization, as defined in the note for guidance on the quality of herbal medicinal products, means adjusting the herbal drug preparation to a defined content of a constituent or group of substances with known therapeutic activity. However, the group further states that in some member states of the European Union the expression is used to describe all measures which are taken during the manufacturing process and quality control leading to a reproducible effect (EMEA, 2000).

The EMEA makes the distinction between constituents with known therapeutic activity, which can be used to standardize to a biological effect, and marker compounds, which allow standardization on a set amount of the chosen compound. Constituents with known therapeutic activity are defined as chemically defined substances that are generally accepted to contribute substantially to the therapeutic activity of a herbal drug or of a preparation. Examples given of known active constituents include the kava pyrones in kava kava (*Piper methysticum* G. Forst.); silymarin in milk thistle [*Silybum marianum* (L.) Gaertn.]; and aescin in horse chestnut (*Aesculus hippocastanum* L.) (EMEA, 2000).

The EMEA defines marker compounds as chemically defined constituents of a herbal drug which are of interest for control purposes, independent of whether they have any therapeutic activity or not. Examples of markers are the valerenic acids in valerian (*Valeriana officinalis* L.), ginkgolides and flavonoids in ginkgo (*Ginkgo biloba* L.), and flavonoids, hypericin, and hyperforin in St. John's wort (*Hypericum perforatum* L.) (EMEA, 2000).

In Europe, herbal preparations with known actives are standardized in reference to the pharmacopoeial monograph. Where the active compound is not known, the whole preparation is considered to be the active principle. In this case the monograph sets quality guidelines and measurement of marker compounds as a means of quality control.

Both the *European* and *United States Pharmacopoeias* set lower and upper limits for chemical constituents in an extract. As an example, the *European Pharmacopoeia* defines standardized senna leaf

(*Senna alexandrina* Mill.) extract as containing 5.5 to 8.0 percent hydroxyanthracene glycosides, calculated as sennosides (Ph Eur, 2002b). Since the level of active sennosides has been defined, the monograph can reasonably recommend a dose of the whole extract that is expected to produce the declared laxative effect.

In the United States, compliance with pharmacopoeial standards is required for drugs but is optional for dietary supplements.

SITUATION IN THE MARKETPLACE

Assumptions have been made about what the term standardized means when applied to herbal products. It is often incorrectly assumed that botanicals are similar to single-entity drugs, e.g., aspirin, in which one chemical listed on the label is responsible for the activity. This assumption has led consumers, retailers, and even extract manufacturers to presume that controlling the levels of a chemical constituent is equivalent to controlling the physiological effect. Furthermore, when examining the label of a botanical dietary supplement marketed in the United States, it is not possible to distinguish the listing of active constituents of a botanical preparation from marker compounds that may either be inactive or possess pharmacological activity unrelated to the therapeutic application.

Because of the assumed correlation with pharmaceutical agents with identified active ingredients, U.S. manufacturers and consumers often assumed that "more is better." This attitude has prevailed regardless of whether the identified chemical is an active component or a marker compound. On the market, ginseng product labels frequently claim anywhere from 2 to 10 percent ginsenosides. However, no evidence suggests that the effects are increased with higher levels of ginsenosides. In fact, one clinical study suggests that no additional increase in physical work capacity occurs when the ginsenoside content is increased from 4 to 7 percent (Forgo and Kirchdorfer, 1982).

Thus, enrichment of a chemical constituent does not necessarily result in an increase in potency. Even in the case of identified active constituents, other components of the botanical may be present which either increase or complement that action. Or components may decrease or oppose the principal action. The matrix of components in the botanical may also affect the bioavailability of the preparation by enhancing solubility, absorption, and/or stability. These complex interactions are not well understood. Therefore, the entire plant material or herbal preparation should be regarded as the active substance.

Efforts to increase the amount of marker compounds used for standardization are usually driven by market forces and reveal a lack of understanding of the complexity of the issue. The only exception is when this increase is backed by product-specific clinical data and an established link to efficacy or consumer benefit has been identified.

When a preparation differs from the traditional or pharmacopoeial guidelines by enriching the concentration of a select constituent, it must be considered a novel preparation. As a new preparation, appropriate efficacy and safety data need to be collected. The product ought to be tested clinically. Data from established products demonstrating efficacy and tolerability do not necessarily apply to other products. For example, safety and efficacy data collected on kava products containing 30 to 40 percent kavalactones may not apply to products containing twice that percentage, and vice versa.

PERSPECTIVE

Regulatory requirements for the quality of botanical products vary depending on the country and the regulatory category. The same herbal product can be marketed as a drug in Germany and as a dietary supplement in the United States. In Germany, medicinal plant products are produced to quality standards typical for pharmaceutical products. This is especially true for potent herbals in which the active ingredients are defined, contribute substantially to the therapeutic activity, and allow standardization to a biological effect. Specifications for these products include standardization of a constituent, or constituents, within a set range supported by a pharmacopoeial monograph.

If the active components are not established, then markers are used to assure/measure quality. When there is no established link between the marker compound and consumer benefit or efficacy, the herbal drug or the herbal preparation *in its entirety* is regarded as the active substance.

Individual governments, the World Health Organization, and panels of academic experts and clinicians provide guidelines for manufacturing and quality control, as well as therapeutic use (indication, dose, and possible safety concerns). Many of these guidelines are contained in pharmacopoeial monographs. Compliance with these guidelines is governed by regulations that cover all aspects from manufacturing to labeling and advertising of final products.

In the United States, compliance of dietary supplements to a pharmacopoeial monograph is optional. Therefore, it is difficult for consumers of dietary supplements to make informed decisions about self-medication based upon label information. The level of quality control used by different manufacturers varies widely. Claims of standardization are made without definition of the term, or indication of whether the chemicals used in standardization are responsible for the therapeutic effect. Often no indication is given of which test method was used to determine the marker levels. Without all this information, the consumer commonly makes purchasing decisions based upon price. Thus, regrettably, it appears that price, rather than quality or proven therapeutic effect, drives the market.

REFERENCES

Blumenthal M, Busse W, Hall T, Goldberg A, Grünwald J, Riggins C, Rister S, eds. (1998). *The Complete German Commission E Monographs: Therapeutic Guide to Herbal Medicines.* Trans. S Klein. Austin, TX: American Botanical Council.

Court WA, Reynolds B, Hendel JG (1996). Influence of root age on the concentration of ginsenosides of American ginseng (*Panax quinquefolius*). *Canadian Journal of Plant Science* 76 (4): 853-855.

Dentali S (1997). *Herb Safety Review of Kava,* Piper methysticum *Forster f.* Boulder, CO: Herb Research Foundation.

European Agency for the Evaluation of Medicinal Products (EMEA) (2000). Note for guidance on specifications: Test procedures and acceptance criteria for herbal drugs, herbal drug preparations, and herbal medicinal products. CPMP/QWP/2820/00.

European Pharmacopoeia (Ph Eur) (2002a). Belladonna Leaf Dry Extract standardized. *European Pharmacopoeia,* Fourth Edition. Strasbourg Cedex, France: Council of Europe, p. 700.

European Pharmacopoeia (Ph Eur) (2002b). Senna Leaf Dry Extract standardized. *European Pharmacopoeia,* Fourth Edition. Strasbourg Cedex, France: Council of Europe, p. 1885.

Forgo I, Kirchdorfer AM (1982). The effect of different ginsenoside concentrations on physical work capacity. *Notabene Medici* 12 (9): 721-727.

Lang F, Stumpf H (1999). Considerations on future pharmacopoeial monographs for plant extracts. *Pharmeuropa* 11: 268-275.

Upton R, Graff A, Williamson E, Bunting D, Gatherum DM, Walker EB, Butterweck V, Liefländer-Wulf U, Nahrstedt A, Wall A, et al. (1997). *St. John's Wort, Hypericum perforatum. Quality Control, Analytical and Therapeutic Monograph. American Herbal Pharmacopoeia and Therapeutic Compendium.* Ed. R Upton. Santa Cruz: American Herbal Pharmacopoeia.

U.S. Pharmacopeia (USP) (2004a). Belladonna Extract. *US Pharmacopoeia and National Formulary,* USP 27, NF 22: 211. Rockville, MD: U.S. Pharmacopeial Convention.

U.S. Pharmacopeia (USP) (2004b). Digitalis monograph. *US Pharmacopoeia and National Formulary,* USP 27, NF 22: 610. Rockville, MD: U.S. Pharmacopeial Convention.

Chapter 5

The Importance and Difficulty in Determining the Bioavailability of Herbal Preparations

Anton Biber
Friedrich Lang

Bioavailability is an important issue to consider in the evaluation of the therapeutic effects of a botanical (herbal) product. The biological effect of any substance is influenced by the extent to which it is absorbed into the body, metabolized (e.g., by gut flora and/or liver enzymes), distributed throughout the body, and finally excreted. A diverse array of factors influence bioavailability, including the route of administration (oral, IV, or topical), the age of the person, his or her particular genetics, other foods or drugs taken at the same time, whether the person smokes, and any relevant disease pathologies. The pharmacological effect of the drug can occur only if the drug, or an active metabolite, reaches and sustains an adequate concentration at the appropriate site of action in the body.

Studies on bioavailability are an integral part in the development of conventional drugs. One of the most basic considerations in determining bioavailability is the formulation of the drug. Formulation in liquid or solid form (pills, capsules, tablets) and with special coatings (e.g., delayed release) will influence the absorption of the product. The ability of solid products to dissolve is studied in disintegration and dissolution tests using solutions that mimic the conditions in the stomach or intestine. A disintegration test measures the extent to which the solid dosage form dissolves. A dissolution test is designed to detect the presence and quantity of the active principal in the dissolved media. Disintegration and dissolution tests for specific products are described in U.S. Pharmacopeia (USP) monographs. Pharmacokinetic studies measure the metabolism, distribution, and excretion of the active substance in the bodies of animals and humans. Disintegration, dissolution, and pharmacokinetic data are required for most pharmaceutical drugs before marketing. These studies are important because the beneficial effects will not occur if doses are too small, and toxic effects can occur if doses are too large or if the drug accumulates in the body.

Data on the bioavailability of herbal medicinal products are not as common as they are for chemically defined synthetic drugs. Although disintegration studies would be fairly easy to carry out, dissolution and pharmacokinetics studies are inherently difficult. The reason for the difficulty is that these assays require the detection and quantification of isolated constituents. It is often difficult to decide which component(s) of a botanical should be used in these assays. Often the constituents responsible for the therapeutic activity are unknown or there is no scientific agreement on the probable active constituent(s). In this case, a surrogate, or marker compound, is chosen as a measuring tool. However, the extent to which the active constituent(s) is known determines the relevance of the bioavailability studies to the therapeutic effect.

Even when the active ingredient is established, it is often present in low concentrations, making quantification in plasma difficult. However, in the past ten years, sophisticated analytical techniques, such as high performance liquid chromatography (HPLC) or gas chromatography (GC) with sensitive detectors, including ultraviolet (UV), fluorescence, electrochemical (ECD), and mass spectrometry (MS), have become available. As a result, more pharmacokinetic data on herbal medicinal products have been published recently (De Smet and Brouwers, 1997). Some examples of studies are listed in Table 5.1.

In most cases in Europe, no pharmacokinetic data are necessary for the approval for marketing an herbal medicinal product as a drug. At present, dissolution tests are required only for standardized extracts in which the constituents solely responsible for the clinical efficacy have been identified. No data are required for nonstandardized extracts or extracts in which no constituent(s) is acknowledged as being solely responsible for the therapeutic effect (European Medicines Evaluation Agency [EMEA], 1999). Recently, however, it has been acknowledged that biopharmaceutic and pharmacokinetic aspects should be involved in the development of all herbal medicinal prod-

TABLE 5.1. Pharmacokinetic data on humans after administration of herbal medicinal products

Extract/product administered	Substance analyzed	Method	Reference
Horse chestnut, *Aesculus hippocastanum* L.	Aescin	Radioimmunoassay	Oschmann et al., 1996
Ginkgo, *Ginkgo biloba* L.	Ginkgolides A, B, bilobalide	GC/MS	Fourtillan et al., 1995
Milk thistle, *Silybum marianum* (L.) Gaertn.	Silibinin	HPLC	Schulz et al., 1995
Myrtle, *Myrtus communis* L.	Cineol	GC	Zimmermann et al., 1995
St. John's wort, *Hypericum perforatum* L.	Hypericin Hyperforin	HPLC/Fluorescence LC/MS/MS	Kerb et al., 1996; Biber et al., 1998
Buckwheat, *Fagopyrum esculentum* Moench	Quercetin	HPLC/ECD	Graefe et al., 2001

ucts (Blume and Schug, 2000). In this regard, the Herbal Medicinal Products working group of the FIP (Federation Internationale Pharmaceutique/International Pharmaceutical Federation) published recommendations on the biopharmaceutical characterization of herbal medicinal products (Lang et al., 2003).

In the United States, the U.S. Pharmacopeia Subcommittee on Natural Products produced a draft guideline suggesting that dissolution testing should be an integral part of the public standard for botanicals marketed as dietary supplements (USP Committee of Revision, 2000b). The USP Committee proposes that disintegration testing be only an interim standard for botanical formulations in which no dissolution test is feasible (USP Committee of Revision, 2000a). The members acknowledge that the index compound(s) or marker compounds selected for demonstration of dissolution may not be responsible for the therapeutic effect.

For companies applying for approval to market their botanicals as drugs in the United States, the Food and Drug Administration (FDA) *Guidance for Industry: Botanical Drug Products* requests that bioavailability data be submitted when the companies file Investigational New Drug Applications (IND) (FDA/CDER, 2000).

Factors influencing the importance and ease of conducting bioavailability studies include the type of therapeutic activity and the extent to which the active constituents have been identified. Common sense tells us that bioavailability studies are more important for botanicals with immediate and strong activity. For those botanicals with mild or tonic actions (with a wide safety margin), fewer studies may be required (De Smet and Brouwers, 1997).

In the *European Pharmacopoeia,* botanical preparations are divided into three categories depending upon the degree to which the active components are known. In the first category (A) are extracts containing constituents (single compounds or families of compounds) with known and acknowledged therapeutic activity deemed solely responsible for the clinical efficacy. Extracts in this category are standardized by adjusting the amounts of the active constituents within acceptable minimum and maximum levels. This adjustment is achieved by mixing the extract with inert materials or by blending batches of extracts. Examples of category A botanicals in the *European Pharmacopoeia* are aloe dry extract, buckthorn bark dry extract, senna leaf dry extract, and belladonna leaf dry extract. Examples in the *German Pharmacopoeia* are ipecacuanha dry extract, rhubarb dry extract, milk thistle fruit dry extract, and horse chestnut seed dry extract (Lang et al., 2003).

In the second category (B) are extracts containing chemically defined constituents (single or groups) possessing relevant pharmacological properties that are likely to contribute to the clinical efficacy. However, proof that they are solely responsible for the clinical efficacy has not been provided. Quantified extracts are prepared by adjusting select constituents to defined upper and lower tolerance levels by blending batches of extracts. As there may be unidentified constituents with clinical efficacy in the extract, the use of inert material to standardize preparations is not appropriate. Examples of category B botanicals are ginkgo leaf dry extract and St. John's wort dry extract, listed in the *German* and *European Pharmacopoeia,* respectively (Lang et al., 2003).

Extracts that do not contain any constituents regarded as being responsible for the therapeutic activity are placed in category C. For these botanicals, chemically defined constituents (markers) may be used for quality control purposes to monitor good manufacturing practices or to determine the contents in the product. These extracts are essentially defined by their production process specifications (e.g., the state of the herbal material to be extracted, the solvent, the extraction conditions, plant to extract ratio, etc.). An example of a category C botanical in the *German Pharmacopoeia* is valerian root dry extract (Lang et al., 2003).

In the European Medicines Evaluation Agency's "Note for guidance on the investigation of bioavailability and bioequivalence," it is stated that the bioavailability of an active substance from a pharmaceutical product should be known and be reproducible. This is especially the case if one product is to be substituted for another. Bioequivalence studies should be performed for all oral immediate release products intended for systemic action, unless in vitro data are sufficient (EMEA, 2001). This concept, originally developed for synthetic compounds, may be transferred to type A extracts without any modification.

In principle two parameters from in vitro data are essential in this context: solubility (the ability to dissolve as predicted through dissolution tests) and permeability through the intestinal wall according to the Biopharmaceutical Classification System (BCS) (a predictor of absorption rates) (Amidon et al., 1995). If both the solubility and permeability of a substance are good, there should be no problems with bioavailability. However, if one or the other is poor, bioavailability may be compromised. That is, if solubility is good (the rate of dissolution is relatively quick) and permeability is poor, then absorption is the limiting step for the appearance of drug substances in the blood. In this case, bioavailability would not be predicted by the in vitro dissolution rate. However, if the solubility is poor and permeability is good, then bioavailability will depend upon the in vitro dissolution rate and the substance will be absorbed as soon as it dissolves.

For example, Schulz and colleagues (1995) described the pharmacokinetics of silibinin after administration of different milk thistle extract-containing formulations with different dissolution profiles. As silibinin has a low solubility according to the BCS (Ihrig, Dedina, and Möller, 2000), there was, as expected, a correlation between the dissolution rate and the plasma levels. As seen in Figures 5.1 and 5.2, after administration of a product with a high dissolution rate (M9) higher plasma levels were achieved as compared to products M1 and

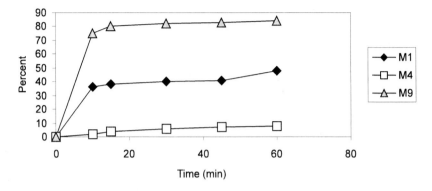

FIGURE 5.1. In vitro dissolution of silibinin from three different milk thistle extract-containing products (*Source:* Adapted from Schulz et al., 1995.)

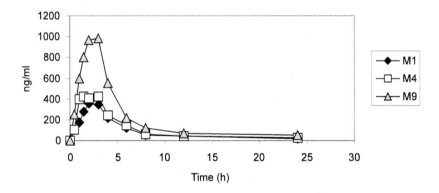

FIGURE 5.2. Plasma concentration of silibinin after oral administration of the products M1 to M4 (*Source:* Adapted from Schulz et al., 1995.)

M4 for which the dissolution rate was considerably lower (Schulz et al., 1995).

In consideration of these studies, the *United States Pharmacopeia–National Formulary* monographs on capsules and tablets containing milk thistle extract include the criteria for in vitro dissolution, that no less than 75 percent of the labeled amount of silymarin must be dissolved under specified conditions (United States Pharmacopeial Convention, 2002). This is especially important if another brand of product is substituted for a clinically tested brand of herbal medicinal product containing low-solubility substances. In these cases, bioavailability studies in human subjects should be performed, to the extent that is possible. However, certain restrictions may apply due to technical difficulties in measuring the desired marker compound(s).

For type B extracts, the solubility of both the markers likely to contribute to the clinical efficacy and the total extract should be studied in the pH of the gastrointestinal tract (pH 1 to 6.8). If the solubility of the extract and of the markers is good (>90 percent soluble from the highest dose strength), no problems with permeability through the intestinal wall and bioavailability are to be expected. If the solubility of the total extract and/or the markers is poor (<90 percent), bioavailability studies or clinical studies should be performed before bioequivalence with a clinically tested product can be determined.

A correlation between solubility and bioavailability was demonstrated for the ginkgolides (A, B) and bilobalide in two different ginkgo extract preparations. The reference preparation had an in vitro dissolution rate at pH 1 and 4.5 of over 99 percent after 15 minutes. In contrast, the test preparation had an in vitro dissolution rate of less than 33 percent after one hour. Bioavailability (plasma levels of constituents) of the two preparations was measured in 12 healthy volunteers in a crossover design. The reference preparation caused statistically significant greater maximum plasma concentrations and areas under the curve (amounts measured in the plasma) for all three constituents compared to the test preparation. Statistical analysis, using 90 percent confidence intervals, showed that these two products, with apparently similar chemical profiles, were not bioequivalent (Kressmann et al., 2002).

In the case of type C extracts, in which the constituents responsible for the therapeutic activity are unknown, no bioavailability problems are to be expected if solubility of the extract is high. In the theoretical case of poorly soluble type C extracts, clinical studies should be conducted on a case-by-case basis.

In bioavailability studies containing type B or C extracts, it would be desirable to measure not only (active) markers but also the total active principle of the extract. Chemical assays measure only a small percentage of botanical components, and in the case where the active components are not determined, they may not predict the pharmacological activity of the preparation. Therefore, bioassays that measure biological activity (pharmacodynamic effects) may be more suitable end points. Recently, biochemical assays have been proposed for several plant extracts, as depicted in Table 5.2 (Rininger et al., 2000). An ideal bioassay would be a measurement that correlated with the therapeutic activity of the extract. However, this ideal is difficult to achieve. In most cases biochemical assays do not reflect therapeutic effects as a whole but only selected pharmacological aspects caused by individual active markers. A disadvantage of biochemical assays is that they are generally not as reproducible as chemical analytical methods, and the variability in results may complicate evaluation of the bioavailability studies. Nevertheless, bioassays or biochemical assays may play an important role for future pharmacokinetic approaches if intelligent strategies can be found.

It should not be taken for granted that different brands of botanicals are equivalent in their bioavailability. The presence or absence of substances in the product other than the active ingredients may prevent, prolong, or enhance absorption. In the scramble to differentiate products in the U.S. dietary supplement market, some manufacturers have adopted novel delivery systems and/or innovative formulations. These innovations may be beneficial, but they need to be tested to determine the bioavailability of the ingredients.

In summary, further research is needed into the bioavailability of herbal products. This research is complicated by the need for identification of active constituents. However, technical advances have helped in this process, and there is movement toward the establishment of standards for the disintegration, dissolution, and bioavailability of herbal products.

TABLE 5.2. Bioassays for plant extracts

Extract	Extract type	Bioassay
Hypericum	B	Serotonin and dopamine reuptake inhibition
Ginkgo	B	Free-radical scavenging activity
Ginseng	C	Induction of corticosterone
Echinacea	C	TNF (tumor necrosis factor)-alpha production
Saw palmetto	B	5-alpha-reductase inhibition

REFERENCES

Amidon GL, Lennernäs H, Shah VP, Crison JR (1995). A theoretical basis for a biopharmaceutical drug classification: The correlation of in vitro drug product dissolution and in vivo bioavailability. *Pharmaceutical Research* 12 (3): 413-420.

Biber A, Fischer H, Römer A, Chatterjee SS (1998). Oral bioavailability of hyperforin from *Hypericum* extracts in rats and human volunteers. *Pharmacopsychiatry* 31 (Suppl. 1): 36-43.

Blume HH, Schug B (2000). Biopharmaceutical characterisation of herbal medicinal products: Are in vivo studies necessary? *European Journal of Drug Metabolism and Pharmacokinetics* 25 (1): 41-48.

De Smet PAGM, Brouwers RBJ (1997). Pharmacokinetic evaluation of herbal remedies. *Clinical Pharmacokinetics* 32 (6): 427-436.

European Medicines Evaluation Agency (EMEA) (1999). Note for Guidance on Specifications: Test procedures and acceptance criteria for herbal drugs, herbal drug preparations and herbal medicinal products. EMEA/HMPWP/19/99.

European Medicines Evaluation Agency (EMEA) (2001). Note for Guidance on the Investigation of Bioavailability and Bioequivalence. Draft. EMEA CPMP/EWP/QWP/1401/98.

Food and Drug Administration Center for Drug Evaluation and Research (FDA/CDER) (2000). Guidance for industry. Botanical Drug Products. Draft guidance. U.S. Department of Health and Human Services, August. Internet: <http://www.fda.gov/cder/guidance/index.htm>.

Fourtillan JB, Brisson AM, Girault J, Ingrand I, Decourt JPh, Jouenne Ph, Biber A (1995). Proprietes pharmacocinetique du bilobalide et des ginkgolides A et B chez le sujet sain apres administrations intraveineuses et orales d'extrait de *Ginkgo biloba* (EGb761). *Therapie* 50 (2): 137-144.

Graefe EU, Wittig J, Mueller S, Riethling AK, Uehleke B, Drewelow B, Pforte H, Jacobasch G, Derendorf H, Veit M (2001). Pharmacokinetics and bioavailability of quercetin glycosides in humans. *Journal of Clinical Pharmacology* 41 (5): 492-499.

Ihrig M, Dedina E, Möller H (2000). Empfehlung einer einheitlichen Spezifikation für Silymarin-Fertigarzneimittel. *Pharmazeutische Zeitung* 145: 2861-2870.

Kerb R, Brockmöller J, Staffeldt B, Ploch M, Roots I (1996). Single-dose and steady-state pharmacokinetics of hypericin and pseudohypericin. *Antimicrobial Agents and Chemotherapy* 40 (9): 2087-2093.

Kressmann S, Biber A, Wonnemann M., Schug B, Blume HH, Müller WE (2002). Influence of pharmaceutical quality of active components from *Ginkgo biloba* preparations. *Journal of Pharmacy and Pharmacology* 54 (11): 1507-1514.

Lang F, Keller K, Ihrig M, van Oudtshoorn-Eckard J, Moller H, Srinivasan S, He-ci Y (2003). Biopharmaceutical characterization of herbal medicinal products: FIP discussion paper, Part 1. *Die Pharmazeutische Industrie* 65 (6): 547-550. Part 2. *Die Pharmazeutische Industrie* 65 (7): 640-644. Also published in one document in *Pharmacopeial Forum* 29 (4): 1337-1346.

Oschmann R, Biber A, Lang F, Stumpf H, Kunz K (1996). Pharmakokinetik von beta-Aescin nach Gabe verschiedener Aesculus-Extrakt enthaltender Formulierungen. *Die Pharmazie* 51 (8): 577-581.

Rininger JA, Franck Z, Wheelock GD, Hughes B, Mclean A (2000). The value of bioassay in assessing the quality of botanical products. *Pharmacopoeial Forum* 26 (3): 857-864.

Schulz HU, Schürer M, Krumbiegel G, Wächter W, Weyenmeyer R, Seidel G (1995). Untersuchungen zum Freisetzungsverhalten und zur Bioäquivalenz von Silymarin-Präparaten. *Arzneimittel-Forschung/Drug Research* 45 (1): 61-64.

United States Pharmacopeia Committee of Revision (2000a). Headquarters column. *Pharmacopeial Forum* 26 (3): 579-581.

United States Pharmacopeia Committee of Revision (2000b). Nutritional Supplements General Chapter 2040: Disintegration and dissolution of nutritional supplements. *Pharmacopeial Forum* 26 (3): 838-842.

United States Pharmacopeial Convention (2002). *United States Pharmacopeia 26, National Formulary 21* (USP-NF). Rockville, MD: The United States Pharmacopeial Convention, Inc.

Zimmermann T, Seiberling M, Thomann P, Karabelnik D (1995). Untersuchungen zur relativen Bioverfügbarkeit und zur Pharmakokinetik von Myrtol standardisiert. *Arzneimittel-Forschung/Drug Research* 45 (11): 1198-1201.

Chapter 6

"Borrowed Science" and "Phytoequivalence": Can Two Herbal Products Be Judged Equivalent?

Marilyn Barrett

When is it appropriate for a clinical trial conducted on one herbal preparation to be applied to another herbal preparation so as to support the indication of the second product? That is, when can a trial conducted on one ginkgo product be used to establish the efficacy of another ginkgo product? This is the question behind the concept known popularly as "borrowed science." The manufacturers of the second product "borrow" the clinical studies conducted on the first product to establish the efficacy of and to promote their own product.

The first issue to address in borrowed science is product equivalency, i.e., does the second product have the same therapeutic value as the clinically proven product? Substituting one product for another product with an apparently similar description appears reasonable. However, what about products made from different species, plant parts, or manufacturing processes? Often in the United States an herbal preparation is not specified beyond the common name of the plant. Simply "valerian," "echinacea," or "garlic" is used to describe the preparation. That might suffice if all valerian products were equivalent, all echinacea products were equivalent, and all garlic products were equivalent, but they are not. For example, valerian root preparations are available as teas (aqueous extracts) and aqueous alcoholic extracts (70 percent ethanol with an herb-to-extract ratio of 4 to 7:1). These two preparations are not chemically equivalent. It is also common to lump echinacea products together, but can it really be assumed that a preparation made from the expressed juice of *Echinacea purpurea* flowering tops is equivalent to an aqueous alcoholic extract of the roots of *Echinacea angustifolia* roots? Garlic is available raw, dried, aged, and as an oil. None of these preparations are chemically equivalent.

It seems a first step in comparing products is to recognize the source of the knowledge regarding efficacy. For many herbs, the foundation of the evidence comes from traditional use. This evidence may or may not be supported by more recent pharmacological and/or clinical studies. In a few instances, products have been developed, apart from traditional uses or preparations, using pharmacological, toxicological, and clinical experiments.

Once the source of knowledge regarding efficacy has been identified, then the form of the material used to provide that evidence must be considered. Is the evidence regarding efficacy based upon raw plant material, a tea, a traditional tincture or other liquid preparation, or a solid oral formulation containing a dried or semipurified extract?

Duplication of each of these types of products raises slightly different issues. The quality of the raw material is dependent upon the identity and selection of the plant material as well as agricultural and/or harvesting practices. The chemical profile of an extract is, in addition, dependent upon processing methods.

The most common practice of borrowing science in the United States occurs when U.S. companies use the scientific data from European manufacturers to support statements regarding the benefit of their product. In other words, the reason for borrowing science is to aid in marketing and to support an allowable statement regarding the benefit of the product (a structure/function statement allowable under the Dietary Supplement Health and Education Act [DSHEA] of 1994). As noted in Chapter 10, "Motives for Conducting Clinical Trials on Botanicals in Europe," German manufacturers who wish to sell their herbal products as drugs or traditional medicines must provide documentation of efficacy and safety, or their product must conform to the quality specifications of a published monograph. Under DSHEA, dietary supplement structure/function statements must have evidence that the statement is truthful and not misleading. However, the extent of that evidence, and the strength of the link to the dietary supplement itself, have not been fully defined.

The practice in the United States of borrowing science allows for products to be sold more cheaply compared to their European counterparts, as the U.S. manufacturers are not forced to invest substantial amounts of money into researching efficacy or safety. Consumers, for the most part, are unaware of which products have been tested in clinical studies and which have not. Thus price becomes the deciding factor in their purchase.

However, a rational approach to evaluating the phytoequivalence of herbal products does exist. An international group, the Herbal Medicinal Products Working Group of the FIP (Federation Internationale Pharmaceutique/International Pharmaceutical Federation) has taken such an approach in producing guidelines to be used in evaluating the equivalence of herbal medicinal products sold as solid oral formulations (Lang et al., 2003). This group declared that a medicinal product is essentially similar to an original product when it has the same qualitative and quantitative composition in terms of active ingredients, has the same pharmaceutical form, and has demonstrated bioequivalence (similar bioavailability of active ingredients).

CHEMICAL OR PHARMACEUTICAL EQUIVALENCY

In determining whether borrowing science is acceptable, the first issue to examine is whether the two products are pharmaceutically equivalent. Two products are pharmaceutically equivalent if they contain the same active ingredient, the same strength of that active ingredient, the same dosage form, and are intended for the same route of administration and labeled for the same conditions of use (United States Pharmacopeial Convention, 2002).

In the case of drugs that are single-entity chemicals, pharmaceutical equivalence is relatively easy to determine. Chemical analysis of most single-entity chemical ingredients is fairly straightforward. In fact, the idea of equivalency is the basis for the promotion of, usually cheaper, generic drugs. It is relatively easy to identify and quantify the acetylsalicylic acid in Walgreens generic aspirin and determine it to equivalent to that in Bayer Aspirin.

But what of botanical preparations that contain hundreds of chemical components? For a few herbs, the active components have been identified. For those herbs, it is accepted that the defined constituents are responsible for the therapeutic activity, independent of the other components in the herb. The *European Pharmacopoeia* places extracts of aloe, buckthorn, senna, and belladonna in this category, while the *German Pharmacopoeia* includes extracts of ipecacuanha, rhubarb, horse chestnut, and milk thistle in this category (Lang et al., 2003). For these herbs characterization of the active ingredients is sufficient to establish chemical or pharmaceutical equivalency.

What about those herbs that contain several chemical components which are thought to contribute to the activity but do not necessarily account for all of the activity? St. John's wort and ginkgo standardized extracts are placed in this second category by the *European Pharmacopoeia* and *German Pharmacopoeia,* respectively (Lang et al., 2003). What about those herbs for which there is no agreement as to the active component(s)? The *German Pharmacopoeia* places valerian extracts in this third category (Lang et al., 2003). As all the active ingredients have not been identified in the herbs in these latter categories, theoretically all components in the preparations should be congruent for the products to be considered equivalent. However, this is impractical and difficult to demonstrate. Not all constituents may be identified, and even if identified, it would be difficult to quantify all of them. Practical steps in this direction would be to assure that the identities and qualities of the raw material, as well as the manufacturing processes, are similar. For extracts, the processing details would include the plant to extract ratio, the principal extraction solvent, and the extraction method.

BIOEQUIVALENCY OR THERAPEUTIC EQUIVALENCY

As described earlier, pharmaceutical equivalence is achieved if two products contain the same amount of the same active ingredient(s) in the same quantities in the same dosage form. However, chemical equivalence does not imply bioequivalence. Differences in the excipients and/or final formulation of the capsules or tablets may lead to faster or slower dissolution (release of chemical constituents) and/or absorption into the body.

For drugs, the disintegration of the tablet or capsule and the dissolution of chemical constituents are specified in pharmacopoeial monographs. U.S. federal law mandates that drugs comply with monograph specifications published in the *United States Pharmacopeia (USP).* Thus Walgreens aspirin must meet the same disintegration and dissolution specifications as Bayer Aspirin.

Measuring the disintegration of herbal tablets or capsules can be achieved using similar guidelines as those for drugs. However, measuring the dissolution (release of the active chemical constituents) of herbal preparations becomes problematic if the active ingredients are unknown. For those few herbs in which the active ingredients are known, dissolution guidelines are beginning to be drafted into the *United States Pharmacopeia–National Formulary (USP–NF)*. For example, the *USP–NF* monographs on capsules and tablets containing milk thistle extract include criteria for in vitro dissolution of silymarin (United States Pharmacopeial Convention, 2002). However, these guidelines are not in place for the majority of herbs on the market, and no mandatory compliance to the specifications that do exist is enforced.

Once the dissolution of the active components is assured, absorption into the body is the next step. Measurement of the active component(s) or metabolite(s) in the plasma and/or urine is an indication of bioavailability. A bioequivalence study compares the bioavailability of two products. According to the FIP Herbal Medicinal Products Working Group, a bioequivalence study is the most widely accepted means of demonstrating that any apparent differences in the two products being compared have no impact on the rate of absorption and the extent of absorption. The working group adds the caveat that the products contain only excipients which are generally recognized as not having an influence on safety or efficacy (Lang et al., 2003).

APPLICATION OF THE CONCEPTS, GINKGO AS AN EXAMPLE

Ginkgo extracts meeting the specifications of the German Commission E monograph have been approved for use in cases of dementia syndromes, improvement of pain-free walking distance in peripheral arterial occlusive disease, vertigo, and tinnitus (Blumenthal et al., 1998). The product specifications for this indication are a dry extract of the dried leaf that is manufactured using acetone/water with subsequent purification steps, without addition of concentrates or isolated ingredients, and with a drug/extract ratio of 35 to 67:1, on average 50:1. The extract is characterized as containing 22 to 27 percent flavonol glycosides; 5 to 7 percent terpene lactones, of which approximately 2.8 to 3.4 percent consists of ginkgolides A, B, and C and 2.6 to 3.2 percent bilobalide; and ginkgolic acids below 5 mg/kg. This detailed description of approximately 24 percent flavonol glycosides and 6 percent terpene lactones still accounts for only 30 percent of the extract, providing little information on the remaining 70 percent. Other components, yet unidentified, may also contribute to clinical efficacy. The variability of these unidentified components can be minimized using consistent agricultural and manufacturing practices.

Many U.S. dietary supplement products are sold with claims based upon the German Commission E monograph. However, studies have found that not all of them conform to the quality specifications of the monograph (ConsumerLab, 2000; Kressmann, Müller, and Blume, 2002). Analysis of 26 ginkgo products sold in health food stores and supermarkets in the United States found that 16 products conformed to the flavone glycoside specification but only nine and seven conformed to the terpene lactone and ginkgolic acid specifications, respectively. A further breakdown of the lactone content revealed that four conformed to the suggested level of total ginkgolides and nine to the bilobalide level (Kressmann, Müller, and Blume, 2002). It must be noted that this level of detail was not on the label of the tested products, so most manufacturers were not in violation of truthful ingredient labeling. However, questions arise as to whether the products on the market provide the same therapeutic benefit as the extract specified by the Commission E monograph.

Kressmann, Müller, and Blume (2002) further compared the in vitro dissolution of the ginkgo products. The dissolution rates of terpene lactones, specifically ginkgolide A, B, and C, as well as bilobalide, were tested. The dissolution rates for the products were comparable, with most brands releasing over 75 percent of the terpene lactones within 30 minutes. Only one product stood out, as it released merely 10 percent of its terpene lactone content in 30 minutes. (It should be noted here that the Commission E monograph does not specify dissolution parameters.)

Another study by this group compared the bioavailabilities of two ginkgo extracts, both characterized on their labels as containing 24 percent flavone glycosides and 6 percent terpene lactones. The reference product was Ginkgold, manufactured by Dr. Willmar Schwabe GmbH & Co. of Germany and distributed by Nature's Way Products, Inc. (Springville, Utah) in the United States. The extract in this product, EGb 761, is the basis of a total of 32 controlled clinical studies reviewed in this book and is the basis for the Commission E monograph. Ginkgold was compared to "Ginkgo biloba extract" distributed by Whitehall-Robins Healthcare (Madison, New Jersey). Previous dissolution studies had indicated that the Whitehall-Robins product released less than 33 percent of its terpene lactone content in 60 minutes, whereas Ginkgold released over 99 percent in 15 minutes. These two products were given to 12 healthy volunteers using a crossover trial design, and the concentrations of ginkgolides A, B, and bilobalide were measured in their blood. The result of the study was that EGb 761 caused statistically significant greater maximum plasma concentrations and areas under the curve (amounts measured in the plasma) for ginkgolides A, B, and bilobalide compared to the test preparation. Statistical analysis, using 90 percent confidence intervals, showed that these two products were not bioequivalent (Kressmann et al., 2002).

META-ANALYSES

Another situation in which it is helpful to determine whether products are similar in therapeutic efficacy is in the pooling of clinical trials conducted on different products. A meta-analysis is a statistical review of multiple trials. It is a systematic way to pool data, often from numerous, small, randomized controlled studies, and examine the significance of their findings as a whole. But what is the significance of pooling data from different botanical preparations, possibly with different chemical profiles and without established bioequivalence?

Certainly there is a basis for comparing studies conducted on different powdered garlic products, but powdered garlic products do not have the same chemical profile as aged garlic or garlic oil. The Agency for Healthcare Research and Quality, an agency in the U.S. Department of Health and Human Services, sponsored a systematic review of garlic through one of its Evidence-Based Practice Centers (EPC). The evidence report separately summarized the effects of garlic on cardiovascular-related factors/disease and cancer. Studies on preparations ranging from dehydrated garlic, aged garlic extracts, and garlic oil macerates to distillates, raw garlic, and combination tablets were all pooled together (Mulrow et al., 2000). This practice of attempting to collectively determine the evidence regarding an herb's efficacy by pooling all products, regardless of their different specifications, provides misleading results. It reinforces the idea that all garlic products are alike, a concept not supported by chemical analysis.

PERSPECTIVE

The appropriateness of borrowed science is not only a question regarding truthful advertising but also a question regarding therapeutic benefit for health practitioners and consumers. Often health practitioners and patients uncritically substitute one herbal product for another. The consequence of this action could be a lack of the expected therapeutic benefit.

For this situation to change, consumers and health care practitioners would need to be aware of the source of the information regarding the efficacy of a product. Is the source of evidence traditional use of a tea or tincture, or is it several clinical studies conducted on a specific type of extract? The next question is, does the form of the product being sold match that of the product with the direct evidence? Of course, certain differences may not influence efficacy, and further research is needed to determine what differences are acceptable or unacceptable. Further, health practitioners and consumers would have to be aware enough of the complexity of herbal preparations to realize that a generic form may provide the same activity, but it also may not. Without evidence of equivalency, health practitioners and consumers would have to be able to distinguish clinically researched products from those that have no direct evidence to support their claims.

At the moment, no regulatory pressure has been placed on manufacturers to conduct either their own efficacy studies or equivalency tests. Without additional regulation, it is unlikely that most manufacturers will invest money into such research.

As outlined in this chapter, the concept of herbal product equivalence can be approached in a rational and scientific manner. The FIP Herbal Medicinal Products Working Group is exploring the means to do just that. The examination of chemical equivalency is determined by the extent of knowledge regarding the active components. For most herbs, it begins with comparison of the botanical identities, the plant parts, and agricultural practices and extends to manufacturing practices. Determination of in vitro disintegration and dissolution are first steps toward determining bioequivalency, which ultimately must be determined clinically. It is important to remember that the extent to which the active constituents are known will determine the degree of correlation between dissolution and bioequivalence tests and efficacy.

Until health practitioners and consumers demand more information on the source of the evidence for efficacy, or until additional regulation is in place, the current problem of borrowed science will continue in the United States. In other words, many U.S. companies will inappropriately attribute science conducted on other products as pertaining to their own.

REFERENCES

Blumenthal M, Busse W, Hall T, Goldberg A, Gruenwald J, Riggins C, Rister S, eds. (1998). *The Complete German Commission E Monographs: Therapeutic Guide to Herbal Medicines*. Trans. S Klein. Austin, TX: American Botanical Council.

ConsumerLab (2000). Product review: Ginkgo biloba and huperzine A—Memory enhancers. <http://www.consumerlab.com/results/ginkgobiloba.asp>.

Kressmann S, Biber A, Wonnemann M., Schug B, Blume HH, Müller WE (2002). Influence of pharmaceutical quality of active components from *Ginkgo biloba* preparations. *Journal of Pharmacy and Pharmacology* 54 (11): 1507-1514.

Kressmann S, Müller WE, Blume HH (2002). Pharmaceutical quality of different *Ginkgo biloba* brands. *Journal of Pharmacy and Pharmacology* 54 (5): 661-669.

Lang F, Keller K, Ihrig M, van Oudtshoorn-Eckard J, Möller H, Srinivasan S, He-ci Y (2003). Biopharmaceutical characterization of herbal medicinal products: FIP discussion paper, Part 1. *Die Pharmazeutische Industrie* 65 (6): 547-550. Part 2. *Die Pharmazeutische Industrie* 65 (7): 640-644. Also published in one document in *Pharmacopeial Forum* 29(4): 1337-1346.

Mulrow CD, Lawrence V, Ackermann R, Ramirez G, Morbidoni L, Aguilar C, Arterburn J, Block E, Chiquette E, Gardener C, et al. (2000). Garlic: Effects on cardiovascular risks and disease, protective effects against cancer and clinical adverse effects. Evidence Report/Technology Assessment No. 20, October, AHRQ Publication No. 01-E023. Rockville, MD: Agency for Healthcare Research and Quality.

United States Pharmacopeial Convention (2002). *United States Pharmacopeia 26, National Formulary 21* (USP-NF). Rockville, MD: The United States Pharmacopeial Convention, Inc.

Chapter 7

Determining Efficacy
of Herbal Preparations

Tieraona Low Dog

Herbal medicine has been used since prehistoric times and gave birth to the sciences of botany, pharmacology, and, in part, chemistry. The initial evidence for the efficacy of these medicines was derived from direct human experience and observation. Some of the most effective medicines in our recent past originated from plants, including aspirin (salicylic acid from willow bark and meadowsweet), quinine (from cinchona bark), digoxin (from foxglove), and morphine (from opium poppy). Although many health care practitioners recognize that a number of other botanicals may be of therapeutic benefit, there is an undeniable sense of skepticism given the amount and quality of information currently available.

New information about the safety and efficacy of botanicals is becoming available on a daily basis. For this reason, both patients and providers utilize the Internet to gather health information; 52 million American adults have used the Web for this purpose (Pew Internet and American Life Project, 2000). Most users like the convenience of using the Web and the fact that they can do their research anonymously, yet 86 percent of those using the Internet for medical information worry about getting information from unreliable sources. The Federal Trade Commission (FTC) is charged with enforcing laws that ban "unfair or deceptive acts or practices." In 1998, the FTC held a "health claims surf day," during which 80 organizations from 25 countries searched the Internet for treatment and/or cures for cancer, arthritis, heart disease, AIDS, diabetes, and multiple sclerosis. Unfortunately, during this one afternoon of searching they found 400 sites making unfounded claims (Rusk, 2001).

So how does a health care provider determine what evidence is available regarding a specific botanical product? How does one assess the strength and weight of the existing evidence and apply that to a given patient? Evidence on the efficacy of herbal medicines ranges from historical use data, pharmacological studies, case reports, and uncontrolled clinical studies to the gold standard of randomized, double-blinded, placebo-controlled clinical studies. The strengths and weaknesses of each type of evidence and the criteria for a quality clinical trial are presented in this chapter.

A long history of traditional use of an herb can be an important source of information about safety and efficacy, especially if the information is corroborated by similar uses in multiple cultures which have apparently discovered that use independently. Objective pharmacological measurements using isolated tissue or cell culture is a well-accepted first step for understanding the biological activity of a particular substance. Animal studies are often used, as they permit generous control over a number of variables and can help to explain potential mechanisms of action. In vitro and animal data can provide important information about both the effectiveness and the safety of an herb; however, they are limited in their ability to accurately predict physiological effects in humans. Special attention must be paid to the experimental concentrations used in in vitro studies. These amounts should correlate with the concentrations expected in the plasma (blood) following human use. Similar attention should also be paid to the doses used in animal studies. In addition, caution must be used in the extrapolation of an activity produced with an isolated constituent of a plant to the activity expected with a whole plant preparation. Especially in the case of in vitro studies, one must determine if the components in the plant material being studied are altered by gut flora, transported across the intestinal wall, or altered by hepatic first pass metabolism. In addition, any physiological effects due to secondary metabolites must be considered.

OBSERVATIONAL MEDICINE

Decision making in medicine, until very recently, has been based primarily upon observation, personal experience, and intuition. Early physicians observed the patterns of illness and effects of treatment, and many wrote extensively about their findings. Information based upon personal observation by an individual is referred to as anecdotal. However, observations are seldom neutral, as they are based upon the preconceptions of the observer. Realizing the inevitable problem with anecdotal information, Aristotle called for the systematic observation of nature more than 20 centuries ago. Observational information was still an important source of information in early twentieth-century medical journals, and uncontrolled studies remained popular in the literature until their frequency diminished over the past 20 years. Uncontrolled studies do not include randomized groups, blinding of investigators, or a control group. Anecdotal information and uncontrolled studies can provide valuable hypothesis-generating information and assist in the identification of adverse events; however, they are extremely vulnerable to both bias and confounders. Thus, although helpful, these types of evidence should be considered supportive, not primary.

"EVIDENCE-BASED" MEDICINE

The decision-making process in medicine has been undergoing a dramatic shift toward "evidence-based" medicine that is based upon reviews of randomized, placebo-controlled, double-blinded studies which can be used to determine the degree of treatment effect, or lack thereof, of a particular intervention (Evidence-based medicine, 1995). Deciding what determines a high-quality study is complex and is the subject of great debate among researchers in conventional and complementary/alternative medicine. It is well recognized that certain study designs are more persuasive than others because they are less subject to bias. Although not a perfect mechanism for judging all interventions, at this time no other single study design provides a better level of safeguards against bias than a quality randomized, controlled trial (RCT). Three basic design protocols should always be considered when reviewing an RCT: randomization, blinding, and accounting of all participants, including those who withdraw or drop out.

An adequate randomization process assigns subjects that are similar to one another to either receive or not receive an intervention. Allocation of treatments can be either computer generated or through the use of a table of random numbers. The use of hospital numbers, date of admission, date of birth, or alternating numbers is not considered adequate. Selection bias is avoided by not preferentially selecting for the intervention arm those subjects most likely to experience a favorable outcome in the study. Every study participant must have an equal chance of receiving each intervention, and the investigators must not be able to predict which treatment a given participant will receive. Researchers have shown that trials with inadequately concealed allocation yielded larger treatment effects compared to trials in which the intervention assignments were hidden from all study participants (Schulz et al., 1995).

Blinding is achieved by matching the appearance of the placebo or standard treatment to the test substance. This may be somewhat problematic when studying liquid botanical products, as replication of taste and flavor with inert substances can be difficult. Masking of the treatment received by individual subjects (blinding) is adequate when neither the participants, the individuals doing the intervention, outcome assessors, nor the data analysts are able to identify which intervention is being assessed. This is the case for double-blind studies, but not for single-blind studies in which only the participants are blinded. Evidence should be provided that demonstrates successful blinding, and a detailed description of the characteristics of the product or treatment should be provided in the report (Schulz et al., 1996).

All participants included in the study must be properly accounted for at the conclusion of the trial. Those who fail to complete the trial, or who are not included in the analysis, must be described. The number of subjects that withdraw and reasons for withdrawal should be clearly stated. If participants in the active group drop out due to adverse events or because they perceived the treatment wasn't working, this information needs to be conveyed in the reporting of the trial. Many researchers now advocate for an intention-to-treat (ITT) analysis to be included in all randomized clinical trials. The ITT analysis is a strategy for analyzing data in which all participants are included in the group to which they were assigned, whether they completed the intervention given to the group or not (Begg et al., 1996). The ITT approach maintains the randomization originally sought at the beginning of the trial by fully accounting for all participants in both groups. Hollis and Campbell (1999) provide a clear example of the risk of not using an ITT approach. In a trial comparing medical and surgical treatment for stable angina pectoris, some patients allocated to surgical intervention died before being operated on. If these deaths were not attributed to surgical intervention using an intention-to-treat analysis, the surgical intervention would appear to have a falsely low mortality. In addition, it is normal for some patients to discontinue treatment or fail to adhere to prescribed treatment, thus allowing studies with an ITT analysis to more accurately parallel routine clinical practice.

In addition to appropriate randomization, blinding, and accounting of participants, RCTs should state the estimated effect of the intervention on outcome measures. The treatment effect observed in the clinical trial is called the point estimate and provides the best estimate of the true effect size in the study. This statistical measurement (relative risk, reduction in relative risk, absolute risk reduction) is heavily emphasized in the research report, as clinicians and patients are most interested in the question, "What was the difference in outcome between the treatment group and the control group?" The point estimate is the best estimate of the true size of the effect demonstrated in the study and applicable to the larger population that the trial's randomized sample is meant to represent.

The paper should also include an adequate description of the statistical methods used and how they were applied, with the data summarized in a fashion which allows others to perform alternative analyses. One must be careful to limit the risk of an alpha error, the determination that a treatment is effective when it actually is not. Thus, the sample size must be large enough to provide statistical power to detect a significant, i.e., clinically relevant, effect.

The appropriate application of inclusion/exclusion criteria is also an important factor when considering the strength of a study. The criteria for the inclusion and exclusion of subjects must be clearly explained and relevant to the clinical condition being studied. For instance, a study for a cold treatment should clearly list appropriate exclusions for those with chronic illness and those taking antibiotics or over-the-counter cold/cough medications.

Due to the complex nature of botanicals, variation in constituents between species, plant part, and preparation, it is essential that authors clearly provide an adequate description of the product used in the clinical trial. Descriptions should include identification (Latin binomial and authority), plant part (root, leaf, seed, etc.), and type of preparation (tea, tincture, extract, oil, etc.). Tincture and extract descriptions should include the identity of the solvent and the ratio of solvent to plant material. If the preparation is standardized to a chemical constituent, then that information should also be included. Precise and clear dose and dosage form should be provided. Papers that say, "three tablets of *Echinacea purpurea* were given two times per day" are simply unacceptable. How many milligrams were in each tablet? What part of the plant was used? How was it extracted? However, if a commercial product is used in a clinical trial, then information on preparation may be publicly available. Even so, characterization of the product is helpful as specifications can change over time.

Recently, the clinical evidence for efficacy of many herbal treatments has been subjected to systematic reviews (Ernst, 1999). These include reviews of garlic (Ackermann et al., 2001), kava (Pittler and Ernst, 2000a), ginkgo (Pittler and Ernst, 2000b), and St. John's wort (Linde and Mulrow, 2003), to name a few. A systematic review is a method of reviewing multiple clinical trials using a process that minimizes bias. The review includes all existing trials of a predefined quality, such as double-blind and controlled. If possible, statistical analyses are conducted on the end points of the trials, and a broad conclusion may be reached regarding efficacy and/or safety. These systematic literature reviews are becoming extremely important, as practitioners are overwhelmed with unmanageable amounts of information. Single studies are not usually sufficient for providing definitive answers to clinical questions. Recently two systematic reviews were published by the governmental Agency for Healthcare Research and Quality on garlic and milk thistle. These are available online at <http://www.ahrq.gov/clinic/epcix.htm>. Another excellent resource is the Cochrane Database of Systematic Reviews available online at <www.cochrane.org/reviews/index.html>.

SUMMARY

Decision making in medicine, until very recently, has been based primarily upon observation, personal experience, and intuition. Much of the historical information available on herbs is based upon these types of evidence. While recognizing that this type of evidence is valuable and certainly should not be discarded, decision making in medicine is undergoing a shift toward evidence-based medicine, based upon reviews of well-done randomized, placebo-controlled, double-blind studies which can be used to determine the degree of treatment effect, or lack thereof. Herbal preparations can also be evaluated in this manner. Clinical trials included in this book have been reviewed for their level of evidence according to a template included in the methods section. These levels of evidence provide the reader with an assessment of the strength of the evidence presented in the trial.

REFERENCES

Ackermann RT, Mulrow CD, Ramirez G, Gardner CD, Morbidoni L, Lawrence VA (2001). Garlic shows promise for improving some cardiovascular risk factors. *Archives of Internal Medicine* 161 (6): 813-824.

Begg C, Cho M, Eastwood S, Horton R, Moher D, Olkin I, Pitkin R, Rennie D, Schulz KF, Simel D, Stroup DF (1996). Improving the quality of reporting of randomized controlled trials: The CONSORT statement. *JAMA* 276: 637-639.

Ernst, E (1999). The clinical efficacy of herbal treatments: An overview of recent systematic reviews. *The Pharmaceutical Journal* 262: 85-87.

Evidence-based medicine, in its place (1995). *The Lancet* 346 (8978): 785.

Hollis S, Campbell F (1999). What is meant by intention to treat analysis? Survey of published randomised controlled trials. *British Medical Journal* 319: 670-674.

Linde K, Mulrow CD (2003). St. John's wort for depression (Cochrane Methodology Review). The Cochrane Library, Issue 4. Chichester, UK: John Wiley & Sons, Ltd.

Pew Internet and American Life Project (2000). The online health care revolution: How the Web helps Americans take better care of themselves. Available online at <http://www.pewinternet.org/reports/pdfs/PIP_Health_Report.pdf>.

Pittler MH, Ernst E (2000a). Efficacy of kava extract for treating anxiety: Systematic review and meta-analysis. *Journal of Clinical Psychopharmacology* 20 (1): 84-89.

Pittler MH, Ernst E (2000b). Ginkgo biloba extract for the treatment of intermittent claudication: A meta-analysis of randomized trials. *American Journal of Medicine* 108 (4): 276-281.

Rusk, M (2001). FTC Advertising Law and the Marketing of Complementary and Alternative Therapies and Products. Statement of Michelle

Rush before the White House Commission on Complementary and Alternative Medicine Policy, March 26.

Schulz KF, Chalmers I, Grimes DA, Altman DG (1995). Empirical evidence of bias: Dimensions of methodological quality associated with estimates of treatment effects in controlled trials. *JAMA* 273 (5): 408-412.

Schulz KF, Grimes DA, Altman DG, Hayes RJ (1996). Blinding and exclusions after allocation in randomized controlled trials: Survey of published parallel group trials in obstetrics and gynaecology. *British Medical Journal* 312 (7003): 742-744.

Chapter 8

Evaluating Safety of Herbal Preparations

Ezra Béjar
Joseph M. Betz
Marilyn Barrett

A substance is generally considered to be safe if it does not cause harm or risk of harm. Unfortunately, nothing is *absolutely* safe, and substances ingested for their beneficial effect may in some cases also be expected to exhibit undesirable effects. There is an amount (dose or concentration) and time interval (duration) beyond which we should not consume any substance, even one as safe as water. The sixteenth-century alchemist Paracelsus put it best when he stated that the dose makes the poison. Safety is thus a relative term best evaluated in terms of expected benefit weighed against the likelihood the substance will cause harm and the severity of the expected harm.

Undesirable effects can occur at recommended (therapeutic) doses and are called adverse reactions or side effects. The terms adverse reaction and side effect are not synonymous. *Adverse reaction* is used to describe undesirable effects that are not extensions of the known pharmacology of the substance. Adverse reactions may, or may not, be attributed to the product in question. They are usually unexpected until their origin is understood. A typical mild adverse effect is nausea and vomiting after taking a product. *Side effects* are undesirable effects that could be predicted or described based on the known pharmacology of the substance. Examples of side effects are dry mouth observed after taking decongestants such as pseudoephedrine and sleeplessness after taking ephedra. Aspirin may have the side effect of causing direct gastric damage by topical irritant effects and indirect damage via systemic inhibition of cyclooxygenase enzymes and microcirculation injury. An adverse reaction to aspirin may be hives or even anaphylaxis caused by unpredictable hypersensitivity in certain individuals. Both adverse effects and side effects can be mild, moderate, or severe.

If an undesirable effect occurs at a much higher dose than the therapeutic dose, it is considered an intoxication. An example of a toxic effect is a poisonous condition caused by too great a dose of salicylate. Salicylates are ubiquitous in nature and occur in low levels in a range of plants used as foods and flavorings. High blood levels can be obtained through ingestion of large amounts of aspirin (acetylsalicylic acid). Salicylism is characterized by rapid breathing, vomiting, headache, irritability, low blood sugar, and, in severe cases, convulsions and breathing problems. These poisonous effects disappear once the dose is reduced.

Some degree of toxicity is acceptable if the expected benefit is great. For example, the toxicity expected for agents used for cancer chemotherapy is tolerable given the potential of these substances to eliminate fatal cancers. However, if the remedy is a tonic used by otherwise healthy patients, then toxicity is not acceptable.

The goal of this chapter is to discuss ways of evaluating safety, monitoring and cataloging of undesirable effects (adverse reactions and side effects), categorizing herbal products according to their degree of safety, the importance of product quality as a determinant of safety, situations in which certain products are contraindicated, and potential drug-herb interactions. Finally, we will suggest ways we can improve our knowledge of the safety of herbal preparations.

EVALUATION OF SAFETY

A well-established system is used to evaluate the safety of prescription (Rx) and over-the-counter (OTC) drugs. Studies exploring safety begin with in vitro (test tube) and animal laboratory procedures, and then progress to human clinical trials. Animal toxicity procedures determine the lethality of different doses of a drug when administered orally, intraperitoneally, or intravenously to different species of mammal. Clinical observations and laboratory examinations of the animals are performed after one dose (acute) or after many days (chronic) of administering the drug. If a drug appears reasonably safe, these findings are corroborated using human subjects in clinical trials which have been specifically designed to evaluate safety (and later in clinical trials designed to assess therapeutic efficacy).

In the United States, drug manufacturers sponsor the safety studies which the Food and Drug Administration (FDA) reviews before allowing a drug to be sold to the public. Once on the market, systems are in place to monitor possible adverse reactions to the drugs. If concerns arise regarding the safety of a product, then the product is removed from the market or the directions for use are modified.

This well-established procedure is followed for those few herbal products sold as Rx or OTC drugs. However, the bulk of herbal products in this country are not sold as drugs but as dietary supplements. According to the Dietary Supplement Health and Education Act (DSHEA) passed by the U.S. Congress in 1994, botanical ingredients on the market prior to 1994 are considered safe by definition (Blumenthal and Israelsen, 1998). Manufacturers are required to notify the FDA of their intention to market a new dietary ingredient (one brought on the market after the enactment of DSHEA) at least 75 days before the ingredients are introduced into the marketplace. When making the notification, manufacturers must provide documentation to the FDA that the new ingredient is safe. The level of evidence needed to demonstrate the safety of these new ingredients is much less rigidly defined and less rigorous than that required for new foods or drugs. Under DSHEA, manufacturers of dietary supplements are responsible for the safety of their products, but the burden of proving a product already on the market poses a significant or unreasonable risk of injury or illness lies with the FDA. In other words, the FDA reviews safety only after products are on the market (and generally only after adverse reactions are reported).

In spite of the lack of premarket safety review by the FDA for many botanical ingredients, the public generally assumes that herbal products will be nontoxic and free of side effects. Many botanicals marketed as dietary supplements have a long history of use. Therefore, one might expect that any potential adverse reaction would be well documented. This is generally true, but several caveats are worth consideration.

Traditional practitioners and their patients are likely to recognize immediate signs of toxicity, but they are less likely to detect effects due to long-term exposure. These subtle long-term effects may result in cancer or damage to internal organs, such as the liver and/or kidneys. The examples often used to support this viewpoint are the length of time it took to recognize the link between tobacco smoking and lung cancer, or between alcohol and fetal alcohol syndrome.

Another consideration in evaluating safety is that many herbal products in the modern marketplace are not made in the traditional manner. In addition, they are freely available over the counter and are thus used by consumers without the advice of a practitioner. In an effort to establish a position in the market, many manufacturers of dietary supplements attempt to distinguish their products as being unique. Manufacturers may process the herb so that the products are more concentrated, selectively enhance certain constituents of the herb, or combine herbs and other ingredients in a unique (and nontraditional) manner. If products do not share the chemical composition or the dose level of the traditional preparation, or if they contain unique ingredients, they may not have the same safety profile. Furthermore, if the form (liquid, solid) or formulation (sole ingredient, one product in a mixture, capsule, tablet, delayed release, etc.) of the product is changed, the availability of the ingredient to the body's tissues (bioavailability) may also be changed. In all of these instances, the past experiences of traditional practitioners may not be relevant.

If a product has not been marketed previously, or if the formulation and composition have changed substantially, it is appropriate to conduct cell-based and/or animal toxicological procedures as mentioned previously. Once such a product is on the market, its safety record can be monitored using individual case reports, postmarket surveillance, and adverse-event reporting systems.

ADVERSE REACTIONS

According to the World Health Organization's (WHO) International Drug Monitoring Program, an adverse drug reaction (ADR) is defined as a response to a drug that is noxious and unintended, which occurs at doses normally used in humans for the prophylaxis, diagnosis, or therapy of disease, or for the modification of physiological function (WHO, 1972). Untoward reactions that result from ingesting excessive amounts of a substance can best be described as intoxications rather than adverse reactions. It should be noted, however, that the difference between a recommended or therapeutic dose and a toxic dose is very small in some cases.

In evaluating ADRs, it is important to determine whether the product in question actually caused the observed effect and if this effect was caused at the usual dose. The same criteria apply to this determination as those used in evaluating the efficacy of a product. The adverse reaction must first be linked with consumption of the product. The ingredients in the product should also be identified in some manner (chemically if at all possible), as it is not sufficient to rely on the ingredient declaration on the label. Several of the most well-known adverse reactions to botanical products have occurred because the wrong plant somehow ended up in the bottle. A clinician who reports an adverse reaction without performing, or directing, an independent check on the identity of the material can cause considerable confusion. In addition, the product must be examined for contaminants (pesticides, heavy metals, mycotoxins, pathogens) to rule them out as causes of the adverse reaction. Finally, a reaction may sometimes be product specific (linked to a particular product prepared in a specific manner) and may not be attributable to any particular individual botanical ingredient found in other preparations.

Even when a botanical or product is generally considered safe, it is possible for an adverse reaction to occur due to intolerance or an allergic reaction. Individual sensitivity can be responsible for a reaction of uncharacteristic or unpredictable nature and may not reflect any particular hazard to the general population. Although rare, individuals who are allergic to ragweed pollen may find themselves reacting when they consume Roman chamomile flower tea since both plants are members of the same family, the Asteraceae (Der Maderosian and Liberti, 1988).

ADVERSE-EVENT REPORTING SYSTEMS

Reporting systems have been designed to collect ADRs at the national level within the Food and Drug Administration and on the international level within the World Health Organization.

MedWatch is the reporting program for health professionals who wish to notify the FDA of serious reactions and problems with medical products such as drugs and medical devices. In 1993, the FDA Special Nutritionals Adverse Event Monitoring System (SN/AEMS) was established to monitor dietary supplements. This system, which received reports of adverse reactions from FDA's MedWatch program, FDA field offices, other federal, state, and local public health agencies, as well as from letters and phone calls from consumers and health professionals, is now in the process of revision. A major limitation to the system was that many reports were not investigated to determine whether there was a causal link to the suspected substance. In addition, all ingredients in a multiple-ingredient product were listed as causal agents regardless of the quantity present in the formula and the likelihood of their being the actual causative agent.

The WHO maintains the international drug information system (INTDIS) database for ADRs, which is housed in the Uppsala Monitoring Centre in Sweden. Information is gathered from government agencies of countries that are members of the WHO International Drug Monitoring Program. Until recently this program lacked the structure to report ADRs for herbs and herbal ingredients, as they were not suspected of causing ADRs (Olsson and Edwards, 2000). To remedy this deficiency, the Uppsala Monitoring Centre created a special computerized herbal substance register within the INTDIS in the fall of 2001 (Fucik, Backlund, and Farah, 2002). This program is designed to analyze the reported ADR information for a possible causal relationship between the reaction and the botanical. Depending upon the seriousness of the reaction, the quality of the information, and the number of reports, an alert may be generated. Once this system is fully implemented, some of the old ADR reports for herbal products may be reevaluated and compared with other ADR profiles to identify differences and similarities between different herbal product categories, such as crude botanical drugs (infusions, decocotions, or herbal teas considered traditional preparations), refined herbal preparations including phytopharmaceuticals (OTC and prescription herbal drugs), and allopathic prescription drugs based on botanicals (such as digoxin).

It is clear that the pharmacovigilance programs for herbal medicines are in their nascent stage, still being developed both by the U.S. FDA and the WHO.

CATEGORIZATION ACCORDING
TO THE DEGREE OF SAFETY

Botanical ingredients vary widely in their degree of safety. Some herbs are used as spices and are essentially food, others are only used for their therapeutic value, and a few are toxic and their consumption should be avoided. Botanicals in commerce have been categorized by their degree of safety in a publication by the American Herbal Products Association titled *Botanical Safety Handbook*. In this book, the editors have divided botanicals into four categories. The first category (class 1) consists of those botanicals that can be safely consumed when used appropriately. The second category (class 2) contains herbs for which certain restrictions apply. Included in the third category (class 3) are botanicals for which warnings are appropriate, and in the fourth (class 4) are those botanicals for which insufficient data are available to classify them. As examples, valerian is listed as class 1, devil's claw is rated as class 2d (contraindicated for gastric and duodenal ulcers), and digitalis, which contains glycosides with potent stimulant action on the heart, is rated as class 3 (McGuffin et al., 1997). The *Botanical Safety Handbook* does not include culinary herbs, nor does it include poisonous herbs with restricted medicinal use because of their potential toxicity and small margin of safety. The categories are listed in the book as guidance for readers and are not found on product labels.

The U.S. Department of Agriculture (USDA) classification for plants uses three acronyms: GRAF (generally recognized as food); GRAP (generally recognized as poisonous or medicinal); and GRAS (generally recognized as safe). Some herbs can fall into all three categories depending on the plant part and the type of preparation (Duke, 1992).

In considering the safety of a botanical preparation, the mode of preparation of the botanical, the route of administration, the dose, and the duration of administration are very important. Even if a toxin is present in the plant, it may not necessarily be biologically available. Indigenous peoples have used this concept to their advantage, and many potentially poisonous, even deadly, plants have been used in folk medicine or as food (e.g., cassava). Extraction procedures that destroy or neutralize a toxin have been employed, and careful attention is paid to the dose. For example, in traditional Chinese medicine (TCM), the highly toxic roots of aconite, *Aconitum japonicum* Thunb., are processed at 120°C for 40 minutes before administration. This process hydrolyzes the poisonous aconite alkaloids (aconitine, etc.) into compounds that are less toxic (Croom, 1983).

Bioavailability is also affected by route of administration (topical, oral, or intravenous). For example, the pyrrolizidine alkaloids contained in comfrey, *Symphytum officinale* L., roots (and in the leaves in to a lesser extent) are known to be liver toxins. Therefore, the American Herbal Products Association does not recommend oral administration of comfrey preparations. However, topical administration is acceptable due to the minimal absorption following application of comfrey preparations to unbroken skin (McGuffin et al., 1997).

Many poisonous, even deadly, plants have been used in folk medicine. Examples are jimsonweed, *Datura stramonium* L., for asthma, American mistletoe, *Phoradendron serotinum* (Raf.) MC Johnson, for hypotension, and poke roots, *Phytolacca americana* L., for fever, arthritis, and dysentery. In order for these plants to be used safely, their administration must be carefully monitored by experienced practitioners (Croom, 1983).

PRODUCT QUALITY AS AN ASPECT OF SAFETY

As noted, when evaluating adverse events, it is important to examine the product to rule out adulteration or contamination as a source of the reaction. An ADR or even a toxicity observed only with high doses may result from either substitution or contamination of the declared ingredients with a toxic plant (De Smet, 1996).

As an example, a relatively young woman who had taken a product containing plantain and 13 other herbs was admitted to a hospital for treatment of nausea, vomiting, dizziness, and disorientation. Unexplained cardiac arrhythmias were discovered at the hospital, and a subsequent investigation revealed the substitution of the leaves of plantain, *Plantago major* L. with those of *Digitalis lanata* Ehrh. (Slifman et al., 1998). Whereas plantain leaves are considered safe, those of digitalis contain potent cardiac glycosides that can be fatal when consumed in sufficient quantity (Hardman et al., 1996).

Contamination of plant materials with biological pathogens (e.g., bacteria, viruses, parasites), pharmaceuticals, naturally occurring toxins (e.g., mycotoxins), pesticide residues (e.g., dioxins), toxic metals (e.g., lead, mercury), filth (e.g., insect fragments), and/or radioactivity may also be the cause of an ADR.

CONTRAINDICATIONS

Limited information on contraindications (restriction of use) for botanicals is available. Some information can be found in individual monographs that focus on the therapeutic aspects of botanicals. General consensus exists within the medical community that drugs should be given cautiously to patients with certain chronic medical conditions (e.g., diabetes and heart disease), as well as pregnant and lactating women. This same common sense approach should be applied to herbal products. Because some medicinal plants have also been used as foods, the contraindication is often a relative restriction based upon the size of the dose, the extent of its use, and the type of preparation (Brinker, 2001).

DRUG-HERB INTERACTIONS

Herbs may potentially affect the action of drugs or other herbs when the two are taken concurrently. An herbal product may act as an enhancer or inhibitor of another agent at the site of action. Or it may modify absorption, distribution, metabolism, and/or elimination of that agent.

Little reliable information is available on this topic. A few drug-herb interactions have been documented in human studies or case reports, while others have been observed only in animal studies. However, most proposed interactions are based on in vitro assays and speculation about the theoretical mode of action of the herb or its chemical constituents. Knowledge regarding the mode of interaction of the herb is often extrapolated from in vitro studies using individual chemical component(s) of the herb. This logic assumes that the purified, isolated chemical component or components is biologically available and that plasma concentrations reached following consumption by a human are commensurate with those used in the study.

Although assumptions about the mode of action of a botanical have provided useful leads in investigations of drug-drug interactions and some drug-herb interactions, they also lead to erroneous conclusions. Reports of drug-herb interactions often do not take into consideration product differentiation (i.e., garlic powder versus garlic oil). They often do not consider the dose of the herb or the drug, the duration of treatment, and other critical variables defined for drug-drug interactions, such as the age and genetic profile of the subject. Even so, lists of potential drug-herb interaction are useful as a basis for further study. Potential interactions have been reviewed in a number of publications (Ernst, 2000; Fugh-Berman, 2000; Brinker, 2001).

Key to many of the drug-herb interactions is the cytochrome P450 family of enzymes. These enzymes are particularly concentrated in the liver but are also present in other tissues, especially the gut. The P450 enzymes metabolize many drugs, essentially clearing them from the body. Many foods and drugs have been found to either stimulate or inhibit these enzymes. Stimulation or inhibition of these enzymes will cause the body to eliminate a drug too quickly or to prevent elimination of the drug, thus allowing the drug to build up in the body. These actions are especially a concern with pharmaceuticals whose plasma levels must be tightly controlled to ensure safety and/ or efficacy.

One of the few herbs for which solid human clinical data on herb-drug interactions exist is St. John's wort. The issue was first raised by an HIV researcher who administered the protease inhibitor indinavir to healthy volunteers in conjuction with St. John's wort and found that the herb caused indinavir levels to drop to levels below those required for drug efficacy (Piscitelli et al., 2000). Other reports published around the same time indicated that the same phenomenon might be responsible for acute rejection in organ transplant patients who had used St. John's wort (Ruschitzka et al., 2000; Barone et al., 2000). Clinical experiments soon revealed that a St. John's wort product taken at 300 mg three times daily for 14 days stimulated the activity of a P450 isoenzyme called CYP3A4 (Roby et al., 2000). However, the story may be more complicated, as plasma levels of the anticonvulsant drug carbamazepine, which is also thought to be primarily metabolized via CYP3A4, were not affected by the addition of St. John's wort (Burstein et al., 2000).

Recent attention has also been paid to the effects of herbs on an inducible transport system that moves substrates out of cells. The pump, termed P-glycoprotein (Pgp), is a determinant of the oral bioavailability of many drugs. Here, too, it has been suggested that St. John's wort extract increases intestinal expression of Pgp, and, as a result, it is expected that 900 mg extract per day would decrease digoxin concentrations in heart patients after ten days of use (Durr et al., 2000;

Johne et al., 1999). Digoxin is a cardiac glycoside used in the treatment of a number of heart conditions including cardiac insufficiency. This drug is particularly problematic since it has a narrow therapeutic index, meaning that blood levels must be carefully controlled. As with the P450 enzymes, the story with St. John's wort is complex, as recent clinical experiments have revealed that a St. John's wort extract with a different chemical profile (low levels of hyperforin), but also clinically effective against depression, was demonstrated not to alter digoxin levels (Brattström, 2002).

The possibility that herbal preparations can affect the delicate balance of patients on anticoagulation agents is another concern. The discovery of the anticoagulant warfarin followed reports of cattle having hemorrhagic disorders following ingestion of sweet clover stored in silos (Vickery and Vickery, 1980; Bruneton, 1999). It was revealed that the hemorrhagic effect was due to the conversion of coumarins present in clover to the anticoagulant, bishydroxycoumarin (dicoumarol), by fungi growing on the clover. This background led numerous authors to pose an anticoagulant alert for any botanicals that contain coumarins. However, most natural coumarin derivatives found in plants do not ordinarily possess anticoagulant activity. Indeed, a few natural coumarins, such as esculetin and osthole, may affect platelet aggregation but do not have a similar mechanism of action as warfarin (Brinker, 2001). Therefore, the anticoagulant action of plants containing coumarins is not a certainty, as some reference books indicate (Miller and Murray, 1998; Barnes, Anderson, and Phillipson, 2002).

Until we know more about the modes of action of herbal products and their possible interactions with drugs, sensitive populations such as the elderly, chronically ill, and those with compromised immune systems would be well advised to be cautious when combining herbs and drugs.

IMPROVING OUR KNOWLEDGE OF SAFETY

Improvement in quality control for herbal products will help to assure the safety of herbal products. Conducting postmarketing surveillance studies and refining adverse-event reporting systems will certainly improve our knowledge of adverse reactions attributable to herbs. More research into potential drug-herb interactions using animal models will help to separate fact from fiction and may yield an unexpected bonus use of herbs as pharmaceutical adjuncts that allow the doses of synthetic drugs to be lowered (i.e., a "good" herb-drug interaction). Pharmacokinetic studies can help us gain information as to the bioavailability of components of a preparation. Certainly our knowledge of the safe use of herbs will continue to expand as we extend to them the same level of scientific scrutiny given other health-related products.

REFERENCES

Barnes J, Anderson LA, Phillipson JD, eds. (2002) *Herbal Medicine: A Guide for Health Care Professionals,* Second Edition. London: Pharmaceutical Press.

Barone GW, Gurley BJ, Ketel BL, Lightfoot ML, Abul-Ezz SR (2000). Drug interaction between St. John's wort and cyclosporine. *The Annals of Pharmacotherapy* 34 (9): 1013-1016.

Blumenthal M, Israelsen LD (1998). The history of herbs in the United States: Legal and regulatory perspectives. In *Herbal Medicinals: A Clinicians Guide.* Eds. LG Miller and WJ Murray. Binghamton, NY: Pharmaceutical Products Press, pp. 325-353.

Brattström A (2002). Der johanniskrautextrakt Ze 117 (Saint John's wort extract Ze 117). *Deutsche Apothekar Zeitung* 142 (30): 97-101.

Brinker F (2001). *Herb Contraindications and Drug Interactions,* Third Edition. Sandy, OR: Eclectic Medical Publications.

Bruneton J (1999). *Pharmacognosy, Phytochemistry, Medicinal Plants,* Second Edition. London: Intercept Ltd.

Burstein AH, Horton RL, Dunn T, Alfaro RM, Piscitelli SC, Theodore W (2000). Lack of effect of St. John's wort on carbamazepine pharmacokinetics in healthy volunteers. *Clinical Pharmacology and Therapeutics* 68 (6): 605-612.

Croom EM (1983). Documenting and evaluating herbal remedies. *Economic Botany* 37 (1): 13-27.

De Smet PAGM (1996). Quality Control Overview. Lecture given at DIA (Drug Information Association) Workshop "Botanical Quality: Workshop on Identification and Characterization," Washington, DC, April 10.

Der Maderosian A, Liberti L (1988). *Natural Product Medicine, a Scientific Guide to Foods, Drugs, Cosmetics.* Philadelphia: George F. Stickley Co.

Duke J (1992). *Handbook of Phytochemical Constituents of GRAS Herbs and Other Economical Plants.* Boca Raton, FL: CRC Press.

Durr D, Stieger B, Kullak-Ublick GA, Rentsch KM, Steinert HC, Meier PJ, Fattinger K (2000). St. John's wort induces intestinal P-glycoprotein/ MDR1 and intestinal and hepatic CYP3A4. *Clinical Pharmacology and Therapeutics* 68 (6): 598-604.

Ernst E (2000). Possible interactions between synthetic and herbal medicinal products: Part 1. A systematic review of the indirect evidence. *Perfusion* 13: 4-15.

Fucik H, Backlund A, Farah M (2002). Building a computerized herbal substance register for implementation and use in the World Health Organization International Drug Monitoring Programme. *Drug Information Journal* 36: 839-854.

Fugh-Berman A (2000). Herb-drug interactions. *Lancet* 355 (9198): 134-138.

Hardman JG, Limbird LE, Molinoff PB, Ruddon RW, Goodman-Gillman A (1996). *Goodman & Gilman's the Pharmacological Basis of Therapeutics,* Ninth Edition. New York: McGraw-Hill.

Johne A, Brockmoller J, Bauer S, Maurer A, Langheinrich M, Roots I (1999). Pharmacokinetic interaction of digoxin with an herbal extract from St. John's wort *(Hypericum perforatum). Clinical Pharmacology and Therapeutics* 66 (4): 338-345.

McGuffin M, Hobbs C, Upton R, Goldberg A (1997). *American Herbal Products Association's Botanical Safety Handbook.* New York: CRC Press.

Miller LG, Murray WJ (1998). Specific toxicologic considerations of selected herbal products. In *Herbal Medicinals: A Clinicians Guide.* Eds. LG Miller and WJ Murray. Binghamton, NY: Pharmaceutical Products Press, pp. 307-322.

Olsson S, Edwards IR (2000). The WHO International Drug Monitoring Programme. *Side Effects Drugs* 23: 524-529.

Piscitelli SC, Burstein AH, Chaitt D, Alfaro RM, Falloon J (2000). Indinavir concentrations and St. John's wort. *The Lancet* 355 (9203): 547-548.

Piscitelli SC, Formentini E, Burstein AH, Alfaro R, Jagannatha S, Falloon J (2002). Effect of milk thistle on the pharmacokinetics of indinavir in healthy volunteers. *Pharmacotherapy* 22 (5): 551-556.

Roby CA, Anderson GD, Kantor E, Dryer DA, Burstein AH (2000). St. John's wort: Effect on CYP3A4 activity. *Clinical Pharmacology and Therapeutics* 67 (5): 451-457.

Ruschitzka F, Meier PJ, Turina M, Luscher TF, Noll G (2000). Acute heart transplant rejection due to St. John's wort. *Lancet* 355 (9203): 548-549.

Slifman NR, Obermeyer WR, Aloi BK, Musser SM, Correll WA Jr., Cichowicz SM, Betz JM, Love LA (1998). Contamination of botanical dietary supplements by *Digitalis lanata. New England Journal of Medicine* 339: 806-811.

Vickery M, Vickery B (1980). Coumarins and related compounds in members of the Connaraceae. *Toxicology Letters* 5 (2): 115-118.

World Health Organization (WHO) (1972). *WHO Technical Report.* 498: 9. Geneva, Switzerland: WHO.

Chapter 9

Conducting Clinical Trials on Herbal Dietary Supplements in North America: Commercialization, Confidence, and Conflicts

Anthony L. Almada

Query most executives of dietary supplement marketing companies with, "Why don't you sponsor randomized controlled trials on one or more of your products?" and you're likely to receive volleys such as these:

"They cost too much."
"We do the pioneering work and then everyone benefits from it."
"Why should we? We've been successful *without* them."
"We have stacks of testimonials—we *already* know it's safe and effective."
"What if the study shows our product *doesn't* work, or is *un-safe*?"

Despite the shortcomings and imperfections of randomized controlled trials (RCTs), they appear to be the best available tool to objectively assess the safety and especially the efficacy of prophylactic, therapeutic, and biological response-modifying agents, which effectively can describe botanical supplements. However, the primary incentives for undertaking research—namely, a rather exclusive position in the marketplace (by virtue of the competitor products almost categorically lacking independent validation of safety and effectiveness) and a consumer confidence-inspiring marketing message—do not appear to be attractive enough to many companies.

This chapter will explore and illustrate why a paucity of ingredient- and product-specific RCTs exist, the advantages and disadvantages of sponsoring RCTs, and both current and future thrusts to invite and recruit a greater commitment to specific, branded products that have been shown to be safe and effective.

THE SPIRIT TO SPONSOR:
IS THERE AN ADEQUATE ECONOMIC INCENTIVE
TO FUND RESEARCH?

Both short-term (tax incentives, marketing message, public relations campaign) and long-term (increased consumer confidence, market distinction, higher likelihood of being acknowledged by medical professionals, increased corporate value) economic incentives exist for the company that invests in clinical trials in the United States. However, if we examine the profiles of empowered dietary supplement company executives, i.e., CEOs, presidents, and COOs, we uncover a dearth of individuals who have biomedical research training and experience. The path to the pole position in the corporate structure of natural products companies is typically via scaling the sales and/or the marketing ladder. It is understandable to expect such a corporate leader to be challenged by the idea of embracing or even understanding the mechanics of *research and development* versus the norm of *search and duplicate*. Science and research is a wholly different language.

In contrast, if we focus the innovation telescope upon the biotechnology/life sciences communities, it is almost the norm for a leader to have a PhD, an MD, or even a combination of degrees. In the drug pathway, Food and Drug Administration (FDA) regulations mandate the performance of both "test tube" (in vitro) and animal studies (collectively known as preclinical studies), followed up by clinical (human) studies. The barrier to entry here is a compelling safety and efficacy evidence package.

However, unless a dietary supplement is a new botanical ingredient (either singly or in combination) being introduced to the market, *no* scientific evidence is required. The barrier to entry is at ground level. If a company seeks to introduce a new botanical ingredient, i.e., one that was not in commerce in the United States before passage of the 1994 Dietary Supplement Health and Education Act (DSHEA) (the FDA's rules governing dietary supplements) then one needs to submit only adequate safety or human consumption data, *not* efficacy data. Although safety data are of critical importance, the consumer ultimately may purchase a product that is safe but innocuous—completely without efficacy (independent from the placebo effect).

Afforded the luxury of hyperbole, every company has the same product, makes the same soft efficacy and structure/function claims, and asserts their product(s) is the best, fastest acting, or most "synergistic." My colleagues and I have estimated that less than 0.01 percent of all the different products in commerce fly within the rarefied air accorded those with *product-specific science.*

Hard Costs: Softening the Reality

The challenge confronting botanical dietary supplements, from the perspective of both companies which market them and consumers who use them, is developing a cost-effective manner in which independent RCTs could be initiated. It is also to provide both a return on investment for the companies taking the risk and prescription drug-like confidence among individual consumer buyers. When I was directing research and development (R&D) for a medium-sized dietary supplement company in the early 1990s, I was told by one of the vice presidents that RCTs cost "six figures to half a million." Having previously been involved in a few clinical trials at the University of California, San Francisco, I knew that they *could* meet or exceed that figure, but they absolutely didn't *have to.* Yes, some studies have been done on botanical products to the tune of two million dollars plus. For example, Lichtwer Pharma sponsored a four-year study assessing the influence of its Kwai garlic upon atherosclerotic lesions in otherwise healthy adults (Koscielny et al., 1999).

Assuming one could design an RCT that was a fraction of this cost, do magnetic economic incentives exist to compel action? In other words, are there up front tax benefits for making the investment, back end advantages over the competition, and the promise of greater consumer demand if and when the product is introduced for sale and is marketed?

Manufacturers may not be aware that the execution of RCTs on botanical products is very much within the reach of most companies, even those in their first years of business. If one initially abandons the notion that an RCT must enroll 100 or more subjects, involve supplementation for a year or longer, and employ a battery of expensive diagnostic and invasive measures, then one can envision the fiscal possibility of conducting a study. RCTs can be done for as low as $15,000, with incremental costs being mostly a function of the number of patients/subjects, the number of times the subjects are evaluated for changes, and the actual measures that are being performed. An RCT budgeted at $15,000 likely will not have more than 12 to 14 subjects and two low-cost measurements. Measurements of weight loss, blood total cholesterol, or knee pain, for example, could be made before supplementation and after supplementation ("pre-post"). A rule of thumb to apply is $1,200 to $1,500 per subject enrolled in a study in which simple measures of efficacy are performed and limited to pre-post frequency.

As a case in point, in 1994 my associates and I sponsored a collaborative study at an acknowledged and respected private research center. We collaborated with a cardiologist and a PhD student. We had an ample and motivated patient population (dyslipidemic men and women), a motivated and interested research team, and a willingness to engage in creative budgeting. We completed a 12-week RCT with 33 subjects, presented (Almada, Mitchell, and Earnest, 1996; Earnest, Almada, and Mitchell, 1996b; Mitchell, Almada, and Earnest, 1996) and published the data in a noted peer-reviewed journal (Earnest, Almada, and Mitchell, 1996a), and filed and prosecuted a patent (Almada and Byrd, 1997), all for less than $15,000 (including *all* of the legal fees). Although this was all conducted with a biochemical (creatine), one could apply the same template to a botanical product. Putting this in perspective, this amount is somewhat to far less than many companies' advertising budgets over a fiscal quarter, or sometimes even a month. This raises the question for companies marketing botanical dietary supplements as to how to allocate resources: exclusively for sales, marketing, advertising, and promotions, or accommodating a clinical research budget that grows with the company?

The exceptional RCT example cited is intended to serve as an impetus to readers to create both an awareness of the economic possibility and an earnest interest in pursuing research as a tool to create distinction and enhanced consumer desirability amid a sea of products that all claim to be "safe and effective." Similar collaborative research opportunities exist, in both the academic and the private sectors. One simply needs a skillful and experienced navigator (in-house or outsourced) to identify and harness them. The tacit dogma of a CEO's directives does not exclude identifying and constructing strategic research and development alliances and networks. The savvy CEO can inspire her or his management team with a mission of finding and developing cost-effective research alliances that serve the corporate goals and aim to provide consumers with safe and effective products.

Tax Tasking

Another salient message to communicate is that R&D expenditures enjoy special tax treatments. This includes expenditures associated with filing and prosecuting a patent (legal fees) related to a specific invention. Super allowances and tax credits exist for R&D expenditures, which are best identified by a tax professional with relevant experience. If a company is engaged in collaborative contract research, i.e., conducting research in alliance with another outside entity, they can enjoy a higher (75 percent) tax credit. Research qualifies if it simply is technological in nature and is expected to be useful in developing new or improved products for the company in question. Most important, the research can fail and one can *still* use the tax credit. Finding an individual or company who has expertise in this area—research tax credits and incentives—could instantly add to the bottom line. Such tax strategies can be applied both prospectively and retroactively, i.e., filings from previous years.

EXTRACTING VALUE FROM SCIENCE

If one can attach an umbilical cord from a specific branded ingredient or product to its complementary, well-designed and executed RCT data one now has assembled a multifaceted, bow-tied "package," boasting the following features:

- *Regulatory insulation:* Having one or more RCTs on a product, revealing safety and efficacy data, puts a manufacturer in good stead in the event either the FDA or the FTC (Federal Trade Commission) seeks to challenge label or off-label/advertising claims.

- *Off-label marketing communications:* Press releases and press conferences can lead to medium to big media pickup, resulting in free, credible advertising. This may be the most potent tactical tool to generate significant awareness about independent clinical research confirming safety and efficacy of a company's unique botanical product. If the data are first communicated through the forum of a national or international scientific research meeting, the chances of obtaining the interest of a prominent health journalist are augmented manyfold.
- *Competitive advantage:* Entering or existing in the market with product-specific clinical research, which is artfully communicated to the consumer and retailer, can generate immediate distinction for one's own product while creating doubt about other competitor products that claim to be safe and effective but lack any independent, specific evidence. In this era it is likely that the majority of the competition has *no* comparable studies on their actual ingredient or finished good.
- *Competitive insulation/intellectual property:* Even in the absence of a patent, data on a complex ingredient or entity is a form of intellectual property (IP) and provides specific rights to exclude competitors. In some ways branded product-specific science is superior to a patent in that it never expires, is instantly available for use (to exclude others), and is far more expensive for others to duplicate. In contrast, a company must wait for a patent to be issued before it can exclude competitors from practicing the same invention. Regrettably, the strength of a patent is often dependent upon the resources spent defending it.

COMPETITOR KEVLAR: PREVENTING PIRACY OF PRODUCT-SPECIFIC DATA

Perhaps the greatest challenge confronting the natural products industry today is the "borrowing of science," what I prefer to call *data piracy.* Not unlike unfettered *biopiracy*—the theft of natural products from lesser-developed/IP-unsophisticated countries by scientists and attorneys from other countries—these properties are taken and never returned, and no "use tax" is paid. These are *not* books checked out with a library card, destined to be returned. The best examples are illustrated by specific innovator botanical extracts, which were created, developed, and ultimately researched by European phytophar-maceutical houses but rendered generic by a spate of other companies who have enjoyed a research-free balance sheet.

Although the transferability of data is not yet proven, companies use clinical research done on other companies' products to prove safety/efficacy of their own products. Do two botanical extracts man-ufactured by different companies show biological and pharmacologi-cal equivalence in humans? An element to the assumption is that the chemical marker compounds comprise most or *all* of the bioactive constituents in the plant. A striking illustration of this is St. John's wort, in which less than 4 percent of the extract composition is com-prised of known marker compounds. No data exist to support the as-sumption that the remaining 96 percent have no bearing upon the bio-logical activity of the extract in humans.

In the face of different chemical compositions between ostensibly identical botanical extracts (no two botanical handprints are identical, even if using the same biomass, unless they are processed identi-cally), how can one logically argue that a generic *Ginkgo biloba* ex-tract is pharmacoequivalent to the patented extract produced by Schwabe (EGb 761) until demonstrated as such? Indeed, one clinical investigation exploring the acute pharmacodynamic effects of three different standardized *Ginkgo* extracts found only one, the innovator product (EGb 761), to demonstrate "superior" central nervous system (CNS) bioactivity in humans (Itil and Martorano, 1995). Although this study used a specific research test to assess bioactivity (quantita-tive electroencephalography [EEG] readings) which may not be pre-dictive of clinical efficacy, e.g., improved cognitive function, it does offer evidence to strongly suggest that different botanical products claiming to be chemically similar indeed are *not* identical and may differ in their biological activity. Whether this difference in biological activity is related to chemical composition or to bioavailability, me-tabolism, distribution in body fluids, or transformation by and entry into "target" tissues remains enigmatic.

What about protecting the value invested in an RCT on a propri-etary product or ingredient? Let's see how intellectual property can be protected. Company X creates two product compositions, one consisting of (i.e., made solely of) and one containing (i.e., made of, in addition to one or more additional bioactive ingredients) a pine tree-derived extract containing 15 percent phytosterols by weight.

Company X sponsors one RCT on each product, presents the data at a few biomedical research conferences, and even gets one of the studies written up and published in a reviewed journal. After each RCT was completed, company X began to market, sell, promote, and advertise the respective product. Company Y notices one of X's products (and that it is enjoying strong sales growth) and creates its own pine tree-derived 15 percent phytosterol mixture. However, company Y never sponsors an RCT on its product. In its own marketing, promotional, or advertising materials, company Y cites the biomedical conference abstract (published in a supplement of a certain reviewed journal) and the full-length article that appeared in a different reviewed journal, both linked to one of company X's phytosterol products. Company X gets wind of these activities and consults their IP attorney. They then claim "Foul!" and file a lawsuit. Company Y retains its own attorneys, their day in court arrives, and the gavel strikes resoundingly. *Company Y is forever prevented from referring to company X's studies and attributing them to their (company Y's) product.* Is this a fantasy? This is anchored in federal law, but it is rarely invoked.

One such case was decided in Utah Federal District Court in April 1999. The parties were Pharmanex (Utah), then marketers of the proprietary (polymolecular) red yeast rice extract Cholestin, and HPF, LLC (Pennsylvania). The latter marketed a different red yeast rice product called Cholestene. Only Cholestin enjoyed product-specific preclinical and clinical research, but HPF attributed Pharmanex's studies to its own product. As a result, HPF was permanently prevented from making these false attributions, which were asserted by Pharmanex to be violations of the Lanham Act, a federal law in effect since 1947.

Undergoing numerous amendments since its introduction, the Lanham Act is the most potent weapon with which to seek redress for false advertising and attribution. It is an expensive undertaking, but if the measured or forecasted erosion of sales merits such an investment, the marketplace implications are very powerful.

In contrast, if a company sued one or more companies who were claimed to infringe on a patent, the costs would likely be even greater. Patent litigation costs, which proceed to trial, average around $500,000 per case. This enormous economic onus typically would overshadow, or dwarf, Lanham Act litigation.

A much less costly avenue to pursue is the National Advertising Division of the Council of Better Business Bureaus (NAD/CBBB). This independent body serves as a self-regulatory forum for the advertising industry and employs a variety of attorneys who assess complaints submitted by companies from a variety of business interests. The benefits of using this venue include greatly reduced costs (the filing fee is $1,000 to $2,000), a decision within 60 to 70 business days, and the exceptionally high degree of compliance among companies that are ultimately found to have unsubstantiated claims. Advertising in the eyes of the NAD includes labeling nationally advertised vehicles, which would include a Web site. If a product is simply offered for sale on the shelf and is *not* advertised the NAD does nothing. Advertising is subject to review if any person or entity submits a petition to the NAD. If a company fails to respond to a challenge submitted to the NAD, it will be the subject of a press release indicating such, with the possibility of the claim being referred to a federal agency, e.g., the FDA or the FTC. Numerous companies have used the NAD to settle disputes. The entity's Web site is <www.nadreview.org>.

The use of product- or ingredient-specific data to thwart and exclude others from making similar claims is akin to the Coca-Cola strategy, with the "experience" being systemic rather than gustatory. The secret recipe that makes this cola beverage "Coca-Cola" is known by less than a handful of individuals and enjoys more security than the FBI's most classified files. The "efficacy" of this polymolecular syrup is defined by the reproducible, high-fidelity taste experience enjoyed by global users of this product. All attempts to duplicate this recipe have failed. If one can extend the "efficacy" to a systemic process, e.g., deep venous circulation, or skin physiology, e.g., mitigation of inflammatory cell recruitment and cytokine expression in psoriatic lesions, then the user of such a product will enjoy reproducible efficacy. The ultimate objective of investing in clinical research on botanical products is to compel the consumer to try the proven brand and then, through the consumer's experience being positive (the product works), becoming a loyal, enduring customer. The bottom line is making consumers care enough to buy science-backed products versus the cheapest, "prettiest" things on the shelf.

HOW MUCH DATA IS ENOUGH?

How much data is enough to substantiate structure/function benefit claims for dietary supplements? The unwritten rule, voiced by both FDA and the FTC officials, is that two randomized, placebo-controlled clinical trials using state-of-the-art methods, the actual product in question, and statistical analysis yielding a statistically significant difference compared to placebo are required to show efficacy. For consumers, the amount of data required to show efficacy is a highly individualized question—some may say that one study is enough whereas more skeptical consumers would seek or require several studies, and perhaps even some long-term (one year or longer) studies before they would offer it to their children. For health professionals, again the quantity of data required to show efficacy would cover a broad range. A medical doctor may demand several hundred-person studies lasting up to two years (similar to that for prescription drugs) whereas a naturopath or chiropractor may be satisfied with one to two RCTs with a duration of only four to eight weeks.

My colleagues and I have found most prospective sponsors of clinical trials to be confronted with the *designing for dollars* conundrum: they want a great study, worthy of publication in a high-impact factor journal, with stunning statistics, and yet at a bargain-basement price. When asked about how many subjects they had in mind, for some obscure reason the reply most commonly is 60 subjects. For the first foray into sponsored clinical research, my colleagues and I recommend focusing upon the budget rather than the sample size.

Power calculations, which provide researchers with a ballpark estimate of how many persons would be needed in a study to measure a difference between two or more groups, are nice and desirable to perform. The calculated sample sizes depend upon (1) the study hypothesis or "what are we proposing to test"; (2) the amount of variability in measurement of what is expected to change, e.g., blood antioxidant activity or bone density; and (3) an estimate of a clinically meaningful and significant difference compared to presupplementation values and/or a placebo. However, if the sample size estimated via power calculations is prohibitively large, e.g., 84 subjects, does one close the research checkbook? As botanical product marketers do not have billions of dollars in revenue like drug companies, it is an economic impossibility for the majority of them to sponsor RCTs that enroll hundreds (or even one hundred) subjects. In our experience, a study conducted with two groups of 12 to 15 or more subjects is noteworthy and provides a starting point, a foundation upon which other evidence can be based.

Strategy in product indication and clinical outcome parameter selection assume preeminent importance in designing a clinical study. Because the overwhelming majority of sponsored research is conducted with a return on investment in mind, if the results are not *consumer relevant* and *consumer compelling* why do the trial? For both ingredient and finished product marketing companies, the real selling target is the end user. Does a drop in interleukin-1ß or altered expression of uncoupling protein II mean anything, compared to a decrease in pain or a reduction in body fatness? Consumers and most health professionals will be compelled to read further and inquire into use of the product if the outcome measure(s) encompass at least one clinically meaningful measure, i.e., one that assesses a widely recognized and/or symptomatic or physical feature or attribute. Lowering of diastolic blood pressure, reduction of waist size or body weight, increased head hair growth, elevation of HDL cholesterol, or a reduction in fasting blood sugar, insulin, or hemoglobin A1C are examples of relevance and import to persons seeking to achieve these outcomes.

If the product or ingredient of interest requires a duration of use greater than 30 to 60 days the likelihood of extracting a robust return on investment is slim *or* it will require a string of studies, effectively and repetitively communicated through the media and through advertising, e.g., vitamin E, garlic, and echinacea.

It would appear prudent to choose investigators who have a demonstrated expertise in clinical research, especially in relation to the parameters intended to be assessed, i.e., a family practice physician would unlikely be skilled in assessing a population of osteoarthritic men and women being assessed for responses to a botanical formula purported to modify joint pain and disease progression (unless he or she had done similar research before). In addition, the use of investigators that lack material interests in the product or company marketing the product would be strongly encouraged. Given the policy of many journals and companies to not provide full disclosure of the interests of scientific investigators, many such relationships are opaque to consumers, clinicians, and regulators. Researchers and marketers are earnestly encouraged to offer full disclosure of any interests, from consultancy fees and honoraria to travel and lodging to equity and stock options.

Mitigation of economic risk in research with innovative, "new to the world" compositions or those enjoying only preclinical (in vitro and animal studies) or anecdotal "validation" may involve taking a path that initially diverges from a phase II study approach. Phase II studies are small-scale RCTs done at a single research center where evaluating the efficacy of a product is the primary interest and the dose range is already established. Thus for a product where the dose response is unknown, it may be financially *imprudent* undertaking a phase II RCT. My associates and I often suggest that manufacturers do an open-label pilot study (six to ten participants) with applications that are much less prone to strong placebo responses, e.g., *not* chronic pain conditions, weight loss or appetite reduction, or mood disorders. Alternatively, employing a small sample size (three to five participants) with a conservative washout period and a crossover offers more statistical rigor, albeit at the expense of greater than doubling the time to completion of the study. These tactics can bolster confidence in going forward with phase II-type studies and still augment the "package" that encloses an ingredient or product invention.

Assuming one has an idea of a dose response or is willing to make the investment in a phase II study, we recommend the sponsored research investment to be dictated by both the budgetary restraints and reality—an RCT (adhering to the guidelines discussed) for $10,000 is unrealistic, as is one with 12 participants (that is, it will carry little weight). A safe number to start with is a sample size of at least 20 subjects, coupled with a power calculation done prior to the study. Although one may not be able to afford a properly powered study in the first round, one can obtain valuable preliminary evidence and, if the product outperforms expectations, achieve both a clinically and statistically significant result. Inevitably subjects drop out, for a myriad of reasons. One does not need to have a larger population to achieve *statistical* nirvana, as the magnitude of "effectiveness" dictates what is or is not statistically significant. For example, if a combination botanical product being tested for its ability to reduce the severity and size of psoriasis-related lesions (represented as a lesional sum score) shows a very large score reduction after four weeks of supplemen- tation, compared to a very small score reduction in the placebo group, the difference between the two groups (indicative of the effectiveness of the product) will be large. As long as there is not large variability between subjects in both groups, this result will manifest as both a statistically and clinically significant outcome. If the product in question has moderate to dramatic bioactivity or efficacy in vivo, this can likely override variability within and between groups and any psychogenic/placebo effects. Many preliminary drug studies have been published, with an RCT design, "favorable" statistics, and a sample size of only 20 to 30 subjects. This is a start, and a distinctive start indeed. If the results are promising and they are appropriately translated to the customer, incremental revenues can self-fund additional, larger studies, of even longer duration.

WE HAVE DATA—NOW WHAT?

There does not appear to be a need to present or publish the data emanating from sponsored studies, but one cannot underestimate the economic and brand-augmenting value from doing so. Product-specific clinical research that endures the scrutiny of the scientific peer review process and enters into the pages of a medium or high impact peer-reviewed journal brings instant clout to a product and also serves as independent third party evidence of safety and effectiveness. If the publication of such a study is coupled with a strategic media/public relations campaign, the possibility of this news entering a regional or national daily newspaper or even local or national network TV broadcast is imminently higher than if it never had been published. Moreover, the FTC shows favor upon studies that have been published in reviewed journals, viewing such data as having endured some independent scrutiny. Finally, omission of data that are contrary to what is being promoted can position a national marketing and advertising campaign within the central visual and auditory field of the regulatory agencies. The platform of two RCTs supporting the safety and efficacy of *Alpinia galanga* for rheumatoid arthritis will buckle if two or more other studies contravene these findings. Not unlike the blinded patron of justice, the overall weight of the evidence is what is assessed, not only the favorable evidence.

In the rush to begin extracting commercial value from the execution of a clinical research study on a botanical product, many companies are confronted with the challenge of patience. They can either wait for a scientific meeting (if they are even aware of such an opportunity and strategy) or seek an audience of peers who would likely buy the product on site, i.e., a trade show. One of the most distressing observations is witnessing a company who has sponsored research on a proprietary product or ingredient disseminating the results via presentation at a trade show, or via a press release with a dateline other than from a scientific conference or reviewed publication. The drive to disseminate the data and exploit it often engenders myopic activities such as these, in which the resulting impact is mired in the endemic bog of trade communications. Although this is a facet of data translation that should not be overlooked, what continues to be the onus of the natural products industry is the scrutiny and scoffing originating within the biomedical community. If one can get attention within this "esteemed" community, even without initial acceptance, such dialogue can foster interest and perhaps, with a continued commitment to research investigations, acknowledgement and adoption. Limiting the leverageability of data by avoiding the media-accepted audience of the academic and biomedical research communities diminishes the return on investment and attenuates the promise of greater consumer adoption. However, the allure of being able to both present to the trade (retailers, health professionals) and write orders afterward is hard for many to withstand and may prove irresistible. For some companies the instant gratification and reduced expenditures accompanying presentation of clinical research results at a trade convention may prove ideal.

The astute company plans a communication strategy in which they use the data to drive consumer demand via obtaining media coverage and reinforcing the brand message (not garlic extract but Allipin garlic—fictitious brand) with its own promotions, advertising, and marketing. My colleagues and I believe the best platform from which to obtain the loudest microphone is the national or international biomedical research conference/meeting. These range from the American Heart Association to Experimental Biology to Digestive Disease Week to the American Urological Association. If one such research story is picked up by even a regional newspaper or local TV network affiliate, the ensuing coverage in smaller consumer and trade media vehicles (magazines, local and regional newspapers, health and medicine Web sites) is usually quite robust and the broad downstream cascade is invaluable.

WHO HAS SCIENCE
AND HOW DID THEY ACQUIRE IT?

For consumers and health professionals, an appropriate question to ask of any botanical product marketer is simply for copies of any and all studies that support the *actual product being marketed*. If clinical research is provided, one needs to ascertain that indeed the entire product was the subject of the research, not just one ingredient. Last, ask if any of the researchers that conducted the clinical trial have received, are receiving, or will receive any financial or stock compensation for their involvement with the company, or if they happen to be an inventor of a patent related to the product.

CONCLUSION

Sponsoring and completing clinical research on botanical dietary supplements is an achievable reality for many product marketers, offering both direct (sales, marketshare, distinction) and indirect (tax benefits) economic incentives without the need to spend inordinately large amounts. For product consumers and "influencers," e.g., health professionals, the selection and recommendation of products that enjoy specific clinical research provides a degree of confidence in safety and efficacy largely absent from the majority of products on the market. Because proprietary botanical extracts are almost without exception unique recipes, the performance of clinical trials on a specific product confers upon it a form of intellectual property and competitive insulation that has valuable features distinctly different from that of a patent or untested trade secret. One hopes that both consumer purchase selection and corporate direction will steer the botanical dietary supplement industry into the realm of greater confidence and evidence circumscribed by the implementation of rigorous clinical research tools.

REFERENCES

Almada A, Byrd E (1997). Method for reduction of serum blood lipids or lipoprotein fraction. U.S. Patent 5,627,172, May 6.

Almada A, Mitchell T, Earnest C (1996). Impact of chronic creatine supplementation on serum enzyme concentrations. *The FASEB Journal* 10: A791.

Earnest CP, Almada AL, Mitchell TL (1996a). High-performance capillary electrophoresis-pure creatine monohydrate reduces blood lipids in men and women. *Clinical Science* 91 (1): 113-118.

Earnest C, Almada A, Mitchell T (1996b). Influence of chronic creatine supplementation on hepatorenal function. *The FASEB Journal* 10: A790.

Itil T, Martorano D (1995). Natural substances in psychiatry (*Ginkgo biloba* in dementia). *Psychopharmacology Bulletin* 31 (1): 147-158.

Koscielny J, Klubendorf D, Latza R, Schmitt R, Radtke H, Siegel G, Kiesewetter H (1999). The antiatherosclerotic effect of *Allium sativum*. *Atherosclerosis* 144 (1): 237-249.

Mitchell T, Almada A, Earnest C (1996). Creatine reduces blood lipid concentrations in men and women. *The FASEB Journal* 10: A521.

Chapter 10

Motives for Conducting Clinical Trials on Botanicals in Europe: A Focus on Germany

Joerg Gruenwald
Stefan Spiess

In the past two decades approximately 80 percent of the clinical research on botanical products has been conducted in Europe or on European products. Though other medicinal systems, such as the Ayurvedic medicine of India and traditional medicine of China, have extensive documentation of the use of botanicals, their use of classic Western preclinical and clinical research methods has been limited.

Several incentives exist for manufacturers in Europe to conduct clinical trials. One reason is to comply with regulatory requirements for product registration. For example, both Germany and France regulate botanical products mainly as drugs. Other incentives for conducting clinical studies include appeal to health care professionals, eligibility for reimbursement by medical insurance, product differentiation, and patent protection.

In order for a botanical product to be classified as a drug in Germany, it must be registered with the German Federal Institute for Drugs and Medical Devices (BfArM or Bundesinstitut für Arzneimittel und Medizinprodukte, <www.bfarm.de>). The product (and/or the ingredients) must comply with a monograph in the *European Pharmacopoeia,* or a pharmacopoeia from another European country—provided that such a monograph exists. Registration requirements are the same as those for synthetic drugs, including full chemical, pharmaceutical, preclinical (animal and in vitro testing), and clinical documentation, along with expert reports evaluating that documentation. Both the preclinical and clinical documentation can be based on existing scientific literature or on recent research conducted on the product in question. Therapeutic claims for the prevention and cure of a disease that are supported by documentation are allowed. Botanical drugs are sold mostly in pharmacies, and their cost to the patient is often reimbursed by medical insurance. Insurance reimbursement of botanicals is common in Germany, France, Austria, and Switzerland, and, to a smaller extent, in the Netherlands, Belgium, and Greece.

Some botanicals are registered as "traditional" herbal medicines, a subcategory of the drug category. In Germany, a traditional herbal medicine must have been on the market in that country for at least 30 years. Proposed European guidelines would require traditional herbal medicines to be on the market for 30 years, with only 15 of those required to be in Europe. As traditional medicines are drugs, they require full pharmaceutical-quality documentation. In this category, products are allowed to make mild therapeutic claims (e.g., as tonics) that are defined in lists published by the government. Proof of efficacy is not required for these drugs. They often contain multiple ingredients and lower concentrations of botanicals than standard botanical drugs. Some products are combinations of botanicals and non-botanicals such as vitamins, minerals, or amino acids. Traditional herbal medicines are not reimbursable by medical insurance and often are sold outside of pharmacies in supermarkets, drugstores (German "drugstores" do not contain pharmacies), health food stores, and via mail order.

Other regulatory categories for botanicals are dietary supplements and functional foods. The dietary supplement category in Europe is quite different from that in the United States, as it does not include the typical botanical medicines. The category includes vitamins and minerals as well as some herbal ingredients, such as lycopenes, flavonoids, and broccoli extracts. The dietary supplement category in Europe does not allow for any claims related to health or illnesses.

The system for registration of botanical drugs in Germany has a long history and is based mainly on existing clinical literature. These existing studies are the basis for general monographs of drug preparations in the *German* and *European Pharmacopoeias*. The pharmacopoeial monographs specify manufacturing details, such as the extraction parameters (plant to solvent ratios, solvent, etc.), as well as analytical methods for monitoring quality. Applicable therapeutic claims and dosage information are not usually listed in the pharmacopoeial monographs. However, they are present in monographs produced by the German Commission E, the European Scientific Committee on Phytotherapy (ESCOP), and the World Health Organization (WHO) (Blumenthal et al., 1998; ESCOP, 1999; WHO, 1999).

Some European manufacturers produce their botanical drugs according to existing monographs. In doing so, they have to follow the quality guidelines listed in the monograph. Products in accordance with such monographs are regarded as complying with the standard and therefore do not need additional clinical studies for registration.

The incentive for many companies to perform clinical trials on their products is to differentiate them from the rest of the products on the market. They can do this by changing the dosage form or the extraction media. They can also develop a new indication (one that is not supported by established literature) or a new combination of ingredients. Changes of this sort require the company to conduct its own clinical studies before it can register its product as a drug. For example, in the Commission E monograph for St. John's wort, the upper dosage is four grams herb or one milligram total hypericin. This dose was usually delivered in a dose of 300 mg extract containing 0.3 percent hypericin. However, following clinical research, dosages of extract were increased to include up to 900 mg extract containing 2.7 mg total hypericin in three divided doses (Schulz, 2002). In addition, data from clinical studies that confirmed efficacy, and did not demonstrate additional side effects, allowed the usual three-times-a-day split dose to be converted to a once-a-day dose (Rychlik et al., 2001).

As mentioned previously, botanical products in some European countries are eligible for insurance reimbursement. Recently, the German system for insurance reimbursement changed so that only those products which have solid clinical documentation are eligible. Products produced under traditional guidelines whose efficacy is not established using clinical trials are mostly no longer eligible for reimbursement. This is a new interpretation of the existing law § 93 "Sozialgesetzbuch." This change provides yet another incentive for German manufacturers to conduct scientific studies on their products.

Another incentive to document the efficacy of a product with clinical studies is to appeal to health care professionals. Half of the products in the drug category are recommended by doctors either through private prescription (not reimbursed by health insurance) or prescription with reimbursement. The other half of products in the drug category are purchased for self-medication, either directly requested by the patient or recommended by a pharmacist (Schwabe and Paffrath, 2001). In order for health care professionals to prescribe or recommend a product, it is essential for that product to have well-accepted scientific backing. For this reason, some manufacturers have chosen to document the efficacy of their products by performing double-blind, placebo-controlled trials. Examples of companies that perform these types of trials are Bionorica Arzneimittel, Dr. Willmar Schwabe Pharmaceuticals, Lichtwer Pharma AG, Madaus AG, Max Zeller Sohne AG, and Schaper & Brümmer GmbH.

Based on this approach, several herbal products that previously had only a small role in the market have become major players. This increase in popularity has occurred not only locally in Europe, but also internationally. In the past 20 years, completely new markets were created for botanicals based upon scientific support. Two good examples are garlic for reduction in cholesterol levels and St. John's wort for relieving depression. For both botanicals, there were already German Commission E approved monographs for these indications. However, several companies chose to develop these products by conducting additional good-quality clinical research. As a result, they have developed a worldwide market for garlic and St. John's wort in the range of approximately 300 and 500 million U.S. dollars in annual retail sales, respectively (Gruenwald, 2002). In a similar example, solid scientific data have enabled Indena S.p.A., an extraction company based in Italy, to become an internationally preferred source for numerous manufacturers.

Another incentive for the development of proprietary versions of botanicals and new combinations of botanicals is that of patent protection. However, patents for botanical preparations are often easier to circumvent than synthetic pharmaceuticals, as their specifications are often broad. In addition, obtaining the patent is only the first step, as the strength of a patent often depends upon the effort spent to support it. An example of a strong patent, with a combination of unique manufacturing specifications for upper and lower limits for several ingredients and broad clinical documentation, is that for Schwabe's ginkgo extract, EGb 761. As a result of this extensive documentation, the Commission E monograph for ginkgo is written according to specifications for EGb 761 (Blumenthal et al., 1998), and Schwabe has established an almost exclusive market for its product in Germany. Many clinical trials are not performed to receive a new registration or patent for a product; rather, they are conducted to promote and maintain existing registrations and for marketing purposes. For the majority of European manufacturers, clinical trials are used as additional marketing tools to improve their products' image in the eyes of the consumers. This concept of conducting trials for marketing purposes and to promote individual product recognition is developing internationally. Almost all of the successful botanical products in Europe have several well-controlled trials to support their use.

Top manufacturers follow the requirements for pharmaceutical drug clinical trials, i.e., they perform randomized, placebo-controlled or comparison trials with competitive products and follow good clinical practice (GCP) standards. However, a number of other forms of clinical trials are also common, including open (not blinded) trials, drug-monitoring trials, and small pilot studies. These trials can be used successfully for marketing and public relations purposes.

In addition, trials have been performed in order to expand population likely to use a product. As an example, manufacturers of some products with a record of safe use in adults are seeking to extend their products' use to children. In the past, administration to children was common, but only a few trials with children under 12 have been conducted. As a result of a review of existing data, the number of products allowed for use in children in Germany and in Europe has diminished tremendously (Gruenwald, 2002). For this reason, a political initiative has begun that urges manufacturers to perform trials on children in order to confirm the safety and efficacy of certain products for that population. For example, a multicenter, postmarketing surveillance study was carried out with 101 children aged one through twelve years assessing the use of St. John's wort (extract LI 160) for depression and psychovegetative disorders (Hubner and Kirste, 2001).

Conducting clinical trials also allows manufacturers to expand their worldwide distribution. For example, most European botanical products enter the U.S. market as dietary supplements. These products may be produced entirely by the European manufacturer. Alternatively, the raw materials or extracts from Europe can be reformulated and/or packaged by American manufacturers. However, a number of European companies (along with American companies) are in the process of applying to the U.S. Food and Drug Administration (FDA) for drug status for their products in the United States. In order to comply with the FDA drug requirements, clinical trials need to be performed according to the scientific rigor of good clinical practice, i.e., placebo-controlled, double-blind studies.

A disincentive for the investment of companies into studies on botanical medicines is the financial risk involved in what may possibly be a negative clinical trial. Another disincentive is the limited exclusivity that manufacturers obtain with their clinical trial data. Even if a patent is obtained, it can require substantial investment to defend. In addition, if a clinical study is published, competitors may use that data to support their own products. This phenomenon, often called "borrowed science," is common in the United States.

In summary, the incentives for European manufacturers to conduct clinical studies include registration of a product as a new drug or registration for a new indication. Additional incentives include marketing advantages that come from differentiation from other products on the market, appeal to health care professionals, and patent protection. Further, experience indicates that conducting clinical trials can lead to expansion of the market and the population likely to take the product. Finally, conduction of clinical research and tight regulation of quality have allowed botanical products in Germany to be part of the mainstream health system.

REFERENCES

Blumenthal M, Busse W, Hall T, Goldberg A, Gruenwald J, Riggins C, Rister S, Eds. (1998). *The Complete German Commission E Monographs: Therapeutic Guide to Herbal Medicines.* Trans. S Klein. Austin, TX: American Botanical Council.

European Scientific Cooperative on Phytotherapy (ESCOP) (1999). *Monographs on the Medicinal Uses of Plant Drugs.* Exeter, UK: European Scientific Cooperative on Phytotherapy.

Gruenwald J (2002). Phytopharm Herbal Market Report (unpublished).

Hubner WD, Kirste T (2001). Experience with St. John's wort *(Hypericum perforatum)* in children under 12 years with symptoms of depression and psychovegetative disturbances. *Phytotherapy Research* 15 (4): 367-370.

Rychlik R, Siedentop H, von den Driesch V, Kasper S (2001). St. John's wort extract WS 5572 in mild to moderate depression: Efficacy and tolerability of 600 and 1200 mg active ingredient/day. *Fortschritte der Medizin* 119 (3-4): 119-128.

Schulz V (2002). Clinical trials with hypericum extracts in patients with depression—Results, comparisons, conclusions for therapy with antidepressant drugs. *Phytomedicine* 9 (5): 468-474.

Schwabe U, Paffrath D, Eds. (2001). *Arzneiverordnungs-Report.* Berlin: Springer Verlag.

World Health Organization (WHO) (1999). *WHO Monographs on Selected Medicinal Plants,* Volume 1. Geneva, Switzerland: World Health Organization.

Chapter 11

Pharmacopoeias
and Botanical Monographs

Marilyn Barrett
Roy Upton
V. Srini Srinivasan

In order to ensure both the safety and efficacy of conventional and herbal drug products, quality control standards are required. Once the character, quality, and strength of the product are specified, then guidelines for therapeutic use can be established. These standards and guidelines are provided in texts known as pharmacopoeias (also spelled pharmacopeia, the spelling used by the United States Pharmacopeial Convention) or compendia. A pharmacopoeia is a collection of monographs that contain technical information on specific medicinal agents, including botanical and pharmaceutical drugs as well as inert additives used in the formulation of drugs. Some pharmacopoeias, and hence their monographs, are made official through governmental recognition. In this instance, compliance with the specifications in the monograph is enforced by governmental regulation. Monographs are of three basic formats. They contain information on quality, therapeutic use, or both.

Monographs that focus on quality contain information, assays, and specifications useful in assuring identity and purity. For botanical agents, these monographs include the plant names (common name and Latin binomial), plant part, and criteria or definition of the substance, as well as descriptions of the whole and ground plant material, along with chemical constituents. The *United States Pharmacopeia, European Pharmacopoeia, British Herbal Pharmacopoeia, Pharmacopoeia of Japan,* and *Ayurvedic Pharmacopoeia of India* contain monographs of this sort.

Therapeutic monographs vary greatly in scope and detail. They typically include information on therapeutic indication, dose, dosage forms, pharmacology, contraindications, drug interactions, side effects, and toxicology. Examples include the monographs of the *United States Pharmacopeia—Drug Information,* German Commission E, European Scientific Cooperative on Phytotherapy, and *British Herbal Compendium.*

The American Herbal Pharmacopoeia and the World Health Organization produce monographs that combine both quality control standards and therapeutic information.

UNITED STATES PHARMACOPEIA
AND NATIONAL FORMULARY (USP-NF)

The *United States Pharmacopeia–National Formulary (USP-NF)* is the officially recognized standard for drugs in the United States. The first version of the pharmacopoeia was published in 1820 by the United States Pharmacopeial Convention, a private, nonprofit organization. The pharmacopoeia was revised every ten years from 1820 to 1942, every five years until 2000, and, following the 2002 edition, it will be revised every year. In 1975, the USP acquired the National Formulary and started to publish both of them in a single volume, titled the *United States Pharmacopeia–National Formulary (USP-NF,* 2004). In a separate publication, the *United States Pharmacopeia— Dispensing Information (USP-DI)* provides a review of the clinical and pharmacological data, dosage recommendations, and safety assessments to assist health professionals and consumers in the appropriate use of drugs (USP-DI, 2003). In addition, the USP organization provides the reference standards to be used in the methods described in its monographs.

The *USP-NF* is recognized in several statutes and regulations, including the U.S. Federal Food, Drug, and Cosmetic Act and its amendments. These regulations stipulate that if a drug does not conform to *USP* standards for strength, quality, and purity, it is considered adulterated. The *USP* also has official governmental recognition outside the United States in over 40 countries, both developing and industrialized (*USP-NF,* 2004).

The *USP-NF* contains approximately 4,000 monographs containing tests and standards for assuring the strength, quality, and purity of drug substances and products (*USP-NF,* 2004). In general, monographs for active ingredients and preparations appear in the *USP* section of the book and the *NF* contains botanical dietary supplements and excipients (ingredients that aid in the formulation of drugs). With the publication of the 2004 edition, a new section was created in the *USP* for dietary supplements. Previously, monographs for botanicals marketed as dietary supplements were published in the *NF* as they are not subject to premarket approval by the FDA.

In the first edition of the *USP,* approximately 600 botanicals and botanical preparations were recognized. By the turn of the twentieth century, only 169 botanicals remained. Many of the original plant drugs were removed and supplanted by synthetic compounds and their preparations. By 1990 the USP was estimated to contain only 25 botanical drug preparations (Grady, 1994). At that time, the USP resolved to expand its scope to include monographs on nutritional supplements containing vitamins and minerals. In 1995, the USP adopted a resolution to once again develop monographs for botanicals currently being sold as dietary supplements. Since then the USP has proceeded with the development of a number of monographs for raw plant materials, extracts, and final formulations.

The primary goal of the USP regarding botanicals is to develop monographs for those widely used by the American public and constituting 90 percent of the monetary sales in the U.S. market (approximately 25 botanicals). Aside from market share, other criteria are applied in the identification and prioritization of botanicals for monograph development. These include evidence for historical use in traditional medicines; safety; availability of literature documenting pharmacological activity; identity and chemical constituents; and availability of reference standards used to document compliance with specifications for identity and quality.

Information monographs, containing therapeutic information, were prepared for inclusion in the *USP-DI* on ginger rhizome, valerian root, feverfew leaf, St. John's wort flowering plant, and saw palmetto berry. In addition, a negative monograph was published on comfrey, discouraging its use for safety reasons. In 2000 the USP established criteria for levels of evidence for judging the safety and efficacy of botanical dosage forms and published these in the USP Web site (www.usp.org).

The USP continues to develop and establish monographs defining standards of quality for botanicals and their preparations. However, the development of information monographs on botanicals has been discontinued.

AMERICAN HERBAL PHARMACOPOEIA (AHP) AND THERAPEUTIC COMPENDIUM

The American Herbal Pharmacopoeia (AHP) is a private, non-profit organization founded in 1995. The purpose of the AHP is to develop quality control standards and to critically review the therapeutic data for botanical supplements sold in the United States. Although lacking official government recognition, *AHP* monographs are considered authoritative and are accepted as compendial standards by many organizations.

AHP monographs cover botanicals with their origins in traditional Ayurvedic, Chinese, and Western herbal traditions. They provide a synthesis of traditional and scientific information.

The monographs are published individually, with the first *AHP* monograph published in 1997 on St. John's wort (Upton et al., 1997). As of the beginning of 2004, a total of 18 monographs had been finalized and another 30 were in development. The goal is to develop a total of 300 monographs.

The quality control section of each *AHP* monograph includes nomenclature standards, several methods of identification, purity standards, several methods of qualitative and quantitative chemical assessment, as well as guidelines for proper harvesting, storage, and processing of botanicals. Unlike all other pharmacopoeias, the *AHP* includes detailed graphics for use in raw material identification and detection of potential adulterants. The analytical methods are carefully chosen following an extensive review and are then subjected to trial and validation by a minimum of two independent laboratories.

The *Therapeutic Compendium,* another section of *AHP* monographs, provides a detailed and critical assessment of the currently available clinical and pharmacological literature. This enables the reader to determine the level of evidence available for specific therapeutic applications of each medicinal plant. Recommendations for dose are provided from both the traditional and scientific literature. Also included is a detailed review of safety aspects including side effects, contraindications, drug interactions, use in pregnancy and lactation, mutagenicity, and toxicology.

Each monograph contains many separate sections written by experts in those particular areas of botanical medicine. Once compiled, the monographs are subjected to an extensive peer review process. The reviewers are a multidisciplinary committee of medicinal plant experts worldwide, including botanists, chemists, herbalists, pharmacists, pharmacologists, and physicians.

EUROPEAN PHARMACOPOEIA (EP)

The *European Pharmacopoeia (EP)* was founded by eight states (Belgium, France, Germany, Italy, Luxembourg, Netherlands, Switzerland, United Kingdom) in 1964. It has since expanded to many other nations both within and outside the European Union. The pharmacopoeia is published by the Directorate for the Quality of Medicines of the Council of Europe (EDQM) in accordance with the Convention on the Elaboration of a European Pharmacopoeia (European Treaty Series No. 50). It is an official compendium for establishing the quality control standards, replacing the old national pharmacopoeias for member nations. It is currently in its fourth (2002) edition, and the fifth edition will be effective in January 2005. The pharmacopoeia contains specific monographs governing the quality of specific herbal products and it also contains general monographs that apply to all unspecified extracts, herbal drug preparations, herbal drugs, and herbal teas (Ph Eur, 2002).

BRITISH HERBAL PHARMACOPOEIA (BHP) *AND* BRITISH HERBAL COMPENDIUM (BHC)

The *British Herbal Pharmacopoeia (BHP)* is published by the British Herbal Medicine Association and written by the members of its Scientific Committee. The *BHP* monographs do not have official government recognition. *BHP* monographs establish standards of quality control and purity for botanical raw materials but not for final product forms. The first monographs were published in 1971. A pharmacopoeia, with 232 monographs containing both quality and therapeutic information, was published in 1983. A subsequent edition with revised format emphasizing quality standards covering 84 botanicals was published in 1990 (*BHP,* 1996). Therapeutic and regulatory information were published separately in 1992 in a volume called the *British Herbal Compendium (BHC)* (Bradley, 1992). In 1996, an expanded version of the *BHP* incorporating an additional 85 monographs was published, thus providing quality standards for 169 botanicals (*BHP,* 1996).

GERMAN COMMISSION E

The German Commission E is an independent scientific committee of experts established in 1978 by the German Federal Health Agency for the evaluation of the therapeutic use of herbal remedies. The committee evaluated information on the safety and efficacy of crude herbal drug preparations and gave either a positive or negative assessment in a published monograph. In the case of a positive finding, the monograph was structured as a package insert, providing precise directions for use, including dosage, approved actions, side effects, drug interactions, contraindications, and chemical constituents. In the case of a negative decision, the monograph explains why the botanical was perceived to lack benefit. Monographs were first published as drafts for public comment, and then the final version appeared in the *Federal Gazette,* or *Bundesanzeiger.* Approximately 300 monographs were published before the Commission suspended monograph writing in August 1994. The Commission E monographs have been translated into English and published by the American Botanical Council (Blumenthal et al., 1998). When the Commission was actively writing monographs, those monographs formed the primary basis for approval of health or disease claims on botanical products in Germany. However, due to the availability of new scientific data, the Commission E monographs are no longer considered to be sufficient for governmental approval of therapeutic claims. The current focus of the Commission is to review the registration of botanical drugs in Germany.

EUROPEAN SCIENTIFIC COOPERATIVE ON PHYTOTHERAPY (ESCOP)

The European Scientific Cooperative on Phytotherapy (ESCOP) was formed in 1989 with the purpose of advancing the scientific status of phytomedicines and to assist in the harmonization of their regulatory status in Europe. ESCOP members include associations from the majority of countries within the European Union and from a number of non-European Union countries. ESCOP monographs are therapeutically oriented and do not include information on quality.

Monographs are initially written by individuals with professional backgrounds such as medical doctors, phytotherapists, pharmacognosists, and regulatory specialists. The drafts are then circulated to members of ESCOP's Scientific Subcommittees for review and discussion. The subcommittee prepares a second draft, which is reviewed by a board of supervising editors consisting of academic experts in phytotherapy and medicinal plant research. This process ensures that each monograph that is developed is reflective of many national viewpoints and the advice of many authorities on the subject. The final document is published and submitted to the Committee on Proprietary Medicinal Products of the Commission of the European Community (EEC). Between 1996 and 1999, six fascicles, each containing ten monographs, were published. More recently these original monographs were revised and twenty monographs added to produce a publication containing 80 monographs (ESCOP, 2003). The monographs are recognized by the European Medicines Evaluation Agency of the Council of Europe.

CHINESE PHARMACOPOEIA

The *Pharmacopoeia of the People's Republic of China* is now in its seventh edition, also known as the *Chinese Pharmacopoeia 2000* or *Ch.P.2000*. The People's Republic of China's Ministry of Public Health first published the *Chinese Pharmacopoeia* in 1953. The current pharmacopoeia is published in both English and Chinese and contains two volumes. Volume I includes 992 monographs of Chinese materia medica (botanicals and other crude drugs of natural sources) and traditional Chinese patent medicines (specified formulations). As many as 602 botanical monographs in Volume I specify thin-layer chromatography for identification, and about 300 monographs specify quantitative analytical techniques (liquid or gas chromatography) for chemical constituents. Volume I also contains actions and indications of the botanicals and other crude drugs of natural sources. Volume II contains monographs on chemicals, antibiotics, biochemicals, radiopharmaceuticals, and biological agents (The Pharmacopoeia Commission of PRC, 2000).

AFRICAN PHARMACOPOEIA

The *African Pharmacopoeia* was published in English, French, and Arabic in a collaborative effort by the Council of Ministers of the Organization of African Unity (OAU) with the United Nations Industrial Development Organization, World Health Organization, and other donor agencies. This effort established the African Center for Traditional Medicines. Publication of the first edition of the *African Pharmacopoeia* was in two volumes. Volume I was published in 1985 and Volume II in 1986. Volume I includes 95 monographs containing names, botanical descriptions, uses, and geographical distributions of herbal drugs. Volume II is a companion to the first volume and contains general methods of quality control analysis (Inter African Committee, 1985-1986). Copies of the *African Pharmacopoeia* are difficult to locate and publication has not continued.

THE PHARMACOPOEIA OF JAPAN

The *Pharmacopoeia of Japan*, Fourteenth Edition, was published in 2001, in two parts. Included in the *Pharmacopoeia* are quality guidelines for crude drugs obtained from plants, animals, and minerals. The *Pharmacopoeia* contains guidelines for purity and identity for over 165 raw herbs used in traditional Kampo medicines. Kampo medicines, which are based mostly on decoctions of herbs, are indicated by prescription and reimbursed by Japan's national health insurance program (*The Pharmacopoeia of Japan*, 2001).

THE PHARMACOPOEIAS OF INDIA

The Ayurvedic Pharmacopoeia of India is the legal document of standards for the quality of single drugs of plant origin. The Ayurvedic Pharmacopoeia Committee was formed in 1963 to write monographs detailing identity, purity, and strength. Volume I, first published in 1986 by the Department of Health, Government of India, contains 80 monographs. Recently the Controller of Publications in Delhi has reprinted Volume I (2001), along with Volumes II (1999) and III (2001). Volume II contains 78 monographs, and Volume III contains 100, for a total of 258 single plant drugs in the three volumes. Volume IV is under preparation. A total of 636 combination formulas are described in *The Ayurvedic Formulary of India* (Volumes I and II contain 444 and 192 formulas, respectively), published by the Government of India (*The Ayurvedic Formulary of India,* 2001).

Another traditional form of medicine in India is Unani. The Unani Pharmacopoeial Committee in the Ministry of Health and Family Welfare, India, has recently prepared Part I of the *Unani Pharmacopoeia of India* containing 45 monographs on single drugs of plant origin. However, there is no official publication yet by the government of India.

WORLD HEALTH ORGANIZATION (WHO)

The World Health Organization (WHO) has had a long tradition of supporting the appropriate use of botanicals in the health care systems of both developed and developing nations (Akerele, 1993). The WHO is currently publishing model monographs in order to facilitate the proper use of high-quality herbal medicines in WHO member states (countries). The goal is to provide a model for assisting member states in developing their own monographs and to facilitate information exchange. The monographs are presented in two parts. Part 1 focuses on quality assurance, botanical features, geographic distribution, identity tests, purity requirements, and a listing of chemical constituents. Part 2 summarizes clinical applications, pharmacology, posology (dosage), contraindications, precautions, and potential adverse reactions. The monographs are prepared under the direction of the WHO Collaborative Center at the University of Illinois–Chicago. Volume I, containing 28 monographs, was published in 1999, and Volume II containing an additional 30 monographs, was published in 2002 (WHO, 1999-2002). Volume III with 31 monographs is to be released soon, and IV is in development.

OTHER PHARMACOPOEIAS

In addition to the compendia described herein, the majority of nations have either official or unofficial pharmacopoeias. Although some are available in English, most are published only in their native languages. Numerous other books containing profiles of medicinal plants are considered to be authoritative and may be used by governmental agencies. The degree of accuracy and depth of information in these texts is variable.

SUMMARY AND PERSPECTIVE

The pharmacopoeias described offer a number of authoritative sources for information regarding the quality of botanicals. In addition, but not described in this chapter, both national and international standards for manufacturing of botanical products also exist. Together, the monographs and manufacturing standards have been developed to assure a level of quality and consistency for therapeutic products. Once the quality and consistency of products are assured, then guidelines may be established for therapeutic use.

In the United States, compliance with quality standards set by the USP for products sold as drugs is mandatory. Under current federal regulations, compliance for products sold as dietary supplements is voluntary. However, dietary supplements are not without regulation, as federal law dictates that botanical products sold as dietary supplements accurately disclose their ingredients, be free of pathogenic microbes and other contaminants, and be truthful regarding any claim regarding health benefits. Only if the USP name is put on the label of the product must the product conform to USP specifications. The AHP also provides guidelines for assurance of identity and quality, and the same rules apply. Seals of quality have begun to appear on dietary supplements, which vary in meaning depending upon their certification process. Both the USP and NSF International, a Michigan-based company, have begun to offer seals based on manufacturing site inspections as well as product quality testing. Until these and other mechanisms of assuring quality are more widespread, consumers and health professionals must take an active role in investigating the quality of botanical supplements they are contemplating consuming or prescribing.

SOURCES OF PHARMACOPOEIAS

American Herbal Pharmacopoeia and Therapeutic Compendium
P.O. Box 66809
Scotts Valley, CA 95067
Tel: 831-461-6318
FAX: 831-475-6219
Web site: www.herbal-ahp.org

American Botanical Council
P.O. Box 144345
Austin, TX 78714
Tel: 512-926-4900
FAX: 512-926-2345
Web site: www.herbalgram.org
(Source for *British Herbal Pharmacopoeia* and ESCOP monographs)

United States Pharmacopeia
12601 Twinbrook Parkway
Rockville, MD 20852
Tel: 301-881-0666
Fax: 301-816-8374
Web site: www.usp.org

REFERENCES

Akerele O (1993). Summary of World Health Organization (WHO) guidelines for the assessment of herbal medicines. *HerbalGram* 28: 13-20.

Ayurvedic Formulary of India, The (2001). Delhi: The Controller of Publications.

Ayurvedic Pharmacopoeia of India, The (1999-2001). Volumes I, II, III. Delhi: The Controller of Publications.

Blumenthal M, Busse W, Hall T, Goldberg A, Gruenwald J, Riggins C, Rister S, eds. (1998). *The Complete German Commission E Monographs: Therapeutic Guide to Herbal Medicines.* Trans. S Klein. Austin, TX: American Botanical Council.

Bradley PR, ed. (1992). *British Herbal Compendium: A Handbook of Scientific Information on Widely Used Plant Drugs,* Volume 1. Dorset, UK: British Herbal Medicine Association.

British Herbal Pharmacopoeia (BHP) (1996). Fourth Edition. Exeter, UK: British Herbal Medicine Association.

European Scientific Cooperative on Phytotherapy (ESCOP) (2003). *ESCOP Monographs: The scientific foundation for herbal medicinal products,* Second Edition. Exeter, UK: ESCOP, in collaboration with Stuttgart, Germany: Goerg Thieme Verlag.

Grady LT (1994). Worldwide Harmonization of Botanical Standards: A Pharmacopeial View. Presented at the National Institutes of Health Conference on Botanicals, Washington, DC, December 15-17.

Inter African Committee on Medicinal Plants and African Traditional Medicine (1985-1986). *African Pharmacopoeia.* Lagos: Organization of African Unity, Scientific, Technical and Research Commission.

Ph Eur (2002). *European Pharmacopoeia,* Fourth Edition. Strasbourg Cedex, France: Council of Europe.

Pharmacopoeia Commission of PRC, The (2000). *Pharmacopoeia of the People's Republic of China,* Volumes I and I (English Edition). Beijing, China: Chemical Industry Press.

Pharmacopoeia of Japan, The (2001). Fourteenth Edition (English Version). Tokyo: Society of Japanese Pharmacopoeia.

United States Pharmacopeia Dispensing Information (USP-DI) (2003). Twenty-third Edition. Greenwood Village, CO: Micromedex.

United States Pharmacopeia 27, National Formulary 22 (USP-NF) (2004). Rockville, MD: The United States Pharmacopeial Convention, Inc.

Upton R, Graff A, Williamson E, Bunting D, Gatherum DM, Walker EB, Butterweck V, Liefländer-Wulf U, Nahrstedt A, Wall A, et al. (1997). St. John's wort, *Hypericum perforatum:* Quality control, analytical and therapeutic monograph. American Herbal Pharmacopoeia and Therapeutic Compendium. Ed. R Upton. Santa Cruz: American Herbal Pharmacopoeia.

World Health Organization (WHO) (1999-2002). *WHO Monographs on Selected Medicinal Plants,* Volumes I and II. Geneva, Switzerland: World Health Organization.

PART II:
METHODS

Chapter 12

Methods of Product and Trial Inclusion and Evaluation

Marilyn Barrett

This chapter describes the methods used in generating the second half of this book. A description of how the information on products and clinical studies was collected is included. Also described are the selection criteria for both products and trials. The origin of the system used to evaluate clinical trial quality is also explained. Some of the main challenges encountered during the selection of products and the evaluation of the clinical studies are discussed. The criteria for evaluating the quality of the clinical trials are provided in Chapter 13, "Clinical Trial Reviewer's Guidance and Checklist."

GATHERING INFORMATION ON PRODUCTS AND TRIALS

We used two approaches to gathering products and clinical trial publications for inclusion in the book. The first approach was to contact manufacturers in the United States to ask if they had any products that had been evaluated in clinical studies. The second approach was to identify products from clinical studies published in the scientific literature. Once a product was identified from the literature, the manufacturer was contacted for further information.

In the first approach, manufacturers were contacted in letters sent out in July 1999. These letters were followed up with e-mails and telephone calls. The list of manufacturers was compiled from membership lists of American Herbal Products Association (AHPA), Council for Responsible Nutrition (CRN), and National Nutritional Foods

Association (NNFA). Approximately 200 manufacturers were contacted. Manufacturers were asked for copies of product labels and for reprints of the corresponding clinical literature.

In the second approach, clinical literature was identified through searches of Medline and Embase literature databases in the summer of 2000. Clinical trial reports were also identified through perusal of the author's personal files as well as from reference lists in books and review articles. Clinical trial literature was obtained from local libraries or requested from manufacturers. Translations of literature in Italian, German, and French were commissioned in a few instances. More often the manufacturer supplied the translation.

The list of botanicals to be included in the book was set in December 2000. At that time, we began to send the clinical literature to reviewers for evaluation of the quality of the trials. In the spring and summer of 2002, searches of Medline and Embase were repeated, and more recent trials were added to the original set. New trials were generally included if the botanical product used in the study was already included in the book.

Selection Criteria: Products and Trials

Selection Criteria for Products

- Products containing powdered plant material, teas, juices, oils, tincture, extracts (either simple or semipurified), etc., were evaluated for entry. Formulas containing multiple botanical ingredients were also evaluated for entry. Products containing only purified chemicals derived from plants were excluded.
- Products assessed in controlled clinical trials were evaluated for entry. Products assessed in studies without a control (placebo or other medication) were not included.
- Products sold in the United States were included as a first priority. However, products not for sale in the United States were also included. The purpose of including products sold outside the United States was to complete the profile of a botanical or formula that was already included and/or to supplement the understanding of the activity of that botanical. In a few instances, products that were for sale in the United States when originally included are no longer for sale in the United States. They are still included in the book.

- Products with raw material ingredients (i.e., extracts) that have been clinically tested, but whose final formulation has not, were included (see comments in the subsection regarding challenges in the selection process). If the final formulation included additional active ingredients, then that product was not included.
- Generic (unbranded) preparations tested clinically were included in many instances to help with the understanding of the activity of a botanical already included.

Selection Criteria for Clinical Trials

- Trials that included either a placebo or alternate medication as a comparative control were evaluated for entry. If a product or botanical was already selected for entry, then comparative dosage studies were allowed.
- Trials were generally not included if the test product was not described in sufficient detail as to allow for replication of the study. Leeway was granted for proprietary products, as it was assumed that more information could be obtained from other sources (see comments in the subsection regarding challenges in the selection process).
- Trials published after 1980 were given priority over those published earlier.
- Published and unpublished studies were accepted.
- Trials not easily translated or obtained in the English language were not profiled and were not reviewed as to their level of evidence.
- Full clinical papers were required for inclusion. Study abstracts were not sufficient to be included.
- Epidemiological studies, postmarketing surveillance studies, systematic reviews of clinical trials, and meta-analyses of clinical studies are mentioned in the botanical summary evaluations but are not profiled in detail and were not reviewed as to their level of evidence.

Challenges in the Selection Process

At the beginning of the book project, the product entry criteria were broader than they ended up being. I thought that if I included only products directly tested in clinical studies, then I would necessarily be selecting for European products. I was therefore originally prepared to include products manufactured in the United States with specifications equivalent to those of products tested in clinical studies. In other words, I was ready to include products containing an extract or extracts made to the same specifications as a product tested in a trial. Specifications were to include the plant part, extraction method, extraction solvent, standardization parameters, and recommended dose. However, I found that this process of judging equivalency was not feasible. Even if products appeared to be chemically equivalent from the information available to me at the time, there was no guarantee of therapeutic equivalency (see Chapter 6 on borrowed science). In addition, I found in practice it was very difficult to obtain sufficient information to determine chemical equivalency. Also, manufacturers that had conducted clinical studies on their product(s) were, understandably, not eager to participate in a program that assisted their competition in "borrowing" their scientific studies. I therefore decided to include only products that had been directly tested clinically.

The only caveat to this rule is that I decided to include products containing extracts which had been tested clinically, even if the final product formulation had not been tested clinically. I made this decision for a number of reasons. First, some trials were conducted on extracts and did not name a final product. Second, I knew there was no way that I could determine if the final formulation had changed since the time of the trial. In addition, if a European extract was formulated in the United States, that formulation might be expected to be different from its European equivalent.

As an example, a few trials mentioned the ginkgo extract EGb 761 but gave no product name. Nevertheless, the book ties all the trials on EGb 761, whether a product was named or not, with two products in the United States that contain the EGb 761 extract: Ginkgold (Nature's Way Products, Inc.) and Ginkoba (Pharmaton Natural Health Products). These products differ in the excipients used in the final formulation. Another example is the St. John's wort extract Ze 117, manufactured by Zeller AG of Switzerland which is made available in two different final formulations by General Nutrition Corporation and Rexall Sundown.

Another consideration is the case of an Italian extract manufacturer, Indena S.p.A., who makes many extracts that have been tested clinically. Indena sells extracts to manufacturers around the world, who then formulate them into their own products. Some of those manufacturers have conducted clinical trials on their final formulation, while others have not. For those who did not conduct their own trials, we relied on verification from Indena that the manufacturers' product(s) did indeed contain the Indena extract(s) that have been clinically tested. These products are listed separately from those that have been tested in their final form. As an example, listed separately are several products available in the United States that contain the Indena St. John's wort extract (St. John Select), namely, St. John's Wort Extract by Enzymatic Therapy, Hyper-Ex by Thorne Research, and Hypericum perforatum II by Hypericum Buyers Club. With the exception of the Hypericum Buyers Club product, which has been used in two drug interaction studies, these products have not been tested clinically in their final formulation. Listed in the main summary table are the U.S. product Kira and the European Union (EU) product Jarsin, both manufactured by Lichtwer Pharma AG, Germany. The clinical trials have been conducted either with the Lichtwer product final formulation or the Lichtwer extract LI 160. LI 160 is supplied by Indena and also known as St. John Select.

It is also difficult to determine whether the products on the market today are equivalent to the products tested in the clinical studies. Products with the same name may change in composition. For example, there have been changes in the extraction solvent used in the preparation of Remifemin (Schaper & Brümmer GmbH & Co. KG, Germany), a black cohosh product; however, these changes do not appear to have affected activity (see the black cohosh summary). Changes to the coating on Kwai (Lichtwer Pharma AG, Germany) garlic tablets, however, may have changed the bioavailability of the contents, resulting in a change in activity (see the garlic summary). An even more interesting example is the red yeast rice product, Cholestin. The U.S. version of the product no longer contains red yeast rice, due to a federal order. A formula with an alternate active ingredient is now marketed under the same name (see the red yeast rice summary). More problematic are complex formulas whose ingredients may have changed over time. In many cases, there is insufficient detail in the description in the study report to determine whether the product sold today is the same as the one used in the trial.

The lack of an adequate product description in the clinical study was often a problem. Ideally, the scientific name of the plant, the plant part, preparation details, as well as commercial name and manufacturer should be included. My assistants and I found many cases of inadequate descriptions of products, and the most egregious were not accepted into the book. If a product was described using a proprietary name, I decided to accept that description as adequate, the rationale being that the product details would be available from the manufacturer. However, I also realize that it is important to keep in mind the caveats listed previously.

Products that were provided by contract manufacturers under a private label were not included in the book. This is because the manufacturer and source of the raw material remain a secret and thus there is no assurance of continuity or uniformity of these products over time. As an example, a study conducted with a ginkgo product provided by Walgreens Co., Deerfield, Illinois, was not included. Walgreens is a retail pharmacy that does not manufacture botanicals. The product it offers is obtained via a private labeling contract that enables it to put its name on the contract manufacturer's product. The contract manufacturer is not named on the label and may change from time to time. Even if Walgreens continues to use the same contract manufacturer, the raw material supplier for that manufacturer may change.

In a few cases in which the trial was negative, the product was not described by brand name, instead being replaced by a seemingly generic description. Sometimes further research on our part would determine the true identity of the material. Sometimes, it would not.

A good deal of the information regarding the European products has come from the trials themselves. Not much detail regarding usage guidelines was easily available in English. Also, I do not know if they are still offered for sale or have changed names.

DATA ON PRODUCTS AND TRIALS

Product Information

Product information included in the book is almost entirely from the product labels. In some instances, the label information is supplemented with facts from clinical studies, product information supplied by the manufacturer in promotional leaflets, company Web pages, and direct communication with the manufacturer.

When possible, the information on the botanical ingredients includes the name, the plant part, whether the material in the product was dried plant material or an extract, the quantity of that material, processing details, the name of the extract (if any), and standardization criteria.

In addition, information is included regarding the manufacturer of the product or extract, the distributor of the product in the United States, formulation (liquid, capsule, tablet), recommended dose, indications as to use (Dietary Supplement Health and Education Act [DSHEA] structure/function statements, unless otherwise noted), cautionary statements, other ingredients, miscellaneous comments, and the source(s) of the information.

Challenges in Product Information

The biggest challenge to the inclusion of the product information is keeping up with the changes in the market. While this book was being compiled some products were taken off the shelves. In a few instances the distribution of the product was transferred to another company. The end result is that some of the product information listed in the book may not be up to date.

Trial Information

Clinical trial information included in the book has been abstracted from the full clinical paper. The clinical study information includes the bibliographic reference, a summary of the product description (botanical name, product name, extract name, and manufacturer), and the therapeutic indication tested in the study. Information regarding the trial design includes a summary description, duration, dose, route of administration, randomization, blinding, and whether a placebo or another agent was present for comparison. Also included is information on the site of the study. The number of subjects enrolled and the number completing the study are presented. Details as to their age, sex, and inclusion and exclusion criteria are outlined. The end points of the study, measurements that were used to determine efficacy or clinical benefit, are also presented. The results of those end points, along with any side effects, are noted. Also included are any comments that the author(s) of the study have made regarding the meaning of the study. Finally, the ratings and comments made by an independent reviewer regarding the quality of the study are presented. Further details on the review process and rating scales are provided in the following section, Evaluation of Clinical Trial Quality, and in the next chapter.

Botanical Summaries

Summaries of information on products and their trials were grouped by botanical or formula. Both common and Latin names are cited with reference to the American Herbal Products Association's *Herbs of Commerce* (McGuffin et al., 2000). The summaries were written by me, Marilyn Barrett, with reference to comments made by the trial reviewers. The summaries include an "at-a-glance" table of the products, manufacturers, U.S. distributors (if any), product characteristics, the dose used in the trials, indication, number of trials, and the ratings as to therapeutic benefit and evidence level (see the section Evaluation of Clinical Trial Quality for more information on rating of the studies).

The summary table is followed by a summary of the preparations used in the reviewed clinical studies. This is followed by a summary of the reviewed clinical studies. Following that is any additional information, when available, from meta-analyses, systematic reviews, or epidemiological studies. Next, obtainable information regarding adverse reactions, side effects, or clinical information concerning drug-herb interactions is presented. (*Author's note:* Many cautionary statements regarding drug-herb interactions are based on theoretical modes of action of the herb. I have not included that information in this book. I have included only drug-herb interactions that have been demonstrated clinically.)

Finally, information from published therapeutic monographs from select pharmacopoeias is included. Those sources include the *American Herbal Pharmacopoeia, United States Pharmacopeia, United States Pharmacopeia—Drug Information, British Herbal Compendium,* European Scientific Cooperative on Phytotherapy (ESCOP), German Commission E, and the World Health Organization.

EVALUATION OF CLINICAL TRIAL QUALITY

Development of the "Levels of Evidence" for the Clinical Studies

Tieraona Low Dog, MD, developed the "Levels of Evidence" used to rank the clinical studies included in this book (see the following chapter). The purpose of the ranking is to enable the reader to quickly and accurately assess the validity of the clinical trial. The levels of evidence imply a hierarchy of quality and/or strength of scientific evidence. Trials of the highest scientific quality are classed as Level I. Those trials of moderate quality are classed as Level II, and trials with insufficient strength in their methodology or write-up to support their conclusions are classed as Level III.

The levels of evidence are based on a score generated by the Reviewer's Checklist. The first half of the checklist includes criteria to minimize bias on the part of either the participants or the researchers. These criteria, established by Dr. Jadad and colleagues (1996), emphasize the importance of blinding the study participants and the investigators, random allocation of patients into study groups, and a complete accounting of all patients that discontinue the study.

The second half of the checklist is comprised of criteria provided by Dr. Low Dog. These include the quality of the data summary, statistical methods, and a clear definition of the outcome measures. In addition, descriptions of the botanical preparation, the inclusion and exclusion criteria for the participants, and the appropriateness of the number of participants are evaluated.

Dr. Low Dog compiled the second half of the levels of evidence used in this book following reference to the United States Pharmacopeia Botanical Information Experts Committee (USP, 2000), the World Health Organization, and the United States Agency for Health Care Policy and Research.

Selection of MD Reviewers

An effort was made to have physicians or PhDs with expertise in the clinical indication of the study determine the trial quality. For example, a physician with expertise in the area of immunology and infectious diseases reviewed clinical studies evaluating the efficacy of echinacea to treat the common cold. In a few cases, the reviewer is also an author of a study he or she reviewed.

Review Process

Physician reviewers were sent packages that included the clinical studies and guidelines for ranking the quality of the studies. Points were given to each trial based upon an 11-point questionnaire (see the following chapter). A recommended level of evidence was given based upon the number of points. In addition, the reviewers assessed whether any therapeutic benefit was determined by the study and commented on the study in general.

Individual Trial Summaries

Included in each trial summary report is the level of evidence (I, II, or III) according to the reviewer's determination. Also included is a determination of therapeutic benefit (Yes, Trend, No, Undetermined). A designation of Yes meant the results were clearly in support of the therapeutic indication and the statistical analysis was strong. A Trend toward a positive benefit was designated when the results were generally positive but weak, in that they lacked sufficient statistical analysis or not all the analyses were positive. No therapeutic benefit was assigned when the results were clearly negative and the statistical analysis was strong. A designation of Undetermined was made if the results did not adequately address the therapeutic question.

A paragraph with the reviewer's comments is provided. At the end of this paragraph is the numerical score from the reviewer's checklist. This score is separated into two parts as described previously. The first score uses the Jadad criteria with a total of five points possible. The second score is derived from the second half of the checklist with a total of six points possible (see the reviewer's checklist in the following chapter for more detail).

Challenges in Clinical Trial Evaluation

The evaluation and ranking system that we used focuses more on the quality of the trial description than the true quality of the trial. The trial may have been of good quality, but if the write-up or translation were inadequate, then the trial would not score well.

In addition, a trial may be ranked high in terms of its level of evidence, being well conducted and well described, without giving any direct indication of therapeutic benefit. Our level of evidence evaluation system does not take the therapeutic utility of the trial into account in its ranking system. For example, the trial end points may not be directly connected with a disease state. It is often more convenient to measure intermediate outcomes, and these outcomes can offer useful information if there is a good correlation with the therapeutic end point. As an example, hypertension and high cholesterol levels are the intermediate outcomes that correlate well with the therapeutic outcomes of heart attack and stroke. However, measured antioxidant activity does not necessarily indicate a benefit for those with heart disease or any other disease, as no direct connection is established.

If the purpose of the trial was to establish tolerance of the preparation, it was difficult, if not inappropriate, to evaluate a trial as to whether it established a therapeutic benefit. For example, studies with kava and valerian preparations studying reaction times or possible additive effects due to alcohol would end up as being rated as therapeutic benefit "Undetermined," as this is not their purpose. However, the numerical scoring system still gives valuable information about the quality of the trial, e.g., whether one should believe a trial claiming that a botanical is safe or unsafe.

If the purpose of the trial was to explore the mode of action of the preparation, it was also inappropriate to evaluate a trial as to whether it established a therapeutic benefit. In place of the therapeutic benefit assessment, these studies were designated MOA (mode of action).

Controlled studies include a group given a comparison treatment of placebo or another therapeutic agent, or both. If the comparison agent is an established therapeutic agent, recognized as effective by today's standards, then some reviewers felt that the study did not need a placebo arm. If, however, the comparison treatment is not established, then the benchmark is insufficient and a placebo arm is required. In the final analysis, this seems to be an issue addressed on an individual basis, depending upon the treatment and the opinion of the reviewer. In cases in which the reviewer thought a placebo arm was needed but not present, the trial was rated as therapeutic benefit "Undetermined." On the other hand, if the reviewer thought the comparison agent was adequate and the placebo arm was not needed, then the trial might be rated as therapeutic benefit "Trend," "Yes," or "No."

The trial evaluations were reviewed and checked for agreement with guidelines by the editors. In order to achieve consistency among reviewers, the level of evidence score was occasionally adjusted up or down by the editors to match the reviewer's guidelines. We found that according to their own personal experience, each reviewer focused on slightly different aspects of the trials, and some were more harsh than others in their judgment. Some reviewed the trials according to their previous experience, without strictly sticking to our guidelines. Some missed information in the trial reports, as several of the European trials include methods information in places other than the methods section of the paper. In addition, some reviewers commented on the "take home" message of the trial while others did not. We have included these comments if they are different from those included in the results section of the trial report.

REFERENCES

Jadad AR, Moore RA, Carroll D, Gavaghan DJ, McQuay HJ (1996). Assessing the quality of reports of randomized clinical trials: Is blinding necessary? *Controlled Clinical Trials* 17 (1): 1-12.

McGuffin M, Kartesz JT, Leung AY, Tucker AO (2000). *The American Herbal Products Association's Herbs of Commerce,* Second Edition. Silver Spring, MD: American Herbal Products Association.

United States Pharmacopeial Convention, Inc., The (USP) (2000). Saw Palmetto (sawpalmetto.pdf). <www.usp.org>. Accessed: December 3, 2002.

Chapter 13

Clinical Trial Reviewer's Guidance and Checklist

Tieraona Low Dog

LEVELS OF EVIDENCE

When reviewing individual trials it is important for the reader to be able to accurately assess the trials' validity. Levels of evidence describe an implied hierarchy of quality and/or strength of scientific evidence. In order to evaluate the probable effect of therapy, the reviewer must know if the allocation to treatment was random, if participants and investigators were blind to the allocation, and if all participants were accounted for. Statistical methods must be adequately stated and the data summarized in a fashion that permits alternative analyses and replication. The botanical preparation must be adequately described.

These levels of evidence used to rank the clinical trials were derived from the workings of the U.S. Pharmacopeia Botanical Experts Committee, the World Health Organization, and the U.S. Agency for Health Care Policy and Research.

Level I: Trials of the Highest Scientific Quality

A Level I study is a randomized, controlled trial that is adequately powered to show a treatment effect versus placebo, or an appropriate active or historical control. The study describes in detail the methods of blinding and randomization, accounts for all withdrawals and dropouts from the study, and describes the statistical methods employed. A study at this level does not have any methodological flaws sufficient to undermine the conclusions of the study.

Level II: Trials of Moderate Scientific Quality

A Level II study is also a randomized, controlled trial that is adequately powered to show a treatment effect versus placebo, or an appropriate active or historical control. However, a study at this level suffers from technical flaws or an inadequate description of the methods or analyses such that the study cannot meet the full criteria for Level I. The flaws in a Level II study are not serious enough to negate the results or conclusions of the study.

Level III: Nonexperimental Designs and Anecdotal Evidence of Uncertain Quality

This level includes studies not meeting the criteria for Levels I or II. It includes nonrandomized trials, efficacy studies lacking an appropriate control group, randomized studies with serious methodological flaws, or studies that are too small or of insufficient duration to be of value. There is insufficient strength in the methodology or write-up of a Level III study to support its conclusions; however, this does not mean that those conclusions are necessarily invalid.

GUIDELINES FOR REVIEWER CHECKLIST: PART I

Part I uses the Jadad scoring system whose purpose is to evaluate the potential for bias in the trial. It asks questions about randomization, blinding, and subject withdrawals or dropouts. For example, if one can predict which group an individual belongs to, bias can be introduced on the part of the investigator and/or the participant. If one group drinks tea and the other receives a tablet, it is apparent to the participant which group they belong to. If 200 participants begin the trial, but only 126 are included in the analysis without any discussion of the dropouts, there is a serious risk of bias in the trial. Did 74 people drop out of the trial because the intervention made them ill, didn't work, etc.?

The total possible score is five. A score of four or five indicates that the trial is relatively free of bias.

Question 1. Was the Study Randomized?

If the author describes the study in the article as randomized, random, or randomly give one point. If not, give zero.

Examine questions 1a and 1b together; only one of them applies.

Question 1a. Was the Randomization Process Adequately Described and Appropriate?

Add one point if the method of randomization is described and is appropriate (for instance: computer generated, table of random numbers, etc.). The trial should describe the methods used to generate the allocation schedule and concealment. Each study participant must have the same chance of receiving each intervention, and the investigators must not be able to predict which treatment will be next.

Question 1b. Was the Randomization Process Not Described or Inadequate?

Deduct one point, effectively making the score for question 1 zero, if the author fails to describe the method for randomization or the method described is inappropriate. Allocation should not be determined by hospital numbers, date of admission, date of birth, or alternating numbers.

Question 2. Was the Study Double-Blind?

If the author describes the trial as "double-blind" give one point. If not, give zero.

Examine questions 2a and 2b together; only one of them applies.

Question 2a. Was the Double-Blinding Described and Was It Appropriate?

Add one point if the double-blinding was described *and* appropriate. To be considered appropriate, neither the participants nor the investigators should be able to identify which intervention is being assessed (identical placebo, dummy, active placebo, etc.).

Question 2b. Was the Double-Blinding Not Described or Inappropriate?

Deduct one point, effectively making the score for question 2 zero, if the author fails to describe the double-blinding or if the description indicates the method was inappropriate (tablets differ in appearance, injection versus capsule, etc.).

Question 3. Was There a Description of All Withdrawals and Dropouts?

Participants who were included in the study but did not complete the trial and/or were not included in the analysis must be accounted for. The reasons for withdrawal must be clearly stated. Every participant must be accounted for. If there were no dropouts, this should be clearly stated. If the withdrawals/dropouts are not adequately described *or* if this item is not mentioned in the article, give zero points. If withdrawals are appropriately accounted for, give one point.

GUIDELINES FOR REVIEWER CHECKLIST: PART II

This part is designed to review the article for quality and is scored separately from the Jadad scoring system in Part I. A total of six points are possible. A score of five or six points indicates a likelihood of a good-quality study. Scores of three or less indicate that the quality of the study may be poor.

Question 4. Were the Data Summarized in Sufficient Detail to Permit Alternative Analyses and Replication?

Give one point if the data are summarized in a fashion that allows others to perform alternative analyses. This means error bars on plotted graphs, data presented in a complete and concise manner, clear description how the data were collected, etc. If the paper does not provide these, zero points are given.

Question 5. Were Statistical Methods Adequately Described and Applied?

Give one point if the paper states the estimated effect of the intervention on outcome measures including a point estimate and measure of precision. The paper should include an adequate description of the statistical methods used and how they were applied. If the paper does not provide these, zero points are given.

Question 6. Was the Botanical Preparation Adequately Described?

Due to the complex nature of botanicals, variation in the chemical composition between species, plant part, and preparation, it is essential that authors clearly provide an adequate description of the preparation used in the clinical trial. Descriptions should include identification (Latin binomial and authority), plant part (root, leaf, seed, etc.), and type of preparation (tea, tincture, extract, oil, etc.). Tincture and extract description should include the identity of the solvent and the ratio of solvent to plant material. If the preparation is standardized to a chemical constituent, then that information should also be included. If the trial substance is a proprietary product for which a detailed description is available from the manufacturer and/or product literature, then this is considered adequate. One point is given for an adequate description of the botanical, zero points if not.

Question 7. Were the Inclusion/Exclusion Criteria Adequate and Appropriate?

The inclusion and exclusion criteria should be clearly stated and relevant to the clinical condition being studied. For instance, a study for a cold treatment should clearly list appropriate exclusions for those with chronic illness and those taking antibiotics or over-the-counter cold/cough medications. One point is given for adequate description of inclusion/exclusion criteria, zero points if not.

Question 8. Was the Sample Size Appropriate?

Was a power calculation done? The study must be of appropriate size to generate meaningful results. If the trial included adequate numbers but did not describe a power calculation, one point should still be given. If the trial was very small (fewer than 40 subjects), zero points should be given.

Question 9. Were the Outcome Measures Clearly Defined?

Outcome measurements should be clearly stated using validated methods. If adequately described give one point, zero points if not.

SCORING

After reviewing the trials and answering the previous questions, the study must be ranked according to the levels of evidence as either a category I, II, or III. Studies given the rank of Level I must be of outstanding quality and have scored a total number of ten or eleven points. Studies of good quality with flaws that are unlikely to change the outcome of the study should be placed in Level II. Level III is reserved for those trials with severe risk of bias (three or less on the Jadad scale) and/or questionable quality (scoring three or less in Part II).

Please include a few sentences under "Reviewer's Comments" noting the major strengths or flaws observed in the trial. These comments are intended as rationale for the assigned level of evidence.

Checklist for Evaluation of Clinical Trial

Please fill out one sheet for every trial you review.

Reviewer: _____ Botanical: _____

Trial Number: _____ First Author: _____

Name of Trial: _____

Descriptor	**Points**
Part I	
Was the study randomized?	0 or 1
Was the randomization process adequately described and appropriate?	+1
Was the randomization process not described or inappropriate?	−1
Was the study double-blinded?	0 or 1
Was the double-blinding described and appropriate?	+1
Was the double-blinding not described and/or inappropriate?	−1
Was there a description of all withdrawals and dropouts?	0 or 1
Total	/5
Part II	
Were data summarized in sufficient detail to permit alternative analyses and replication?	0 or 1
Were statistical methods adequately described and applied?	0 or 1
Was the botanical preparation adequately described?	0 or 1
Were the inclusion/exclusion criteria adequate and appropriate?	0 or 1
Was the sample size appropriate?	0 or 1
Were the outcome measures clearly defined?	0 or 1
Total	/6

Reviewer's Comments:

_____

_____

_____

Recommended Level of Evidence: _____

Therapeutic Benefit? (circle one):   Yes   Trend   No   Undetermined

Comments on the Dose of Either the Botanical or Comparison Treatment (if any):

_____

_____

_____

Comments on the Length of Treatment:

_____

_____

_____

Adverse Effects Noted with Intervention:

_____

_____

_____

PART III:
BOTANICAL PROFILES—
PRODUCT AND CLINICAL TRIAL
INFORMATION
(Artichoke–Ginseng)

SINGLE HERBS

Artichoke

Other common names: **Cynara, globe artichoke**
Latin name: ***Cynara scolymus* L.** [Asteraceae]
Plant part: **Leaf**

PREPARATIONS USED
IN REVIEWED CLINICAL STUDIES

Artichokes were greatly valued by the ancient Greeks (fourth century B.C.) for treating digestive disorders. Clinical studies have been conducted on aqueous extracts of the leaves. The extracts characteristically contain caffeoylquinic acid derivatives, including caffeic acid, chlorogenic acid, and cynarin (1,5-dicaffeoylquinic acid) (Kraft, 1997).

Cynara-SL™ contains 320 mg per capsule of a dried aqueous extract called LI 120, with an herb-to-extract ratio of 3.8 to 5.5:1. It is manufactured in Germany by Lichtwer Pharma AG and distributed in the United States by Lichtwer Pharma U.S., Inc. This extract is marketed in Europe as Hepar-SL forte®.

Valverde Artischocke, which is manufactured by Novartis Consumer Health GmbH in Germany, is not provided in the United States. The tablets contain 450 mg of a dried aqueous extract called CY-450 with a ratio of 25 to 35:1.

ARTICHOKE SUMMARY TABLE

Product Name	Manufacturer/ U.S. Distributor	Product Characteristics	Dose in Trials	Indication	No. of Trials	Benefit (Evidence Level-Trial No.)
Cynara-SL™ (US), Hepar-SL forte ® (EU)	Lichtwer Pharma AG, Germany/ Lichtwer Pharma U.S., Inc.	Aqueous extract (LI 120)	6 capsules, 1.92 g (intraduoden-ally)	Choleresis (bile secretion)	1	MOA (III-1)
Valverde Artischocke (EU)	Novartis Consumer Health GmbH, Germany/None	Aqueous extract (CY450)	2 tablets twice daily (1.8 g extract/day)	Hyper-lipo-proteinemia (elevated cholesterol levels)	1	Yes (I-1)

SUMMARY OF REVIEWED CLINICAL STUDIES

Artichoke preparations may relieve digestive complaints through increases in the formation and flow of bile. The increased flow of bile is called choleresis. Bile is excreted from the liver, stored in the gallbladder, and released into the intestine. Bile acids form a complex with dietary fats in the intestine and thereby assist in their digestion and absorption (Kraft, 1997).

In addition, stimulation of bile production results in reduced serum cholesterol, as cholesterol is pulled from the blood to be converted into bile acids. The increased flow of bile may also be beneficial for patients with irritable bowel syndrome (IBS) (Walker, Middleton, and Petrowicz, 2001).

Cynara-SL (LI 120)

Choleresis (Bile Secretion)

A mode of action study using the Lichtwer product Cynara-SL (Hepar-SL) demonstrated that artichoke extract increased the flow of bile. Administration of six capsules (1.92 g) intraduodenally caused a peak increase (100 to 150 percent compared to baseline) in bile one hour later (Kirchhoff et al., 1994). According to our reviewer, Dr. David Heber, this study inferred, but did not clearly demonstrate, therapeutic benefit for dyspepsia; the one-day study was too short, was not conducted on subjects with dyspepsia, and the product was not delivered orally.

Valverde Artischocke

Hyperlipoproteinemia (Elevated Cholesterol Levels)

A study with the Novartis product Valverde Artischocke on 131 patients with elevated cholesterol (total serum cholesterol greater than 280 mg/dl) reported a 20.2 percent decrease in cholesterol, compared to 7.2 percent in the placebo group. The product was given in a dose of 900 mg, twice daily, before meals, for six weeks (Englisch et al., 2000). This well-conducted trial indicates efficacy of Valverde Artischocke in the treatment of elevated cholesterol.

POSTMARKETING SURVEILLANCE STUDIES

A review of metabolic, pharmacological, and clinical studies described two postmarketing surveillance studies (Kraft, 1997). The first study, reported by Held (1991), included 417 patients with hepatic and biliary tract disease who were treated for four weeks with artichoke leaf extract (product not named). Prior to the study, the average duration of symptoms of abdominal pain, bloating, meteorism, constipation, lack of appetite, and nausea was four months. Elimination of these symptoms occurred in 65 to 77 percent of patients after one week, and in 52 to 82 percent of patients after four weeks.

The second postmarketing surveillance study was published by Fintelmann (1996) and Fintelmann and Menssen (1996). It included 553 subjects with dyspepsia who were administered the Lichtwer product Hepar-SL. The authors reported a clinically impressive and statistically significant improvement for 87 percent of patients within six weeks of treatment. In a subset of 302 patients for whom cholesterol values were routinely determined, serum cholesterol and serum triglyceride concentrations dropped significantly ($p < 0.001$). For this group of subjects, the average daily dose was approximately 1.5 g extract and treatment extended to an average of 43.5 days (six weeks) (Kraft, 1997).

Walker, Middleton, and Petrowicz (2001) reported an analysis of another patient subset with key symptoms of irritable bowel syndrome (279 in number). These patients experienced significant reductions in symptoms (71 percent) after six weeks of treatment with six capsules per day, with improvement noted within ten days. Although the initial survey by Fintelmann and Menssen (1996) did not include all the diagnostic criteria for IBS, patients were included if they had at least three of five key symptoms.

ADVERSE REACTIONS OR SIDE EFFECTS

No adverse reactions or side effects were reported in the clinical studies described. The Fintelmann (1996) postmarketing study reported that 1.3 percent of 553 subjects experienced mild reactions, such as flatulence, feeling of weakness, and hunger.

INFORMATION FROM PHARMACOPOEIAL MONOGRAPHS

Source of Published Therapeutic Monographs

German Commission E

Indications

The German Commission E approves the use of fresh or dried artichoke leaf for dyspeptic problems due to its choleretic action (Blumenthal et al., 1998).

Doses

Fresh or dried leaf: 6 g per day (Blumenthal et al., 1998)

Contraindications

The Commission E mentions the following contraindications: known allergies to artichokes and other composites and obstruction of bile ducts. It also suggests that in case of gallstones, use only after consulting with a physician (Blumenthal et al., 1998).

Adverse Reactions

The Commission E lists no known adverse reactions (Blumenthal et al., 1998).

Drug Interactions

The Commission E lists no known drug interactions (Blumenthal et al., 1998).

REFERENCES

Blumenthal M, Busse W, Hall T, Goldberg A, Gruenwald J, Riggins C, Rister S, eds. (1998). *The Complete German Commission E Mono-*

graphs: Therapeutic Guide to Herbal Medicines. Trans. S Klein. Austin, TX: American Botanical Council.

Englisch W, Beckers C, Unkauf M, Ruepp M, Zinserling V (2000). Efficacy of artichoke dry extract in patients with hyperlipoproteinemia. *Arzneimittel-Forschung/Drug Research* 50 (3): 260-265.

Fintelmann V (1996). Antidyspeptische und lipidsenkende Wirkungen von Artischockenextrakt: Ergenbnisse klinischer Untersuchungen zur Wirksamkeit und Verträglichkeit von Hepar-SL forte an 553 Patienten. *Zeitschrift fur Allgemeinmedizin* 72 (Suppl. 2): 3-19. Cited in Kraft K (1997). Artichoke leaf extract—Recent findings reflecting effects on lipid metabolism, liver and gastrointestinal tracts. *Phytomedicine* 4 (4): 369-378.

Fintelmann V, Menssen HG (1996). Aktuelle Erkenntnisse zur Wirkung von Artischockenblätterextrakt als Lipidsenker und Antidyspeptikum. *Deutsche Apotheker-Zeitung* 136: 1405. Cited in Kraft K (1997). Artichoke leaf extract—Recent findings reflecting effects on lipid metabolism, liver and gastrointestinal tracts. *Phytomedicine* 4 (4): 369-378.

Held C (1991). Artischoke bei Gallenwegsdyskinesien: Workshop "Neue Aspekte zur Therapie mit Choleretika." *Kluvensiek* 2: 9. Cited in Kraft K (1997). Artichoke leaf extract—Recent findings reflecting effects on lipid metabolism, liver and gastrointestinal tracts. *Phytomedicine* 4 (4): 369-378.

Kirchhoff R, Beckers CH, Kirchhoff GM, Trinczek-Gartner H, Petrowicz O, Reimann HJ (1994). Increase in choleresis by means of artichoke extract. *Phytomedicine* 1: 107-115. (Also published in *Arzneimittel-Forschung/Drug Research* 1993; 40 [1]: 1-12.)

Kraft K (1997). Artichoke leaf extract—Recent findings reflecting effects on lipid metabolism, liver and gastrointestinal tracts. *Phytomedicine* 4 (4): 369-378.

Walker AF, Middleton RW, Petrowicz O (2001). Artichoke leaf extract reduces symptoms of irritable bowel syndrome in a post-marketing surveillance study. *Phytotherapy Research* 15 (1): 58-61.

DETAILS ON ARTICHOKE PRODUCTS AND CLINICAL STUDIES

Product and clinical study information is grouped in the same order as in the Summary Table. A profile on an individual product is followed by details of the clinical studies associated with that product. In some instances a clinical study, or studies, supports several products that contain the same principal ingredient(s). In these instances, those products are grouped together.

Clinical studies that follow each product, or group of products, are grouped by therapeutic indication, in accordance with the order in the Summary Table.

Index to Artichoke Products

Product	Page
Cynara-SL™	157
Valverde Artischocke	160

Product Profile: Cynara-SL™

Manufacturer	**Lichtwer Pharma AG, Germany**
U.S. distributor	Lichtwer Pharma U.S., Inc.
Botanical ingredient	**Artichoke leaf extract**
Extract name	**LI 120**
Quantity	320 mg
Processing	Plant to extract ratio 3.8-5:1, aqueous extract
Standardization	No information
Formulation	Capsule

Recommended dose: For regular longer-term use to help maintain a healthy liver and digestive system and to support the normal cleansing process of the liver take one to two capsules daily. For nutritional support, take one to two capsules shortly before or after eating or drinking too much. Up to six capsules may be taken per day. Effects can be noticed as soon as 30 to 60 minutes.

DSHEA structure/function: Clinically proven to help maintain a healthy liver and digestive system; clinically proven to provide fast and effective herbal support for the digestive system when eating or drinking too much; supports the normal cleansing process of the liver.

Cautions: If taking prescription medicine, are pregnant, nursing a baby, or administering to children under the age of 12, consult a health care professional before using this product.

Other ingredients: Lactose, gelatin, magnesium stearate, silicon dioxide, talc, titanium dioxide, sodium lauryl sulphate, FD&C blue no. 1, yellow no. 5.

Comments: Sold in Europe as Hepar-SL forte®.

Source(s) of information: Kirchhoff et al., 1994; product packaging; information provided by distributor (11/2/99).

Clinical Study: Hepar-SL forte®

Extract name	LI 120
Manufacturer	Sertürner Arzneimittel GmbH, Germany (Lichtwer Pharma AG, Germany)
Indication	**Choleresis** (bile secretion)
Level of evidence	**III**
Therapeutic benefit	**MOA**

Bibliographic reference
Kirchhoff R, Beckers CH, Kirchhoff GM, Trinczek-Gartner H, Petrowicz O, Reimann HJ (1994). Increase in choleresis by means of artichoke extract. *Phytomedicine* 1: 107-115. (Also published in *Arzneimittel-Forschung/Drug Research* 1993; 40 [1]: 1-12.)

Trial design
Crossover. Eight-day pretrial period to establish case histories and clinical and laboratory parameters. One-day treatment periods were separated by an eight-day washout period.

Study duration	1 day
Dose	Single dose of 6 capsules (1.92 g artichoke extract)
Route of administration	Intraduodenal
Randomized	Yes
Randomization adequate	No
Blinding	Double-blind

Blinding adequate	No
Placebo	Yes
Drug comparison	No
Site description	Single center
No. of subjects enrolled	20
No. of subjects completed	18
Sex	Male
Age	Mean: 26 years

Inclusion criteria
Subjects with acute or chronic metabolic disorders with previous gastro-enterological and chemical examination.

Exclusion criteria
Subjects with upper abdominal problems lasting more than four weeks, intolerance of fatty foods, irregular bowel movements with changes in feces color, heavy smokers (>10 cigarettes per day), or heavy coffee drinkers (>4 cups per day). Ingestion of metabolically active drugs not permitted two weeks prior to start of test.

End points
On days of the investigation, capsule contents were dissolved in 50 ml water and administered via an intraduodenal probe. Measurement of intraduodenal bile secretion began 30 minutes after substances were administered and continued for up to four hours using multichannel probes.

Results
Increases in bile secretion in the active group were 127.3 percent after 30 minutes, 151.5 percent after 60 minutes, and 94.3 percent after 90 minutes, each in relation to the initial value. These measurements were significantly different from placebo, $p < 0.01$. The most significant increase after administration of placebo was 39.5 percent after 30 minutes. At later times of 120 and 150 minutes the volume of bile secreted under the active treatment was still significantly higher than under placebo ($p < 0.05$).

Side effects
None reported.

Authors' comments
Results indicate that artichoke extract can be recommended for the treatment of dyspepsia, especially when the cause may be attributed to dyskinesia of the bile ducts or disorder in the assimilation of fat.

Reviewer's comments
This study was flawed by the small sample size and the short duration of treatment. (0, 5)

Product Profile: Valverde Artischocke

Manufacturer	**Novartis Consumer Health GmbH, Germany**
U.S. distributor	None
Botanical ingredient	**Artichoke leaf extract**
Extract name	**CY450**
Quantity	450 mg
Processing	Plant to extract ratio 25-35:1, aqueous extract of fresh leaves
Standardization	No information
Formulation	Tablet

Source(s) of information: Englisch et al., 2000.

Clinical Study: Valverde Artischocke

Extract name	CY450
Manufacturer	Novartis Consumer Health GmbH, Germany
Indication	**Hyperlipoproteinemia** (elevated blood lipid levels)
Level of evidence	**I**
Therapeutic benefit	**Yes**

Bibliographic reference
Englisch W, Beckers C, Unkauf M, Ruepp M, Zinserling V (2000). Efficacy of artichoke dry extract in patients with hyperlipoproteinemia. *Arzneimittel-Forschung/Drug Research* 50 (3): 260-265.

Trial design
Parallel.

Study duration	6 weeks
Dose	2 x 450 mg twice daily, before meals
Route of administration	Oral
Randomized	Yes
Randomization adequate	Yes
Blinding	Double-blind
Blinding adequate	Yes

Placebo	Yes
Drug comparison	No
Site description	3 hospitals
No. of subjects enrolled	143
No. of subjects completed	131
Sex	Male and female
Age	35-69 years

Inclusion criteria
Patients between 18 and 70 years old with total cholesterol of >7.3 mmol/l (>280 mg/dl) in plasma or serum. During participation in the study, patients were not allowed to take other cholesterol-lowering drugs or any antibiotic treatments.

Exclusion criteria
Patients who had taken lipid-lowering drugs within two weeks of enrollment.

End points
After enrollment, patients were seen on days 7, 14, 28, and 42. At each visit, blood samples were drawn and patient conditions noted. Blood samples were tested for total cholesterol, low-density lipoprotein (LDL cholesterol), high-density lipoprotein (HDL cholesterol), triglycerides, liver enzymes (gamma-glutamyl transferase, glutamic oxaloacetic transaminase, glutamic pyruvic transaminase, and glutamate dehydrogenase), and glucose.

Results
Artichoke extract was significantly superior to placebo in decreasing total cholesterol (18.5 percent versus 8.6 percent, $p = 0.001$), LDL cholesterol (22.9 percent versus 6.3 percent, $p = 0.001$), and LDL/HDL ratio (20.2 percent versus 7.2 percent). There was a slight decrease in gamma-GT levels in both groups from baseline to end of study, with no significant difference between groups. There were no changes to glucose levels in either group.

Side effects
No drug-related adverse events.

Authors' comments
This prospective study could contribute clear evidence to recommend artichoke extract CY450 for treating hyperlipoproteinemia and, thus, prevention of atherosclerosis and coronary heart disease.

Reviewer's comments
Well-conducted and well-designed study with positive and significant results. (5, 6)

Bilberry

Other common names: **European blueberry; huckleberry; whortleberry**
Latin name: *Vaccinium myrtillus* **L.** [Ericaceae]
Plant part: **Fruit**

PREPARATIONS USED
IN REVIEWED CLINICAL STUDIES

Both the leaves and fruits of bilberry (European blueberry) have been used medicinally. Most commercial preparations are standardized to contain a percentage of flavonoids, specifically anthocyanidins or anthocyanins (anthocyanidins with sugars attached). These molecules are natural pigments responsible for the blue to purple color of the fruit. They also have strong antioxidant activity (Upton et al., 2001).

Most of the clinical studies on bilberry have been conducted with a product called Tegens® produced by Inverni della Beffa, Italy. Tegens contains an extract named Myrtocyan® (now called MirtoSelect™) that is manufactured by Indena S.p.A., Milan, Italy. It is characterized as containing 36 percent anthocyanins or 25 percent anthocyanidins. This extract is available in the United States in a product called Bilberry Extract produced by Enzymatic Therapy® and in a product named Vacimyr® produced by Thorne Research. The Indena extract is available in other products as well, but only single-ingredient products are included here. Products including other active ingredients are not included unless those ingredients have been studied in combination in a clinical trial.

FAR-1 is manufactured in Italy by Ditta Farmigea S.p.A.; it is not sold in the United States. FAR-1 is also characterized as containing 25 percent anthocyanidins.

BILBERRY SUMMARY TABLE

Product Name	Manufacturer/ U.S. Distributor	Product Characteristics	Dose in Trials	Indication	No. of Trials	Benefit (Evidence Level-Trial No.)
Tegens® (EU)*	Inverni della Beffa, Indena S.p.A, Italy*	Contains the extract MirtoSelect™, formerly Myrtocyan®, with 25 % anthocyanidins	160 mg 2-3 times daily	Diabetic retinopathy	2	Trend (II-1) Undetermined (III-1)
				Varicose veins	1	Trend (III-1)
				Dysmenor-rhea (painful menstrua-tion)	1	Undetermined (III-1)
			80 mg 3 times daily	Pupillary reflex	1	MOA (III-1)
FAR-1 (EU)	Ditta Farmigea S.p.A., Italy/None	Extract contains 25% anthocyanidins	180 mg 2 times daily +Vit E	Senile cataracts	1	Trend (II-1)

*The following products, sold in the United States, contain the Indena extract (MirtoSelect) as a single ingredient; the extract in these products has been tested clinically but the final formulation has not.

Product Name **Manufacturer/Distributor**
Bilberry Extract (U.S.) Enzymatic Therapy®
Vacimyr® (U.S.) Thorne Research

SUMMARY OF REVIEWED CLINICAL STUDIES

Bilberry products have been used to treat circulatory disorders, namely fragility and altered permeability of blood vessels that is either primary or secondary to arterial hypertension, arteriosclerosis, or diabetes. In vitro studies have shown that bilberry extracts have antioxidant activity, inhibit platelet aggregation, prevent degradation of collagen in the extravascular matrix surrounding blood vessels and joints, and have a relaxing effect on arterial smooth muscle. These actions have been described as vasoprotective, increasing capillary resistance and reducing capillary permeability (Morazzoni and Bombardelli, 1996). We report here a total of six studies with treatments for diabetic and hypertensive retinopathy, senile cataracts, pupillary reflex, varicose veins, and primary dysmenorrhea (painful menstruation).

Retinopathy is an eye disorder that results from changes to the blood vessels in the retina. It is characterized by an increase in vascular permeability and decrease in resistance of the vessels, resulting in microaneurisms, edema, and eventually hard exudates (Perossini et al., 1987). Varicose veins are blood vessels that have become twisted and swollen when their one-way valves begin to leak or when the vein wall weakens. The symptoms include edema in the legs and ankles, sensation of pressure, cramps, and tingling or "pins and needles" sensations (Gatta, 1988). Although the cause of primary dysmenorrhea is unknown (unlike secondary dysmenorrhea, it is not caused by an observable abnormality), it is characterized by pelvic pain, nausea and vomiting, diarrhea, headache, swollen breasts, and a sensation of heaviness in the legs and feet (Colombo and Vescovini, 1985).

Tegens (MirtoSelect)

Diabetic Retinopathy

Two studies on diabetic retinopathy, using a dose of 160 mg Tegens twice daily, demonstrated a trend toward improvement in mild cases of the disease. The first study was a one-month, placebo-controlled study that included 36 subjects, a few of which had hypertensive retinopathy. At the end of the month, 10 of 13 patients in the

Tegens group with opthalmoscopically detectable retinal abnormalities (microaneurisms, hemorrhagic foci, exudates) were improved, while all 15 patients with these abnormalities in the placebo group remained unchanged. A similar trend was observed among those patients with fluoroangiographic abnormalities (Perossini et al., 1987). The second study lasted one year and included 40 subjects who were given Tegens or placebo in addition to the usual therapy for retinopathy. As a result, in 50 percent of patients given bilberry, the retinal lesions and associated edema were improved, compared to 20 percent in the control group (Repossi, Malagola, and De Cadilhac, 1987). According to our reviewer, Dr. David Heber, the first study was relatively well designed and supported a trend toward efficacy. The second, although seemingly positive, was deemed undetermined due to the poorly described methodology. The evidence of both studies was limited by small sample sizes.

Varicose Veins

Symptoms of varicose veins were improved with 160 mg Tegens, three times daily for one month, in a placebo-controlled trial with 60 participants (Gatta, 1988). Determination of therapeutic benefit was hampered by the short length of the study and by poor methodology.

Dysmenorrhea (Painful Menstruation)

In a placebo-controlled trial with 30 females with primary dysmenorrhea, significant relief compared to placebo was reported for the symptoms of pelvic and lumbar-sacral pain, swollen breasts, and heaviness in the lower limbs following treatment with a dose of 160 mg Tegens, twice daily for two menstrual cycles (Colombo and Vescovini, 1985). The evaluation criteria in this trial were considered highly subjective, and the methodology was inadequately described. Thus, it was difficult to assess the potential benefit of this treatment.

Pupillary Reflex

A mechanistic study using Myrtocyan examined changes in pupillary reflexes to light following a single high dose of 240 mg anthocyanosides or placebo in 40 healthy volunteers. The study was conducted to explore the use of bilberry in work situations where exposure to high light intensities dampens pupillary reflexes and leads to vision fatigue. The authors of the study suggested that the pigments in bilberry might increase sensitivity to light and improve blood flow in the capillaries of the eye. Improvement in pupillary reflexes was observed in both groups, with the improvement in the treatment group being only slightly better than that in the placebo group (Vannini et al., 1986). Dr. Heber judged the benefit to be undetermined.

Additional controlled clinical studies, which were not available to us for critical review, are summarized elsewhere (Morazzoni and Bombardelli, 1996; Upton et al., 2001).

FAR-1

Senile Cataracts

A mixture of vitamin E and bilberry (FAR-1) showed a trend toward prevention of senile cataracts after four months of 180 mg twice daily. When the placebo group was changed from placebo to the bilberry preparation, and the trial continued for an additional four months, there was no statistical difference between the two groups. The rationale for this study was previous indications that antioxidants might prevent the development of senile cataracts (Bravetti, Fraboni, and Maccolini, 1989).

ADVERSE REACTIONS OR SIDE EFFECTS

No side effects were reported in the clinical studies described. In a 1987 postmarketing surveillance study with 2,295 subjects, only 94 subjects (4.1 percent) complained of minor side effects, most of which involved the gastrointestinal tract. Most of the subjects took 160 mg Tegens twice daily for one to two months (Eandi, 1987). No details were given in the review that cited this study as to the efficacy of the treatment, which was given for lower limb venous insufficiency (24 percent), disorders due to fragile or permeable capillaries (21 percent), functional changes in retinal microcirculation (10 percent), hemorrhoids (7 percent), and other reasons (Morazzoni and Bombardelli, 1996).

INFORMATION FROM PHARMACOPOEIAL MONOGRAPHS

Sources of Published Therapeutic Monographs

American Herbal Pharmacopoeia (AHP)
German Commission E

Indications

The dried, ripe fruit is approved by the German Commission E for treatment of nonspecific, acute diarrhea and mild inflammation of the mucous membranes of the mouth and throat (Blumenthal et al., 1998). The *American Herbal Pharmacopoeia* lists the following medical indications supported by clinical trials: vascular insufficiency and its associated symptoms (edema, varicosities, pain, paraesthesias, and cramping); capillary fragility and the associated tendency to bruising; pain, itching, and burning associated with hemorrhoidectomy and hemorrhoids; postoperative hemorrhagic complications (reducing the incidence and severity) when administered prior to ear, nose, and throat surgeries; and disorders of the eye (slows progression), including the early stage of diabetic and hypertensive retinopathy (Upton et al., 2001).

Doses

Dried, ripe fruit: 20 to 60 g per day (Blumenthal et al., 1998)
Decoction: 1 cup four to six times per day (Upton et al., 2001)
Extract: 160 to 960 mg powdered extract (standardized to 25 percent anthocyanin glycosides) per day in divided doses (Upton et al., 2001)
External: 10 percent decoction or equivalent preparations (Blumenthal et al., 1998)

Contraindications

The Commission E and the *AHP* list no known contraindications (Blumenthal et al., 1998; Upton et al., 2001).

Adverse Reactions

While the Commission E mentions no known adverse reactions, the *AHP* lists gastric pain, nausea, and pyrosis (Blumenthal et al., 1998; Upton et al., 2001).

Precautions

The *AHP* states no precautions, but the Commission E suggests if diarrhea persists for more than three to four days, a physician should be consulted (Upton et al., 2001; Blumenthal et al., 1998).

Drug Interactions

The Commission E lists no known drug interactions (Blumenthal et al., 1998).

REFERENCES

Blumenthal M, Busse W, Hall T, Goldberg A, Gruenwald J, Riggins C, Rister S, eds. (1998). *The Complete German Commission E Monographs: Therapeutic Guide to Herbal Medicines*. Trans. S Klein. Austin, TX: American Botanical Council.

Bravetti GO, Fraboni E, Maccolini E (1989). Preventive medical treatment of senile cataract with vitamin E and *Vaccinium myrtillus* anthocyanosides: Clinical evaluation. *Annali di Ottalmologia e Clinica Oculistica* 115 (2): 109-116.

Colombo D, Vescovini R (1985). Studio clinico controllato sull'efficacia degli antocianosidi del mirtillo nel trattamento della dismenorrea essenziale. *Giornale Italiano di Ostetricia e Ginecologia* 7 (12):1033-1038.

Eandi M (1987). Post marketing investigation on Tegens® preparation with respect to side effects. Data on file. Cited in Morazzoni P, Bombardelli E (1996). *Vaccinum myrtillus* L. *Fitoterapia* 67 (1): 3-29.

Gatta L (1988). *Vaccinium myrtillus* anthocyanosides in the treatment of venous stasis: Controlled clinical study on sixty patients. *Fitoterapia* 59 (Suppl. 1): 19-26.

Morazzoni P, Bombardelli E (1996). *Vaccinum myrtillus* L. *Fitoterapia* 67 (1): 3-29.

Perossini M, Chiellini S, Guidi G, Siravo D (1987). Diabetic and hypertensive retinopathy therapy with *Vaccinium myrtillus* anthocyanosides
(Tegens) double-blind placebo-controlled clinical trial. *Annali di Ottalmologia e Clinica Oculistica* 113 (12): 1173-1190.

Repossi P, Malagola R, De Cadilhac C (1987). The role of anthocyanosides
on vascular permeability in diabetic retinopathy. *Annali di Ottalmologia
e Clinica Oculistica* 113 (4): 357-361.

Upton R, Graff A, Länger R, Sudberg S, Sudberg E, Miller T, Reich E,
Bieber A, Roman M, Ko R, et al. (2001). *Bilberry Fruit,* Vaccinum
myrtillus *L.* American Herbal Pharmacopoeia and Therapeutic Compendium: Standards of Analysis, Quality Control, and Therapeutics. Eds. R
Upton, A Graff, C Petrone. Santa Cruz, CA: American Herbal Pharmacopoeia.

Vannini L, Samuelly R, Coffano M, Tibaldi L (1986). Study of the pupillary reflex after anthocyanoside administration. *Bollettino d'Oculistica*
65 (Suppl. 6): 569-577.

DETAILS ON BILBERRY PRODUCTS
AND CLINICAL STUDIES

Product and clinical study information is grouped in the same order as in the Summary Table. A profile on an individual product is followed by details of the clinical studies associated with that product. In some instances a clinical study, or studies, supports several products that contain the same principal ingredient(s). In these instances, those products are grouped together.

Clinical studies that follow each product, or group of products, are grouped by therapeutic indication, in accordance with the order in the Summary Table.

Index to Bilberry Products

Product Profile: Tegens®

Manufacturer	**Inverni della Beffa, Italy (Indena S.p.A., Italy**
U.S. distributor	None
Botanical ingredient	**Bilberry fruit extract**
Extract name	**Myrtocyan®** (now named Mirto Select)
Quantity	160 mg
Processing	Plant to extract ratio 100:1
Standardization	25% anthocyanidins
Formulation	Capsule

Source(s) of information: Perossini et al., 1987; Colombo and Vescovini, 1985; Indena USA, Inc., product information; and personal correspondence with Indena USA, Inc.

Product Profile: Bilberry Extract

Manufacturer	**Enzymatic Therapy® (Indena S.p.A., Italy)**
U.S. distributor	**Enzymatic Therapy®**
Botanical ingredient	**Bilberry fruit extract**
Extract name	**MirtoSelect™**
Quantity	80 mg
Processing	Plant to extract ratio 100:1
Standardization	25% anthocyanosides calculated as anthocyanidins
Formulation	Capsule

Recommended dose: Two capsules three times daily.

DSHEA structure/function: Dietary supplement to support healthy eye function.

Other ingredients: Cellulose, gelatin, magnesium stearate, titanium dioxide color.

Source(s) of information: Product label; information provided by Indena USA, Inc.

Product Profile: Vacimyr®

Manufacturer	**Thorne Research (Indena S.p.A., Italy)**
U.S. distributor	**Thorne Research**
Botanical ingredient	**Bilberry fruit extract**
Extract name	**MirtoSelect™**
Quantity	80 mg
Processing	Plant to extract ratio 100:1
Standardization	25% anthocyanosides
Formulation	Capsule

Cautions: If pregnant, consult a health care practitioner before using this or any other product.

Other ingredients: Cellulose capsule. May contain one of the following hypoallergenic ingredients to fill space—magnesium citrate, silicon dioxide.

Source(s) of information: Product label; information from Indena USA, Inc.

Clinical Study: Tegens®

Extract name	Myrtocyan®
Manufacturer	Inverni della Beffa, Italy (Indena S.p.A., Italy)

Indication	**Diabetic and hypertensive retinopathy**
Level of evidence	**II**
Therapeutic benefit	**Trend**

Bibliographic reference
Perossini M, Chiellini S, Guidi G, Siravo D (1987). Diabetic and hypertensive retinopathy therapy with *Vaccinium myrtillus* anthocyanosides (Tegens) double-blind placebo-controlled clinical trial. *Annali di Ottalmologia e Clinica Oculistica* 113 (12): 1173-1190.

Trial design
Parallel. After the one-month placebo-controlled parallel study, placebo patients whose retinopathy was unchanged, worsened, or only slightly improved (all placebo patients) continued in the study for an additional month receiving bilberry extract; patients originally receiving bilberry did not continue the study.

Study duration	1 month
Dose	1 (160 mg) capsule twice daily
Route of administration	Oral
Randomized	Yes
Randomization adequate	Yes
Blinding	Double-blind
Blinding adequate	Yes
Placebo	Yes
Drug comparison	No
Site description	Not described
No. of subjects enrolled	40
No. of subjects completed	36
Sex	Male and female
Age	19-78 years (mean: 59.5)

Inclusion criteria
Patients with diabetic or hypertensive vascular retinopathy.

Exclusion criteria
Patients with advanced or irreversible retinal lesions (stage IV); patients with

severe metabolic disorders, hyperproteinemia, decompensated diabetes, or severe liver deterioration; patients with severe systemic arterial hypertension or malignant hypertension; patients with glaucoma or opacification of the refractive media. Patients not permitted to take any therapeutic agents likely to exert an antiexudative, antiedemic, anti-inflammatory, vasoprotective, or hemorheological action.

End points

Before admission to the trial, and after 30 days (and 60 days for placebo patients continuing), patients underwent ophthalmoscopic examination and fluoroangiographic assessment. Blood pressure, heart rate, blood glucose, and glycosylated hemoglobin were recorded at the same time.

Results

Of the 36 subjects completing the trial, 33 had diabetes and three had arterial hypertension. At baseline, 28 subjects had opthalmoscopically detectable retinal abnormalities, 13 in the treatment group and 15 in the placebo group. After the placebo-controlled study, 10 of the patients taking bilberry were improved, whereas none showed any change in the placebo group. Also at baseline, after a fluoroangiographic exam, 17 patients taking bilberry and 18 taking placebo were found to have abnormalities. In the bilberry group, 13 showed improvement, whereas in the placebo group only one patient showed improvement, 14 had no change in their condition, and three showed deterioration. After the initial one-month study, patients originally taking placebo were given bilberry for an additional month. After this treatment, 12 of the 15 patients with opthalmoscopic abnormalities showed improvement, and 17 of the 18 with fluoroangiographic abnormalities showed improvement. There were no clinically relevant changes in blood pressure, blood glucose, or glycosylated hemoglobin values during the study.

Side effects

One mild epigastric complaint which cleared without discontinuing treatment.

Authors' comments

Tegens appears to be a safe and effective therapy for diabetic or hypertensive vascular retinopathy.

Reviewer's comments

Relatively well-designed and well-conducted trial. The study was limited by the small sample size. (5, 4)

Clinical Study: Tegens®

Extract name	Myrtocyan®
Manufacturer	Inverni della Beffa, Italy (Indena S.p.A., Italy)
Indication	**Diabetic retinopathy**
Level of evidence	**III**
Therapeutic benefit	**Undetermined**

Bibliographic reference

Repossi P, Malagola R, De Cadilhac C (1987). The role of anthocyanosides on vascular permeability in diabetic retinopathy. *Annali di Ottalmologia e Clinica Oculistica* 113 (4): 357-361.

Trial design

Parallel. Patients continued with their usual therapy for retinopathy (not described).

Study duration	1 year
Dose	1 (160 mg) capsule twice daily
Route of administration	Oral
Randomized	No
Randomization adequate	No
Blinding	Not described
Blinding adequate	No
Placebo	Yes
Drug comparison	No
Site description	Not described
No. of subjects enrolled	40
No. of subjects completed	40
Sex	Not given
Age	Not given

Inclusion criteria

Diabetic patients with retinopathy in a relatively initial phase, showing at the back pole some hard exudates distributed or in circinate form, but not involving the macular region.

Exclusion criteria

Patients with hard exudates affecting the macular region of the eye were eliminated.

End points

All patients were examined by fluoroangiography before the trial and after 12 months. Opthalmoscopic evaluations were conducted every three months. Hard exudation was used as an index of alteration of capillary permeability to evaluate the integrity of the hematoretinal barrier.

Results
Of patients showing hard exudates in the back pole, 50 percent improved, 30 percent remained the same, and 20 percent worsened with treatment with anthocyanosides. In the placebo group, 20 percent improved, 45 percent remained the same, and 35 percent worsened.

Of patients showing circinate deposits of the hard exudates, 15 percent improved, 60 percent remained the same, and 25 percent worsened with treatment with anthocyanosides. In the placebo group, 10 percent improved, 50 percent remained the same, and 40 percent worsened.

Side effects
No short- or long-term side effects.

Authors' comments
The results obtained with the group of patients treated with anthocyanosides for a period of 12 months are significant. The results point out that the highest efficacy is gained with very early diagnosis and immediate therapy.

Reviewer's comments
This study was limited by several flaws: the sample was not randomized; there is no description of blinding; and there is no description of withdrawals or dropouts. (Translation reviewed) (0, 1)

Clinical Study: Tegens®

Extract name	Myrtocyan®
Manufacturer	Inverni della Beffa, Italy (Indena S.p.A., Italy)
Indication	**Varicosis** (varicose veins)
Level of evidence	**III**
Therapeutic benefit	**Trend**

Bibliographic reference
Gatta L (1988). *Vaccinium myrtillus* anthocyanosides in the treatment of venous stasis: Controlled clinical study on sixty patients. *Fitoterapia* 59 (Suppl 1): 19-26.

Trial design
Parallel.

Study duration	30 days
Dose	3 (160 mg) capsules daily
Route of administration	Oral
Randomized	Yes
Randomization adequate	Yes
Blinding	Double-blind
Blinding adequate	No
Placebo	Yes
Drug comparison	No
Site description	Outpatients
No. of subjects enrolled	60
No. of subjects completed	60
Sex	Male and female
Age	19-66 years (mean: 44)

Inclusion criteria
Subjects with various forms of the varicose syndrome.

Exclusion criteria
None mentioned.

End points
Parameters chosen for the assessment of efficacy were the following symptoms: sensation of pressure in the legs, cramplike pains, paresthesias. Observations were also made of stasis edema and leg girth 2 cm above the medial malleolus and 12 cm below the patella. Blood flow graphs were also taken before and after 30 days of treatment in the patients treated with bilberry.

Results
Bilberry was superior to placebo in the reduction of symptoms: leg and ankle edema, sensation of pressure, and cramps ($p < 0.01$), as well as for paresthesias (tingling or "pins and needles" sensation) ($p = 0.05$). Reduction of leg and ankle circumference, although small, was statistically significant ($p < 0.001$). After treatment with placebo, the circumference values were practically unchanged. In the bilberry group, venous stasis, indicated in rheographic tracing, was significantly lower after treatment compared to baseline ($p = 0.05$).

Side effects
No undesirable effects attributable to the treatment.

Authors' comments
Based on this blind clinical trial, *Vaccinium myrtillus* anthocyanosides are of definite therapeutic value in the management of venous diseases.

Reviewer's comments
The study was limited by the inadequate length of treatment (too short), the inadequately described inclusion/exclusion criteria, and the small sample size. (Translation reviewed) (2, 3)

Clinical Study: Tegens®

Extract name	Myrtocyan®
Manufacturer	Inverni della Beffa, Italy (Indena S.p.A., Italy)
Indication	**Chronic primary dysmenorrhea** (painful menstruation)
Level of evidence	**III**
Therapeutic benefit	**Undetermined**

Bibliographic reference
Colombo D, Vescovini R (1985). Studio clinico controllato sull'efficacia degli antocianosidi del mirtillo nel trattamento della dismenorrea essenziale. *Giornale Italiano di Ostetricia e Ginecologia* 7 (12):1033-1038.

Trial design
Patients were treated over two consecutive menstrual cycles. Therapy began on the third day before the start of the cycle and continued for five days.

Study duration	2 menstrual cycles
Dose	1 (160 mg) capsule twice daily
Route of administration	Oral
Randomized	Yes
Randomization adequate	Yes
Blinding	Double-blind
Blinding adequate	Yes
Placebo	Yes
Drug comparison	No
Site description	Not described
No. of subjects enrolled	30
No. of subjects completed	30
Sex	Female
Age	17-30 years

Inclusion criteria
Females suffering from chronic primary dysmenorrhea for at least one year (average 4.7 years).

Exclusion criteria
Females suffering from secondary dysmenorrhea (endomitriosis/adenomiosis, pelvic inflammatory diseases, vaginal/hymenal malfunctions, cervical stenosis, and ovarian cysts).

End points
The subjective symptoms of primary dysmenorrhea (pelvic and lumbar pain, mammary tension, headache, nausea and vomiting, heaviness of the lower limbs) were recorded before the study, on the first day of the cycle, and after treatment.

Results
Symptomatic relief occurred in patients taking bilberry, while the placebo was ineffective. After two menstrual cycles, the difference between the effects of bilberry and placebo were highly significant for pelvic and lumbar-sacral pain, swollen breasts, and heaviness in the lower limbs ($p < 0.002$). The benefit was less pronounced for nausea and vomiting ($p < 0.05$) and not significant for headache.

Side effects
None attributable to the therapy.

Authors' comments
Anthocyanosides, natural derivatives basically lacking any side effects, demonstrated results that were superior to expectations. Further studies are necessary to confirm these data and explore dosing requirements.

Reviewer's comments
The study was flawed by the highly subjective evaluation criteria for dysmenorrhea; therefore, it is difficult to assess the botanical's benefit. The treatment length was also inadequate, and there is no description of withdrawals or dropouts. (Translation reviewed) (4, 1)

Clinical Study: MirtoSelect™ (Myrtocyan®)

Extract name	Myrtocyan
Manufacturer	Indena S.p.A., Italy
Indication	**Pupillary reflex**
Level of evidence	**III**
Therapeutic benefit	**MOA**

Bibliographic reference
Vannini L, Samuelly R, Coffano M, Tibaldi L (1986). Study of the pupillary reflex after anthocyanoside administration. *Bollettino d'Oculistica* 65 (Suppl. 6): 569-577.

Trial design
Parallel.

Study duration	1 day
Dose	3 (80 mg anthocyanosides w/25 percent anthocyanidins) capsules
Route of administration	Oral
Randomized	No
Randomization adequate	No
Blinding	Double-blind
Blinding adequate	Yes
Placebo	Yes
Drug comparison	No
Site description	Not described
No. of subjects enrolled	40
No. of subjects completed	40
Sex	Male and female
Age	15-35 years (mean: 25.5)

Inclusion criteria
Volunteers who were internally and ophthalmologically normal.

Exclusion criteria
None mentioned.

End points
A computerized infrared videopupillograph was used to assess light reflex (amplitude of pupillary contraction, latency time, total contraction time, contraction velocity, dilation velocity, and acceleration of contraction). A baseline pupillographic recording was taken, then the drug or placebo was administered, and pupillographic tests were conducted after 1, 1.5, 2, and 4 hours.

Results
Fifteen of the 20 subjects who took bilberry extract showed an improvement in pupillary dynamics. With a constant latency time, the response of the pupil to light showed greater and faster movement, greater acceleration and in less time. The greatest improvement in pupillary dynamics occurred two hours after administration of bilberry. Thirteen of the 20 patients taking placebo showed improvement in pupillary dynamics. Contraction velocity and maximum acceleration improved and the total contraction time decreased, but the degree of contraction was unchanged.

Side effects
None mentioned in paper.

Authors' comments
Anthocyanosides may be used in healthy subjects who work in strong light, where the light reflex presumably wanes more easily, and who need a more efficient response to light due to fatigue.

Reviewer's comments
Mechanistic study. (Translation reviewed) (3, 5)

Product Profile: FAR-1

Manufacturer	**Ditta Farmigea S.p.A., Italy**
U.S. distributor	None
Botanical ingredient	**Bilberry fruit**
Extract name	None given
Quantity	180 mg
Processing	No information
Standardization	25% anthocyanidins
Formulation	Capsule

Other ingredients: DL-tocopherol (vitamin E, 100 mg).

Source(s) of information: Bravetti, Fraboni, and Maccolini, 1989.

Clinical Study: FAR-1

Extract name	None given
Manufacturer	Ditta Farmigea S.p.A., Italy
Indication	**Senile cataracts**
Level of evidence	**II**
Therapeutic benefit	**Trend**

Bibliographic reference
Bravetti GO, Fraboni E, Maccolini E (1989). Preventive medical treatment of senile cataract with vitamin E and *Vaccinium myrtillus* anthocyanosides: Clinical evaluation. *Annali di Ottalmologia e Clinica Oculistica* 115 (2): 109-116.

Trial design
Parallel, double-blind trial for four months. Then the trial was continued openly for another four months, with both groups receiving active treatment.

Study duration	4 months
Dose	2 (100 mg DL-tocopherol acetate, 180 mg anthocyanosides w/25 percent anthocyanidins)
Route of administration	Oral
Randomized	Yes
Randomization adequate	Yes
Blinding	Double-blind
Blinding adequate	Yes
Placebo	Yes
Drug comparison	No
Site description	Not described
No. of subjects enrolled	59
No. of subjects completed	50
Sex	Male and female
Age	48-81 years (mean: 67)

Inclusion criteria
Patients had central visual acuity for distant objects (with best correction) between 4/10 and 8/10.

Exclusion criteria
Patients could have no other ocular or systemic pathologies that might affect the purpose of the trial.

End points
Assessments of central visual acuity (measured with Snellen charts) both with and without correction, crystalline opacity, and subjective impression of patient of his or her vision were made prior to trial, as well as after four and eight months.

Results
After four months, 31 eyes remained unchanged and one worsened in the treated group. In placebo group, 23 eyes remained unchanged and seven worsened. There were no "improved" eyes. After eight months, the treatment group had 29 unchanged eyes and three worsened eyes, while the former-placebo group had 21 unchanged eyes and nine worsened eyes. At four months, there was a statistical significance between groups, $p < 0.05$. At eight months, when both groups had been receiving treatment, there was no statistical difference between the two.

Side effects
None found or reported.

Authors' comments
The validity of the trial is hindered by the lack of an objective, precise, and repeatable technique for detecting lenticular opacities in vivo. The observed data suggest, however, that the mixture of vitamin E and anthocyanosides can prevent the progression of senile cataracts.

Reviewer's comments
There was a 62 percent incidence of cataracts and no improved eyes after eight months. The study was limited by the outcome measures not being clearly defined. (Translation reviewed) (5,4)

Black Cohosh

Other common names: **Black bugbane, black snakeroot, rheumatism weed**
Latin name: *Actaea racemosa* **L.** [Ranunculaceae]
Latin synonyms: *Cimifuga racemosa* **(L.) Nutt.**
Plant parts: **Root, rhizome**

PREPARATIONS USED IN REVIEWED CLINICAL STUDIES

Black cohosh is native to North America. Native Americans used the rhizomes and roots as a gynecological remedy as well as for treatment of rheumatic conditions and hives. Black cohosh was also used for its sedative and pain-relieving properties. Dried plant material, hydroalcoholic liquid, and dried extracts are available commercially. The underground parts contain cycloartane-type triterpene glycosides, which are measured for quality control purposes (Flannery et al., 2002).

Clinical research has been conducted on a commercial preparation called Remifemin®, which is manufactured by Schaper & Brümmer in Germany and distributed in the United States by GlaxoSmithKline. Remifemin is available in tablet form, and each tablet contains black cohosh root extract equivalent to 20 mg root/rhizome. Over time, the formulation has changed from a solution to tablets, and the medium of extraction has changed from ethanolic alcohol (60 percent by volume) to isopropyl alcohol (40 percent by volume). The preparations are standardized to contain 1 mg total triterpene saponins (expressed as 27-deoxyactein) in each dose, equivalent to 20 mg root/rhizome. Recent analysis of the structure of 27-deoxyactein has determined that it is actually 26-deoxyactein (Chen et al., 2001).

BLACK COHOSH SUMMARY TABLE

Product Name	Manufacturer/ U.S. Distributor	Product Characteristics	Dose in Trials	Indication	No. of Trials	Benefit (Evidence Level-Trial No.)
Remifemin®	Schaper & Brümmer GmbH & Co. KG, Germany/ GlaxoSmithKline	Isopropanolic extract	1 or 2 tablets twice daily (equivalent to 40 mg root/day)	Menopausal symptoms	6	Yes (II-I) No (II-I) Undetermined (III-3) MOA (III-I)

SUMMARY OF REVIEWED CLINICAL STUDIES

Black cohosh root extracts have been used for treating menopausal symptoms. Menopause is the cessation of menstruation, which generally occurs when women reach age 50. The physical symptoms of menopause include hot flashes, sweating, cardiovascular complaints, fatigue, vertigo, muscle and joint pain, urinary incontinence, vaginal dryness, and atrophy of the vaginal epithelium. Psychological symptoms include irritability, forgetfulness, anxiety, depression, sleep disturbances, and reduced libido. Menopause is thought to occur when no eggs are left in a woman's ovaries. The resulting decline in ovarian function causes a reduced production of estrogen and progesterone and a corresponding increase in follicle-stimulating hormone (FSH) and luteinizing hormone (LH) (Murray and Pizzorno, 1999).

Remifemin

Menopausal Symptoms

We reviewed six clinical studies that examined the effects of Remifemin on menopause. The studies ranged in duration from two to six months. Measured end points included hormone levels, symptoms evaluated using the Kupperman Menopausal Index (an older scale that includes hot flashes, insomnia, and depression, but does not include vaginal dryness), and a battery of psychometric tests. Two tablets twice daily (8 mg extract, equivalent to 40 mg root/rhizome per day) was the common dose, although one trial used 40 drops twice daily of a liquid preparation (also equivalent to 40 mg root/rhizome).

In a comparison trial, 55 women with menopausal symptoms were randomly assigned to receive Remifemin (40 drops twice daily), conjugated estrogens (0.6 mg), or diazepam (2 mg) for three months. All treatments reduced symptoms according to the Kupperman index and the clinical global impression (CGI) scale. Treatment with Remifemin and estrogens caused changes in vaginal cytology from the forth to sixth week onward. As expected, the psychotropic drug (diazepam) had no effect on this end point (Warnecke, 1985). Our reviewer, Dr. Tieraona Low Dog, determined that the efficacy of Remifemin was not established in this trial due to poor methodology. Another study with 64 menopausal women compared Remifemin (two tablets twice daily) with low-dose estrogen (0.6 mg) and placebo. After three months of treatment, all three groups improved. There was no improvement in the estrogen group compared to placebo, indicating that the dose was too low. However, the Kupperman index for the Remifemin group was significantly lower compared to the other two groups, indicating greater improvement for the black cohosh group. This group also uniquely exhibited positive changes in vaginal tissue, showing signs of increased proliferation of the vaginal epithelium (Stoll, 1987). The strength of the trial was reduced by the loss of 16 out of 80 women, including 12 of those in the estrogen group, during weeks five to eight due to perceived lack of efficacy.

In another study, also deemed poor quality, women who had undergone hysterectomy were given estriol (1 mg/day), conjugated estrogen (1.25 mg/day), combination therapy (estradiol 2 mg/day and norethisterone acetate 1 mg/day), or Remifemin. The authors reported similar reductions compared to baseline in all treatment groups in a modified Kupperman index at 4, 8, 12, and 24 weeks (Lehmann-Willenbrock and Riedal, 1988).

A dose-response study with 123 peri- and postmenopausal women compared the usual dose equivalent to 40 mg root to a tripling of the dose, equivalent to 127 mg root. Both doses caused a reduction in the Kupperman index and the self-depression scale over six months. Neither dose altered vaginal cytology or affected hormone levels (17-beta-estradiol, FSH, LH, prolactin, and sex hormone binding globulin) (Liske et al., 2002). This study did not include a placebo arm but was useful for safety data and indicated an absence of estrogenic effects even at the high dose.

A recent study with breast cancer survivors reported a comparable reduction in hot flashes and other menopausal symptoms following administration of Remifemin (two tablets per day) or placebo for two months. The only difference in favor of the treatment was a greater reduction in the amount of sweating. No effect on hormones FSH and LH was noted. It may be significant that approximately 70 percent of the women in this study were concurrently taking tamoxifen, an antiestrogenic agent (Jacobson et al., 2001).

Studies provide conflicting data regarding the potential estrogenic activity of this preparation of black cohosh root, as measured by suppression of LH and changes in vaginal cytology. A placebo-controlled study with 110 women with menopausal symptoms reported a reduction in LH, but not FSH, following a dose of 8 mg extract (equivalent to 40 mg root) for two months (Duker et al., 1991). However, three other trials showed no significant effects on LH or FSH following treatment for two to six months with doses equivalent to 40 to 127 mg root (Lehmann-Willenbrock and Riedel, 1988; Liske et al., 2002; Jacobson et al., 2001). Two trials reported changes in vaginal cytology and increases in proliferation and maturation of vaginal epithelium following doses equivalent to 40 mg root for three months. These effects were comparable to those observed in the control groups given low-dose estrogens (0.6 mg per day) (Warnecke, 1985; Stoll, 1987). However, another study comparing doses of 40 mg root to 127 mg root found no such effect after the same three-month time period (Liske et al., 2002).

In general, the reviewed studies indicate that Remifemin may improve vasomotor symptoms and mood associated with menopause. However, Dr. Low Dog considered that the poor quality of the trials made it impossible to say with conviction that black cohosh extract given at the doses used in these trials is effective in alleviating menopausal symptoms and/or has any inherent estrogenic activity.

POSTMARKETING SURVEILLANCE STUDIES

A postmarketing surveillance study reported on 704 menopausal women who were treated with a dose of 40 drops Remifemin twice daily (equivalent to 40 mg root/rhizome) for six to eight weeks. Symptoms of hot flashes and profuse sweating improved, as did mood, in 75 percent of 629 women after four weeks (Stolze, 1982).

ADVERSE REACTIONS OR SIDE EFFECTS

No significant adverse reactions or side effects were reported in the clinical trials. Stolze's (1982) postmarketing surveillance study reported good tolerability for 93 percent of women with a dose of 40 drops twice daily. Mild and transitory symptoms, commonly gastrointestinal complaints, were reported in 7 percent.

Treatment of menopausal symptoms with estrogens is generally contraindicated for breast cancer survivors, due to a concern over increased risk of cancer. A two-month study with 85 breast cancer survivors reported no evidence of harm from using black cohosh. The authors suggested that treatment with Remifemin for hot flashes might be more acceptable than conventional hormone replacement therapy (HRT) due to its lack of estrogenic effects (Jacobson et al., 2001).

INFORMATION FROM PHARMACOPOEIAL MONOGRAPHS

Sources of Published Therapeutic Monographs

German Commission E
British Herbal Compendium (BHC)
American Herbal Pharmacopoeia (AHP)

Indications

Preparations of fresh or dried rhizome with attached roots are approved by the German Commission E for premenstrual discomfort, dysmenorrhea, or climacteric (menopausal) neurovegetative ailments; actions are listed as estrogen-like, binding to estrogen receptors, and suppression of luteinizing hormone (Blumenthal et al., 1998).

The *British Herbal Compendium* states that black cohosh is used to treat menopausal disorders, uterine spasm, muscular rheumatism, rheumatoid arthritis, and tinnitus; actions include endocrine (pituitary, oestrogen-mimetic) activity, emmenagogue, and antirheumatic (Bradley, 1992).

The *American Herbal Pharmacopoeia* lists the following indications supported by clinical trials of black cohosh extract: menopausal complaints, including outbreaks of sweating, anxiety, and hot flashes. The *AHP* also lists the following traditional indications for black cohosh: nervous disorders (chorea, nyalgia, epilepsy, hysteria, neuralgia, depression, anxiety and nervousness, and sciatica); cardiovascular disorders (hypertension and arrythmia due to vascular or nervous tension); various infectious diseases; and gynecological disorders (amenorrhea, leukorrhea, dysmenorrhea, atony of the uterus, premature labor, cramps during pregnancy, postpartum pain or hemorrhage, and pelvic pain). The traditional actions listed are anxiolytic; antispasmodic; emmenagogue; nervine; uterine relaxant; partus prepara-tory; and uterine tonic (Flannery et al., 2002).

Doses

Dried rhizome and root: 40 to 200 mg or by decoction (Bradley, 1992); 1 g up to three times daily (Flannery et al., 2002)

Tincture: (1:10, 60 percent ethanol) 0.4 to 2 ml (Bradley, 1992); (1:10, 40 to 60 percent alcohol v/v) 0.4 ml daily (Flannery et al., 2002)

Extract: (alcohol 40 to 60 percent v/v) corresponding to 40 mg drug (Blumenthal et al., 1998; Flannery et al., 2002)

Treatment Period

The Commission E recommends that treatment should not last lon-ger than six months (Blumenthal et al., 1998).

Contraindications

The Commission E lists no known contraindications, while the *BHC* lists pregnancy and lactation (Blumenthal et al., 1998; Bradley, 1992). The *AHP* states that a conclusive determination about contra-indications cannot be made with the available data (Flannery et al., 2002).

Adverse Reactions

According to the Commission E, gastric discomfort occurs occa-sionally (Blumenthal et al., 1998). The *AHP* also lists mild gastroin-testinal upset as the most frequent adverse event and lists several other minor adverse events (headache, vertigo, mastalgia, weight gain, heavy feeling in the legs, and a stimulant effect) (Flannery et al., 2002).

Precautions

The *AHP* warns that since the long-term use of black cohosh for menopausal symptoms is a new indication, women using black cohosh for menopausal symptoms, or those with a history of breast cancer, should first consult a health care professional (Flannery et al., 2002). The *AHP* also suggests that black cohosh should not be used during pregnancy (except after consultation with a health care professional) or by children.

Drug Interactions

The Commission E and the *AHP* state there are no known drug interactions (Blumenthal et al., 1998; Flannery et al., 2002).

REFERENCES

Blumenthal M, Busse W, Hall T, Goldberg A, Gruenwald J, Riggins C, Rister S, eds. (1998). *The Complete German Commission E Monographs: Therapeutic Guide to Herbal Medicines.* Trans. S Klein. Austin, TX: American Botanical Council.

Bradley PR, ed. (1992). *British Herbal Compendium: A Handbook of Scientific Information on Widely Used Plant Drugs,* Volume 1. Dorset, UK: British Herbal Medicine Association.

Chen SN, Li WK, Fabricant DS, Santarsiero BD, Mesacar A, Fitzloff JF, Fong HHS, Farnsworth NR (2001). Isolation, structure elucidation and absolute configuration of 26-deoxyactein from *Cimifuga racemosa* and clarification of nomenclature associated with 27-deoxyactein. *Journal of Natural Products* 65 (4): 601-605.

Duker E, Kopanski L, Jarry H, Wuttke W (1991). Effects of extracts from *Cimicifuga racemosa* on gonadotropin release in menopausal women and ovariectomized rats. *Planta Medica* 57 (5): 420-424.

Flannery MA, Bencie R, Graff A, Hartung T, Länger R, Nagarajan M, Thiekoetter K, Reich E, Brown P, Takahashi R, et al. (2002). *Black Cohosh Rhizome,* Actea racemosa *L. syn.* Cimifuga racemose *(L.) Nutt.* American Herbal Pharmacopoeia and Therapeutic Compendium: Standards of Analysis, Quality Control, and Therapeutics. Eds. R Upton, A Graff. Santa Cruz, CA: American Herbal Pharmacopoeia.

Jacobson JS, Troxel AB, Evans J, Klaus L, Vahdat L, Kinne D, Lo KMS, Moore A, Rosenman PJ, Kaufman EL, et al. (2001). Randomized trial of black cohosh for the treatment of hot flashes among women with a history of breast cancer. *Journal of Clinical Oncology* 19 (10): 2739-2745.

Lehmann-Willenbrock E, Riedel HH (1988). Clinical and endocrinologic examinations concerning therapy of climacteric symptoms following hysterectomy with remaining ovaries. *Zentralblatt fur Gynakologie* 110: 611-618.

Liske E, Hänggi W, Henneicke-von Zeppelin HH, Boblitz N, Wüstenberg P, Rahlfs VW (2002). Physiological investigation of a unique extract of black cohosh (*Cimicifugae racemosae* rhizoma): A 6-month clinical study demonstrates no systemic estrogenic effect. *Journal of Women's Health and Gender-Based Medicine* 11 (2): 163-174. (Also published as Liske E, Boblitz N, Henneicke-von Zepelin H-H [2000]. Therapie Klmakterischer Beschwerden mit *Cimicifuga racemosa:* Daten zur Wirkung und Wirksamkeit aus einer randomisierten Kontrollierten Doppelblindstudie. In *Phytopharmaka VI.* Eds. Rietbrock N, Donath MF, Loew D, Roots I, Schulz V. Darmstadt: Verlag Steinkopft, pp. 247-257.)

Murray MT, Pizzorno JE (1999). Menopause. In *Textbook of Natural Medicine.* Eds. Pizzorno JE, Murray MT, Second Edition, Volume 2. Edinburgh: Churchill Livingstone, pp. 1387-1396.

Stoll W (1987). Phytotherapy influences atrophic vaginal epithelium. *Therapeuticon* 1: 23-31.

Stolze H (1982). Der andere weg, klimaterische beschwerden zu behandeln. *Gyne* 3: 14-16.

Warnecke G (1985). Influencing menopausal symptoms with a phytotherapeutic agent. *Die Medizinische Welt* 36: 871-874.

DETAILS ON BLACK COHOSH PRODUCTS
AND CLINICAL STUDIES

Product and clinical study information is grouped in the same order as in the Summary Table. A profile on an individual product is followed by details of the clinical studies associated with that product. In some instances a clinical study, or studies, supports several products that contain the same principal ingredient(s). In these instances, those products are grouped together.

Clinical studies that follow each product, or group of products, are grouped by therapeutic indication, in accordance with the order in the Summary Table.

Product Profile: Remifemin®

Manufacturer	**Schaper & Brümmer GmbH & Co. KG, Germany**
U.S. distributor	**GlaxoSmithKline**
Botanical ingredient	**Black cohosh root and rhizome extract**
Extract name	None given
Quantity	Equivalent to 20 mg root and rhizome
Processing	Isopropanol extract (40 percent v/v). Plant to extract ratio 0.78-1.14:1; 0.018-0.026 ml liquid extract in tablet
Standardization	Triterpene glycosides content (calculated as 27-deoxyactein)
Formulation	Tablet

Recommended dose: Take one tablet in the morning and one tablet in the evening, with water. Improvements can be expected within a few weeks with full benefits after using Remifemin twice a day for 4 to 12 weeks.

DSHEA structure/function: Clinically shown to reduce menopausal symptoms (including hot flashes, night sweats, mood swings, irritability, and related occasional sleeplessness).

Cautions: This product should not be used by women who are pregnant or considering becoming pregnant or are nursing. For a few consumers, gastric discomfort may occur but should not be persistent. If gastric discomfort persists, discontinue use and see a health care

practitioner. This product does not contain estrogen. Remifemin is not meant to replace any drug therapy.

Other ingredients: Lactose, cellulose, potato starch, magnesium stearate, and natural peppermint flavor.

Source(s) of information: Product packaging (©2000 SmithKline Beecham); Liske et al., 2002; information provided by Enzymatic Therapy; Remifemin® Scientific Brochure (Schaper & Brümmer GmbH & Co. KG, Germany, 1997).

Clinical Study: Remifemin®

Extract name	None given
Manufacturer	Schaper & Brümmer GmbH & Co. KG, Germany
Indication	**Menopausal symptoms**
Level of evidence	**III**
Therapeutic benefit	**Undetermined**

Bibliographic reference
Warnecke G (1985). Influencing menopausal symptoms with a phytotherapeutic agent. *Die Medizinische Welt* 36: 871-874.

Trial design
Parallel. Three-arm study: 20 women received Remifemin, 20 were treated with 0.6 mg conjugated estrogens, and 20 were given 2 mg diazepam per day.

Study duration	3 months
Dose	40 drops twice daily
Route of administration	Oral
Randomized	Yes
Randomization adequate	No
Blinding	Open
Blinding adequate	No
Placebo	No
Drug comparison	Yes
Drug name	Conjugated estrogens or diazepam
Site description	1 gynecology practice
No. of subjects enrolled	60
No. of subjects completed	55

Sex   Female
Age   45-60 years (mean: 54)

Inclusion criteria
Women between the ages of 45 and 60 with no or only irregular bleeding and menopausal symptoms that did not require high-dose hormone treatment or therapy with psychotropic drugs.

Exclusion criteria
Contraindications against one of the trial treatments, hormone treatment within the past four to six weeks, and surgery within the past six months.

End points
Patients were evaluated at the beginning of the study and after 2, 4, and 12 weeks of treatment. Neurovegetative symptoms were evaluated using the Kupperman index. Psychological symptoms were quantified using the Hamilton Anxiety Scale (HAMA) and the Self-Assessment Depression Scale (SDS). Vaginal epithelial calls were examined microscopically for changes. The clinical global impression scale assessed the outcome of therapy.

Results
All three forms of therapy had a comparably good effect on menopausal symptoms according to the Kupperman index and CGI. Remifemin and estrogens caused changes in vaginal cytology from the fourth to sixth week onward. The psychotropic drug, as expected, had no effect on these changes.

Side effects
None mentioned.

Author's comments
Long-term and consistent therapy with *Cimifuga* monoextract (Remifemin) yields at least equivalent rates of success against menopausal symptoms as low-dose conjugated estrogen and is better than therapy with psychotropic drugs.

Reviewer's comments
This study is limited by several flaws, including a lack of randomization and blinding, and an inadequate power calculation for the sample size. (1, 2)

Clinical Study: Remifemin®

Extract name   None given
Manufacturer   Schaper & Brümmer GmbH & Co. KG, Germany

Indication	**Menopausal symptoms**
Level of evidence	**III**
Therapeutic benefit	**Undetermined**

Bibliographic reference
Stoll W (1987). Phytotherapy influences atrophic vaginal epithelium. *Therapeuticon* 1: 23-31.

Trial design
Parallel. Three-arm study: Remifemin (30 women), low-dose estrogen (30 women, 0.625 mg), and placebo (20 women).

Study duration	3 months
Dose	2 (2 mg extract) tablets twice daily
Route of administration	Oral
Randomized	No
Randomization adequate	No
Blinding	Double-blind
Blinding adequate	Yes
Placebo	Yes
Drug comparison	Yes
Drug name	Estrogen
Site description	Not described
No. of subjects enrolled	80
No. of subjects completed	64
Sex	Female
Age	46-58 years

Inclusion criteria
Women suffering from (1) neurovegetative complaints: hot flushes (at least three per day), sweating, and palpitation; (2) psychic complaints: anxiety, insomnia, and depression; and (3) somatic disorders such as vaginal dryness and menstrual disorders.

Exclusion criteria
Bilateral ovariectomy, castration, contraindication for hormone treatment, osteoporosis due to menopause, hormone therapy within the past four weeks, antihypertensive medications, menopausal complaints due to other causes.

End points
The Kupperman Menopausal Index (neurovegetative symptoms) and the Hamilton Anxiety Scale (HAMA) (psychological complaints) were assessed

every four weeks. The proliferative status of vaginal epithelium was measured at the beginning of the study and after 12 weeks.

Results

After three months of treatment, the Kupperman index showed a decrease for all three groups, but the Remifemin group was significantly lower than both estrogen and placebo groups, $p < 0.001$. The index for the Remifemin group fell from over 30 to under 15, an indication that treatment is no longer needed. The HAMA score also fell for all three groups, but again the Remifemin group was significantly lower, $p < 0.001$. The degree of proliferation of the vaginal epithelium improved in the Remifemin group, but there was no change for the other groups. The difference was significant, $p < 0.01$.

Side effects

Twelve of the Remifemin patients reported minor side effects.

Author's comments

Remifemin is suited as the drug of first choice to treat menopausal failure, particularly if a hormone therapy is only indicated on reflection or not wanted by the patient.

Reviewer's comments

The study is limited by several flaws: lack of randomization; risk of attrition bias due to the loss of 12 out of 30 women in the estrogen group between weeks five through eight because of perceived lack of efficacy; and FSH was not used as inclusion/exclusion criteria to determine menopausal status. (3, 4)

Clinical Study: Remifemin®

Extract name	None given
Manufacturer	Schaper & Brümmer GmbH & Co. KG, Germany
Indication	**Menopausal symptoms** in hysterectomized patients
Level of evidence	**III**
Therapeutic benefit	**Undetermined**

Bibliographic reference

Lehmann-Willenbrock E, Riedel HH (1988). Clinical and endocrinologic examinations concerning therapy of climacteric symptoms following hysterectomy with remaining ovaries. *Zentralblatt fur Gynakologie* 110: 611-618.

Trial design
Parallel. Patients were divided into four treatment groups: group 1 was given estriol (Ovestin) one tablet containing 1 mg; group 2 received conjugated estrogens (Presomen) one tablet containing 1.25 mg; group 3 received estrogen-gestagen (Trisequens) one tablet a day; and group 4 received Remifemin.

Study duration	6 months
Dose	2 (2 mg extract) tablets twice daily
Route of administration	Oral
Randomized	Yes
Randomization adequate	No
Blinding	Open
Blinding adequate	No
Placebo	No
Drug comparison	Yes
Drug name	Estriol, conjugated estrogens, and estrogen-gestagen therapy
Site description	Not described
No. of subjects enrolled	60
No. of subjects completed	60
Sex	Female
Age	Under 40 years

Inclusion criteria
Patients who had undergone hysterectomy between 1975 and 1984 and had at least one intact ovary. Patients also had climacteric symptoms, predominantly consisting of hot flushes and sweating.

Exclusion criteria
Women unable to undergo hormone therapy because of chronic hepatitis, deep vein thrombosis, postoperative state following mastocarcinoma, or uncontrollable diabetes mellitus were excluded. Patients refusing any hormone therapy at all were also excluded.

End points
Women assessed their severity of a list of symptoms on a modified Kupperman index at baseline and 4, 8, 12, and 24 weeks after starting the study. Blood was taken to measure concentrations of prostaglandin E2, progesterone, FSH, and LH.

Results
Compared to the initial severity of symptoms, results in patients taking

estriol or conjugated estrogens were significantly different after 8, 12, and 24 weeks. In patients taking Remifemin or estrogen-gestagen complex, symptom severity after 4, 8, 12, and 24 weeks also differed significantly from severity at the beginning of the trial. There were no significant differences in LH or FSH levels in any of the groups.

Side effects
None discussed in paper.

Authors' comments
Alleviation of menopausal symptoms due to ovarial deficiency following hysterectomy may be successfully treated by all four treatment schemes (estriol, conjugated estrogen, estrogen-gestagen complex, or Remifemin). If osteoporosis prevention is intended, conjugated estrogen or estrogen-gestagen is recommended.

Reviewer's comments
This trial was flawed by the lack of blinding and placebo control. There was also no power calculation to determine the appropriateness of the sample size. (1, 4)

Clinical Study: Remifemin®

Extract name	None given
Manufacturer	Schaper & Brümmer GmbH & Co. KG, Germany
Indication	**Menopausal symptoms**
Level of evidence	**II**
Therapeutic benefit	**Yes**

Bibliographic reference
Liske E, Hänggi W, Henneicke-von Zeppelin HH, Boblitz N, Wüstenberg P, Rahlfs VW (2002). Physiological investigation of a unique extract of black cohosh (*Cimicifugae racemosae* rhizoma): A 6-month clinical study demonstrates no systemic estrogenic effect. *Journal of Women's Health and Gender-Based Medicine* 11 (2): 163-174. (Also published as Liske E, Boblitz N, Henneicke-von Zepelin H-H [2000]. Therapie Klmakterischer Beschwerden mit *Cimicifuga racemosa:* Daten zur Wirkung and Wirksamkeit aus einer randomisierten kontrollierten Doppelblindstudie. In *Phytopharmaka VI*. Eds. Rietbrock N, Donath MF, Loew D, Roots I, Schulz V. Darmstadt: Verlag Steinkopft, pp. 247-257.)

Trial design
Parallel. The trial had a 12-week treatment period with extension to 24 weeks.

Study duration	6 months
Dose	39 mg or 127.3 mg root daily
Route of administration	Oral
Randomized	Yes
Randomization adequate	Yes
Blinding	Double-blind
Blinding adequate	Yes
Placebo	No
Drug comparison	No
Site description	4 gynecological clinics
No. of subjects enrolled	152
No. of subjects completed	123
Sex	Female
Age	42-60 years (mean: 50)

Inclusion criteria
Peri- and postmenopausal volunteers aged 42 to 60 who had a Kupperman Menopausal Index of at least 20 were included in this study.

Exclusion criteria
Serious gynecological, internal, or psychiatric diseases were exclusion criteria, as well as all other circumstances that could interfere with the study.

End points
The primary assessment of the degree of menopausal symptoms and of possible therapeutic effects was the Kupperman Menopausal Index. The self-depression scale (SDS), as well as the clinical global impressions scale, were secondary parameters. Assessments were carried out at baseline and after 2, 4, 8, 12, 16, 20, and 24 weeks. Hormone tests (17 beta estradiol, lutenizing hormone, follicle-stimulating hormone, prolactin, and sex hormone-binding globulin) and studies of vaginal cytology were also conducted. Physiological parameters were evaluated at baseline and at weeks 4, 12, and 24.

Results
Both doses of black cohosh extract lowered the Kupperman index. Seventy percent of the standard-dose (39 mg) group were responders, as were 72 percent of the high-dose (127.3 mg) group. The median score on the SDS also decreased for both groups (from 44.5 to 37 and from 44 to 36, respec-

tively). A large majority of both groups rated the global assessment of efficacy after 12 weeks as "very good" or "good" (78.4 percent and 78.6 percent, respectively). Neither treatment was significantly better than the other for any of the efficacy criteria. Black cohosh did not alter the vaginal cytology measures in the 12-week study, and no significant differences were observed in hormone levels.

Side effects
The incidence of adverse events was statistically equal in both groups. Most of the adverse events were mild or moderate and included the following organ classes: gastrointestinal, CNS, breast/genitals, and other. Biochemical or hematological laboratory findings were not affected by either dose.

Authors' comments
The findings indicate that this *C. racemosa* formulation offers an alternative for menopausal complaints when HRT is either contraindicated or refused.

Reviewer's comments
The exclusion criteria is vague; no mention is made of medications, other botanicals, soy, etc. This study suffers from the lack of a placebo arm, but it provides useful safety data on endometrial effects, hormonal effects, and adverse events. (5, 5)

Clinical Study: Remifemin®

Extract name	None given
Manufacturer	Schaper & Brümmer GmbH & Co. KG, Germany
Indication	**Menopausal symptoms;** hot flashes in women treated for breast cancer
Level of evidence	**II**
Therapeutic benefit	**No**

Bibliographic reference
Jacobson JS, Troxel AB, Evans J, Klaus L, Vahdat L, Kinne D, Lo KMS, Moore A, Rosenman PJ, Kaufman EL, et al. (2001). Randomized trial of black cohosh for the treatment of hot flashes among women with a history of breast cancer. *Journal of Clinical Oncology* 19 (10): 2739-2745.

Trial design
Parallel. Patients were either taking tamoxifen (59) or no tamoxifen (26), and these groups were then randomized to receive either placebo or black

cohosh. Subjects were allowed to use nonhormonal medications during the study but were instructed not to begin new therapy for hot flashes.

Study duration	2 months
Dose	1 tablet twice daily
Route of administration	Oral
Randomized	Yes
Randomization adequate	Yes
Blinding	Double-blind
Blinding adequate	Yes
Placebo	Yes
Drug comparison	No
Site description	Medical center
No. of subjects enrolled	85
No. of subjects completed	69
Sex	Female
Age	>18 years

Inclusion criteria
Women over 18 years who were previously treated for breast cancer, completed primary therapy, including radiation therapy and chemotherapy, at least two months before the trial start, and experienced hot flashes daily

Exclusion criteria
The use of hormonal replacement therapy for hot flashes, pregnancy, major psychiatric illness, or known recurrent or metastatic breast cancer.

End points
Patients recorded the intensity and number of hot flashes for three days before beginning treatment, on days 27 to 30, and again on days 57 to 60. Subjects also completed a detailed menopausal symptom index and a visual analog scale rating overall health and well-being before starting treatment and at the end of the study. The first 41 subjects were asked to supply a blood sample at the first and last visits. Follicle-stimulating hormone and luteinizing hormone levels were examined for the first 37 and 18 women, respectively (of those who provided blood samples).

Results
Both groups reported a decline in the number of hot flashes; from baseline to the trial end this decline was about 27 percent. The differences between treatment groups at the trial end were not significant. Both groups also experienced a decline in hot flash intensity, but the difference between groups was not significant. Improvements in menopausal symptoms and the global

ratings of well-being and health were seen in both the treatment and placebo groups, but the treatment group reported only a significantly greater improvement for sweating ($p = 0.04$). For those samples tested, the changes in FSH and LH were small and not statistically significant in any group.

Side effects

Three serious adverse events were reported (one in placebo/tamoxifen group and two in treatment/tamoxifen group), including hysterectomy, breast cancer recurrence, and appendectomy. Ten minor adverse events were also reported (six in treatment/tamoxifen group, two in placebo/tamoxifen group, and two in placebo/no tamoxifen group). None of the adverse events appeared to be related to treatment with black cohosh.

Authors' comments

In short, for breast cancer survivors, these data provide little evidence of either harm or benefit from using black cohosh to control hot flashes, although a reduction in sweating may be important to patients.

Reviewer's comments

The dose of black cohosh extract was not given, and the identity of the product was obtained through credits to the manufacturer. Soy or other medications that may affect hot flashes (selective serotonin reuptake inhibitors, clonidine, etc.) were not excluded. The sample size was also too small for women not on tamoxifen. (5, 4)

Clinical Study: Remifemin®

Extract name	None given
Manufacturer	Schaper & Brümmer GmbH & Co. KG, Germany
Indication	**Menopausal symptoms;** gonadotropins (LH and FSH release) in menopausal women
Level of evidence	**III**
Therapeutic benefit	**MOA**

Bibliographic reference

Duker E, Kopanski L, Jarry H, Wuttke W (1991). Effects of extracts from *Cimicifuga racemosa* on gonadotropin release in menopausal women and ovariectomized rats. *Planta Medica* 57 (5): 420-424.

Trial design
Parallel.

Study duration	2 months
Dose	2 (2 mg extract) tablets twice daily
Route of administration	Oral
Randomized	No
Randomization adequate	No
Blinding	Open
Blinding adequate	No
Placebo	Yes
Drug comparison	No
Site description	Single center
No. of subjects enrolled	110
No. of subjects completed	Not given
Sex	Female
Age	Mean: 52 years

Inclusion criteria
Patients who had received no steroid replacement therapy for at least six months and complained about climacteric (menopausal) symptoms.

Exclusion criteria
None mentioned.

End points
After two months of treatment, blood samples were drawn. LH and FSH were measured in blood samples.

Results
LH, but not FSH, levels were significantly reduced in patients receiving the *Cimicifuga* extract compared with placebo ($p < 0.05$).

Side effects
None mentioned.

Authors' comments
Data demonstrate for the first time that a commercially available extract (Remifemin) selectively suppresses LH secretion in menopausal women, which points to an estrogenic effect of *Cimifuga racemosa* preparations.

Reviewer's comments
This trial is limited by several flaws: trial was not blinded or randomized; no exclusion criteria were provided; and no description of dropouts was given. (0, 3)

Boxwood

Latin name: ***Buxus sempervirens*** **L.** [Buxaceae]
Plant part: **Leaf**

PREPARATIONS USED
IN REVIEWED CLINICAL STUDIES

The leaves of the boxwood tree were formerly used as a botanical remedy in Europe for "purifying the blood" and for rheumatism (*PDR*, 1998). The preparation used in this clinical study is called SPV_{30}^{TM} and contains boxwood leaf powder. It is manufactured by Arkopharma Laboratoires Pharmaceutiques in France and distributed by the U.S. division (Health from the Sun/Arkopharma) in Bedford, Massachusetts.

SUMMARY OF REVIEWED CLINICAL STUDIES

Human immunodeficiency virus (HIV) infection usually leads to AIDS (acquired immune deficiency syndrome) or AIDS-related symptoms. One indication of the progression of the disease is the number of CD4 T-lymphocytes (a type of white blood cell) in the blood. The idea for the use of boxwood in HIV disease came from an anecdotal report backed by laboratory data. It was noticed that an individual's intake of a boxwood product, $SPV_{30,}$ appeared to correlate with an increase in lymphocyte (CD4) cell count.

SPV_{30}

Human Immunodeficiency Virus

A well-designed, placebo-controlled study was designed to explore the use of SPV_{30} in 135 asymptomatic HIV patients who had

BOXWOOD SUMMARY TABLE

Product Name	Manufacturer/ U.S. Distributor	Product Characteristics	Dose in Trials	Indication	No. of Trials	Benefit (Evidence Level-Trial No.)
SPV$_{30}$™	Arkopharma Laboratoires Pharmaceutiques, France/Health from the Sun/ Arkopharma	Powdered leaves	2 (165 mg) capsules every 8 hours (990 mg per day)	HIV	1	Yes (I-1)

not previously taken any antiretroviral or immunomodulating medicines. There was a significant benefit compared with placebo in patients given a dose of two (165 mg each) capsules every eight hours. Benefit was seen as fewer decreases in CD4 cell counts, fewer increases in viral load, and a slower overall rate of disease progression. Less benefit was seen in the group given a higher dose of two (330 mg) capsules every eight hours (Durant et al., 1998). In spite of the positive outcome with the lower dose, our reviewer, Dr. Richard O'Connor, questioned the utility of the preparation due to the availability of highly effective modern antiretroviral therapy.

ADVERSE REACTIONS OR SIDE EFFECTS

No severe side effects were reported in the trial reviewed, and there was no significant difference in adverse reactions between the treatment and placebo groups.

No health hazards or side effects are reported with the proper administration of designated therapeutic dosages of boxwood leaf preparations in general. However, toxic effects, such as diarrhea, vomiting, severe clonic spasms, and ultimately signs of paralysis followed by fatal asphyxiation, can occur if taken in large doses (e.g., for dogs: 5 to 10 g/kg body weight) (*PDR*, 1998). This toxicity has been reported in cows, horses, and pigs that have eaten clippings left in the pasture (Bruneton, 1999).

REFERENCES

Bruneton J (1999). *Toxic Plants Dangerous to Humans and Animals.* Paris, France: Lavoisier Publishing.

Durant, J, Chantre Ph, Gonzales G, Vandermander J, Halfon Ph, Rousse B, Guedon D, Rahelinirina V, Chamaret S, Montagnier L, Dellamonica P (1998). Efficacy and safety of *Buxus sempervirens* L. preparations (SPV$_{30}$) in HIV-infected asymptomatic patients: A multicentre, randomized, double-blind, placebo-controlled trial. *Phytomedicine* 5 (1): 1-10.

PDR for Herbal Medicines (1998). Montvale, NJ: Medical Economics Co.

DETAILS ON BOXWOOD PRODUCTS
AND CLINICAL STUDIES

Product and clinical study information is grouped in the same order as in the Summary Table. A profile on an individual product is followed by details of the clinical studies associated with that product. In some instances a clinical study, or studies, supports several products that contain the same principal ingredient(s). In these instances, those products are grouped together.

Clinical studies that follow each product, or group of products, are grouped by therapeutic indication, in accordance with the order in the Summary Table.

Product Profile: SPV$_{30}$™

Manufacturer	**Arkopharma Laboratoires Pharmaceutiques, France**
U.S. distributor	**Health from the Sun/Arkopharma**
Botanical ingredient	**Boxwood leaf**
Extract name	**SPV$_{30}$**
Quantity	330 mg
Processing	Powdered plant material
Standardization	No information
Formulation	Capsule

Recommended dose: Take one capsule three times per day with a glass of water.

DSHEA structure/function: Nutritional support for the body's immune system. Strengthens immune function by maintaining a healthy immune cell count.

Cautions: If taking any medications or are pregnant or lactating, consult a physician before taking this product.

Other ingredients: Cellulose derivative (capsule shell).

Source(s) of information: Product package and leaflet.

Clinical Study: SPV$_{30}$™

Extract name	SPV$_{30}$
Manufacturer	Arkopharma Laboratoires Pharmaceutiques, France

Indication	**Human immunodeficiency virus**
Level of evidence	I
Therapeutic benefit	**Yes**

Bibliographic reference

Durant J, Chantre Ph, Gonzales G, Vandermander J, Halfon Ph, Rousse B, Guedon D, Rahelinirina V, Chamaret S, Montagnier L, Dellamonica P (1998). Efficacy and safety of *Buxus sempervirens* L. preparations (SPV$_{30}$) in HIV-infected asymptomatic patients: A multicentre, randomized, double-blind, placebo-controlled trial. *Phytomedicine* 5 (1): 1-10.

Trial design

Parallel. Two doses of SPV$_{30}$ compared to placebo. The study was designed to last 18 months. However, it was stopped early due to the decision that it was unethical to carry on the trial with a placebo group. Therefore the median treatment duration for placebo was 37 weeks (range 8 to 64), for SPV$_{30}$ 990 mg 37 weeks (range 4 to 64), and for SPV$_{30}$ 1980 mg 38 weeks (range 4 to 64).

Study duration	4 to 64 weeks (median 37 weeks)
Dose	2 (165 mg or 330 mg) capsules every 8 hours (990 or 1980 mg/day)
Route of administration	Oral
Randomized	Yes
Randomization adequate	Yes
Blinding	Double-blind
Blinding adequate	Yes
Placebo	Yes
Drug comparison	No
Site description	16 hospitals
No. of subjects enrolled	145
No. of subjects completed	135
Sex	Male and female
Age	Mean: 34 years

Inclusion criteria

Asymptomatic, seropositive HIV, CD4 lymphocyte counts from 250 to 500 ×

$10^6/l$, platelet count $>75 \times 10^9/l$, hemoglobin >9.0 mg/dl, serum transaminases less than five times the upper limit of normal values, serum creatinine <200 µmol/l, Karnofsky performance score at least 90 percent, and age at least 18 years.

Exclusion criteria
Patients who had previously taken antiretroviral or immunomodulating medicines, and pregnant women. The following concomitant medication was not allowed during the study: anti-HIV therapy (AZT, DDI, D4T, 3TC, DDC); any drug under investigation; cancer chemotherapy; systemic corticosteroids (>7 days); and immunomodulator and immunosuppressive treatments.

End points
Patients were evaluated every four weeks for adverse events, signs, and symptoms of HIV disease. Body weight and Karnofsky performance scores were recorded and blood was taken. Therapeutic failures were defined by occurrence of AIDS, AIDS-related complex, or decrease of CD4 cell count below $200 \times (10^6)/l$ twice.

Results
There was a statistically significant difference in therapeutic failures between groups in favor of the 990 mg group, including decreases of CD4 cell count and/or number of clinical aggravations. The treatment groups differed statistically in the rate of disease progression in favor of 990 mg/day. Fewer patients receiving 990 mg/day had an increase in viral load greater than 0.5 log at the end ($p = 0.029$). The higher-dose group did not experience an overall benefit.

Side effects
No severe side effects observed.

Authors' comments
From these results, SPV_{30} 990 mg per day has beneficial effects in HIV asymptomatic patients and appears to delay the progression of HIV disease.

Reviewer's comments
A well-designed, well-described study. Institutional review board (IRB) approval and informed consent from subjects were obtained. HIV seropositive patients were not receiving antiretroviral therapy in this study. The effectiveness seen in the low-dose group did not occur in the high-dose group, but the utility of SPV_{30} seems unlikely with the availability of highly active antiretroviral therapy (HAART) that is now used. (5, 6)

Butterbur, Purple

Other common names: **Petasites, sweet coltsfoot**
Latin name: *Petasites hybridus* **(L.) P. Gaertn. et al.**
[Asteraceae]
Latin synonyms: *Petasites officinalis* **Moench**
Plant part: **Root**

PREPARATIONS USED
IN REVIEWED CLINICAL STUDIES

Purple butterbur, or petasites, rhizomes (underground parts) have been traditionally used in Europe for their antispasmodic and analgesic activity. The active chemical constituents are thought to be a group of sesquiterpenes, the petasins (Grossmann and Schmidramsl, 2000).

Petadolex™ contains a liquid carbon dioxide extract of butterbur root (plant/extract ratio 30:1) standardized to contain at least 7.5 mg petasin and isopetasin. The commercial product contains 50 mg extract per capsule, and the recommended dose is one capsule twice daily. It is manufactured by Weber & Weber International GmbH & Co. KG in Germany and distributed by Weber & Weber USA in Manson, Washington.

ZE 339 is manufactured in Switzerland by Zeller AG. It is a carbon dioxide extract standardized to 8.0 mg total petasins per tablet. It is not sold in the United States.

BUTTERBUR SUMMARY TABLE

Product Name	Manufacturer/ U.S. Distributor	Product Characteristics	Dose in Trials	Indication	No. of Trials	Benefit (Evidence Level-Trial No.)
Petadolex™	Weber & Weber Intl. GmbH & Co. KG, Germany/ Weber & Weber USA	Liquid carbon dioxide extraction	2 (25 mg) capsules twice daily	Migraine prevention	1	Yes (I-1)
ZE 339	Zeller AG	Liquid carbon dioxide extraction (ZE 339)	1 tablet four times daily	Allergic rhinitis (hay fever)	1	Yes (II-1)

SUMMARY OF REVIEWED CLINICAL STUDIES

Petadolex

Migraine Prevention

The cause of migraine headaches is largely unknown; however, the cause may be a combination of a constriction of blood vessels and an inflammation affecting the nerves in the brain. A well-designed and well-conducted study on the prevention (prophylaxis) of migraine headaches was conducted using 60 patients. A dose of 50 mg twice daily was given for three months. Patients taking Petadolex had significantly fewer migraine attacks and comparatively fewer migraine days per month compared to those given placebo (Grossmann and Schmidramsl, 2000).

ZE 339

Allergic Rhinitis (Hay Fever)

A trial was conducted comparing ZE 339 to cetirizine which included 124 adults with a history of seasonal allergic rhinitis (hay fever) with the symptoms of runny nose, nasal congestion, and itchy nose or eyes. Cetirizine reduces allergy symptoms through blocking histamine activity (Hardman et al., 1996). In a double-placebo design, subjects were given either ZE 339 (one tablet four times daily) or cetirizine (one 10 mg tablet daily) for two weeks. At the end of the treatment period, there was no difference in the two groups according to a questionnaire they filled out covering physical and emotional function, vitality, mental health, general health, physical activity, social functioning, and pain. There was also no difference in a clinical global impression scale (CGI) evaluated by attending physicians (Schapowal, 2002). Our reviewer, Dr. Richard O'Connor, commented that the study lacked a placebo group, which is essential in hay fever trials in which response rates of 40 to 50 percent have been reported. Also, it would have been preferable to examine hay fever symptoms as an end point and not just quality-of-life measures.

ADVERSE REACTIONS OR SIDE EFFECTS

No adverse effects were reported by patients taking Petadolex during the trial. In the trial with ZE 339, the incidence of side effects was similar to those with cetirizine (16 to 17 percent). In the butterbur group, the most commonly reported effects were fatigue and headache.

INFORMATION FROM PHARMACOPOEIAL MONOGRAPHS

Source of Published Therapeutic Monographs

German Commission E

Indications

The dried roots (underground parts) are approved by the German Commission E as supportive therapy for acute spastic pain in the urinary tract, particularly if stones exist. The action is antispasmodic. The leaf is not approved for use, as the effectiveness is not well documented, and the leaves may contain toxic pyrrolizidine alkaloids. However, the leaves are used for nervous cramplike states and associated pain, colic, headaches, as well as to stimulate the appetite (Blumenthal et al., 1998).

Doses

Root: preparations equivalent to 4.5 to 7 g per day (Blumenthal et al., 1998)

Treatment Period

The Commission E suggests that treatment periods not last longer than four to six weeks per year (Blumenthal et al., 1998).

Contraindications

Pregnancy and nursing are contraindicated while taking butterbur according to the Commission E (Blumenthal et al., 1998).

Adverse Reactions

The Commission E lists no known adverse reactions (Blumenthal et al., 1998).

Drug Interactions

The Commission E lists no known drug interactions (Blumenthal et al., 1998).

REFERENCES

Blumenthal M, Busse W, Hall T, Goldberg A, Gruenwald J, Riggins C, Rister S, eds. (1998). *The Complete German Commission E Monographs: Therapeutic Guide to Herbal Medicines.* Trans. S Klein. Austin, TX: American Botanical Council.

Grossmann M, Schmidramsl H (2000). An extract of *Petasites hybridus* is effective in the prophylaxis of migraine. *International Journal of Clinical Pharmacology and Therapeutics* 38 (10): 430-435. (Also published in Grossmann W [1996]. *Der Freie Arzt* 3 [May/June].)

Hardman JG, Limbird LE, Molinoff PB, Ruddon RW, Gilman AG (1996). *Goodman and Gillman's The Pharmacological Basis of Therapeutics,* Ninth Edition. New York: McGraw-Hill.

Schapowal A (2002). Randomized controlled trial of butterbur and cetirizine for treating seasonal allergic rhinitis. *British Medical Journal* 324 (7330): 144-146.

DETAILS ON BUTTERBUR PRODUCTS
AND CLINICAL STUDIES

Product and clinical study information is grouped in the same order as in the Summary Table. A profile on an individual product is followed by details of the clinical studies associated with that product. In some instances a clinical study, or studies, supports several products that contain the same principal ingredient(s). In these instances, those products are grouped together.

Clinical studies that follow each product, or group of products, are grouped by therapeutic indication, in accordance with the order in the Summary Table.

Index to Butterbur Products

Product Profile: Petadolex™

Manufacturer	**Weber & Weber International GmbH & Co. KG, Germany**
U.S. distributor	**Weber & Weber USA**
Botanical ingredient	**Butterbur root extract**
Extract name	None given
Quantity	50 mg
Processing	Plant to extract ratio 30:1, liquid carbon dioxide extraction
Standardization	At least 7.5 mg of petasin and isopetasin
Formulation	Capsule

Recommended dose: One capsule twice daily with meals. Discontinue Petadolex after the initial cycle of four to six months. It will maintain its benefits even after taking it. Resume supplementation for another four- to six-month cycle when the number of migraines experienced begins to increase.

DSHEA structure/function: Helps maintain proper muscle tone in cerebral blood vessels; 62 percent reduction of migraine days.

Cautions: If pregnant or nursing a baby, do not use this product.

Other ingredients: Natural coloring: carmine, glycerol, gelatin, titanium-oxide.

Source(s) of information: Product package; Petadolex Caregiver's Guide; Grossmann and Schmidramsl, 2000.

Clinical Study: Petadolex™

Extract name	None given
Manufacturer	Weber & Weber GmbH & Co. KG, Germany
Indication	**Migraine prophylaxis** (prevention)
Level of evidence	**I**
Therapeutic benefit	**Yes**

Bibliographic reference
Grossmann M, Schmidramsl H (2000). An extract of *Petasites hybridus* is effective in the prophylaxis of migraine. *International Journal of Clinical Pharmacology and Therapeutics* 38 (10): 430-435. (Also published in Grossmann W [1996]. *Der Freie Arzt* 3 [May/June].)

Trial design
Parallel. Four-week run-in phase without trial medication, followed by three-month treatment period.

Study duration	3 months
Dose	2 (25 mg) capsules twice daily
Route of administration	Oral
Randomized	Yes
Randomization adequate	Yes
Blinding	Double-blind
Blinding adequate	Yes
Placebo	Yes
Drug comparison	No
Site description	Hospital outpatient clinic
No. of subjects enrolled	60
No. of subjects completed	58
Sex	Male and female
Age	19-38 years (mean: 29)

Inclusion criteria

Outpatients with a minimum of three attacks per month within the past three months prior to the study, and a minimum of two attacks in the four-week run-in phase. Inclusion criteria were as defined by the International Headache Society in 1988.

Exclusion criteria

Exclusion criteria were as defined by the International Headache Society in 1988.

End points

Outcome variables were the frequency, intensity, and duration of migraine attacks as well as accompanying symptoms. Patients recorded migraine attacks and symptoms in a diary. They were seen every four weeks.

Results

Patients taking Petadolex had significantly fewer migraine attacks than the placebo group and comparatively fewer migraine days per month ($p < 0.05$). The difference was noted four weeks after treatment began and continued until the end of the study. Pain intensity of migraines and duration of migraine attacks were lower in Petadolex group, but significant only at the end of the second month (and not at the end of the study).

Side effects

None reported by patients.

Authors' comments

The results suggest that migraine patients can benefit from prophylactic treatment with this special extract. The combination of high efficacy and excellent tolerance emphasizes the particular value that *Petasites hybridus* has for the prophylactic treatment of migraine.

Reviewer's comments

Sixty patients is a relatively small trial. Otherwise, a well-designed study with clearly defined inclusion/exclusion criteria and definitive end points. However, values are provided as mean +/–, but we are not told if the standard error of the mean (SEM) or standard deviation (SD) is used. Length of treatment (12 weeks) was long enough for a clear separation between groups to occur. (5, 5)

Product Profile: ZE 339

Manufacturer	**Zeller AG, Switzerland**
U.S. distributor	None

Botanical ingredient	**Butterbur leaf extract**
Extract name	**ZE 339**
Quantity	20-54 mg extract; 8 mg petasins
Processing	Carbon dioxide extract
Standardization	8.0 mg total petasins per tablet
Formulation	Tablet

Recommended dose: Adults and children over 12 years old should take 1 tablet twice daily during the allergy season. Up to 4 tablets can be taken if exposure to allergen is increased.

DSHEA structure/function: Swiss drug indication is: treatment of all symptoms of allergic rhinitis (hay fever).

Source(s) of information: Schapowal, 2002; communication with Zeller AG.

Clinical Study: ZE 339

Extract name	ZE 339
Manufacturer	Zeller AG, Switzerland
Indication	**Allergic rhinitis** (hay fever)
Level of evidence	**II**
Therapeutic benefit	**Yes**

Bibliographic reference
Schapowal A (2002). Randomised controlled trial of butterbur and cetirizine for treating seasonal allergic rhinitis. *British Medical Journal* 324 (7330): 144-146.

Trial design
Parallel. In a double-dummy design, subjects were given either butterbur extract or cetirizine (one 10 mg tablet daily).

Study duration	2 weeks
Dose	1 tablet 4 times daily (8 mg total petasine per tablet)
Route of administration	Oral
Randomized	Yes
Randomization adequate	Yes
Blinding	Double-blind
Blinding adequate	Yes

Placebo   No
Drug comparison   Yes
Drug name   Cetirizine

Site description   4 outpatient clinics

No. of subjects enrolled   131
No. of subjects completed   124
Sex   Male and female
Age   Mean: 37 years

Inclusion criteria
At least 18 years old with a history of seasonal allergic rhinitis (at least two consecutive years) with the presence of all the following symptoms: rhinorrhea, sneezing, nasal congestion, and itching (nose or eyes). Two or more of these symptoms must have been rated above 2 on a five-point scale (0 = none, 4 = very severe).

Exclusion criteria
Subjects were excluded if they had a history of alcohol or substance abuse; were pregnant or breast-feeding; had a parasitic disease causing an increase in IgE or eosinophil levels; had taken corticosteroids in the past two months, antihistamines in the past six weeks, or anti-inflammatories in the past two weeks; had nonseasonal rhinitis; had received an organ transplant; or had a serious concomitant disease.

End points
Participants were assessed at baseline and at the end of the two weeks of treatment. Assessment consisted of a full medical examination and laboratory tests (hematology and biochemistry). Participants also filled out a medical outcome health survey questionnaire (SF-36), and doctors rated the patients with a clinical global impressions score. The primary end point was the change from baseline to the treatment end of each score on the questionnaire, and the secondary outcome was the change in the clinical global impression score.

Results
Butterbur performed similarly to cetirizine on the primary outcome measure, the health survey questionnaire, which included questions regarding physical and emotional function, vitality, mental health, general health, physical activity, social functioning, and pain. There was also no difference in efficacy between the two treatments on the secondary outcome measure, the clinical global impression score, including the severity of the condition, global improvement, and the risk-to-benefit ratio.

Side effects
The incidence of adverse events was similar in both groups. None in the butterbur group could be specifically tied to the treatment, while two-thirds of the adverse events in the cetirizine group are typical of antihistamines (drowsiness and fatigue).

Author's comments
This randomized, double-blind study showed that the effects of butterbur (ZE 339 extract tablets) are similar to those of cetirizine in patients with seasonal allergic rhinitis. Butterbur did not produce the sedative effects associated with antihistamines and was well tolerated by patients.

Reviewer's comments
This study lacks a placebo group which is essential in trials of allergic rhinitis in which response rates of 40 to 50 percent have been reported. Also, it would have been better to examine clinical symptoms as a primary outcome, not just the quality-of-life measures. (5, 5)

Cat's Claw

Other common names: **Uña de gato**
Latin name: *Uncaria tomentosa* **(Willd.) DC.** [Rubiaceae]
Plant part: **Root**

PREPARATIONS USED
IN REVIEWED CLINICAL STUDIES

Cat's claw, or uña de gato, is a South American vine that has been used widely as a folk remedy. Claims have been made for its effectiveness against viral infections, including human immunodeficiency virus (HIV), as well as cancer, arthritis, and a long list of largely incurable diseases. Following clues from the Asháninka Indians in the Central Peruvian rain forest, it was discovered that there are two chemotypes of *U. tomentosa*. One contains predominately pentacyclic oxindole alkaloids (pteropodine, isopteropodine, isomitraphylline, etc.), which are reported to have immunostimulatory activity. The other chemotype contains primarily tetracyclic oxindole alkaloids (rhynochophylline and isorynchophylline), which are thought to oppose the actions of the pentacyclic oxindole alkaloids. Because these two chemotypes are identical in appearance, commercial cat's claw is usually a mixture of the two. Thus, it is suggested that cat's claw products taken for their immunostimulatory action have no more than 0.02 percent tetracyclic oxindole alkaloids (Schulz, Hänsel, and Tyler, 2001; Reinhard, 1999).

Saventaro® (Krallendorn®) capsules contain 20 mg root extract, which is standardized to 1.3 percent pentacyclic oxindole alkaloids and free of tetracyclic oxindole alkaloids. Saventaro is manufactured by IMMODAL Pharmaka GmbH in Austria and under license in the United States by Enzymatic Therapy, Green Bay, Wisconsin.

CAT'S CLAW SUMMARY TABLE

Product Name	Manufacturer/ U.S. Distributor	Product Characteristics	Dose in Trials	Indication	No. of Trials	Benefit (Evidence Level-Trial No.)
Saventaro® (US) Krallendorn® (EU)	IMMODAL Pharmaka GmbH, Austria/Enzymatic Therapy	Extract containing 1.3 percent pentacyclic oxindole alkaloids	3 (20 mg) capsules daily	Rheumatoid arthritis	1	Trend (III-1)

SUMMARY OF REVIEWED CLINICAL STUDIES

Saventaro

Rheumatoid Arthritis

Saventaro (three 20 mg capsules daily) was given to patients with rheumatoid arthritis stage II and III in a double-blind, placebo-controlled trial that included 40 subjects. After six months, there was a significant reduction in pain but no effect on joint swelling or laboratory indicators of inflammation compared to placebo (Clinical Examinations of Krallendorn Products, 1999). Our reviewer, Dr. John Trimmer Hicks, commented that although significant pain relief was documented, a much larger sample size is needed to prove significant differences in trials on disease-modifying agents for rheumatoid arthritis due to large placebo effects usually seen in these trials.

ADVERSE REACTIONS OR SIDE EFFECTS

The reviewed clinical trial reported no difference in adverse effects for the treatment and placebo groups.

REFERENCES

Clinical Examinations of Krallendorn Products: Double-blind placebo controlled trial in rheumatoid arthritis (1999). Confidential report by IMMODAL Pharmaka GmbH.

Reinhard KH (1999). *Uncaria tomentosa* (Willd.) DC: Cat's claw, *uña de gato*, or Savéntaro. *The Journal of Alternative and Complementary Medicine* 5 (2): 143-151.

Schulz V, Hänsel R, Tyler VE (2001). *Rational Phytotherapy: A Physicians' Guide to Herbal Medicine*, Fourth Edition. Trans. TC Telgar. Berlin: Springer-Verlag.

DETAILS ON CAT'S CLAW PRODUCTS AND CLINICAL STUDIES

Product and clinical study information is grouped in the same order as in the Summary Table. A profile on an individual product is followed by details of the clinical studies associated with that product. In some instances a clinical study, or studies, supports several products that contain the same principal ingredient(s). In these instances, those products are grouped together.

Clinical studies that follow each product, or group of products, are grouped by therapeutic indication, in accordance with the order in the Summary Table.

Product Profile: Saventaro®

Manufacturer	**Enzymatic Therapy® (IMMODAL Pharmaka GmbH, Austria)**
U.S. distributor	**Enzymatic Therapy**
Botanical ingredient	**Cat's claw root extract**
Extract name	None given
Quantity	20 mg
Processing	No information
Standardization	A minimum of 1.3 percent pentacyclic oxindole alkaloids and no tetracyclic oxindole alkaloids
Formulation	Capsule

Recommended dose: One capsule three times daily for the first ten days and one capsule daily thereafter.

DSHEA structure/function: Enhances natural immunity and modifies the acquired immune system.

Other ingredients: Cellulose, calcium carbonate, magnesium stearate, silicon dioxide, and gelatin capsule.

Comments: Sold in Europe as Krallendorn®. Saventaro is a trademark of IMMODAL Pharmaka GmbH, Austria. Enzymatic Therapy is licensed by IMMODAL to manufacture the product in the United States.

Source(s) of information: Product package.

Clinical Study: Krallendorn®

| Extract name | None given |
| Manufacturer | IMMODAL Pharmaka GmbH, Austria |

Indication	**Rheumatoid arthritis**
Level of evidence	**III**
Therapeutic benefit	**Trend**

Bibliographic reference
Clinical Examinations of Krallendorn Products: Double-blind placebo controlled trial in rheumatoid arthritis (1999). Confidential report by IMMODAL Pharmaka GmbH.

Trial design
Parallel. Both treatment and placebo groups also received disease-modifying therapy (salazopyrine or plaquenil) and analgesic therapy (nonsteroidal and steroidal anti-inflammatory drugs) on demand.

Study duration	6 months
Dose	3 capsules daily
Route of administration	Oral

Randomized	Yes
Randomization adequate	No
Blinding	Double-blind
Blinding adequate	No

| Placebo | Yes |
| Drug comparison | No |

| Site description | Hospital outpatient department |

No. of subjects enrolled	40
No. of subjects completed	35
Sex	Male and female
Age	Not given

Inclusion criteria
Patients with rheumatoid arthritis stage II and III.

Exclusion criteria
None mentioned.

End points
Examination of patients was carried out at baseline and at weeks 4, 8, 16, and 24. Primary criteria of efficacy were the number of tender and swollen

joints (ARA Index), the number and severity of joint pain (Ritchie index), and the subjective assessment of the tenderness and swelling of the joints by the patient (visual analog scale). Secondary criteria of efficacy were the degree of physical impairment (Health Assessment Questionnaire), the rating of joint pain by the patient (visual analog scale), the duration of morning stiffness, and the changes in the surrogate markers, erythrocyte sedimentation rate (ESR), corticotropin releasing factor (CRF), and rheumatoid factor.

Results
After six months, the number of tender joints in the active treatment group was significantly lower than in the placebo group ($p = 0.035$). There was no difference in the number of swollen joints, as both groups showed a decrease. The number of painful joints and the severity of the pain was significantly reduced in the active treatment group, compared with the placebo group ($p = 0.004$). No significant differences were found between the two groups in the patients' assessment of the disease activity, physical impairment, or pain. The duration of morning stiffness was significantly shorter in the active group at the end of treatment than in the placebo group ($p = 0.021$). Rheumatoid factor was significantly lower in the active treatment group than in the placebo group ($p = 0.030$).

Side effects
Adverse events were reported for ten patients in both groups. A definite causal relationship with administration of Krallendorn was not established for any of them.

Authors' comments
This study could indicate a positive effect of Krallendorn on the pathological mechanisms underlying rheumatoid arthritis.

Reviewer's comments
A significant analgesic effect was documented, but no significant effect on joint swelling or lab indicators of inflammation were documented. The size of each study group was too small—a much larger sample size is usually needed to prove significant differences between disease-modifying antirheumatic drugs and placebo in rheumatoid arthritis trials because of the large placebo effect in these clinical trials. (1, 3)

Chaste Tree

Other common names: **Vitex, agnus-castus, chasteberry, monk's pepper**
Latin name: *Vitex agnus-castus* L. [Verbenaceae]
Plant part: **Fruit**

PREPARATIONS USED IN REVIEWED CLINICAL STUDIES

Chaste tree is a shrub native to the Mediterranean region. The hard, black, round berries are used medicinally. The dried, ripe fruits are characterized as containing approximately 0.5 percent volatile oil. Also characteristic of the fruits are the iridoid glycosides (agnuside and aucubin), flavonoids (aglycone, casticin), and diterpenes (Schulz, Hänsel, and Tyler, 2001). Although chaste tree preparations are sometimes standardized to the content of the water-soluble iridoid glycosides, lipid-soluble constituents, in particular the bicyclic diterpenes, have been reported in experimental studies to have dopaminergic activity (Stansbury et al., 2001).

Mastodynon® N, manufactured by Bionorica Arzneimittel GmbH in Germany, contains chaste tree tincture (53 percent alcohol) in combination with five homeopathic herbal extracts: *Caulophyllum thalictroides, Cyclamen purpurascens, Strychnos ignatia, Iris versicolor,* and *Lilium tigrinum.* The daily dose of 2 × 30 drops (1.8 ml solution) contains 32.4 mg chaste tree fruit tincture (2 g plant material in 10 g tincture). Mastodynon N is also sold in tablet form. Mastodynon is distributed in the United States by Mediceutix, Inc.

Agnolyt® capsules, produced by Madaus AG, Germany, contain 3.5 to 4.2 mg dry extract (plant/extract ratio 9.58 to 11.5:1, 60 percent ethanol). Agnolyt is also available in liquid form. Agnolyt was previously sold by Nature's Way Products, Inc., as Femaprin, but the formulation of this product has changed and an equivalent of Agnolyt capsules is not currently available in the United States.

231

CHASTE TREE SUMMARY TABLE

Product Name	Manufacturer/ U.S. Distributor	Product Characteristics	Dose in Trials	Indication	No. of Trials	Benefit (Evidence Level-Trial No.)
Mastodynon® N (EU)	Bionorica Arzneimittel GmbH, Germany/Mediceutix, Inc.	Alcoholic tincture	30 drops twice daily	Mastalgia (cyclic breast pain)	3	Yes (II-1) Trend (II-1) Undetermined (III-1)
				Female infertility	1	Trend (II-1)
Agnolyt® (EU)	Madaus AG, Germany/None	Ethanolic extract	1 capsule (3.5-4.2 mg extract)	PMS	1	Yes (II-1)
Cycle Balance™ (US)	Zeller AG, Switzerland/General Nutrition Corporation (GNC)	Ethanolic extract (Ze 440)	1 tablet (20 mg extract)	PMS	1	Yes (II-1)

Ze 440, produced by Zeller AG, Switzerland, is a dried extract made with 60 percent ethanol (plant/extract ratio 6 to 12:1) and standardized to casticin levels. It is retailed in the United States by GNC under the name Cycle Balance™.

SUMMARY OF REVIEWED CLINICAL STUDIES

Clinical studies on chaste tree have explored its use for cyclical mastalgia (breast pain), female infertility, and premenstrual syndrome (PMS). Mild elevation of prolactin levels has been linked with breast tenderness, menstrual irregularities, infertility, and PMS. Chaste tree preparations are thought to reduce prolactin levels in the blood. Prolactin is secreted by the pituitary gland, and that secretion is mediated by dopamine through interaction with D_2 receptors. Chaste tree preparations are thought to act through stimulation of those receptors (Gorkow, Wuttke, and März, 1999).

Mastodynon

Mastalgia (Cyclic Breast Pain)

Three trials studied the use of Mastodynon for the treatment of cyclical mastalgia. The dose was 30 drops twice daily, or one tablet twice daily, taken for three to four menstrual cycles. In the first of two good-quality trials, Mastodynon solution and tablets were compared to placebo in a double-placebo designed trial with 104 women who had breast pain for at least three days in their most recent cycle. At the end of three menstrual cycles, the intensity of breast pain was significantly lower for both forms of Mastodynon compared to placebo. The onset of pain relief was earlier with the solution than with the tablet. The treatment had no effect on plasma levels of progesterone, follicle-stimulating hormone (FSH), or luteinizing hormone (LH). However, estradiol levels decreased and basal prolactin levels fell in comparison with placebo (Wuttke et al., 1997). The second study included 86 women who had breast pain for at least five days in the previous cycle. After the first and second cycles of treatment, pain intensity decreased significantly compared to placebo. After the third cycle, the pain scale level was so low for the Mastodynon group that only slight reductions were possible, and as a result, there was only a borderline difference between the Mastodynon and the placebo group at this time. After three and four cycles, the total number of pain-free days was significantly greater for the Mastodynon group (Halaška et al., 1999).

A third trial compared Mastodynon (30 drops twice daily) and progestin (5 mg twice daily) to placebo in 121 women with severe breast pain. Both treatments were better than placebo. After four cycles, good relief from premenstrual symptoms was reported for 82 percent of those given progestin, 74.5 percent of those given Mastodynon, but only 36.8 percent of those given placebo (Kubista, Muller, and Spona, 1986). Due to several methodological inadequacies, the efficacy of treatments used in this trial was deemed undetermined.

Female Infertility

Another placebo-controlled study with 66 women indicated a possible role for Mastodynon in female infertility due to secondary amenorrhea (cessation of menstruation) and luteal insufficiency. As a result of three months of treatment with Mastodynon, pregnancy occurred more than twice as often as in the placebo group (Gerhard et al., 1998). The outcome was evaluated as a trend toward efficacy. A longer trial, especially for secondary amenorrhea, would be more conclusive.

Agnolyt

Premenstrual Syndrome

A study with 105 women examined the use of Agnolyt (one capsule daily) for PMS with positive results. The study compared Agnolyt, given daily for three menstrual cycles, to pyridoxine (vitamin B_6, 100 mg twice daily), given for only the last 19 days of each cycle. In the pyridoxine group, a placebo was given on days one through 15. The chaste tree preparation was superior to pyridoxine in relieving symptoms as assessed, using a PMS symptom scale, by both patients and doctors (Lauritzen et al., 1997). Our reviewer, Dr. Tieraona Low Dog, suggested that this trial, although basically good, could have been strengthened by the addition of a placebo arm.

Ze 440

Premenstrual Syndrome

An overall good study with 169 women with PMS, comparing Ze 440, one tablet daily for three cycles, to placebo, found a significant improvement in combined PMS symptoms using a self-assessment scale. A 50 percent reduction in symptoms was experienced by 52 percent of women taking Ze 440 and 24 percent given placebo (Schellenberg, 2001).

POSTMARKETING SURVEILLANCE STUDIES

Two drug monitoring surveys were conducted with 1,542 patients with PMS who had been treated with Agnolyt solution for periods of up to 16 years. The mean duration of treatment was approximately five and one-half months. The mean dose was 42 drops daily. Improvement in symptoms was generally seen after 25 days of treatment. The doctors assessed the efficacy of treatment as good to very good in 71 percent of cases and as satisfactory in 21 percent of cases. The patients judged their symptoms as relieved (33 percent), improved (57 percent), or not changed (4 percent), with no data on the remaining 5 percent of patients (Dittmar et al., 1992).

A review cited five postmarketing studies with chaste tree preparations for PMS. In addition to the Dittmar and colleagues (1992) study mentioned previously, there were two more studies on the Agnolyt solution, one on the Mastodynon solution, and another on Femicur capsules supplied by Schaper & Brümmer GmbH and Co. KG, Germany. In general, PMS symptoms were eliminated in about one-third of the women and improved for one-half of the women (Gorkow, Wuttke, and März, 1999).

Another postmarketing study evaluated the effectiveness of Mastodynon solution for treatment of menstrual cycle disorders. Following treatment with 60 drops per day, 31 of 50 women with secondary amenorrhea began menstruating. Cycle lengths were normalized in 187 of 287 women with oligomenorrhea (cycles longer than 35 days), and in 139 of 192 women with polymenorrhea (cycles shorter than 26 days) (Gorkow, Wuttke, and März, 1999).

ADVERSE REACTIONS OR SIDE EFFECTS

Adverse events reported in the trials reviewed were generally mild to moderate, consisting mostly of nausea and gastrointestinal complaints.

Two drug monitoring surveys reported that 32 of 1,542 (2.1 percent) patients treated with a mean dose of 42 drops daily of Angolyt solution for over five months experienced side effects. The most common complaints were nausea, gastric complaints, and acne (Dittmar et al., 1992).

INFORMATION FROM PHARMACOPOEIAL MONOGRAPHS

Sources of Published Therapeutic Monographs

American Herbal Pharmacopoeia (AHP)
German Commission E

Indications

Preparations of the ripe, dried fruits of chaste tree are approved by the German Commission E for irregularities of the menstrual cycle, premenstrual complaints, and mastodynia (Blumenthal et al., 1998). The *American Herbal Pharmacopoeia* lists the following medical indications supported by clinical trials for chaste tree fruit: menstrual irregularities (secondary amenorrhea, oligomenorrhea, polymenorrhea); relief of PMS symptoms; mastalgia; latent hyperprolactinemia; and infertility due to luteal-phase dysfunction. The actions include menstrual cycle regulator; in vitro dopaminergic activity; prolactin release inhibition; and weak binding to opioid receptors in vitro (Stansbury et al., 2001).

Doses

Dried fruit: (powder) 30 to 40 mg once daily (Stansbury et al., 2001)

Tincture: (1:5) 20 drops two to three times daily (each dose equivalent to 36 mg/ml of dried chaste tree fruit (Stansbury et al., 2001)

Extracts: aqueous-alcoholic (50 to 70 percent v/v) from the crushed fruits taken as liquid or dry extract, amount corresponding to 30 to 40 mg fruit (Blumenthal et al., 1998)

Treatment Period

The *AHP* states that menstrual cycle disorders take three to six weeks of treatment to respond (Stansbury et al., 2001).

Contraindications

The Commission E lists no known contraindications, while the *AHP* claims that no authoritative data are available (Blumenthal et al., 1998; Stansbury et al., 2001).

Adverse Reactions

The Commission E states that there is an occasional occurrence of itching, urticarial exanthemas (Blumenthal et al., 1998). The *AHP* also lists the following adverse reactions for chaste tree: occasional minor skin irritations, nausea, acne, pruritis, rashes, headache, fatigue, tachycardia or palpitations, spotting, allergy, alopecia, circulatory problems, cycle changes, dizziness, ear pressure, edema, fibroid growth, hot flash, intraocular pressure, mastalgia, pelvic disease, polyurea, pyrosis, sweating, vaginitis, and weight gain (Stansbury et al., 2001).

Precautions

The Commission E lists no known precautions. However, the Commission E warns that chaste tree is not to be used during pregnancy, and in animal experiments, an influence on nursing (lactation) performance was observed (Blumenthal et al., 1998). The *AHP* also states that chaste tree is not to be used during pregnancy unless otherwise directed by an expert qualified in the use of the described substance. In addition, the *AHP* says that chaste tree should not be used for PMS if the prevailing symptom is depression and that a qualified expert should be consulted before using chaste tree fruit extract for breast-related symptoms (Stansbury et al., 2001).

Drug Interactions

Both the Commission E and the *AHP* state that interactions are unknown. However, in animal experiments, there is evidence of a dopaminergic effect of the drug; thus, with administration of a dopamine-receptor agonist, a reciprocal decrease in effect may occur (Blumenthal et al., 1998; Stansbury et al., 2001).

REFERENCES

Blumenthal M, Busse W, Hall T, Goldberg A, Gruenwald J, Riggins C, Rister S, eds. (1998). *The Complete German Commission E Monographs: Therapeutic Guide to Herbal Medicines*. Trans S. Klein. Austin, TX: American Botanical Council.

Dittmar FW, Bohnert KJ, Peeters M, Albrechr M, Lamertz M, Schmidt U (1992). Premenstrual syndrome, treatment with a phytopharmaceutical. *Klinik und Praxis, TW Gynakologie* 5: 60-58.

Gerhard I, Patek A, Monga B, Blank A, Gorkow C (1998). Mastodynon for female infertility: Randomized, placebo-controlled, clinical double-blind study. *Forschende Komplementarmedizin/Research in Complementary Medicine* 5 (6): 272-278.

Gorkow C, Wuttke W, März RW (1999). Evidence of efficacy of *Vitex agnus castus* preparations. In *Phytopharmaka V, Forschung und klinische Anwendung*. Eds. Loew D, Blume H, Dingermann TH. Darmstadt, Germany: Steinkopff Verlag GmbH & Co. KG, pp. 189-208.

Halaška M, Beles P, Gorkow C, Sieder C (1999). Treatment of cyclical mastalgia with a solution containing a *Vitex agnus castus* extract: Results of a placebo-controlled double-blind study. *The Breast* 8 (4): 175-181. (Also published in Halaška M, Raus K, Beles P, Martan A, Paithner KG [1998]. *Ceskoslovenska Gynekologie* 63 [5]: 388-392.)

Kubista E, Muller G, Spona J (1986). Treatment of mastopathy with cyclic mastodynia: Clinical results and hormone profile. *Gynakologische Rundschau* 26 (2): 65-79.

Lauritzen CH, Reuter HD, Repges R, Bohnert KJ, Schmidt U (1997). Treatment of premenstrual tension syndrome with *Vitex agnus castus:* Controlled, double-blind study versus pyridoxine. *Phytomedicine* 4 (3): 183-189.

Schellenberg R (2001). Treatment for the premenstrual syndrome with agnus castus fruit extract: Prospective, randomized, placebo controlled study. *British Medical Journal* 322 (7279): 134-137.

Schulz V, Hänsel R, Tyler VE (2001). *Rational Phytotherapy: A Physicians' Guide to Herbal Medicine,* Fourth Edition. Trans. TC Telger. Berlin: Springer-Verlag.

Stansbury J, Upton R, Graff A, Bunting D, Länger R, Sudberg S, Sudberg EM, Williamson E, Henklebach K, Hoberg E, et al. (2001). *Chaste Tree Fruit,* Vitex agnus-castus. American Herbal Pharmacopoeia and Therapeutic Compendium: Standards of Analysis, Quality Control, and Therapeutics. Eds. R Upton, A Graff. Santa Cruz, CA: American Herbal Pharmacopoeia.

Wuttke W, Splitt G, Gorkow C, Sieder C (1997). Treatment of a cyclical mastalgia with a medicinal product containing agnus castus: Results of a randomized, placebo-controlled, double-blind study. *Geburtshilfe und Frauenheilkunde* 57 (10): 569-574.

DETAILS ON CHASTE TREE PRODUCTS
AND CLINICAL STUDIES

Product and clinical study information is grouped in the same order as in the Summary Table. A profile on an individual product is followed by details of the clinical studies associated with that product. In some instances a clinical study, or studies, supports several products that contain the same principal ingredient(s). In these instances, those products are grouped together.

Clinical studies that follow each product, or group of products, are grouped by therapeutic indication, in accordance with the order in the Summary Table.

Index to Chaste Tree Products

Product Profile: Mastodynon® N

Manufacturer	**Bionorica Arzneimittel GmbH, Germany**
U.S. distributor	Mediceutix, Inc.
Botanical ingredient	**Chaste tree fruit extract**
Extract name	None given
Quantity	32.4 mg extract in 60 drops
Processing	10 g tincture (53 percent (v/v) alcohol) contains 2 g plant
Standardization	No information
Formulation	Solution

Recommended dose: Take 30 drops with some liquid in the morning and in the evening. Mastodynon N should be taken for at least three months, also during menstrual bleeding. Improvement is usually felt after six weeks.

DSHEA structure/function: German drug indications include menstrual disorders based on a temporary or permanent corpus luteum insufficiency; infertility due to corpus luteum insufficiency; complaints which can appear shortly before the monthly bleeding (premenstrual syndrome), such as mastodynia, psychic lability swellings of feet and hands, constipation, as well as headache or migraine; benign painful affections of the breast (fibrocystic mastopathy).

Cautions: If complaints reappear upon discontinuation of intake, the therapy should be continued after consultation with the attending physician. Mastodynon N is not indicated for treatment of malignant affections of the breasts.

Other ingredients: *Caulophyllum thalictroides* (dil. D4), *Cyclamen purpurascens* (dil. D4), *Strychnos ignatii* (dil. D6), *Iris versicolor* (dil. D2), *Lilium tigrinum* (dil. D3).

Source(s) of information: Halaška et al., 1999; patient information leaflet (Bionorica GmbH).

Clinical Study: Mastodynon®

Extract name	None given
Manufacturer	Bionorica Arzneimittel GmbH, Germany
Indication	**Mastalgia** (cyclic breast pain)
Level of evidence	**II**
Therapeutic benefit	**Yes**

Bibliographic reference
Wuttke W, Splitt G, Gorkow C, Sieder C (1997). Treatment of a cyclical mastalgia with a medicinal product containing agnus castus: Results of a randomized, placebo-controlled, double-blind study. *Geburtshilfe und Frauenheilkunde* 57 (10): 569-574.

Trial design
Mastodynon solution and tablets were compared to placebo with a double-dummy technique, in three parallel groups, over three menstrual cycles. Treatment was preceded by an observation cycle during which the inclusion and exclusion criteria were evaluated.

Study duration	3 menstrual cycles
Dose	30 drops or 1 tablet Mastodynon twice daily
Route of administration	Oral
Randomized	Yes
Randomization adequate	Yes

Blinding	Double-blind
Blinding adequate	Yes
Placebo	Yes
Drug comparison	No
Site description	Multicenter
No. of subjects enrolled	120
No. of subjects completed	104
Sex	Female
Age	Mean: 33 years

Inclusion criteria
Included were patients who had suffered from clinical mastodynia for at least three cycles with breast pain on at least three days in the last cycle prior to the study. During the course of treatment, the use of hormones or treatment with hormonelike medication was not permitted.

Exclusion criteria
Third-degree galactorrhea, purulent/bloody mammary discharge, severe endocrinopathy, malignoma, necessary breast surgery, simultaneous treatment with analgesics or nonsteroidal antiphlogistics, having undergone alcohol withdrawal treatment, pregnancy, and lactation.

End points
Checkups were conducted in the premenstrual week, in cycles 0, 1, 2, and 3. Patients kept a daily pain journal and indicated the intensity of breast pain on the visual, linear analog scale (VAS). Hormone levels were measured in the premenstrual week of cycles 0, 1, 2, and 3. Analysis of prolactin values after metoclopramide stimulation was carried out in cycles 0 and 3.

Results
At the end of the three-cycle treatment period, the VAS values for breast pain were significantly lower for the tablet and solution groups compared to placebo ($p = 0.0067$ and $p = 0.0076$, respectively). The onset of action for patients taking solution occurred after the first treatment cycle, which was faster than the tablet formulation. The treatment had no effect on progesterone, FSH, and LH. Under both active formulations, estradiol-17 beta values decreased. Basal prolactin levels fell significantly in comparison with placebo, $p = 0.039$ solution, $p = 0.015$ tablets. In comparison with placebo, stimulated prolactin levels at the end of treatment tended to be lower under both active formulations.

Side effects
In general, subjective tolerance was good. Adverse events were mostly mild to moderate, consisting of nausea and gastrointestinal complaints. Severe

adverse reactions in three subjects (nausea and punctual, severe breast pain) led to the discontinuation of treatment.

Authors' comments
The solution and the tablets of the preparation containing agnus castus are effective in mastalgia. Basal prolactin levels dropped significantly with both forms of the preparation. The subjective tolerance was good.

Reviewer's comments
Study was randomized and double-blind with the outcome measures clearly defined. However, subjects were not excluded for taking evening primrose oil, B_6, or other phytochemicals. No power calculation was performed, but sample size is likely sufficient. (5, 3)

Clinical Study: Mastodynon®

Extract name	None given
Manufacturer	Bionorica Arzneimittel GmbH, Germany
Indication	**Mastalgia** (cyclic breast pain)
Level of evidence	**II**
Therapeutic benefit	**Trend**

Bibliographic reference
Halaška M, Beles P, Gorkow C, Sieder C (1999). Treatment of cyclical mastalgia with a solution containing a *Vitex agnus castus* extract: Results of a placebo-controlled double-blind study. *The Breast* 8 (4): 175-181. (Also published in Halaška M, Raus K, Beles P, Martan A, Paithner KG [1998]. *Ceskoslovenska Gynekologie* 63 [5]: 388-392.)

Trial design
Parallel. Trial was preceded by one menstrual cycle without treatment in which patients were examined for inclusion and exclusion criteria.

Study duration	4 menstrual cycles
Dose	2 × 30 drops (1.8 ml) daily
Route of administration	Oral
Randomized	Yes
Randomization adequate	No
Blinding	Double-blind
Blinding adequate	Yes
Placebo	Yes

Drug comparison   No

Site description   Single center

No. of subjects enrolled   97
No. of subjects completed   86
Sex   Female
Age   18-45 years

Inclusion criteria
Patients with mastalgia on at least five days in the cycle before treatment began. The minimum cycle duration within the last three cycles before treatment was 25 days; the maximum duration was 35 days. Signs of fibrocystic mastopathic tissue alterations were allowed. Hormonal contraceptives were admitted providing they had been taken for the past six months before treatment and were continued without alteration.

Exclusion criteria
Breast cancer, fibroadenoma, intraductal papilloma, galactorrhea, purulent or bloody nipple discharge, severe endocrinopathies, recent or impending breast surgery, concomitant therapy with analgesics or NSAIDs, and successful alcohol detoxication were exclusion criteria. Pregnancy and lactation were also reasons for exclusion from the study.

End points
Assessment was carried out on day 3 or 4 of cycles 1, 2, 3, and 4 using the visual analog scale score for the intensity of mastalgia. Patients also recorded pain in a daily diary.

Results
After the first and second cycles, there were significant differences in the mean decrease in pain intensity between the Mastodynon group and placebo ($p = 0.018$ and $p = 0.006$, respectively). After three cycles, there was only borderline significance between Mastodynon and placebo in the decrease in pain intensity ($p = 0.064$); in the treatment group after three cycles, the pain scale level was so low that only slight reductions were possible. After three and four cycles, the Mastodynon group had significantly more pain-free days compared with placebo ($p = 0.007$ and $p = 0.014$, respectively).

Side effects
Adverse events were slight; no difference in frequency in the two groups.

Authors' comments
The current study demonstrated that Mastodynon is an effective and well-tolerated treatment for breast pain. The favorable benefit-risk ratio justifies the use of *Vitex agnus-castus*–containing solution for at least three months

in women with severe breast pain, before alternative drugs with a higher rate of side effects are considered.

Reviewer's comments
Although the study was randomized, no description of the randomization process was provided. Subjects were not excluded for taking B_6, evening primrose oil, or other phytochemicals. Sample size was appropriate, and outcome measures were clearly defined. (3, 5)

Clinical Study: Mastodynon®

Extract name	None given
Manufacturer	Bionorica Arzneimittel GmbH, Germany
Indication	**Mastalgia** (cyclic breast pain)
Level of evidence	**III**
Therapeutic benefit	**Undetermined**

Bibliographic reference
Kubista E, Muller G, Spona J (1986). Treatment of mastopathy with cyclic mastodynia: Clinical results and hormone profile. *Gynakologische Rundschau* 26 (2): 65-79.

Trial design
Three parallel groups, Mastodynon compared with a progestin (Lynestrenol 2 x 5 mg from the sixteenth to twenty-fifth day of the cycle) and placebo.

Study duration	4 menstrual cycles
Dose	2 x 30 drops daily
Route of administration	Oral
Randomized	Yes
Randomization adequate	No
Blinding	Double-blind
Blinding adequate	No
Placebo	Yes
Drug comparison	Yes
Drug name	Lynestrenol (a progestin)
Site description	Gynecology and Obstetrics Division, University of Vienna
No. of subjects enrolled	160
No. of subjects completed	121

Sex   Female
Age   Not given

Inclusion criteria
Female patients with severe clinical manifestations of mastopathy with cyclic mastodynia, normal cycles, and nonsuspicious mammographic and thermographic results.

Exclusion criteria
Patients who had taken drugs with effects on prolactin levels.

End points
Before the study and after two and four cycles of treatment, prolactin and progesterone serum levels were measured. The clinical efficacy of treatment was evaluated on a basis of a self-evaluated pain scale. Thermographic and mammographic checks were conducted before and after three months of therapy.

Results
The best clinical result was obtained in the progestin group: 82.1 percent of patients reported a marked improvement of the premenstrual pain and premenstrual tension, compared to 74.5 percent of the Mastodynon group and 36.8 percent of placebo group. The efficacy of Mastodynon was significantly better than placebo ($p < .01$). After two cycles of treatment, prolactin levels increased and progesterone levels fell in the progestin group ($p < 0.01$) relative to the placebo and Mastodynon groups.

Side effects
Mild side effects, consisting mostly of nausea and weight gain, were reported by 7.2 percent of Mastodynon patients compared to 21.4 percent of the progestin group and 10.5 percent of the placebo group.

Authors' comments
Despite their efficacy, long-term therapy with progestins should be applied only after other possibilities of therapy have been exhausted. Therapy with the nonhormonal phytotherapeutic preparation Mastodynon constitutes a reliable alternative to progestins which is low in side effects.

Reviewer's comments
The study had no discussion of randomization. Only Mastodynon and placebo arms appear blinded, not the progestin arm. Although a description of withdrawals and dropouts was provided, adequate inclusion/exclusion details were not given. (1, 4)

Clinical Study: Mastodynon®

Extract name	None given
Manufacturer	Bionorica Arzneimittel GmbH, Germany

Indication	**Female infertility**
Level of evidence	**II**
Therapeutic benefit	**Trend**

Bibliographic reference
Gerhard I, Patek A, Monga B, Blank A, Gorkow C (1998). Mastodynon for female infertility: Randomized, placebo-controlled, clinical double-blind study. *Forschende Komplementarmedizin/Research in Complementary Medicine* 5 (6): 272-278.

Trial design
Parallel. After verification of inclusion and exclusion criteria, patients went through a treatment-free diagnostic cycle.

Study duration	3 months
Dose	2 × 30 drops daily
Route of administration	Oral
Randomized	Yes
Randomization adequate	No
Blinding	Double-blind
Blinding adequate	Yes
Placebo	Yes
Drug comparison	No
Site description	Single center
No. of subjects enrolled	96
No. of subjects completed	66
Sex	Female
Age	Mean: 29 years

Inclusion criteria
Women suffering from secondary amenorrhea (spontaneous menstruation less than once every three months), corpus luteal insufficiency, or idiopathic infertility. Women trying unsuccessfully to become pregnant for about two years. Patency of at least one fallopian tube, positive or not more than restricted Sims-Huhner postcoital test eight to twelve hours after sexual intercourse on the ovulation date or after previous estrogen treatment, and good general health. Male partners were to present a current normal spermio-

gram. Women were to have used no medication at all, and the last hormone treatment was to have taken place at least three months previously.

Exclusion criteria
Anatomical anomalies causing infertility, previous alcohol withdrawal treatment, age under 18 years.

End points
Pregnancy or spontaneous menstruation in women with amenorrhea, pregnancy or improved concentrations of luteal hormones in women with luteal insufficiency or idiopathic infertility. Hormone levels were evaluated at baseline in all women and after three months in the women who did not become pregnant.

Results
The outcome measure was achieved in 31 of 66 women: 57.6 percent of the Mastodynon group compared to 36.0 percent of placebo group. A total of 15 pregnancies occurred, seven patients with amenorrhea, four with idiopathic infertility, and four with luteal insufficiency. Pregnancy occurred more than twice as often in women taking Mastodynon (21 percent) as with placebo (10 percent). There were no significant (5 percent level) hormonal changes due to therapy.

Side effects
One complaint (mastodynia) in the Mastodynon group and three complaints with placebo.

Authors' comments
In women with sterility due to secondary amenorrhea and luteal insufficiency, a treatment with Mastodynon can be recommended over a period of three to six months.

Reviewer's comments
Fairly well-designed and well-conducted study. However, study was of short duration, especially to assess secondary amenorrhea, and the outcome measure is questionable. A trend benefit was seen for women with infertility due to secondary amenorrhea or luteal insufficiency. (3, 5)

Product Profile: Agnolyt®

Manufacturer	**Madaus AG, Germany**
U.S. distributor	None
Botanical ingredient	**Chaste tree fruit extract**

Extract name	None given
Quantity	3.5 to 4.2 mg
Processing	Plant to extract ratio 9.58-11.5:1, ethanol 60 percent
Standardization	No information
Formulation	Capsule

Comments: Also available in liquid form.

Source(s) of information: Personal communication with Roy Upton, 1999; and Lauritzen et al., 1997.

Clinical Study: Agnolyt®

Extract name	None given
Manufacturer	Madaus AG, Germany
Indication	**Premenstrual syndrome**
Level of evidence	**II**
Therapeutic benefit	**Yes**

Bibliographic reference
Lauritzen CH, Reuter HD, Repges R, Bohnert KJ, Schmidt U (1997). Treatment of premenstrual tension syndrome with *Vitex agnus castus:* Controlled, double-blind study versus pyridoxine. *Phytomedicine* 4 (3): 183-189.

Trial design
Parallel. Patients in the Agnolyt group received one capsule of Agnolyt and one capsule of placebo daily. Patients in the pyridoxine group received one capsule of placebo twice daily on days 1 to 15, then one capsule of pyridoxine HCL (100 mg) twice daily on days 16 to 35 of the menstrual cycle.

Study duration	3 menstrual cycles
Dose	1 capsule Agnolyt daily
Route of administration	Oral
Randomized	Yes
Randomization adequate	No
Blinding	Double-blind
Blinding adequate	Yes
Placebo	No
Drug comparison	Yes
Drug name	Pyridoxine (vitamin B_6)

Site description   15 study centers

No. of subjects enrolled   175
No. of subjects completed   105
Sex   Female
Age   18-45 years

Inclusion criteria

Premenstrual tension syndrome (PMTS) symptoms had to correlate with the luteal phase of the menstrual cycle, recur with every cycle, and be sufficiently severe to affect the patient's quality of life. For every menstrual cycle, the patient had to be able to indicate at least one week in which she was free from complaints. In addition, the patient should not have received any drug therapy for the syndrome during the three menstrual cycles preceding the start of the trial.

Exclusion criteria

Depression (not to exceed 10 point score on von Zerssen Depression Scale), premenopausal complaints or marked irregular cycle anomalies, women with idiopathic pregnancy icterus, severe pregnancy pruritus, or Morbus Parkinson were excluded by anamnesis. Women wishing to conceive, pregnant or nursing women, women with a known drug or alcohol abuse problem, psychiatric conditions, neurotic personality, and serious consuming illnesses. Disallowed concomitant medications included a list of drugs, botanical products, and vitamins.

End points

Therapeutic response was assessed using the premenstrual tension syndrome scale (PMTS scale), the recording of six characteristic complaints of the syndrome, and the clinical global impressions scale. After completion of the trial, efficacy was assessed subjectively by the patient and physician. Assessments were made at baseline and in the last seven days of the next three menstrual cycles.

Results

Absolute changes of the PMTS scores were 10.1 points in the Agnolyt group and 6.8 points in the pyridoxine group. This difference was significant, in favor of Agnolyt ($p = 0.037$). Improvement on the CGI scale was also more marked in the Agnolyt group. The benefit-to-risk ratio was more favorable for Agnolyt, as were the subjective ratings by doctors and patients.

Side effects

Mild adverse events (gastrointestinal and lower abdominal complaints, skin manifestations, and transitory headache) occurred in five patients taking pyridoxine and in 12 patients taking Agnolyt.

Authors' comments
At first glance, the effect of pyridoxine appears to be equivalent to that of Agnolyt in the present comparative trial. However, careful evaluation of all available data and scales permits the conclusion that Agnolyt was superior to pyridoxine in the present study.

Reviewer's comments
Although the outcome measures and inclusion/exclusion criteria were defined and appropriate, there was no description of randomization. Study rates Level II as there was no placebo arm, and pyridoxine is a questionable agent to use as a historical control. (3, 6)

Product Profile: Cycle Balance™

Manufacturer	**Zeller AG, Switzerland**
U.S. distributor	**General Nutrition Corporation**
Botanical ingredient	**Chaste tree fruit extract**
Extract name	**Ze 440**
Quantity	40 mg
Processing	Plant to extract ratio 6-12:1, 60 percent (m/m) ethanol
Standardization	0.6 percent casticin = 0.24 mg
Formulation	Tablet

Recommended dose: Take one tablet daily with eight ounces of water or juice.

DSHEA structure/function: May provide monthly support and hormonal balance in women.

Other ingredients: Cellulose, lactose.

Source(s) of information: Schellenberg, 2001; product package.

Clinical Study: Ze 440

Extract name	Ze 440
Manufacturer	Zeller AG, Switzerland
Indication	**Premenstrual syndrome**
Level of evidence	**II**
Therapeutic benefit	**Yes**

Bibliographic reference
Schellenberg R (2001). Treatment for the premenstrual syndrome with agnus castus fruit extract: Prospective, randomized, placebo controlled study. *British Medical Journal* 322 (7279): 134-137.

Trial design
Parallel.

Study duration	3 menstrual cycles
Dose	1 (20 mg extract) tablet daily
Route of administration	Oral
Randomized	Yes
Randomization adequate	Yes
Blinding	Double-blind
Blinding adequate	No
Placebo	Yes
Drug comparison	No
Site description	6 community clinics
No. of subjects enrolled	170
No. of subjects completed	169
Sex	Female
Age	Mean: 36 years

Inclusion criteria
Women 18 years or older, with premenstrual syndrome diagnosed according to the DSM-III-R.

Exclusion criteria
Exclusion criteria were participation in other trials, concomitant psychotherapy, pregnancy or breast-feeding, inadequate contraception, dementia, alcohol or drug dependence, concomitant serious medical condition, hypersensitivity to agnus castus, fever, pituitary disease, and concomitant use of sex hormones except oral contraceptives for which the doses were kept unchanged.

End points
Main efficacy variable: change from baseline to end point (end of third cycle) in women's self-assessment of irritability, mood alteration, anger, headache, breast fullness, and other menstrual symptoms including bloating. Secondary efficacy variables: changes in clinical global impressions (severity of condition, global improvement, and risk or benefit) and responder rate (50 percent reduction in symptoms). Assessment was carried out at baseline (start of the first menstrual cycle) and after the third cycle.

Results
Patients who received agnus castus had a significant improvement in combined symptoms compared with those on placebo according to self-assessment and each of the three global impression items ($p < 0.001$). Responder rates were 52 percent and 24 percent for active group and placebo, respectively.

Side effects
Four subjects in the active group and three in placebo reported adverse effects, but none caused discontinuation of treatment. Complaints included acne, intermenstrual bleeding or early period, and gastric upset.

Author's comments
Dry extract of agnus castus fruit is an effective and well-tolerated treatment for the relief of symptoms of premenstrual syndrome.

Reviewer's comments
A well-done study overall; however, the exclusion criteria did not include pyridoxine, evening primrose oil, or phytoestrogen substances. Women taking oral contraceptives were admitted to the study if the dose remained unchanged, but the author did not describe how long the participants had been on the hormonal therapy. (3, 5)

Cordyceps

Other common names: **Chinese caterpillar fungus, dong chong xia cao**
Latin name: *Cordyceps sinensis* **(Berk.) Sacc.**
[Clavicipitaceae]
Plant part: **Fungal mycelium**

PREPARATIONS USED IN REVIEWED CLINICAL STUDIES

Cordyceps sinensis is a parasitic fungus that grows on several species of caterpillars found in the Tibetan highlands. The traditional remedy is a composite, consisting of the fungal body as well as the caterpillar larva. This natural material known as caterpillar fungus, dong chong xia cao, is rare. Therefore, Chinese scientists have developed a technique for isolating fermentable strains of the fungus. The result is a strain called Cs-4 that has been extensively characterized and its pharmacological actions researched. The active components of cordyceps have yet to be identified; however, cordycepin (3-deoxyadenosine) and cordycepic acid (actually *d*-mannitol) may play a role (Zhu, Halpern, and Jones, 1998a).

CordyMax® Cs-4 is a cordyceps product produced by Pharmanex, LLC, a wholly owned subsidiary of Nu Skin Enterprises, Inc. Each capsule contains 525 mg of fungal mycelium Cs-4. Cs-4 is available in China in a commercial product called JinShuiBao.

SUMMARY OF REVIEWED CLINICAL STUDIES

Cordyceps is reported to have a tonic effect in humans, reducing fatigue, intolerance to cold, dizziness, tinnitus, and memory loss, while increasing respiratory capacity. Treatments with cordyceps are associated with increased libido, lowered levels of blood lipid levels

CORDYCEPS SUMMARY TABLE

Product Name	Manufacturer/ U.S. Distributor	Product Characteristics	Dose in Trials	Indication	No. of Trials	Benefit (Evidence Level-Trial No.)
JinShuiBao (China), CordyMax® Cs-4 (US)	Pharmanex, LLC/ Pharmanex, LLC	Fermented mushroom mycelia (Cs-4)	330 mg 3 times daily	Hyperlipidemia (elevated blood lipid levels)	1	Yes (III-1)
				Asthenia syndrome (symptoms associated with aging)	1	Undetermined (III-1)

and blood sugar levels, as well as improved respiratory function, renal function, liver function, and kidney function (Zhu, Halpern, and Jones, 1998b).

CordyMax Cs-4

We reviewed two controlled studies on cordyceps (JinShuiBao), one exploring the blood lipid-lowering (hypolipidemic) effects and the other exploring the effects on fatigue associated with age.

Hyperlipidemia (Elevated Blood Lipid Levels)

The study on hypolipidemic effects was a large placebo-controlled study completed in China. The study included 273 patients with hyperlipidemia, including 215 with elevated cholesterol and 245 with elevated triglycerides. Patients were treated with three (330 mg mycelium) capsules three times daily for two months. Cordyceps lowered total cholesterol levels by 17.5 percent and trigylcerides by 9.2 percent. High-density lipoprotein levels were increased by 27.2 percent. All changes were statistically significant compared to the placebo group levels (Shao, 1995). Our reviewer, Dr. David Heber, concluded that this clinical effect could be significant and deserves repetition. The trial report was an internal Pharmanex document and did not include details such as the baseline lipid levels for the participants.

Asthenia Syndrome (Symptoms Associated with Aging)

The second trial included 59 men and women, 60 to 84 years old, and studied symptoms of aging known in traditional Chinese medicine as asthenia syndrome (Xu-Zheng). The symptoms included fatigue, intolerance to cold, dizziness, tinnitus, pain in loins, hyposexuality, urinary terminal dribbling, amnesia, alopecia (hair loss), and loosened teeth. After three months of treatment with a dose of three (330 mg mycelium) capsules three times daily, the symptom score was reduced compared with the placebo group. There was improvement in lassitude of loins and legs, intolerance to cold, cold in extremities, dizziness, tinnitus, and frequency of nocturia. There was no change in alopecia, loosened teeth, hyposexuality, or amnesia. Levels of the antioxidant superoxide dismutase (SOD) in red blood cells was increased, and levels of malondialdehyde (MDA) in plasma were decreased, compared to baseline levels (Zhang et al., 1995). Dr. Heber concluded that the therapeutic benefit was undetermined due to the subjective outcome measures and other methodological inadequacies.

ADVERSE REACTIONS OR SIDE EFFECTS

Adverse effects reported in one of the clinical studies were gastrointestinal upset and thirst (Shao, 1995).

INFORMATION FROM PHARMACOPOEIAL MONOGRAPHS

Source of Published Therapeutic Monographs

Chinese Pharmacopoeia

Indications

The *Chinese Pharmacopoeia* states that Chinese caterpillar fungus composite, consisting of the stroma of the fungus parasitized on the larva along with the caterpillar, is indicated for chronic cough and asthma, hemoptysis in phthisis, impotence, and seminal emissions with aching of loins and knees. The action, according to traditional Chinese medicine, is to tonify the lung and kidney meridians, dispel phlegm, and arrest bleeding (Pharmacopoeia Commission of PRC, 1997).

Dose

Crude drug: 3 to 9 g (Pharmacopoeia Commission of PRC, 1997)

REFERENCES

Pharmacopoeia Commission of PRC, The (1997). *Pharmacopoeia of the People's Republic of China.* Beijing: Chemical Industry Press.

Shao G (1995). Clinical report of jinshuibao capsule in treating hyperlipidemia. *Journal of Administration of TCM.* Report# G 076 090 152. (Also published in *Chung hsi i chieh ho tsu chih* [China] 1985; 5 [11]: 652-654.)

Zhang Z, Huang W, Liao S, Li J, Lei L, Lui J, Leng F, Gong W, Zhang H, Wan L, et al. (1995). Clinical and laboratory studies of JinShuiBao capsules in eliminating oxygen free radicals in elderly senescent Xu-Zheng patients. *Journal of Management of Traditional Chinese Medicine* 5 (Suppl): 14-18. (Also published in part by Cao Z, Wen Y [1993], *Journal of Applied Traditional Chinese Medicine* 1: 32-33.)

Zhu JS, Halpern GM, Jones K (1998a). The scientific rediscovery of an ancient Chinese herbal medicine: *Cordyceps sinensis.* Part I. *The Journal of Alternative and Complementary Medicine* 4 (3): 289-303.

Zhu JS, Halpern GM, Jones K (1998b). The scientific rediscovery of an ancient Chinese herbal medicine: *Cordyceps sinensis.* Part II. *The Journal of Alternative and Complementary Medicine* 4 (4): 429-457.

DETAILS ON CORDYCEPS PRODUCTS
AND CLINICAL STUDIES

Product and clinical study information is grouped in the same order as in the Summary Table. A profile on an individual product is followed by details of the clinical studies associated with that product. In some instances a clinical study, or studies, supports several products that contain the same principal ingredient(s). In these instances, those products are grouped together.

Clinical studies that follow each product, or group of products, are grouped by therapeutic indication, in accordance with the order in the Summary Table.

Product Profile: CordyMax® Cs-4

Manufacturer	**Pharmanex, LLC**
U.S. distributor	**Pharmanex, LLC**
Botanical ingredient	**Cordyceps fermented mycelium**
Extract name	**Cs-4**
Quantity	525 mg
Processing	Fermentable mycelial strain isolated from the *Cordyceps sinensis* mushroom
Standardization	No information
Formulation	Capsule

Recommended dose: Take two capsules two to three times daily with food and drink.

DSHEA structure/function: Promotes vitality and stamina. Supports the body's natural ability to adapt to daily dietary, occupational, and environmental stresses. Clinical research supports its ability to promote healthy lung function.

Other ingredients: Gelatin.

Comments: Cs-4 is a specialized strain of cordyceps. It is sold in China as JinShuiBao.

Source(s) of information: Product package.

Clinical Study: JinShuiBao

Extract name	Cs-4
Manufacturer	Pharmanex, LLC
Indication	**Hyperlipidemia** (elevated blood lipid levels)
Level of evidence	**III**
Therapeutic benefit	**Yes**

Bibliographic reference

Shao G (1995). Clinical report of jinshuibao capsule in treating hyperlipidemia. *Journal of Administration of TCM.* Report# G 076 090 152. (Also published in *Chung hsi i chieh ho tsu chih* [China] 1985; 5 [11]: 652-654.)

Trial design

Parallel. Seven days prior to study, other lipid-lowering drugs were stopped. All dietary habits, lifestyle, and activities were kept constant.

Study duration	2 months
Dose	3 (330 mg mycelium) capsules 3 times daily
Route of administration	Oral
Randomized	Yes
Randomization adequate	No
Blinding	Double-blind
Blinding adequate	No
Placebo	Yes
Drug comparison	No
Site description	Several Chinese hospitals
No. of subjects enrolled	273
No. of subjects completed	Not given
Sex	Not given
Age	Not given

Inclusion criteria

Patients with primary hyperlipidemia or hypertriglyceremia with complaints of hypertension or ischemic heart disease and normal blood tests, as well as normal liver and kidney function.

Exclusion criteria

Patients with secondary hyperlipidemia due to diabetes, hypolipidemia, liver and bile disease, and syndromes of renal disease.

End points
Fasting blood specimens were collected to measure blood lipids, both before and after 30 and 60 days of treatment. Patients showing excellent or no response to the drugs were excluded from observation, and treatment continued on patients who showed effective response to cordyceps in the clinical tests. Blood levels of total cholesterol, triglycerides, and if possible high-density lipoproteins were determined. Percent of blood lipid variation was used to determine effectiveness of treatment to compensate for the different analytical methods at different sites.

Results
Cordyceps lowered total cholesterol by 17.5 percent after two months, statistically more than placebo ($p < 0.001$). Also, after two months, triglycerides were lowered by 9.2 percent and high-density lipoprotein levels were increased by 27.2 percent (both $p < 0.05$ compared to placebo). The report did not give baseline lipid levels.

Side effects
Study reported no serious side reactions (adverse effects included thirst, gastrointestinal upset, and nausea). Two patients in both control and test groups had increased serum glutamic pyruvic transaminase (SGPT), and two patients in control and one patient in test group had decreased platelets. Three patients stopped treatment due to somnolence, dizziness, and rash.

Author's comments
The study showed that the effects of JinShuiBao in lowering total cholesterol are trustworthy and can be used in treating hypercholesterolemia. A further study in observing its effects in reducing triglycerides is required.

Reviewer's comments
A significant decrease in cholesterol was documented; however, the study needs to be repeated. Treatment length and sample size were appropriate, and outcome measures were clearly defined. The sex and ages of patients were not mentioned. The numbers of subjects was also different for each variable and time frame. (0, 5)

Clinical Study: JinShuiBao

Extract name	Cs-4
Manufacturer	Jiangxi JinShuiBao Pharmaceutical L.L.C., China (Pharmanex, LLC)

Indication	**Asthenia syndrome** (symptoms associated with aging)
Level of evidence	**III**
Therapeutic benefit	**Undetermined**

Bibliographic reference

Zhang Z, Huang W, Liao S, Li J, Lei L, Lui J, Leng F, Gong W, Zhang H, Wan L, et al. (1995). Clinical and laboratory studies of JinShuiBao capsules in eliminating oxygen free radicals in elderly senescent Xu-Zheng patients. *Journal of Management of Traditional Chinese Medicine* 5 (Suppl): 14-18. (Also published in part by Cao Z, Wen Y [1993]. *Journal of Applied Traditional Chinese Medicine* 1: 32-33.)

Trial design

Parallel. Three-arm study. Elderly patients were treated with either cordyceps or placebo. In addition, 30 college students (age 17 to 20) formed a control group.

Study duration	3 months
Dose	3 capsules (containing 330 mg powder each) 3 times daily
Route of administration	Oral
Randomized	No
Randomization adequate	No
Blinding	Not described
Blinding adequate	No
Placebo	Yes
Drug comparison	No
Site description	Not described
No. of subjects enrolled	59
No. of subjects completed	59
Sex	Male and female
Age	60-84 years

Inclusion criteria

Asthenia syndrome (Xu-Zheng) is a group of major disease conditions according to diagnostic classification of traditional Chinese medicine. Patients with the syndrome who had four or more of the following senescent symptoms: fatigue, intolerance to cold, dizziness, tinnitus (and/or deafness), pain in loins, hyposexuality, urinary terminal dribbling, amnesia, alopecia, and loosened teeth. Patients discontinued other medication for the duration of the study.

Exclusion criteria
Patients suffering from obvious heart, lung, liver, and renal disease, severe diabetes mellitus, stage III hypertension, and hyperthyroidism.

End points
Patients were examined every 15 days, and detailed recordings were made of all changes in symptoms, signs, blood pressure, and heart rate. A total accumulated score of senescent symptoms was obtained by inquiring, observation, and pulse reading. Superoxide dismutase activity in red blood cells as well as lipoperoxide (LPO) and malonaldehyde content in plasma were also measured.

Results
Cordyceps therapy decreased the symptom score by at least two-thirds in five patients, by one-third to two-thirds in 23 patients, and by less than one-third in five patients. In the control group, none of the 30 patients had a decrease in score greater than one-third. Over 80 percent improvement was seen in lassitude of loins and legs, intolerance to cold and cold in extremities, and dizziness. Also improved were tinnitus and frequency of nocturia. No improvement occurred in alopecia, loosened teeth, hyposexuality, or amnesia. JinShuiBao elevated SOD levels and reduced LPO compared with baseline measurement (both $p < 0.01$). SOD levels in the young adults was significantly higher than the pretreatment levels for the elderly, and MDA content was lower (both $p < 0.01$). However, after treatment with cordyceps, SOD levels in the elderly were higher than in young adults and MDA levels were comparable. Four months after completion of the study, SOD levels were back to prestudy levels but MDA levels were still somewhat reduced.

Side effects
None mentioned in paper.

Authors' comments
These data suggest that JinShuiBao (cordyceps) has the capability to increase SOD activity and to decrease MDA content, possibly delaying the senescence process of aging. It may be useful in treatment and/or prevention of elderly senescent Xu-Zhneg.

Reviewer's comments
This is a poorly described and designed study. No definite effect was reported with the cordyceps preparation. (Translation reviewed) (0, 0)

Cranberry

Other common names: **American cranberry, large cranberry**
Latin name: *Vaccinium macrocarpon* **Aiton** [Ericaceae]
Plant part: **Fruit**

PREPARATIONS USED IN REVIEWED CLINICAL STUDIES

Cranberry is native to eastern North America. The shrub produces small, dark-red fruits that are widely consumed as juice and sauce. Cranberries contain anthocyanidins (cyanidin, peonidin), proanthocyanins (condensed tannins), flavonols (predominately myricetin and quercetin), as well as organic acids (predominately quinic acid and citric acid) (Winston et al., 2002).

Cranberry juice concentrate and low-calorie cocktail products, which were studied clinically, are produced by Ocean Spray Cranberries, Inc., of Lakeville, Massachusetts.

A dry extract, Cranberry AF™, marketed by Solaray®, Inc., and manufactured by Nutraceutical Corporation, Park City, Utah, was also tested clinically. The extract is marketed in capsules containing 400 mg extract, under the trade name CranActin®.

SUMMARY OF REVIEWED CLINICAL STUDIES

The three double-blind, placebo-controlled studies on cranberry products we review here address prevention of urinary tract infection (UTI). In vitro studies indicate that cranberry products prevent adhesion of bacteria to the cell walls of the urinary tract, thus preventing infection (Winston et al., 2002). Although some of the study methods in the clinical studies cited could be improved, these studies also suggest a benefit in the prevention of bacteriuria (greater than or equal to

CRANBERRY SUMMARY TABLE

Product Name	Manufacturer/ U.S. Distributor	Product Characteristics	Dose in Trials	Indication	No. of Trials	Benefit (Evidence Level-Trial No.)
Cranberry juice concentrate/ cocktail	Ocean Spray Cranberries, Inc.	Juice or juice concentrate	2 oz concentrate or 300 ml cocktail/day	Urinary tract infection (prevention)	2	Yes (I-1) No (II-1)
CranActin®	Nutraceutical Corp./Solaray®, Inc.	Contains the Cranberry AF™ dry extract	400 mg/day	Urinary tract infection (prevention)	1	Yes (II-1)

266

10,000 colony-forming units per ml) and symptomatic urinary tract infection.

Cranberry Juice Cocktail/Concentrate

Urinary Tract Infection (Prevention)

A well-conducted study with 153 elderly women demonstrated a reduced frequency of bacterial infections compared to placebo after four to eight weeks of administration of 300 ml cranberry juice cocktail per day. Those with bacterial infections, indicated by urine samples containing white blood cells and high concentrations of bacteria, and taking cranberry juice cocktail were only about one-quarter as likely as the placebo group to continue to have an infection the next month (Avorn et al., 1994).

A pilot study including 15 children with neurogenic bladder receiving intermittent catheterization four times a day investigated the effect of cranberry juice cocktail on the frequency of bacteriuria. Administration of 2 oz cranberry juice concentrate, the equivalent of 300 ml cranberry juice cocktail, for three months had no effect on bacterial counts in the urine of these children (Schlager et al., 1999).

CranActin

Urinary Tract Infection (Prevention)

A crossover trial studied ten sexually active women who had a history of urinary tract infections. They were given either 400 mg cranberry extract (CranActin) or placebo daily for three months before switching treatments. The women had significantly fewer infections while taking the cranberry product compared to when they took the placebo (Walker et al., 1997).

ADVERSE REACTIONS OR SIDE EFFECTS

No significant side effects were reported with the use of cranberry juice or extract.

INFORMATION FROM PHARMACOPOEIAL MONOGRAPHS

Source of Published Therapeutic Monographs

American Herbal Pharmacopoeia (AHP)

Indications

The *American Herbal Pharmacopoeia* lists the following indications supported by clinical trials for cranberry products: urinary tract infections and reduction of urinary odor. Actions include bacterial antiadhesion activity, possibly vitamin B_{12} absorption-enhancing effects, and cholesterol-lowering, anticancer, and vasorelaxant effects (Winston et al., 2002).

Doses

Juice: 30 to 300 ml daily (Winston et al., 2002)
Dry extract: 400 to 450 mg cranberry solids twice daily (Winston et al., 2002)

Contraindications

The *AHP* states that no contraindications are cited in the literature (Winston et al., 2002).

Adverse Reactions

The *AHP* lists no known adverse reactions (Winston et al., 2002).

Precautions

The *AHP* suggests that in the treatment of cystitis, conditions such as pyelonephritis must be ruled out before relying on only cranberry (Winston et al., 2002). Also, if urinary tract infection symptoms persist despite use of cranberry, a physician should be consulted.

Drug Interactions

The *AHP* lists no known drug interactions in the literature (Winston et al., 2002).

REFERENCES

Avorn J, Monane M, Gurwitz J, Glynn R, Choodnovskiy I, Lipsitz L (1994). Reduction of bacteriuria and pyuria after ingestion of cranberry juice. *Journal of the American Medical Association* 271 (10): 751-754.

Schlager TA, Anderson S, Trudell J, Hendley JO (1999). Effects of cranberry juice on bacteriuria in children with neurogenic bladder receiving intermittent catheterization. *The Journal of Pediatrics* 135 (6): 698-702.

Walker EB, Barney DP, Mickelsen JN, Walton RJ, Mickelsen RA (1997). Cranberry concentrate: UTI prophylaxis. *The Journal of Family Practice* 45 (2): 167-168.

Winston D, Graff A, Brinckmann J, Länger R, Turner A, Reich E, Bieber A, Howell A, Romm AJ (2002). *Cranberry Fruit,* Vaccinium macrocarpon *Aiton.* American Herbal Pharmacopoeia and Therapeutic Compendium: Standards of Analysis, Quality Control, and Therapeutics. Eds. R Upton, A Graff. Santa Cruz, CA: American Herbal Pharmacopoeia.

DETAILS ON CRANBERRY PRODUCTS AND CLINICAL STUDIES

Product and clinical study information is grouped in the same order as in the Summary Table. A profile on an individual product is followed by details of the clinical studies associated with that product. In some instances a clinical study, or studies, supports several products that contain the same principal ingredient(s). In these instances, those products are grouped together.

Clinical studies that follow each product, or group of products, are grouped by therapeutic indication, in accordance with the order in the Summary Table.

Index to Cranberry Products

Product Profile: Cranberry Juice Cocktail

Manufacturer	**Ocean Spray Cranberries, Inc.**
U.S. distributor	**Ocean Spray Cranberries, Inc.**
Botanical ingredient	**Cranberry fruit juice**
Extract name	N/A
Quantity	2 ounces cranberry concentrate equivalent to 300 ml cranberry juice cocktail
Processing	No information
Standardization	No information
Formulation	Liquid

Recommended dose: Serving size: 8 fl oz; for maintaining urinary tract health: 10 fl oz.

DSHEA structure/function: Food label: helps maintain immune system health; helps maintain healthy bones, teeth, and skin; and helps maintain urinary tract health

Other ingredients: Filtered water, high fructose corn syrup, ascorbic acid.

Source(s) of information: Schlager et al., 1999; product label.

Clinical Study: Cranberry Juice Cocktail

Extract name	N/A
Manufacturer	Ocean Spray Cranberries, Inc.
Indication	**Urinary tract infection; bacterial bladder infections** in elderly women (prevention)
Level of evidence	**I**
Therapeutic benefit	**Yes**

Bibliographic reference
Avorn J, Monane M, Gurwitz J, Glynn R, Choodnovskiy I, Lipsitz L (1994). Reduction of bacteriuria and pyuria after ingestion of cranberry juice. *Journal of the American Medical Association* 271 (10): 751-754.

Trial design
Parallel. One-month run-in with placebo beverage.

Study duration	6 months
Dose	300 ml per day
Route of administration	Oral
Randomized	Yes
Randomization adequate	Yes
Blinding	Double-blind
Blinding adequate	Yes
Placebo	Yes
Drug comparison	No
Site description	Multisite
No. of subjects enrolled	192
No. of subjects completed	153
Sex	Female
Age	Mean: 78.5 years

Inclusion criteria
Subjects in long-term care facility and elderly housing complexes.

Exclusion criteria
Subjects with terminal diseases or severe dementia.

End points
Urine samples were collected at baseline and then monthly (total seven samples). Samples were tested for bacteria and white blood cells. If subjects

were taking antibiotics, collection of urine was cancelled for that month and then resumed the following month. The primary outcome was bacteriuria (greater than or equal to 100,000 organisms per ml urine) and pyuria (white blood cells in the urine).

Results
Effect of cranberries on reducing frequencies of bacteriuria with pyuria in elderly women was not seen until after four to eight weeks with daily cranberry juice intake. Bacteriuria with pyuria was found in 28.1 percent of urine samples in the placebo group, compared to only 15.0 percent in the cranberry group. Those with a bacteriuric-pyuric infected urine sample were only about one-quarter as likely as controls to continue to have an infected sample the next month (odds ratio 0.27, $p = 0.006$).

Side effects
None mentioned in study.

Authors' comments
These findings suggest that use of a cranberry beverage reduces the frequency of bacteriuria with pyuria in older women.

Reviewer's comments
A very good study demonstrating a decrease in bacteriuria and pyuria in older women. Length of treatment was adequate, sample size appropriate, and the outcome measures clearly defined. (4, 6)

Clinical Study: Cranberry Juice Concentrate

Extract name	N/A
Manufacturer	Ocean Spray Cranberries, Inc.
Indication	**Urinary tract infection; bacterial bladder infections** in children with neurogenic bladder (prevention)
Level of evidence	**II**
Therapeutic benefit	**No**

Bibliographic reference
Schlager TA, Anderson S, Trudell J, Hendley JO (1999). Effects of cranberry juice on bacteriuria in children with neurogenic bladder receiving intermittent catheterization. *The Journal of Pediatrics* 135 (6): 698-702.

Trial design
Crossover after three months.

Study duration	3 months
Dose	2 ounces of cranberry concentrate per day (equal to 300 ml of cranberry juice cocktail)
Route of administration	Oral
Randomized	Yes
Randomization adequate	No
Blinding	Double-blind
Blinding adequate	Yes
Placebo	Yes
Drug comparison	No
Site description	Homes
No. of subjects enrolled	15
No. of subjects completed	15
Sex	Male and female
Age	2-18 years

Inclusion criteria
Children with neurogenic bladder receiving clean intermittent catheterization four times a day, living at home, with normal findings on renal ultrasonography and voiding cystourethrogram, and living within a one-hour drive of the hospital.

Exclusion criteria
None mentioned.

End points
Weekly home visits with sample urine from intermittent catherization. The urine was cultured and the frequency of bacteriuria (greater than or equal to 10,000 colony-forming units per mL urine) was determined.

Results
Frequency of bacteriuria in children drinking cranberry concentrate and placebo beverage were both 75 percent. No significant difference was observed in the acidification of urine in the two treatments.

Side effects
None observed.

Authors' comments
The frequency of bacteriuria in children with neurogenic bladder receiving intermittent catherization is 70 percent. Cranberry concentrate had no effect on bacteria counts in this population.

Reviewer's comments
This study demonstrated no beneficial effect of a cranberry concentrate on children with neurogenic bladder. The study is limited by small sample size; however, the treatment length was adequate. (3, 5)

Product Profile: CranActin®

Manufacturer	**Nutraceutical Corporation**
U.S. distributor	**Solaray, Inc.**
Botanical ingredient	**Cranberry fruit extract**
Extract name	**Cranberry AF™**
Quantity	400 mg
Processing	No information
Standardization	Tested for and guaranteed to contain bacterial antiadherence activity
Formulation	Capsule

Recommended dose: One capsule two to four times per day.

DSHEA structure/function: CranActin is intended to provide dietary support to help promote a normal, healthy urinary tract.

Other ingredients: Vitamin C (as ascorbic acid) 30 mg, gelatin (capsule), magnesium oxide, cellulose, magnesium stearate, vegetable juice, silica.

Comments: Also available as CranActin Chewables.

Source(s) of information: Product package.

Clinical Study: CranActin™

Extract name	Cranberry AF
Manufacturer	Solaray, Inc.
Indication	**Urinary tract infection** (prevention)
Level of evidence	**II**
Therapeutic benefit	**Yes**

Bibliographic reference
Walker EB, Barney DP, Mickelsen JN, Walton RJ, Mickelsen RA (1997). Cranberry concentrate: UTI prophylaxis. *The Journal of Family Practice* 45 (2): 167-168.

Trial design
Crossover after three months.

Study duration	3 months
Dose	1 (400 mg) capsule daily
Route of administration	Oral
Randomized	Yes
Randomization adequate	Yes
Blinding	Double-blind
Blinding adequate	Yes
Placebo	Yes
Drug comparison	No
Site description	1 hospital
No. of subjects enrolled	19
No. of subjects completed	10
Sex	Female
Age	28-44 years (median: 37)

Inclusion criteria
Sexually active women between the ages of 18 and 45 years who were generally healthy other than suffering from a demonstrated history of urinary tract infections (four UTIs during the previous year or at least one UTI within the previous 3 months).

Exclusion criteria
Pregnancy.

End points
Symptomatic urinary tract infection with diagnostic culture.

Results
Cranberry concentrate was found to be more effective than placebo in reducing the occurrence of UTI ($p < 0.005$). While taking cranberry, seven of the ten subjects exhibited fewer UTIs, two subjects exhibited the same number, and one subject experienced one more UTI. Of the total 21 incidents of UTIs recorded among the participants during the six months, six UTIs occurred during the time they were taking cranberry. The frequency was calculated to be an average of 2.4 infections per year. In contrast, a total of 15

UTIs occurred while on placebo. This frequency was calculated as an average of 6.0 infections per year.

Side effects
None mentioned.

Authors' comments
Data reveal that daily consumption of powdered cranberry extract as a dietary supplement can help reduce the number of urinary tract infections over a period of three months.

Reviewer's comments
This study demonstrates a reduction in the number of urinary tract infections experienced by women on a cranberry supplement. There are some flaws in the study, however, such as a small number of patients and no definition of a UTI. The study also lacks details regarding the cranberry supplement. (5, 3)

Devil's Claw

Latin name: *Harpagophytum procumbens* (**Burch.**) **DC. ex Meisn.** [Pedaliaceae]
Plant part: **Root**

PREPARATIONS USED IN REVIEWED CLINICAL STUDIES

Devil's claw is a native South African plant with large underground tubers. The chopped and dried tubers have been used traditionally for their tonic, antipyretic, and analgesic properties. Several iridoid glycosides, notably harpagoside, are used to characterize the plant (Schulz, Hänsel, and Tyler, 2001).

Harpadol® capsules, manufactured by Arkopharma Laboratoires Pharmaceutiques in France, contain powdered root. A dose of six (435 mg) capsules per day delivers 57 mg harpagoside. The capsules are sold in the United States as Arkojoint™ by Arkopharma/Health from the Sun in Newport, New Hampshire.

The extract WS 1531 is manufactured by Dr. Willmar Schwabe GmbH & Co. in Germany. The extract has a ratio of 6 to 9:1, and a dose of 600 or 1200 mg per day delivers 50 or 100 mg harpagoside, respectively. This extract is not sold in the United States.

Ardeypharm GmbH in Germany produces an extract with a ratio of 2.5:1. A dose of 800 mg three times daily delivers 50 mg harpagoside. This product is not available in the United States.

SUMMARY OF REVIEWED CLINICAL STUDIES

Devil's claw preparations have been examined for their analgesic (pain relieving) and anti-inflammatory properties (Schulz, Hänsel, and Tyler, 2001). We review three trials here, one for the treatment of osteoarthritis and two for lower back pain. Osteoarthritis is a com-

DEVIL'S CLAW SUMMARY TABLE

Product Name	Manufacturer/ U.S. Distributor	Product Characteristics	Dose in Trials	Indication	No. of Trials	Benefit (Evidence Level-Trial No.)
Arkojoint™ (US), Harpadol® (EU)	Arkopharma Laboratoires Pharmaceutiques, France/Health from the Sun/ Arkopharma	Powdered root	6 (435 mg) capsules/day (57 mg harpagoside/ day)	Osteoarth- ritis	1	Trend (II-1)
(Not sold in US)	Dr. Wilmar Schwabe GmbH & Co., Germany/ None	Root extract (WS 1531)	600 or 1200 mg extract/day (50 or 100 mg harpagoside/ day)	Lower back pain	1	No (I-1)
(Not sold in US)	Ardeypharm GmbH, Ger- many/None	Root extract	800 mg 3 times daily (50 mg har- pagoside)/day	Lower back pain	1	No (I-1)

mon rheumatic disease, characterized by pain, inflammation, and reduced joint function. The cause of back pain is often unknown, but it
has been attributed to several different causes, including weak back
muscles and reduced flexibility of the spine (Chrubasik et al., 1996).

Arkojoint

Osteoarthritis

In a comparison study with 92 patients, Harpadol (Arkojoint) reduced pain due to osteoarthritis of the knee and hip. A dose of six capsules a day (2.6 g root powder) was compared with 100 mg of
diacerhein (an anthraquinone derivative) in this four-month study.
Diacerhein and Harpadol reduced pain to a similar extent, but by the
end of the study, the Harpadol group used significantly fewer analgesics and NSAIDs (nonsteroidal anti-inflammatory drugs) (Chantre
et al., 2000). This was a well-designed and well-conducted study.
However, there was no placebo group, and diacerhein is a relatively
unproven remedy. The choice of a well-documented agent to serve as
the control would have strengthened the study.

WS 1531

Lower Back Pain

A study including 183 subjects with lower back pain compared
two doses of devil's claw extract WS 1531 to placebo. Patients were
given either 600 or 1200 mg extract WS 1531 or placebo for one
month. As a result, there was a trend toward an increase in pain-free
days for the two devil's claw groups during the last week of the study.
However, there was no significant difference from placebo (Chrubasik et al., 1999).

Ardeypharm

Lower Back Pain

Another one-month study with 109 subjects with lower back pain
again showed a trend toward reduction in pain with devil's claw that

was not significantly different from placebo. Reduction in pain was confined to a subgroup whose back pain did not radiate to one or both legs. The devil's claw treatment was 800 mg extract (Ardeypharm GmbH) three times daily (50 mg harpagoside daily) (Chrubasik et al., 1996).

ADVERSE REACTIONS OR SIDE EFFECTS

All three devil's claw products were well tolerated. The only side effects mentioned were diarrhea (Chantre et al., 2000) and mild and infrequent gastrointestinal symptoms (Chrubasik et al., 1999).

INFORMATION FROM PHARMACOPOEIAL MONOGRAPHS

Sources of Published Therapeutic Monographs

British Herbal Compendium (BHC)
European Scientific Cooperative on Phytotherapy (ESCOP)
German Commission E

Indications

Devil's claw root, consisting of the dried, secondary tubers, is approved by the German Commission E and listed by the *BHC* and ESCOP as being used for the treatment of loss of appetite and dyspepsia. It is also indicated for supportive therapy of degenerative disorders of the locomotor system, including painful arthrosis and tendonitis (Blumenthal et al., 1998; Bradley, 1992; ESCOP, 1996). Actions include choleretic (digestive stimulant), antiphlogistic (anti-inflammatory), and mildly analgesic (Blumenthal et al., 1998; Bradley, 1992).

Doses

For Dyspepsia or Lack of Appetite

Tuber: 1.5 g daily (Blumenthal et al., 1998)

Decoction: 0.5 g tuber three times daily (Bradley, 1992; ESCOP, 1996)
Tincture: (1:5, 25 percent ethanol), 1 ml three times daily (Bradley, 1992) or (1:10, 25 percent ethanol) 2 ml three times daily (ESCOP, 1996)

For Painful Arthrosis or Tendonitis

Tuber: 1 to 3 g three times daily (ESCOP, 1996)
Decoction: 1.5 to 3 g tuber three times daily (ESCOP, 1996)
Extracts: hydroalcoholic, equivalent to 1 to 3 g tuber three times daily (ESCOP, 1996)

Other Indications

Tuber: 4.5 g daily (Blumenthal et al., 1998)
Decoction: 1.5 to 2.5 g dried tuber three times daily (Bradley, 1992)
Extract: (1:1, 25 percent ethanol), 1 to 2ml three times daily (Bradley, 1992)

Treatment Period

ESCOP recommends treatment for at least two to three months in the case of arthrosis; if symptoms persist, consult a doctor (ESCOP, 1996).

Contraindications

The Commission E, the *BHC,* and ESCOP list gastric and duodenal ulcers as contraindications (Blumenthal et al., 1998; Bradley, 1992; ESCOP, 1996).

Adverse Reactions

The Commission E lists no known adverse reactions, but ESCOP states that mild gastrointestinal disturbances may occur in sensitive individuals, especially at higher dosage levels (Blumenthal et al., 1998; ESCOP, 1996).

Precautions

The Commission E suggests that with gallstones, use only after consultation with a physician (Blumenthal et al., 1998).

Drug Interactions

The Commission E lists no known drug interactions (Blumenthal et al., 1998).

REFERENCES

Blumenthal M, Busse W, Hall T, Goldberg A, Gruenwald J, Riggins C, Rister S, eds. (1998). *The Complete German Commission E Monographs: Therapeutic Guide to Herbal Medicines.* Trans. S Klein. Austin, TX: American Botanical Council.

Bradley PR, ed. (1992). *British Herbal Compendium: A Handbook of Scientific Information on Widely Used Plant Drugs,* Volume 1. Dorset, UK: British Herbal Medicine Association.

Chantre P, Cappelaere A, Leblan D, Guedon D, Vandermander J, Fournie B (2000). Efficacy and tolerance of *Harpagophytum procumbens* versus diacerhein in treatment of osteoarthritis. *Phytomedicine* 7 (3): 177-183.

Chrubasik S, Junck H, Breitschwerdt H, Conradt Ch, Zappe H (1999). Effectiveness of *Harpagophytum* extract WS 1531 in the treatment of exacerbation of low back pain: A randomized, placebo-controlled, double-blind study. *European Journal of Anaesthesiology* 16 (2): 118-129.

Chrubasik S, Zimpfer Ch, Schütt U, Ziegler R (1996). Effectiveness of *Harpagophytum procumbens* in treatment of acute low back pain. *Phytomedicine* 3 (1): 1-10.

European Scientific Cooperative on Phytotherapy (ESCOP) (1996). *Harpagophyti radix:* Devil's claw. *Monographs on the Medicinal Uses of Plant Drugs.* Fascile 2. Exeter, UK: European Scientific Cooperative on Phytotherapy.

Schulz V, Hänsel R, Tyler VE (2001). *Rational Phytotherapy: A Physicians' Guide to Herbal Medicine,* Fourth Edition. Trans. TC Telger. Berlin: Springer-Verlag.

DETAILS ON DEVIL'S CLAW PRODUCTS AND CLINICAL STUDIES

Product and clinical study information is grouped in the same order as in the Summary Table. A profile on an individual product is followed by details of the clinical studies associated with that product. In some instances a clinical study, or studies, supports several products that contain the same principal ingredient(s). In these instances, those products are grouped together.

Clinical studies that follow each product, or group of products, are grouped by therapeutic indication, in accordance with the order in the Summary Table.

Index to Devil's Claw Products

Product Profile: Arkojoint™

Manufacturer	**Arkopharma Laboratoires Pharmaceutiques, France**
U.S. distributor	**Health from the Sun/Arkopharma**
Botanical ingredient	**Devil's claw secondary roots**
Extract name	None given
Quantity	435 mg
Processing	Powdered root
Standardization	Iridoid glycosides (14.5 mg)
Formulation	Capsules

Recommended dose: Take one to two capsules three times a day with food and a full glass of water. Best results are obtained after one month with continued use.

DSHEA structure/function: Helps maintain healthy, flexible joints.

Other ingredients: Cellulose derivative (capsule shell), vegetal magnesium stearate.

Comments: Sold as Harpadol in Europe.

Source(s) of information: Product package.

Clinical Study: Harpadol®

Extract name	N/A
Manufacturer	Arkopharma Laboratoires Pharmaceutiques, France
Indication	**Osteoarthritis**
Level of evidence	**II**
Therapeutic benefit	**Trend**

Bibliographic reference

Chantre P, Cappelaere A, Leblan D, Guedon D, Vandermander J, Fournie B (2000). Efficacy and tolerance of *Harpagophytum procumbens* versus diacerhein in treatment of osteoarthritis. *Phytomedicine* 7 (3): 177-183.

Trial design

Parallel. Patients in the comparison group took two (50 mg) capsules of diacerhein plus six capsules of placebo per day.

Study duration	4 months
Dose	6 (435 mg) capsules/day (plus 2 capsules placebo/day)
Route of administration	Oral
Randomized	Yes
Randomization adequate	Yes
Blinding	Double-blind
Blinding adequate	Yes
Placebo	No
Drug comparison	Yes
Drug name	Diacerhein
Site description	Multicenter
No. of subjects enrolled	122
No. of subjects completed	92
Sex	Male and female
Age	30-79 years (mean: 62)

Inclusion criteria
Patients suffering from osteoarthritis of the knee and hip. Spontaneous pain intensity rated 50 mm on a 100 mm visual analog scale and a score of at least 4 in the Lequesne Algofunctional Index. Patients also had to show a grade 1, 2, or 3 in Kellgren's scale.

Exclusion criteria
Significant renal, hepatic, hematological, or cardiovascular disease. Inflammatory articular diseases, chondrocalcinosis. Very severe arthritis (unable to walk and/or requiring surgical intervention). Past or present malignancy. Oral, intra-articular, or parenteral corticosteroids within the previous four weeks. Chondroprotective drugs (e.g., glucosamine sulfate, hyaluronic acid, chondroitin sulfate, etc.) within the previous eight weeks. Gastritis and/or gastroduodenal ulcer in active phase. History of allergic reactions to nonsteroidal anti-inflammatory drugs (NSAIDs). Pregnancy or lactation.

End points
Primary end point: visual analog scale was used to record the level of spontaneous pain. Secondary end point: functional disability of movement, Lequesne index score, and amount of diclofenac or paracetamol-caffeine taken as rescue drugs if pain relief was judged by the patient to be inadequate.

Results
Both treatments showed a marked reduction in spontaneous pain index (63.6 to 31.3 in Harpadol patients, 61.6 to 35.8 in diacerhein patients) without significant difference between the two. A similar result was true for the Lequesne functional index scores. At the completion of four months, patients on Harpadol were using significantly fewer NSAIDs and analgesics than patients on diacerhein. In a global assessment of efficacy, 65.3 percent of patients taking Harpadol and 60 percent taking diacerhein were judged as having a positive outcome.

Side effects
Frequency of adverse effects in Harpadol group was lower than in diacerhein group. Diarrhea (most frequently reported side effect) occurred in 8.1 percent of Harpadol patients and in 26.7 percent of diacerhein patients.

Authors' comments
One can argue that without a placebo arm it is difficult to judge effectiveness of the two drugs investigated in this study. However, the importance of placebo effect in osteoarthritis has been recently assessed. The results of the present study confirm the efficacy and the very good tolerance of Harpadol in the treatment of osteoarthritis. Harpadol is at least comparable with diacerhein and is an effective therapeutic agent in osteoarthritis and can be safely administrated to patients.

Reviewer's comments
This is a well-designed and well-conducted study. However, no placebo group was included. The trial is rated as Level II due to the use of diacerhein, an unproven remedy as a control and not a well-documented efficacious agent. (5, 6)

Product Profile: WS 1531

Manufacturer	**Dr. Willmar Schwabe GmbH & Co., Germany**
U.S. distributor	None
Botanical ingredient	**Devil's claw root extract**
Extract name	**WS 1531**
Quantity	200 mg
Processing	Plant to extract ratio 6-9:1
Standardization	17 mg harpagoside (8.3%)
Formulation	Tablet

Source(s) of information: Chrubasik et al., 1999.

Clinical Study: WS 1531

Extract name	WS 1531
Manufacturer	Dr. Willmar Schwabe GmbH & Co., Germany
Indication	**Lower back pain**
Level of evidence	**I**
Therapeutic benefit	**No**

Bibliographic reference
Chrubasik S, Junck H, Breitschwerdt H, Conradt Ch, Zappe H (1999). Effectiveness of *Harpagophytum* extract WS 1531 in the treatment of exacerbation of low back pain: A randomized, placebo-controlled, double-blind study. *European Journal of Anaesthesiology* 16 (2): 118-129.

Trial design
Parallel, three-group study.

Study duration	1 month
Dose	600 mg extract (50 mg harpagoside) or 1200 mg extract (100 mg harpagoside) daily
Route of administration	Oral
Randomized	Yes
Randomization adequate	Yes
Blinding	Double-blind
Blinding adequate	Yes
Placebo	Yes
Drug comparison	No
Site description	Not described
No. of subjects enrolled	197
No. of subjects completed	183
Sex	Male and female
Age	18-75 years

Inclusion criteria
Subjects suffering from low back pain with or without radiation to the legs, at least six months susceptibility to low back pain, a current exacerbation of their complaint affecting both rest and movement, pain greater than a 5 on a 1 to 10 visual analog scale, and expected to require at least four weeks of symptomatic treatment.

Exclusion criteria
Low back pain attributable to identifiable causes such as disc prolapse, hip disease, spondylolisthesis, osteomalacia, or inflammatory arthritis. Participation within 30 days in any other clinical study. Serious organic illness affecting any organ system. A history of drug or alcohol abuse or requirement for psychotherapeutic agents. Pregnancy, actual or possible, or lactation. Known allergy to any of the proposed trial medications. Difficulties with language or anticipated cooperation.

End points
Patient condition was monitored using the Arhus Low Back Pain Index. The primary outcome measure was the number of patients who were pain-free without the permitted rescue medication for five days out of the last week of the study. Subsidiary outcome measures were the change in Arhus Low Back Pain Index relative to baseline and the consumption of rescue medication, tramadol (tramadol was allowed to patients in doses from 50 to 400 mg per day if necessary).

Results
The number of patients who were pain-free without using tramadol for at least five days of last week was three in placebo group, six in H600 group,

and ten in H1200 group. The median overall change in Arhus index was about 20 percent in all three groups. These changes in the three groups were significantly different from baseline, but not significantly different from one another.

Side effects
No evidence for side effects except possibly for mild and infrequent gastrointestinal symptoms.

Authors' comments
Harpagophytum can probably help many of those suffering from low back pain who might also be helped by bed rest, paracetamol, NSAIDs, or manipulation, and back school. Of a wide range of treatments for low back pain, none is convincingly effective in patients suffering from back pain for more than three months. Overall, 10 percent of the patients in this study responded to the primary outcome measures (no pain for five days of last week of study), but most of these responders had had back pain for less than six weeks. One could argue that at least half of the patients who would have responded to anything responded to the treatment (including placebo). The daily contact and interest of the investigators probably provided its own distinct psychotherapeutic benefits in an ailment which is heavily influenced by psychological and social factors.

Reviewer's comments
This is a well-designed study with adequate sample size and inclusion/exclusion criteria. There was a trend toward less need for tramodal in the two devil's claw groups, but no significant differences from the placebo group were seen. (5, 6)

Product Profile: Devil's Claw

Manufacturer	**Ardeypharm GmbH, Germany**
U.S. distributor	None
Botanical ingredient	**Devil's claw secondary roots extract**
Extract name	None given
Quantity	400 mg
Processing	Plant to extract ratio 2.5:1
Standardization	2% harpagoside
Formulation	Tablet

Source(s) of information: Chrubasik et al., 1996.

Clinical Study: Devil's Claw

Extract name	None given
Manufacturer	Ardeypharm GmbH, Germany
Indication	**Lower back pain**
Level of evidence	**I**
Therapeutic benefit	**No**

Bibliographic reference
Chrubasik S, Zimpfer Ch, Schütt U, Ziegler R (1996). Effectiveness of *Harpagophytum procumbens* in treatment of acute low back pain. *Phytomedicine* 3 (1): 1-10.

Trial design
Parallel.

Study duration	1 month
Dose	2 (400 mg) tablets 3 times daily (50 mg harpagoside/day)
Route of administration	Oral
Randomized	Yes
Randomization adequate	Yes
Blinding	Double-blind
Blinding adequate	Yes
Placebo	Yes
Drug comparison	No
Site description	Not described
No. of subjects enrolled	118
No. of subjects completed	109
Sex	Male and female
Age	18-75 years

Inclusion criteria
Patients with at least six months of low back pain not attributable to identifiable causes (e.g., disc prolapse, hip disease, spondylolisthesis, osteomalacia, or inflammatory arthritis). Those suffering from acute increases of pain that affected both rest and movement, who were expected to require at least four weeks of symptomatic treatment.

Exclusion criteria
Participation in other clinical studies within the past 30 days, pregnancy, lactation, or insufficient contraceptive methods, difficulties with language or co-

operation, known allergy to any of the proposed trial medications, a history of drug or alcohol abuse, requirement for psychotherapeutic agents, or serious organic illness affecting any of the organ systems.

End points

Patients given either placebo or devil's claw were allowed to take a rescue medication, tramadol, if pain relief not adequate. Primary measure of effectiveness was amount of tramadol patients took to alleviate back pain in the last three weeks of study. Secondary measures were numbers of totally pain-free patients at the end of treatment and change in Arhus Low Back Pain Index relative to baseline.

Results

Tramadol (rescue drug) consumption during the last three weeks of treatment was 95 mg in the drug group and 102 mg in the placebo group. Average pain score on the Arhus index did not correlate with average tramadol consumption. After four weeks, nine patients in the drug group and one patient in the placebo group were pain-free. Arhus index in both groups improved significantly after four weeks of treatment (20 percent improvement in drug group, 8 percent in placebo group; difference between the groups: $p = 0.059$). Reduction in pain in the drug group was confined to the subgroup of patients whose pain did not radiate to one or both legs.

Side effects

No identifiable clinical, hematological, or biochemical side effects.

Authors' comments

Change in tramadol consumption was chosen as the principal outcome measure on the simplistic assumption that greater pain would lead to greater consumption. That was probably confounded by the fact that most patients prefer a degree of pain to some of the side effects that can accompany most conventional analgesic treatments. Although the design of this study prevents conclusions to be drawn, treatment with devil's claw for four weeks appears to have caused a greater number of patients to become pain-free than did placebo and a greater percentage of pain reduction in the Arhus index.

Reviewer's comments

This study was well designed, but there was really no proven benefit of test drug over placebo. (5, 6)

Dragon's Blood Croton

Other common names: **Sangre de drago**
Latin name: *Croton lechleri* **Müll. Arg.** [Euphorbiaceae]
Plant part: **Sap**

PREPARATIONS USED IN REVIEWED CLINICAL STUDIES

Sangre de drago, meaning dragon's blood, is a common name for closely related species of *Croton* growing in South America. The English term, dragon's blood, is a common name used to describe different genera from Malaya, the Canary Islands, Guyana in the West Indies, and South America. Dragon's blood croton, or *C. lechleri,* is a South American tree whose blood-red latex or sap is a traditional remedy. It is used internally for coughs, flu, "lung problems," diarrhea, and stomach ulcers, and externally for wound healing. The major constituents of the sap are proanthocyanidins, which are also called condensed tannins. The sap also contains taspine (a phenanthrene alkaloid) as well as lignans (Jones, in press; Ubillas et al., 1994).

SP-303™ is an extract from the sap of dragon's blood croton that is high in proanthocyanidin content. The SP-303 extract is manufactured by Shaman Pharmaceuticals, Inc., and is found in two different products: SB-Normal Stool Formula™, distributed by ShamanBotanicals.com; and Bowel Support Formula, distributed by General Nutrition Corporation. Tablets of both products contain 250 mg SP-303 each. SP-303 was studied experimentally under the name Provir.™

DRAGON'S BLOOD CROTON SUMMARY TABLE

Product Name	Manufacturer/ U.S. Distributor	Product Characteristics	Dose in Trials	Indication	No. of Trials	Benefit (Evidence Level-Trial No.)
SB-Normal Stool Formula™; Bowel Support Formula	Shaman Pharmaceuticals, Inc./ ShamanBotanicals. com; General Nutrition Corporation	Extract (SP-303™)	500 mg every 6 hours	Diarrhea in AIDS patients	2	Yes (I-1, III-1)

SUMMARY OF REVIEWED CLINICAL STUDIES

The two trials reviewed here study the use of SP-303 for AIDS-related diarrhea. These studies are relevant, as chronic diarrhea is often a problem for those affected with HIV (human immunodeficiency virus). The incidence of diarrhea caused by infectious organisms has been reduced with the advent of new treatments for HIV. However, many patients continue to have chronic diarrhea even though extensive evaluation has not revealed any pathogenic cause (Holodniy et al., 1999).

SP-303

Diarrhea in AIDS Patients

A well-conducted, placebo-controlled, double-blind study included 45 AIDS patients (HIV-1 infection) with chronic diarrhea. After four days of administration of two (250 mg) capsules every six hours, there was a significant reduction in stool weight and stool frequency compared to placebo (Holodniy et al., 1999).

A subsequent study with 393 AIDS patients with diarrhea compared 250 mg delayed-release tablets, 500 mg delayed-release tablets, and 500 mg delayed-release beads to placebo. The final dose levels were 500 mg or 1000 mg four times daily. A significant reduction in stool weight was observed for the group given 500 mg delayed-release tablets (a total of 4 g per day) compared with placebo. There was also a significant reduction compared to baseline measurements. No other treatment group showed significant changes (Koch, 2000). Unfortunately, this study was not written up in full, and many details of the study methodology were not included in the report we reviewed.

ADVERSE REACTIONS OR SIDE EFFECTS

No serious adverse effects or laboratory abnormalities were observed in either study cited.

REFERENCES

Holodniy M, Koch J, Mistal M, Schmidt JM, Khandwala A, Pennington JE, Porter SB (1999). A double blind, randomized, placebo-controlled phase II study to assess the safety and efficacy of orally administered SP-303 for the symptomatic treatment of diarrhea in patients with AIDS. *The American Journal of Gastroenterology* 94 (11): 3267-3273.

Jones K (In press). "Sangre de drago" *(Croton lechleri):* Clinical and pre-clinical studies of a South American medical tree sap. *Journal of Alternative and Complementary Medicine.*

Koch J (2000). A phase III, double-blind, randomized, placebo-controlled multicenter study of SP-303 (Provir) in symptomatic treatment of diarrhea in patients with acquired immunodeficiency syndrome (AIDS). Unpublished paper.

Ubillas R, Jolad SD, Bruening RC, Kernan MR, King SR, Sesin DF, Barrett M, Stoddart CA, Flaster T, Kuo J, et al. (1994). SP-303, an antiviral oligomeric proanthocyanidin from the latex of *Croton lechleri* (sangre de drago). *Phytomedicine* 1: 77-106.

DETAILS ON DRAGON'S BLOOD PRODUCTS AND CLINICAL STUDIES

Product and clinical study information is grouped in the same order as in the Summary Table. A profile on an individual product is followed by details of the clinical studies associated with that product. In some instances a clinical study, or studies, supports several products that contain the same principal ingredient(s). In these instances, those products are grouped together.

Clinical studies that follow each product, or group of products, are grouped by therapeutic indication, in accordance with the order in the Summary Table.

Index to Dragon's Blood Products

Product Profile: SB-Normal Stool Formula™

Manufacturer	**Shaman Pharmaceuticals, Inc.**
U.S. distributor	**ShamanBotanicals.com**
Botanical ingredient	**Dragon's blood croton sap from bark extract**
Extract name	**SP-303**
Quantity	350 mg
Processing	No information
Standardization	250 mg SP-303
Formulation	Tablet (enteric coated)

Recommended dose: Take one to two tablets, two to four times per day as needed or as directed by a physician. Take with water. Do not break or crush tablets.

DSHEA structure/function: Normalizes excess water flow in the bowel (intestinal tract) and promotes normal stool formation, without causing constipation.

Cautions: This product should not be used for people with bloody diarrhea and high fever. If experiencing these symptoms, consult a physician.

Other ingredients: Microcrystalline cellulose, coating (methacrylic acid copolymer, magnesium silicate, triethyl citrate), glyceryl monostearate, sodium starch glycolate, silicon dioxide.

Comments: Also called Provir.

Source(s) of information: Product label; Holodniy et al., 1999.

Product Profile: Bowel Support Formula

Manufacturer	**Shaman Pharmaceuticals, Inc.**
U.S. distributor	**General Nutrition Corporation**
Botanical ingredient	**Dragon's blood croton sap extract**
Extract name	**SP-303™**
Quantity	350 mg
Processing	No information
Standardization	250 mg of SP-303
Formulation	Tablet

Recommended dose: Take one to two tablets, two to four times a day with water, as needed or as directed by a physician. Do not break or crush tablets.

DSHEA structure/function: Helps manage occasional diarrhea. Normalizes water and chloride secretion in the bowel. Promotes normal stool formation.

Cautions: For occasional diarrhea only. Consult a physician if experiencing persistent diarrhea. Do not use this product if experiencing bloody diarrhea or a fever.

Other ingredients: Microcrystalline cellulose, coating (methacrylic acid copolymer, magnesium silicate, triethyl citrate), glyceryl monostearate, sodium starch glycolate, silicon dioxide.

Comments: Also called Provir.

Source(s) of information: Product package; Holodniy et al., 1999.

Clinical Study: Provir™

Extract name	SP-303
Manufacturer	Shaman Pharmaceuticals, Inc.
Indication	**Diarrhea in AIDS patients**
Level of evidence	**I**
Therapeutic benefit	**Yes**

Bibliographic reference
Holodniy M, Koch J, Mistal M, Schmidt JM, Khandwala A, Pennington JE, Porter SB (1999). A double blind, randomized, placebo-controlled phase II study to assess the safety and efficacy of orally administered SP-303 for the symptomatic treatment of diarrhea in patients with AIDS. *The American Journal of Gastroenterology* 94 (11) 3267-3273.

Trial design
Parallel. Subjects remained in the study unit throughout the 24-hour screening period and treatment period (a total of 96 hours after the first dose).

Study duration	4 days
Dose	2 (250 mg) capsules every 6 hours
Route of administration	Oral
Randomized	Yes
Randomization adequate	No
Blinding	Double-blind
Blinding adequate	No
Placebo	Yes
Drug comparison	No
Site description	2 academic medical centers
No. of subjects enrolled	51
No. of subjects completed	45
Sex	Male and female
Age	21-60 years

Inclusion criteria
AIDS patients with chronic diarrhea between 18 and 60 years of age; HIV-1 infection confirmed by serological screening; a diagnosis of AIDS based on CDC criteria; on a stable medical regimen for treatment of HIV disease and associated conditions for at least two weeks before and during the trial; a history of three or more abnormal stools per day. Subjects were required to discontinue all antidiarrheal medications at least 24 hours before entry into the trial.

Exclusion criteria

Subjects pregnant or nursing; with neutrophil count less than 500 cells/µl; decompensated liver disease; a creatinine clearance of <25 percent of predicted; or if they were previously enrolled in a study within 30 days.

End points

Study personnel recorded the frequency, weight, and consistency of all bowel movements during the treatment period.

Results

The SP-303 treatment group demonstrated a mean reduction from baseline stool weight of 451 g/24 h, compared with 150 g/24 h in the placebo group on day 4 of treatment. A mean reduction in abnormal stool frequency of three abnormal stools in 24 h for the SP-303 group occurred, compared with a reduction of two in 24 h in the placebo group. Daily measures analysis over four days of treatment demonstrated that SP-303 subjects had a significant reduction in stool weight ($p = 0.008$) and an abnormal stool frequency ($p = 0.04$) when compared to placebo-treated subjects.

Side effects

No serious adverse events or laboratory abnormalities.

Authors' comments

SP-303 is safe and well tolerated. These results suggest that SP-303 may be effective in reducing stool weight and frequency in patients with AIDS and diarrhea.

Reviewer's comments

This is a thorough and relevant study, adequate for a phase II trial. The dosage choice was not discussed in the paper or substantiated by reference(s). Given that no adverse effects were noted, a higher dose may have demonstrated greater efficacy. The trial was brief in length, considering that SP-303 is intended for the treatment of chronic, noninfectious, iatrogenic diarrhea. Significant differences from placebo were not present until day 4 in measurements of stool number and chloride, and not until day 3 in measurements of stool weight. Dietary changes made while in the inpatient study unit are a potential confounder. Both placebo and SP-303 showed significant changes in stool weight and number from day 1 onward, suggesting a common underlying factor (e.g., controlled diet) played a role in the observed outcomes. A longer study duration could have allowed for clear resolution of data profile differences between the SP-303 and placebo. (5, 6)

Clinical Study: Provir™

Extract name	SP-303
Manufacturer	Shaman Pharmaceuticals, Inc.
Indication	**Diarrhea in AIDS patients**
Level of evidence	**III**
Therapeutic benefit	**Yes**

Bibliographic reference

Koch J (2000). A phase III, double-blind, randomized, placebo-controlled multicenter study of SP-303 (Provir) in symptomatic treatment of diarrhea in patients with acquired immunodeficiency syndrome (AIDS). Unpublished paper.

Trial design

Parallel. Four groups: two capsules of one of the following four times daily for six days: 250 mg SP-303 delayed-release tablet; 500 mg SP-303 delayed-release beads; 500 mg SP-303 delayed-release tablet; or placebo. Pretrial monitored washout period of 24 hours. After seven-day inpatient study, subjects who had a decrease in stool weight of 50 percent or more compared to baseline were allowed to continue taking the same SP-303 regimen for another 21 days. Nonresponders were discontinued from treatment.

Study duration	6 days
Dose	2 (250 mg) tablets, 2 (500 mg) beads, or 2 (500 mg) tablets, taken 4 times a day
Route of administration	Oral
Randomized	Yes
Randomization adequate	No
Blinding	Double-blind
Blinding adequate	No
Placebo	Yes
Drug comparison	No
Site description	25 academic centers
No. of subjects enrolled	400
No. of subjects completed	393
Sex	Male and female
Age	Mean: 39.5 years

Inclusion criteria

Subjects over 18 years with HIV-1 infection and AIDS diagnosis based on

CDC criteria; stable medical regimen for treatment of HIV disease for at least two weeks; abnormal stool samples (soft or watery) of 300 g or more within the inpatient 24-hour screening period; history of at least one abnormal stool or use of antidiarrheal medication each day for at least 14 days prior to the 24-hour inpatient screening period; cessation of antidiarrheal medication 24 hours prior to admission to the research center.

Exclusion criteria
Subjects who were pregnant or breast-feeding; with neutrophil count less than 500 cells/microliter; decompensated renal or liver disease; frank blood in stool two weeks prior to or during study; enteric infection requiring antimicrobial medication; previously enrolled in a study within 30 days prior to entrance into the study.

End points
The primary efficacy end point was the reduction in the total daily stool weight over the six-day inpatient treatment period. Daily stool weight, frequency, and consistency were measured during the 24-hour screening and 144-hour study period. The daily gastrointestinal index score was assessed by rating and summing seven gastrointestinal complaint measures.

Results
For the 500 mg tablet group, intent-to-treat random regression analysis of the rate of reduction with treatment was significant compared to placebo ($p = 0.033$). An analysis of the reduction rate from baseline to the end of treatment yielded $p = 0.078$. No other treatment group showed significant changes in reduction rate. In subjects with stools weighing 1000 g or more, there was a statistically significant mean change in stool weight between subjects in the placebo and 500 mg groups ($p = 0.008$). In the outpatient phase of the study (continued treatment for patients who had responded to treatment in the first seven days), the 500 mg tablet group saw a sustained effect, and the drug was well tolerated throughout the study.

Side effects
No adverse events or laboratory abnormalities were found among treatment groups.

Author's comments
SP-303 is a safe and effective treatment for diarrhea in subjects with AIDS. Subjects with 1000 g or more in stool weight had statistically significant improvements in diarrhea.

Reviewer's comments
The sample size may have been appropriate; however, no power calculation was presented. Dietary changes made while in the inpatient study unit are a potential confounder, and a pretrial washout period of 24 hours is likely in-

sufficient for certain antidiarrheal agents (e.g., Imodium® or Lomotil®). Safety was mentioned as a primary focus of the study, but it was not described in detail in the results section. Dropouts/withdrawals were also not discussed. The trial period was adequate when the follow-up period is included. Unfortunately, this paper was not written up in full, so methodological details were missing. (0, 3)

Echinacea

Species-specific common names:
E. angustifolia: **Narrow-leaf echinacea, Kansas snakeroot, narrow-leaf purple coneflower**
E. pallida: **Pale-flower echinacea, pale purple coneflower**
E. purpurea: **Purple coneflower**
Latin names:
Echinacea angustifolia **DC. [Asteraceae]**
Echinacea pallida **(Nutt.) Nutt. [Asteraceae]**
Echinacea purpurea **(L.) Moench [Asteraceae]**
Latin synonyms: *E. purpurea = Rudbeckia purpurea* **L.**
Plant parts: **Aerial parts, root**

PREPARATIONS USED IN REVIEWED CLINICAL STUDIES

Echinacea species are plants in the daisy family that have pale (occasionally white) to deep purple flowers and are native to the central plains of North America. Although nine species of echinacea have been identified, only three are commonly used commercially. They are *Echinacea angustifolia, E. pallida,* and *E. purpurea.* Historically, there has been confusion over the identity of the plant material used both commercially and in scientific studies. *Echinacea angustifolia* root has been sold interchangeably with *E. pallida* roots. In addition, *E. purpurea* has been adulterated or substituted with *Parthenium integrifolium* L., a plant also known by the common name snakeroot. Fortunately, modern techniques of botany and chemistry now allow for better determination of identity (Awang and Kindack, 1991).

Many types of echinacea products are available on the market. They differ in species, plant part, and method of preparation. The most common products are the expressed juice of *E. purpurea* and aqueous alcoholic extracts of the roots and/or tops of all three species. Little scientific work has been done on possible differences in the ac-

303

ECHINACEA SUMMARY TABLE

Product Name	Manufacturer/ U.S. Distributor	Product Characteristics	Dose in Trials	Indication	No. of Trials	Benefit (Evidence Level-Trial No.)
Single Ingredient Products						
Echinagard®, Echinacin® (EU); EchinaGuard® (US)	Madaus AG, Germany/Nature's Way Products, Inc.	Juice of *E. purpurea* tops preserved with ethanol (EC31)	24-40 drops three times daily or 4-5 ml twice daily	Cold (treatment)	2	Yes (I-1, II-1)
				Cold (prevention)	1	No (I-1)
				Exercise-induced immuno-suppression (prevention)	1	No (II-1)
				Vaginal candidiasis (prevention)	1	Undetermined (III-1)
Echinaforce®	Bioforce AG, Switzerland/Bioforce USA	Ethanolic extract of *E. purpurea* tops and roots	2 tablets 3 times daily	Cold (treatment)	1	Undetermined (II-1)
				Genital herpes	1	No (II-1)
Generic	None/None	Ethanolic extract of *E. purpurea* roots	180 drops daily (equiv. to 900 mg root)	Flu-type infections (treatment)	1	Undetermined (III-1)

Product	Manufacturer/Source	Components	Dosage	Indication	N	Effective (Grade)
Generic	None/None	Aqueous alcoholic extract of *E. pallida* roots	90 drops daily	Cold (treatment)	1	Yes (II-1)
Generic	None/None	Alcoholic extracts of *E. angustifolia* and *E. purpurea* roots	50 drops (1 ml) twice daily	Cold (prevention)	1	No (I-1)

Combination Products

Product	Manufacturer/Source	Components	Dosage	Indication	N	Effective (Grade)
Esberitox™	Schaper & Brümmer GmbH & Co. KG, Germany/ Enzymatic Therapy	Ethanolic extracts of *E. purpurea* roots, *E. pallida* roots, white cedar, and wild indigo	2-3 tablets 3 times daily	Cold (treatment)	2	Yes (I-1) Undetermined (III-1)
Echinacea Plus®	Traditional Medicinals, Inc./ Traditional Medicinals, Inc.	*E. purpurea* tops, *E. angustifolia* tops, and dry extract of *E. purpurea* root with lemongrass and spearmint	5-6 cups tea down to 1 per day over 5 days	Cold (treatment)	1	Yes (II-1)

tion of these different preparations, although we know them to differ chemically. Further, there is little scientific agreement as to which of the numerous chemical constituents identified in echinacea are responsible for the purported immunostimulatory action. Indeed, the only consensus may be that numerous constituents have activity (Bauer and Wagner, 1991).

The most clinically studied echinacea preparation is made from the expressed juice of *E. purpurea* flowering plants harvested without the roots. The expressed juice preparation contains 22 percent ethanol as a preservative. It is manufactured and sold in Germany by Madaus AG as Echinacin® or Echinagard® and distributed in the United States by Nature's Way Products, Inc. as EchinaGuard®. Echina-Guard is supplied in liquid, capsules, and chewable tablet forms, although only trials on the liquid preparation were reviewed.

Echinaforce® contains an extract of *E. purpurea* made with 65 percent ethanol. It is made from fresh plant material in the ratio of 95 percent herb and 5 percent root. Produced in Switzerland by Bioforce AG, it is distributed in the United States by Bioforce USA, Hudson, New York. It is also marketed in liquid and tablet forms.

One trial was performed with a generic *E. purpurea* root liquid extract made with 55 percent alcohol in a plant to extract ratio of 1:5. Another was performed with a generic extract of the roots of both *E. angustifolia* and *E. purpurea* made with 30 percent alcohol with a plant-to-extract ratio of 1:11. A third was performed with a generic *E. pallida* root liquid extract.

Many products on the market contain echinacea plus other ingredients. Two such products have been tested in clinical studies. The first is Esberitox™, which is manufactured in Germany by Schaper & Brümmer GmbH & Co. KG, and distributed in the United States by Enzymatic Therapy in Green Bay, Wisconsin. It contains root extracts of *E. purpurea* and *E. pallida* made with ethanol in a ratio of 1:1. Esberitox also contains extracts of wild indigo [*Baptisia tinctoria* (L.) R. Br.] root and white cedar (*Thuja occidentalis* L.) leaf.

The second product is a tea formula called Echinacea Plus®, which is manufactured and distributed by Traditional Medicinals in Sebastopol, California. The tea formula contains a blend of *E. purpurea* herb, *E. angustifolia* herb, and a dry extract of *E. purpurea* root (plant-to-extract ratio 6:1), in addition to lemongrass [*Cymbopogon citratus* (DC. ex Nees) Stapf.] leaf and spearmint (*Mentha spicata* L.) leaf. Each tea bag delivers 20 mg of phenolic compounds.

SUMMARY OF REVIEWED CLINICAL STUDIES

Thirteen trials using echinacea products were reviewed, with the majority being focused on the common cold or upper respiratory tract infections. Various organisms cause the cold, the most common being the rhinovirus. An inflammatory response that follows the viral infection is responsible for the characteristic symptoms of sore throat, nasal discharge, cough, headache, and fever (Giles et al., 2000). The clinical studies indicate that echinacea products tend to reduce the severity of the symptoms and length of a cold, if taken when symptoms first appear. However, the studies also indicate that echinacea does not appear to prevent catching a cold when taken on a long-term basis.

EchinaGuard

EchinaGuard (Echinacin) was found to be efficacious in the treatment, but not in the prevention, of colds in three well-conducted studies. Two other trials studied the prevention of exercise-induced immunosuppression and the prevention of recurrence of vaginal candidiasis. Neither trial yielded strongly positive results.

Cold (Prevention and Treatment)

In the first well-conducted, placebo-controlled study, 118 employees of a factory were enrolled at the initial signs of a cold. They were treated for up to ten days with either EchinaGuard (20 drops every two hours for the first day and subsequently three times daily) or placebo. In the EchinaGuard group, only 40 percent experienced a "real" cold with full symptoms, compared to 60 percent of the placebo group. For those who developed a real cold, the time taken to improve was four days compared to eight days for the placebo group (Hoheisel et al., 1997).

Another placebo-controlled trial included 80 subjects with the first signs of a cold and used a dose of 5 ml twice daily for ten days. In this study, the patients evaluated their illness with a scoring system (Jackson score). There was no significant reduction in subjects obtaining a full cold. However, the length of illness was shorter, six days compared to nine days, and the symptom score was reduced in comparison to the placebo group (Schulten et al., 2001).

In the third study, 108 subjects with a history of colds, but otherwise healthy, were given either Echinacin (4 ml twice daily) or placebo for two months. As a result there was no statistically significant difference in the incidence, duration, or severity of colds between the two groups (Grimm and Muller, 1999).

Exercise-Induced Immunosuppression

A trial with EchinaGuard (Echinacin) studying the prevention of exercise-induced immunosuppression included 40 triathletes who were training for a competition. They were given 40 drops three times daily, or a total of 8 ml per day. Small changes in immune parameters were reported in comparison with the placebo group. None of the treatment group developed colds, which were reported in a quarter of the control groups (Berg et al., 1998). In the opinion of our reviewer, Dr. Richard O'Connor, the trial would have benefited from a larger sample size and more clearly described randomization process and outcome measures.

Vaginal Candidiasis

In a study examining the possible benefit of echinacea on recurrent vaginal candidiasis, all patients were given econazole nitrate cream topically, in addition to oral or injectable Echinacin or placebo. The rate of reoccurrence was 60.5 percent for those treated only topically with econazole and 16.7 percent following oral administration of Echinacin, 30 drops three times daily. The reoccurrence rate was even smaller when Echinacin was given subcutaneously (15 percent), intramuscularly (5 percent), or intravenously (15 percent) (Coeugniet and Kuhnast, 1986). However, according to Dr. O'Connor, the trial was so badly designed and described that the benefit was deemed undetermined.

Echinaforce

Echinaforce reduced cold symptoms in a trial in which the quality was insufficient to evaluate benefit and failed to prevent recurrence of genital herpes in another study.

Cold (Treatment)

The effectiveness of Echinaforce in treatment of the common cold was assessed in a controlled, four-arm trial including Echinaforce (extract of 95 percent *E. purpurea* herb and 5 percent root), Echinaforce seven times concentrate, *E. purpurea* root extract (manufacturer and preparation details not given), and placebo. The doses were two tablets three times daily (Echinaforce 40.7 mg extract, Echinaforce concentrate 289.8 mg extract, *E. purpurea* root extract 177.6 mg) for up to seven days. Both Echinaforce and its concentrate significantly reduced cold symptoms compared to placebo, according to the complaint index compiled by the attending doctor. The effect of the *E. purpurea* root extract was not significantly different from placebo (Brinkeborn, Shah, and Degenring, 1999). Although the trial was well designed in many aspects, the analysis of the data was not optimal, and therefore, the extent of benefit could not be determined.

Genital Herpes

A placebo-controlled trial with 30 participants with herpes type II examined the influence of Echinaforce on the recurrence of genital herpes. Participants were given 800 mg extract twice daily or placebo for six months. As a result, there was no difference in the frequency, severity, or duration of recurrences and pain scores in the two groups (Vonau et al., 2001).

Generic Echinacea

Three generic echinacea root extracts were tested in trials. Two trials addressed the treatment of colds, and the other addressed the prevention of colds.

Flu-Type Infections (Treatment)

Patients treated with an *E. purpurea* root extract equivalent to 900 mg dried root per day had a shorter length of illness and reduced symptom score. The study included 180 subjects with flu-like symptoms who were given extract equivalent to 450 mg root, 900 mg root, or placebo. Those given the lower dose of extract did not differ from placebo in symptom scores (Braunig et al., 1992). Dr. O'Connor concluded that the benefit was undetermined as the study was poorly designed and poorly described.

Cold (Treatment and Prevention)

Another study including 160 subjects with symptoms of an upper respiratory tract infection compared an extract of *E. pallida* root (equivalent to 900 mg root) to placebo. When taken for eight to ten days, the extract significantly reduced the length of illness (cold) and symptom scores in comparison with placebo (Dorn, Knick, and Lewith, 1997).

A good-quality study included 289 healthy subjects who took 1 ml root extracts of either *E. angustifolia* or *E. purpurea* or placebo twice daily, Monday through Friday, for 12 weeks. As a result there was no significant difference between the three groups in the time until the first upper respiratory infection. There was also no difference between the groups in the number, severity, or duration of cold symptoms (Melchart et al., 1998).

Esberitox

Cold (Treatment)

The ability of Esberitox to treat colds was studied in two trials. A well-designed, placebo-controlled study included 238 subjects who visited their family doctor for treatment for a cold. The participants were given Esberitox, three tablets three times daily, or placebo for seven to nine days. Compared to placebo, Esberitox was more effective at reducing cold symptoms (rhinitis score, bronchitis score, clinical global impression score, and general well-being), especially for those who started therapy at an early stage of their cold (Henneicke-von Zepelin et al., 1999).

An earlier study, which was limited by design flaws and poorly reported, included 90 subjects with cold symptoms. The subjects were given either Esberitox, two tablets three times daily, or vitamin C for ten days. After three days, the Esberitox group had a significant reduction in symptoms compared to the control group (Vorberg, 1984).

Echinacea Plus

Cold (Treatment)

Another study, which included 95 participants reporting the earliest symptoms of a cold or flu, compared the effects of a tea formula, Echinacea Plus, to the effects of another tea formula on cold symptoms. The dose was five to six cups of tea on the first day of symptoms, tapered down to one cup per day over the next five days. As a result, there was a significant decrease in intensity and duration of symptoms, as measured through a subjective questionnaire, in the Echinacea Plus group compared with the control group (Lindenmuth and Lindenmuth, 2000).

REVIEWS AND META-ANALYSES OF CLINICAL STUDIES

In a clinical review of 13 blinded, placebo-controlled, randomized studies published between 1981 and 1999, the authors concluded that echinacea may be beneficial as early treatment of upper respiratory infections. They also found that very little evidence supports the prolonged use of echinacea for the prevention of such infections. Eight of nine treatment trials reported generally positive results, and three of the four prevention trials reported a marginal benefit. The methodological quality of the trials was modest. A true meta-analysis was not possible due to differences in products, trial methods, and outcome measurements. Due to the variety of products, specific dose recommendations were also problematic. The authors warned of the possibility of publication bias, as the one unpublished report they reviewed had negative results (Barrett, Vohmann, and Calabrese, 1999).

Another systematic review of 17 trials published between 1961 and 1999, which included some of the same studies reviewed previously, also concluded that the studies supported the use of echinacea to treat, but not prevent, upper respiratory tract infections (Giles et al., 2000). An earlier review examined 26 controlled trials conducted on echinacea alone or in combination with other ingredients. Nineteen trials studied the prevention or treatment of infection, four trials studied the reduction of side effects caused by anticancer therapies, and three trials studied the modulation of various laboratory immune parameters. The authors found the quality of most of the studies to be low, with only eight trials of moderate to good quality. The authors concluded that the available published literature provides evidence that products containing echinacea are efficacious immunomodulators, but insufficient evidence existed to make clear therapeutic recommendations as to which preparation to use and at what dose (Melchart et al., 1994).

ADVERSE REACTIONS OR SIDE EFFECTS

Adverse events reported in the trials were mild and transitory and included tiredness, dizziness, headache, and gastrointestinal symptoms. According to a review of clinical studies, echinacea is considered to be relatively safe for short-term use (Barrett, Vohmann, and Calabrese, 1999).

A benefit/risk assessment of Echinacin included clinical reports of therapy for respiratory and gynecological infections. The authors concluded that for all ages of subjects, ranging from infants to adults, oral administration for up to 12 weeks caused few complaints, the most common being an unpleasant taste. The paper cited an unpublished general practice study including 1,231 patients with respiratory or urinary infections who were treated for four to six weeks with Echinacin lozenges, one lozenge three times daily. The incidence of adverse effects was 5.04 percent, and of those complaints, the only one that can be clearly distinguished from symptoms of the infection was that of unpleasant taste (1.7 percent of the total population) (Parnham, 1996).

A prospective, controlled study was conducted on 206 women who had used echinacea during their pregnancy. This group was matched with a control group of women who did not use echinacea. There were no statistical differences between the study and control groups in pregnancy outcome or rates of major or minor malformations. Doses of capsules or tablets ranged from 250 to 1000 mg per day, and doses of tinctures ranged from 5 to 30 drops per day. Duration of use was normally five to seven days continuously. The products included preparations of *E. purpurea* and *E. angustifolia,* with only one patient taking *E. pallida.* Although relatively small in size, this study had an 80 percent chance of detecting a 3.5-fold difference in rate of malformations, and thus the overall conclusion is the use of echinacea by pregnant women is not associated with birth defects (Gallo et al., 2000).

An Australian paper explored hypersensitivity reactions to echinacea by subjects known to be atopic (have an inborn tendency to develop immediate allergic reactions, such as asthma, allergic skin reactions, or hay fever). From 1979 to 2000, there were 26 Australian adverse drug reports suggestive of possible immunoglobulin E-mediated hypersensitivity due to exposure to echinacea. In addition, 20 percent of 100 atopic subjects never previously exposed to echinacea had positive skin prick reactions when tested. The authors also examined five cases of patients with allergic reactions possibly due to echinacea. Three of them had positive skin prick reactions and reported symptoms after repeated exposure to echinacea products. The authors speculated that since echinacea is in the daisy family along with known allergens such as ragweed, there may be some cross reactivity. They suggest, therefore, that atopic patients should use echinacea cautiously (Mullins and Heddle, 2002). It must be noted that the details of the echinacea preparation used in the skin prick test, i.e., species, plant part, extract details, concentration, etc., were not given. Thus, the information from this paper is useful only as a vague cautionary note.

INFORMATION FROM PHARMACOPOEIAL MONOGRAPHS

Sources of Published Therapeutic Monographs

British Herbal Compendium (BHC)
European Scientific Cooperative on Phytotherapy (ESCOP)
German Commission E
World Health Organization (WHO)

Indications

Echinacea angustifolia

The *British Herbal Compendium* lists the uses of *E. angustifolia* root as treating chronic viral and bacterial infections, mild septicaemia, furunculosis, and skin complaints, and it states the following actions: immunostimulant, anti-inflammatory, antibacterial, antiviral, and vulnerary (Bradley, 1992). The German Commission E monograph states that *E. angustifolia* fresh and dried roots as well as aboveground parts, collected at the time of flowering are used to support and promote the body's natural resistant powers, especially in infectious conditions (cold/flu) in the nose and throat, as an alterative in influenza, inflammatory and purulent wounds, abscesses, furuncles, indolent leg ulcers, herpes simplex, inflammation of connective tissue, wounds, headaches, metabolic disturbances, diaphoretic, and as an antiseptic. However, the Commission states that those therapeutic uses cannot be recommended, as they have not been substantiated. The Commission acknowledges that *E. angustifolia* preparations on the market may be incorrectly labeled as *E. pallida,* and it does recommend the use of *E. pallida* root (Blumenthal et al., 1998). The WHO lists the use of *E. angustifolia* root preparations in supportive therapy for colds and infections of the respiratory and urinary tract. The WHO does not distinguish the use of *E. angustifolia* root from that of *E. pallida* root (WHO, 1999). ESCOP has not published a monograph for *E. angustifolia* root but does have one for *E. pallida* root (ESCOP, 1999a).

Echinacea pallida

Echinacea pallida herb (fresh or dried aboveground parts collected at the time of flowering) is used to support and promote the body's natural resistant powers, especially in infectious conditions (cold/flu) in the nose and throat, as an alterative in influenza, inflammatory and purulent wounds, abscesses, furuncles, indolent leg ulcers, herpes simplex, inflammation of connective tissue, wounds, headaches, metabolic disturbances, diaphoretic, and as an antiseptic. The German Commission E monograph states that since the activity of the herb for the conditions listed has not been substantiated, its therapeutic use cannot be recommended (Blumenthal et al., 1998).

The Commission E approves the use of *E. pallida* root, fresh or dried, as supportive therapy for influenza-like infections (Blumenthal et al., 1998). The WHO indicates *E. pallida* root for use as supportive therapy for colds and infections of the respiratory and urinary tract (WHO, 1999). ESCOP indicates the use of *E. pallida* roots as adjuvant therapy and prophylaxis of recurrent infections of the upper respiratory tract (common cold) (ESCOP, 1999a).

Echinacea purpurea

Echinacea purpurea fresh aboveground parts collected at flowering time are approved for internal use in supportive therapy for colds and chronic infections of the respiratory tract and lower urinary tract. They are also approved for external use for poorly healing wounds and chronic ulcerations (Blumenthal et al., 1998; ESCOP, 1999b; WHO, 1999).

ESCOP states that *E. purpurea* fresh or dried roots are indicated for internal use for adjuvant therapy and prophylaxis of recurrent infections of the upper respiratory tract (common cold) (ESCOP, 1999c). The Commission E does not approve *E. purpurea* root for use, as its effectiveness is not documented (Blumenthal et al., 1998). The WHO does not mention *E. purpurea* root (WHO, 1999).

Doses

Echinacea angustifolia *Root*

> Dried root: 1 g three times daily (Bradley, 1992)
> Decoction: 1 g three times daily (Bradley, 1992; WHO, 1999)
> Liquid extract: (1:5, 45 percent ethanol), 0.5 to 1 ml three times daily (Bradley, 1992; WHO, 1999)
> Tincture: (1:5, 45 percent ethanol), 2 to 5 ml three times daily (Bradley, 1992; WHO, 1999)

Echinacea pallida *Root*

> Tincture: (1:5) with 50 percent (v/v) ethanol from native dry extract (50 percent ethanol, 7 to 11:1), corresponding to 900 mg herb (Blumenthal et al., 1998; WHO, 1999; ESCOP, 1999a)

Echinacea purpurea *Herb*

Expressed juice: 6 to 9 ml daily (Blumenthal et al., 1998; ESCOP, 1999b; WHO, 1999)
External: semisolid preparations containing at least 15 percent pressed juice (Blumenthal et al., 1998; ESCOP, 1999b; WHO, 1999)

Echinacea purpurea *Root*

Tincture: (1:5, ethanol 55 percent v/v), 3 × 60 drops equivalent to 3 × 300 mg of crude drug (ESCOP, 1999c)

Treatment Period

The Commission E, ESCOP, and WHO recommend use not to exceed eight successive weeks (Blumenthal et al., 1998; ESCOP, 1999a,b,c; WHO, 1999).

Contraindications

Echinacea angustifolia *Herb and Root*

The Commission E and WHO state that *E. angustifolia* herb and root should not to be used when progressive systemic diseases such as the following exist: tuberculosis, leukosis, collagenosis, multiple sclerosis, AIDS, HIV infection, and other autoimmune diseases (Blumenthal et al., 1998; WHO, 1999). The *BHC* lists no known contraindications (Bradley, 1992). The WHO also lists allergy to plants in the daisy family as a contraindication for the external use of the root (WHO, 1999).

Echinacea pallida *Herb and Root*

The Commission E, ESCOP, and WHO list the following contraindications: not to be used when progressive systemic diseases such as the following exist: tuberculosis, leukosis, collagenosis, multiple sclerosis, AIDS, HIV infection, and other autoimmune diseases (Blumenthal et al., 1998; ESCOP, 1999a; WHO, 1999). The WHO also lists allergy to plants in the daisy family as a contraindication for the external use of the root (WHO, 1999).

Echinacea purpurea *Herb*

The Commission E lists the following contraindications for internal consumption: progressive systemic diseases, such as tuberculosis, leukosis, collagenosis, and multiple sclerosis (Blumenthal et al., 1998). ESCOP lists known hypersensitivity to plants of the daisy family (Compositae) as a contraindication. As with all immunostimulants, echinacea is not recommended in progressive systemic disorders or autoimmune diseases such as tuberculosis, leucosis, collagenoses, multiple sclerosis, AIDS, or HIV infection (ESCOP, 1999b).

The Commission E lists no known contraindications for the external use, but both ESCOP and WHO list allergy to plants in the daisy family (Blumenthal et al., 1998; ESCOP, 1999b; WHO, 1999).

Echinacea purpurea *Root*

ESCOP lists known hypersensitivity to plants of the daisy family (Compositae). As with all immunostimulants, echinacea is not recommended in progressive systemic disorders or autoimmune diseases such as tuberculosis, leukosis, collagenoses, multiple sclerosis, AIDS, or HIV infection (ESCOP, 1999c).

Adverse Reactions

ESCOP and the WHO state that in rare cases hypersensitivity reactions, e.g., skin reactions, may occur (ESCOP, 1999a,b,c; WHO, 1999).

Precautions

The WHO suggests that oral administration is not recommended for children, except on the advice of a physician, and states that no reliable studies have been conducted on use during pregnancy or for nursing mothers (WHO, 1999). The Commission E and ESCOP, however, list no precautions (Blumenthal et al., 1998; ESCOP, 1999a,b,c).

Drug Interactions

The Commission E states that there are no drug interactions (Blumenthal et al., 1998).

REFERENCES

Awang DCV, Kindack DG (1991). Echinacea. *Canadian Pharmaceutical Journal* 124 (11): 512-516.

Barrett B, Vohmann M, Calabrese C (1999). Echinacea for upper respiratory infection. *Journal of Family Practice* 48 (8): 628-635.

Bauer R, Wagner H (1991). Echinacea species as potential immunostimulatory drugs. In *Economic and Medicinal Plant Research,* Volume 5. Eds. H Wagner, R Farnsworth. New York: Academic Press, pp. 253-322.

Berg A, Northoff H, Konig D, Weinstock C, Grathwohl D, Parnham MJ, Stuhlfauth I, Keul J (1998). Influence of Echinacin (EC31) treatment on the exercise-induced immune response in athletes. *Journal of Clinical Research* 1: 367-380.

Blumenthal M, Busse W, Hall T, Goldberg A, Gruenwald J, Riggins C, Rister S, eds. (1998). *The Complete German Commission E Monographs: Therapeutic Guide to Herbal Medicines.* Trans. S Klein. Austin, TX: American Botanical Council.

Bradley PR, ed. (1992). *British Herbal Compendium: A Handbook of Scientific Information on Widely Used Plant Drugs,* Volume 1. Dorset, UK: British Herbal Medicine Association.

Braunig B, Dorn M, Knick E (1992). *Echinacea purpurea* radix for strengthening the immune response in flu-like infections. *Zeitschrift fur Phytotherapie* 13 (1): 7-13.

Brinkeborn RM, Shah DV, Degenring FH (1999). Echinaforce preparations and other echinacea fresh plant preparations in the treatment of the common cold. *Phytomedicine* 6 (1): 1-5.

Coeugniet E, Kuhnast R (1986). Recurrent candidiasis: Adjuvant immunotherapy with different formulations of Echinacin. *Therapiewoche* 36: 3352-3358.

Dorn M, Knick E, Lewith G (1997). Placebo-controlled, double-blind study of *Echinacea pallidae* radix in upper respiratory tract infections. *Complementary Therapies in Medicine* 3 (1): 40-42.

European Scientific Cooperative on Phytotherapy (ESCOP) (1999a). *Echinaceae pallidae* radix: Pale coneflower root. *Monographs on the Medicinal Uses of Plant Drugs.* Fascicle 6. Exeter, UK: European Scientific Cooperative on Phytotherapy.

European Scientific Cooperative on Phytotherapy (ESCOP) (1999b). *Echinaceae purpureae* herba: Pale coneflower herb. *Monographs on the Medicinal Uses of Plant Drugs.* Fascicle 6. Exeter, UK: European Scientific Cooperative on Phytotherapy.

European Scientific Cooperative on Phytotherapy (ESCOP) (1999c). *Echinaceae purpureae* radix: Purple coneflower root. *Monographs on the Medicinal Uses of Plant Drugs.* Fascicle 6. Exeter, UK: European Scientific Cooperative on Phytotherapy.

Gallo M, Sarkar M, Au W, Pietrzak K, Comas B, Smith M, Jaeger TV, Einarson A, Koren G (2000). Pregnancy outcome following gestational exposure to echinacea. *Archives of Internal Medicine* 160 (20): 3141-3143.

Giles JT, Palat CT, Chien SH, Chang ZG, Kennedy DT (2000). Evaluation of echinacea for treatment of the common cold. *Pharmacotherapy* 20 (6): 690-697.

Grimm W, Muller HH (1999). A randomized controlled trial of the effect of fluid extract of *Echinacea purpurea* on the incidence and severity of colds and respiratory infections. *The American Journal of Medicine* 106 (2): 138-143. (Also published in Schoneberger D [1992]. *Forum Immunologie* 8: 2-12.)

Henneicke-von Zepelin HH, Hentschel C, Schnitker J, Kohnen R, Kohler G, Wustenberg P (1999). Efficacy and safety of a fixed combination phytomedicine in the treatment of the common cold (acute viral respiratory tract infection): Results of a randomized, double blind, placebo controlled multicentre study. *Current Medical Research and Opinion* 15 (3): 214-227.

Hoheisel O, Sandber M, Bertram S, Bulitta M, Schafer M (1997). Echinagard treatment shortens the course of the common cold: A double-blind placebo-controlled clinical trial. *European Journal of Clinical Research* 9: 261-268.

Lindenmuth GF, Lindenmuth EB (2000). The efficacy of echinacea compound herbal tea preparation on the severity and duration of upper respiratory and flu symptoms: A randomized double-blind placebo-controlled study. *The Journal of Alternative and Complementary Medicine* 6 (4): 327-334.

Melchart D, Linde K, Worku F, Bauer R, Wagner H (1994). Immuno-modulation with echinacea—A systematic review of controlled clinical trials. *Phytomedicine* 1: 245-254.

Melchart D, Walther E, Linde K, Brandmaier R, Lersch C (1998). Echinacea root extracts for the prevention of upper respiratory tract infections: A double-blind, placebo-controlled randomized trial. *Archives of Family Medicine* 7 (6): 541-545.

Mullins RJ, Heddle R (2002). Adverse reactions associated with echinacea: The Australian experience. *Annals of Allergy, Asthma and Immunology* 88 (1): 42-51.

Parnham MJ (1996). Benefit-risk assessment of the squeezed sap of the purple coneflower *(Echinacea purpurea)* for long-term oral immunostimulation. *Phytomedicine* 3: 95-102.

Schulten B, Bulitta M, Ballering-Brühl B, Köster U, Schäfer M (2001). Efficacy of *Echinacea purpurea* in patients with a common cold. *Arzneimittel-Forschung/Drug Research* 51 (7): 563-568.

Vonau B, Chard S, Mandalia S, Wilkinson D, Barton SE (2001). Does the extract of the plant *Echinacea purpurea* influence the clinical course of recurrent genital herpes? *International Journal of STD and AIDS* 12 (3): 154-158.

Vorberg G (1984). For colds, stimulate the nonspecific immune system; a double-blind study shows: The proven phytotherapeutic Esberitox shortens the duration of symptoms. *Arztliche Praxis* 36 (6): 97-98.

World Health Organization (WHO) (1999). *WHO Monographs on Selected Medicinal Plants,* Volume 1. Geneva, Switzerland: World Health Organization.

DETAILS ON ECHINACEA PRODUCTS AND CLINICAL STUDIES

Product and clinical study information is grouped in the same order as in the Summary Table. A profile on an individual product is followed by details of the clinical studies associated with that product. In some instances a clinical study, or studies, supports several products that contain the same principal ingredient(s). In these instances, those products are grouped together.

Clinical studies that follow each product, or group of products, are grouped by therapeutic indication, in accordance with the order in the Summary Table.

Index to Echinacea Products

Product Profile: EchinaGuard®

Manufacturer	**Madaus AG, Germany**
U.S. distributor	**Nature's Way Products, Inc.**
Botanical ingredient	**Echinacea aerial parts juice**
Extract name	**EC31J0**
Quantity	No information
Processing	Fresh expressed juice of the stem, leaf, and flower of *Echinacea purpurea*. Raw material is pressed, and then the juice is preserved with ethanol
Standardization	At least 10 µg/ml *p*-coumaric acid
Formulation	Liquid

Recommended dose: Maintenance—take 2.5 ml, three times daily for six to eight weeks followed by a two-week break; children under 12 take one-half adult dosage. Intensive—take 2.5 ml, every two hours for the first 48 hours; then 2.5 ml, three times daily for the next eight to nine days. Best if added to water or juice.

DSHEA structure/function: Clinically proven to support the immune system.

Cautions: Not recommended for individuals with autoimmune conditions or allergic to flowers of the daisy family.

Other ingredients: Alcohol, water.

Comments: EchinaGuard is also available in chewable tablets and capsules. Sold as Echinacin® and Echinagard® in Europe.

Source(s) of information: Product label (© Nature's Way Products, Inc., 1999); Grimm and Muller, 1999.

Clinical Study: Echinagard®

Extract name	EC31J0
Manufacturer	Madaus AG, Germany
Indication	**Common cold; upper respiratory tract infection** (treatment)
Level of evidence	**I**
Therapeutic benefit	**Yes**

Bibliographic reference
Hoheisel O, Sandber M, Bertram S, Bulitta M, Schafer M (1997). Echinagard treatment shortens the course of the common cold: A double-blind placebo-controlled clinical trial. *European Journal of Clinical Research* 9: 261-268.

Trial design
Parallel. Subjects were recruited at first sign of a cold.

Study duration	Up to 10 days
Dose	20 drops every 2 hours for the first day and thereafter 3 times daily
Route of administration	Oral
Randomized	Yes
Randomization adequate	Yes
Blinding	Double-blind

Blinding adequate	Yes
Placebo	Yes
Drug comparison	No
Site description	Single center
No. of subjects enrolled	120
No. of subjects completed	118
Sex	Male and female
Age	Mean: 36 years

Inclusion criteria
Employees of a furniture-making factory with a history of recurrent upper respiratory infection. Patients had suffered from at least three respiratory infections within the previous six months and presented with justifiable initial signs of acute respiratory infection.

Exclusion criteria
Subjects who reported acute respiratory infections the week before the start of the study, pregnant or breast-feeding women, subjects with systemic immunological diseases and those on immunotherapy, or with a history of hypersensitivity to plants of the Asteraceae [Compositae] family.

End points
Patients recorded subjective symptoms daily on a diary card and answered a questionnaire at the end of the treatment period. The primary variables were the number of patients who reported that they had had a "real" cold and the time to improvement.

Results
An intention-to-treat analysis revealed that 24/60 patients (40.0 percent) in the Echinagard group, and 36/60 (60.0 percent) in the placebo group, experienced a "real" cold (fully expressed disease). The mean treatment effect was 20 percent (95 percent CI 2.5-37.5 percent, $p = 0.044$). The time taken to improvement was significantly shorter ($p < 0.0001$) in the Echinagard group (median: zero days) than in the placebo group (median: five days). In the subgroup of patients with a "real" cold, the median time taken to improvement was four days (Echinagard, $n = 24$) and eight days (placebo, $n = 36$), respectively. More patients taking Echinagard (31.7 percent) than placebo (18.3 percent) stopped treatment because of improvement. The time taken to stop treatment as a result of improvement in the subgroup of patients with a "real" cold was shorter with Echinagard (median: six days) than with placebo (median: ten days).

Side effects
None were reported.

Authors' comments
The findings of this study show that daily treatment with Echinagard, from the first signs of an upper respiratory infection, on the one hand inhibits the full expression of the disease and on the other, when symptoms have developed fully, leads to more rapid recovery than in patients treated with placebo.

Reviewer's comments
Well-designed and well-conducted study except for failure to obtain informed consent and no mention of institutional review board (IRB) approval. Results suggest that the duration of symptoms was shorter in the patients receiving echinacea versus placebo but that symptom severity was not different. However, 20 drops of Echinagard every two hours in the first day is cumbersome, and patient adherence to such a regimen is doubtful. (5, 6)

Clinical Study: Echinacin®

Extract name	EC31J0
Manufacturer	Madaus AG, Germany
Indication	**Common cold; upper respiratory tract infection** (treatment)
Level of evidence	**II**
Therapeutic benefit	**Yes**

Bibliographic reference
Schulten B, Bulitta M, Ballering-Brühl B, Köster U, Schäfer M (2001). Efficacy of *Echinacea purpurea* in patients with a common cold. *Arzneimittel-Forschung/Drug Research* 51 (7): 563-568.

Trial design
Parallel. Subjects were recruited at first signs of a cold.

Study duration	10 days
Dose	5 ml 2 times daily
Route of administration	Oral
Randomized	Yes
Randomization adequate	Yes
Blinding	Double-blind
Blinding adequate	Yes
Placebo	Yes
Drug comparison	No

Site description   Single center

No. of subjects enrolled	80
No. of subjects completed	77
Sex	Male and female
Age	Mean: 38.8 years

Inclusion criteria
Employees of Madaus AG with first signs of an infection of the upper respiratory tract with the subjective sensation of the following symptoms: sneezing, rhinorrhea, congestion of the nose, sore throat, cough, headache, malaise, and chilliness during the previous 24 hours.

Exclusion criteria
Acute respiratory tract infection during the week preceding the trial, allergy to composites, progressive systemic diseases (e.g., tuberculosis, leukosis, collagenosis, multiple sclerosis, AIDS, HIV infections, or other autoimmune diseases), or pregnancy and lactation. Therapy with immunosuppressants in the week prior to the trial and during participation in the trial, and therapy with immunostimulants (herbal immunostimulants, cytokines, thymus fractions), zinc, or antibiotics during two weeks before the commencement of the trial.

End points
Efficacy was measured by the number of days of illness and the number of patients who had developed a complete picture of a common cold, the duration of the illness, and the area under the curve (AUC) standardized to baseline with regard to the modified Jackson score (the cumulative unweighted sum of eight subjective symptom ratings—documented daily by the patients). A "complete picture of a cold" was a cumulative Jackson score of at least 5, rhinorrhea for three consecutive days, and subjective sensation of a cold. The secondary end points included the patients' subjective assessment of efficacy at the final examination; the AUC of each individual symptom; and the proportion of patients who developed a complete picture of the disease during days one to five.

Results
The median length of illness for the group taking echinacea was 6.0 days compared to 9.0 days for the placebo group; this difference was statistically significant ($p = 0.0112$). Fewer patients taking echinacea (85.4 percent) than placebo (97.4 percent) had a complete picture of the common cold, but this difference was not significant. More patients taking echinacea (61.0 percent) subjectively assessed that their cold was "shorter than usual" than placebo (28.2 percent) ($p = 0.007$). The echinacea group had a smaller AUC for symptom severity than the placebo patients ($p = 0.008$). There were also

statistical differences (favoring the echinacea group) for the following AUCs of single symptoms: sore throat; rhinorrhea; and congestion of the nose.

Side effects
No serious adverse events (AEs) occurred. Six patients in each group (echinacea and placebo) experienced similar AEs. The most frequent AEs were gastrointestinal disorders and respiratory system disorders (may be reactions related to the basic illness).

Authors' comments
In the study of Hoheisel and colleagues (1997) the patients assessed subjectively the presence or a "real" cold, whereas in the current study, the more objective measurement of the Jackson score was used. This study did not evaluate more diagnostic, possibly objectifiable, measures of cold severity, such as tissue counts or nasal mucus weight, because of the impracticability of obtaining these measures in the population of co-workers. The results of this study showed that the time to resolution of all symptoms and the duration of the disease were significantly shorter and less severe in the active treatment group.

Reviewer's comments
Other than the small sample sizes (40 subjects in each group, this is a well-designed, -conducted, and -reported trial. (5, 5)

Clinical Study: Echinacin®

Extract name	EC31J0
Manufacturer	Madaus AG, Germany
Indication	**Common cold; upper respiratory tract infection** (prevention/treatment)
Level of evidence	I
Therapeutic benefit	**No**

Bibliographic reference
Grimm W, Muller HH (1999). A randomized controlled trial of the effect of fluid extract of *Echinacea purpurea* on the incidence and severity of colds and respiratory infections. *The American Journal of Medicine* 106 (2): 138-143. (Also published in Schoneberger D [1992]. *Forum Immunologie* 8: 2-12.)

Trial design
Parallel. Subjects with a history of colds received either echinacea or placebo.

Study duration   2 months
Dose   4 ml extract twice daily
Route of administration   Oral

Randomized   Yes
Randomization adequate   Yes
Blinding   Double-blind
Blinding adequate   Yes

Placebo   Yes
Drug comparison   No

Site description   Single center

No. of subjects enrolled 109
No. of subjects completed 108
Sex   Male and female
Age   23-59 years

Inclusion criteria
Reported more than three common colds or respiratory infections in the preceding year and at least 12 years old.

Exclusion criteria
Acute infections of any kind within one week of recruitment; pregnancy or nursing; use of immunostimulating drugs within four weeks before study entry; known allergy against coneflowers; severe underlying disease of immunosuppression; inability to give informed consent; or unreliability for follow-up as judged by the investigator.

End points
Routine assessments were at baseline and after four and eight weeks. The primary efficacy parameters were incidence and severity of colds and respiratory infections. Patients were asked to come in for unscheduled visits if they experienced symptoms. The severity of each incidence was graded by investigators.

Results
There were no significant differences in the incidence, duration, or severity of colds and respiratory infection in the two groups. During the eight weeks, 35 of the 54 patients in the echinacea group and 40 of 54 patients in the placebo group had at least one cold or respiratory infection [RR = 0.88; 95 percent CI (0.60, 1.22)]. The mean number of colds and respiratory infections per patient was 0.78 in the echinacea group, and 0.93 in the placebo group [difference = 0.15; 95 percent CI (−0.12, 0.41), $p = 0.33$]. Median duration of colds and respiratory infections was 4.5 days in the echinacea group and 6.5 days in the placebo group (95 percent CI −1, +3 days; $p = 0.45$). There were

no significant differences between treatment groups in the number of infections in each category of severity ($p = 0.15$).

Side effects
The adverse events were transient and mild, and included tiredness, dizziness, headache, and gastrointestinal symptoms. They were observed in 11 patients (20 percent) of the echinacea group and in seven patients (13 percent) of the placebo group ($p = 0.44$).

Authors' comments
Eight weeks of follow-up treatment with fluid extract of *Echinacea purpurea* did not decrease the incidence or severity of colds and respiratory infections as compared to placebo. (Study was reevaluated by Grimm and Muller. Previous publication by Schoneberger reported positive results.)

Reviewer's comments
This well-designed trial assessed the prevention of upper respiratory infections and symptom severity. Active treatment was no different than placebo. The sample size was relatively small. (5, 5)

Clinical Study: Echinacin®

Extract name	EC31
Manufacturer	Madaus AG, Germany
Indication	**Exercise-induced immunosuppression**
Level of evidence	**II**
Therapeutic benefit	**No**

Bibliographic reference
Berg A, Northoff H, Konig D, Weinstock C, Grathwohl D, Parnham MJ, Stuhlfauth I, Keul J (1998). Influence of Echinacin (EC31) treatment on the exercise-induced immune response in athletes. *Journal of Clinical Research* 1: 367-380.

Trial design
Parallel. Three-arm double-dummy: Echinacin, Biomagnesin (12 tablets each containing the equivalent of 43 mg Mg^{++}), or placebo.

Study duration	1 month
Dose	40 drops 3 times daily (8 ml total)
Route of administration	Oral
Randomized	Yes

Randomization adequate   No
Blinding   Double-blind
Blinding adequate   Yes

Placebo   Yes
Drug comparison   Yes
Drug name   Biomagnesin

Site description   Not described

No. of subjects enrolled   42
No. of subjects completed   40
Sex   Male
Age   18-47 years (mean: 27.5)

Inclusion criteria
Triathletes who were undergoing regular training for triathlon sprint competition.

Exclusion criteria
Infection during the two weeks before the start of the study.

End points
Fluorescence activated flow cytometry analysis of blood cell populations, serum and urine levels of interleukin 6 (IL-6), and soluble interleukin 2 receptor (sIL-2R) together with clinical chemical and hematological variables were determined at baseline, after 28 days of treatment, and both 1 and 20 hr after the competition (days 29 and 30).

Results
Pretreatment with Echinacin produced slight changes in total peripheral (CD3+) T-lymphocytes, natural killer cells, and CD8+ lymphocyte counts which remained within the range of baseline variation. In comparison to the placebo group, Echinacin markedly decreased sIL-2R in urine before the competition and enhanced the exercise-induced decrease in serum sIL-2R. It further enhanced the exercise-induced increases in urine IL-6 and serum cortisol. None of the Echinacin-treated athletes developed upper respiratory tract infections, which were reported by 3/13 and 4/13 subjects treated with magnesium and placebo, respectively.

Side effects
None reported for the Echinacin group.

Authors' comments
On the basis of these results, it is likely that prophylactic treatment with Echinacin counteracts the immunosuppressive effects of exhaustive exercise and reduces the risk of upper respiratory infections in athletes.

Reviewer's comments
This study is a classic example of overanalysis and overinterpretation of small numbers. However, the study was IRB approved and the inclusion/exclusion criteria appropriate. (3, 3)

Clinical Study: Echinacin®

Extract name	EC31J0
Manufacturer	Madaus AG, Germany
Indication	**Recurrent vaginal candidiasis** (prevention)
Level of evidence	**III**
Therapeutic benefit	**Undetermined**

Bibliographic reference
Coeugniet E, Kuhnast R (1986). Recurrent candidiasis: Adjuvant immunotherapy with different formulations of Echinacin. *Therapiewoche* 36: 3352-3358.

Trial design
Parallel. All patients were given econazole nitrate cream, a topical treatment, for six days. After this, patients were allocated to groups for additional treatment with one of four forms of Echinacin or placebo. The forms of Echinacin were intravenous (IV), subcutaneous (SC) or intramuscular (IM) injection, or oral. Milder cases were put into the oral group.

Study duration	10 weeks
Dose	Ampoules (SC, IM, IV) 0.5 ml increased to 2 ml twice weekly or liquid 30 drops 3 times daily
Route of administration	Oral, injection, intravenous
Randomized	No
Randomization adequate	No
Blinding	Open
Blinding adequate	No
Placebo	Yes
Drug comparison	No
Site description	Single center
No. of subjects enrolled	203
No. of subjects completed	203
Sex	Female
Age	16-65 years

Inclusion criteria
Patients with recurrent candidal colpitis and/or vulvitis confirmed through culturing. The infection was considered recurrent if the inflammation reappeared at least three times after the use of not less than two different antifungal agents or if symptoms recurred within four weeks of the withdrawal of topical treatment.

Exclusion criteria
Not mentioned.

End points
Cell-mediated immunity was assessed in a cutaneous antigen reaction test (Merieux multitest) before the start of treatment and repeated in the second and tenth weeks after initiation of Echinacin treatment. Recurrences of infection within six months of topical treatment were noted.

Results
The incidence of recurrences in patients treated only locally with econazole nitrate (control group) was very high (60.5 percent). This rate was markedly reduced, however, in patients receiving additional nonspecific immunostimulant therapy with Echinacin according to the form of treatment (SC 15 percent, IM 5 percent, IV 15 percent, and oral 16.7 percent). The baseline Merieux skin reactions were small and increased significantly following two weeks of injections or ten weeks of oral treatment ($p < 0.05$).

Side effects
None for oral treatment, both local and systemic with injections.

Authors' comments
The current trial showed that the basic therapeutic principle of immunostimulation with Echinacin represents an important addition to the therapeutic measures available, especially for problem patients whose immunocompetence is likely to be impaired.

Reviewer's comments
This study was not well designed or described. The study was neither randomized nor blinded, and the authors gave no description of statistical methods used. Replication or reanalysis might not be possible due to poor description. IRB review was not obtained. (Translation reviewed) (0, 3)

Product Profile: Echinaforce®

Manufacturer	**Bioforce AG, Switzerland**
U.S. distributor	**Bioforce USA**

Botanical ingredient	**Echinacea aerial parts and root extract**
Extract name	None given
Quantity	6 mg herb and 0.3 mg root (equivalent to 269 mg of fresh material)
Processing	*Echinacea purpurea* aerial parts (95%) and root (5%); plant to extract ratio 9:1, 65% ethanol
Standardization	At least 3 mg cichoric acid and 8 mg alkylamides per 100 g Echinaforce®
Formulation	Tablet

Recommended dose: Adults take one to two tablets three to five times per day. Allow to dissolve slowly in the mouth.

DSHEA structure/function: Supports healthy immune system, natural winter resistance during winter season.

Other ingredients: Lactose, potato starch, magnesium stearate.

Comments: Also available as a liquid.

Source(s) of information: Product label; information supplied by distributor.

Clinical Study: Echinaforce®

Extract name	None given
Manufacturer	Bioforce AG, Switzerland
Indication	**Common cold** (treatment)
Level of evidence	**II**
Therapeutic benefit	**Undetermined**

Bibliographic reference
Brinkeborn RM, Shah DV, Degenring FH (1999). Echinaforce preparations and other echinacea fresh plant preparations in the treatment of the common cold. *Phytomedicine* 6 (1): 1-5.

Trial design
Parallel. Patients received one of four treatments to be taken immediately after the onset of the first symptoms of the common cold. The treatments were Echinaforce (6.78 mg *E. purpurea* extract 95 percent herb and 5 percent root), Echinaforce 7 times concentrate (48.3 mg), *E. purpurea* root extract (29.6 mg), or placebo. Patients were directed to take their treatment until they felt healthy but not longer than seven days.

Study duration	Up to 7 days
Dose	2 tablets 3 times daily
Route of administration	Oral
Randomized	Yes
Randomization adequate	Yes
Blinding	Double-blind
Blinding adequate	Yes
Placebo	Yes
Drug comparison	Yes
Drug name	Other echinacea preparation
Site description	Single center
No. of subjects enrolled	559
No. of subjects completed	246
Sex	Male and female
Age	26-58 years

Inclusion criteria
Older than 18 years and prone to common cold, otherwise healthy.

Exclusion criteria
Participation in another clinical trial during the past four weeks, suffering from chronic diseases which influence the test variables (diabetes mellitus, bronchial asthma, allergy, or autoimmune deficiency), suffering from serious non-related illnesses, especially progressive systemic diseases, and/or taking other medicines which may affect the immune system, such as immunostimulants and antibiotics, or may influence the symptoms, such as nosedrops or anticoughs.

End points
Subjects reported to investigators when they experienced the first symptoms of the common cold. They recorded the progress of their cold daily in a diary and reported to investigators either when they felt healthy or not longer than seven days after beginning treatment. Symptoms were assessed by the investigator at these visits. The primary end point was the relative reduction of the complaint index according to the doctor's record. Secondary end points were the relative reduction of the complaint index according to the patient's diary and assessment of tolerance.

Results
According to the doctor's records, the relative reduction in the complaint index for the Echinaforce concentrate and Echinaforce groups were significantly higher than for the placebo group ($p = 0.003$ and $p = 0.020$, respectively). Results with the *E. purpurea* root extract were not significantly different

from placebo. Similar results were obtained from analysis of the patient's diary. According to the doctors' as well as the patients' judgment, Echinaforce concentrate was more effective than placebo ($p = 0.001$ doctors and $p = 0.002$ patients). The same was true for Echinaforce ($p = 0.035$ doctors and $p = 0.022$ patients). The efficacy of the root extract was not judged as significantly different from placebo by either doctors or patients.

Side effects
The frequency of adverse events was not significantly higher in the echinacea groups than in the placebo group. They were reported in 33 of 246 cases (13 percent), and the majority involved the gastrointestinal tract.

Authors' comments
In summary, Echinaforce and its concentrated preparation represent low-risk and effective alternatives to standard medicine for symptomatic treatment of the common cold.

Reviewer's comments
Overall a well-designed study. However, the use of per-protocol results is not valid since it includes only patients completing the trial and in essence results in "cherry picking" the data. The authors also include the intent-to-treat analysis. They used a one-tailed U test but should have used a repeated measure analysis since the sum score was a composite of 12 different symptoms. (4, 6)

Clinical Study: Echinaforce®

Extract name	None given
Manufacturer	Bioforce AG, Switzerland
Indication	**Genital herpes**
Level of evidence	**II**
Therapeutic benefit	**No**

Bibliographic reference
Vonau B, Chard S, Mandalia S, Wilkinson D, Barton SE (2001). Does the extract of the plant *Echinacea purpurea* influence the clinical course of recurrent genital herpes? *International Journal of STD and AIDS* 12 (3): 154-158.

Trial design
Crossover. Patients received six months each of placebo and echinacea extract.

Study duration   6 months
Dose   800 mg extract twice daily
Route of administration   Oral

Randomized   Yes
Randomization adequate   Yes
Blinding   Double-blind
Blinding adequate   Yes

Placebo   Yes
Drug comparison   No

Site description   Single center

No. of subjects enrolled 49
No. of subjects completed 30
Sex   Male and female
Age   22-72 years (mean: 36.5)

Inclusion criteria
Subjects with culture-proven genital herpes or serology-proven HSV type 2 antibody positivity, no suppressive acyclovir or similar drugs within 14 days of study entry, a minimum of four recurrences in the previous 12 months or prior to suppressive acyclovir.

Exclusion criteria
Subjects who were pregnant or not using effective contraception during the study period, immunosuppression or severe cardiovascular disease, liver disease, renal disease, inability to communicate sufficiently or comply with the study protocol, or a known lactose intolerance.

End points
At baseline, patients had a physical examination and the following assessments and measurements were taken: visual analog scales (VAS) recorded the average pain, impairment of the quality of life, and the impairment of sex life experience during a recurrence; psychological assessment included a Hospital Anxiety and Depression (HAD) scale and an Eysenck Personality Questionnaire (EPQ); and laboratory parameters were taken, including blood count, urea and electrolytes, liver function tests, and HSV serology. During study, patients were evaluated monthly and within 72 hours of the start of a recurrence. The main end point was the frequency, severity, and duration of each recurrence and a pain score using a VAS. Patients also kept a daily diary of symptoms, compliance, and adverse events. At the crossover and at the final visit, biochemistry measurements and the HAD scale were repeated.

Results

There were no statistically significant differences between the echinacea treatment and the placebo for any of the outcomes measured.

Side effects

One patient withdrew due to severe diarrhea while taking the active therapy (may be due to lactose intolerance). Four patients taking echinacea and two on placebo experienced nausea.

Authors' comments

In conclusion, no statistically significant benefit of the plant and root extract of *Echinacea purpurea* (Echinaforce) was shown in the treatment of frequently recurrent genital herpes. Given that there are safe and efficacious alternatives, the value of further studies into its benefits for this indication seems unjustified.

Reviewer's comments

This is a well-designed trial in culture-proven patients. My only criticism is the relatively small sample size. (5, 5)

Product Profile: *Echinacea purpurea* (Generic)

Manufacturer	None
U.S. distributor	None
Botanical ingredient	**Echinacea purpurea root extract**
Extract name	None given
Quantity	450 mg per 90 drops
Processing	Plant to extract ratio 1:5, 55% ethanol
Standardization	No information
Formulation	Liquid

Source(s) of information: Braunig, Dorn, and Knick, 1992.

Clinical Study: *Echinacea purpurea* (Generic)

Extract name	None given
Manufacturer	None

Indication	**Flu-type upper respiratory tract infection** (treatment)
Level of evidence	**III**
Therapeutic benefit	**Undetermined**

Bibliographic reference
Braunig B, Dorn M, Knick E (1992). *Echinacea purpurea* radix for strengthening the immune response in flu-like infections. *Zeitschrift fur Phytotherapie* 13 (1): 7-13.

Trial design
Parallel. Three treatment groups: two doses *E. purpurea* root extract and placebo.

Study duration	8-10 days
Dose	90 drops extract (2 droppersful, 450 mg root) or 180 drops extract (4 droppersful, 900 mg root) daily
Route of administration	Oral
Randomized	Yes
Randomization adequate	No
Blinding	Double-blind
Blinding adequate	No
Placebo	Yes
Drug comparison	No
Site description	General practice
No. of subjects enrolled	180
No. of subjects completed	180
Sex	Male and female
Age	18-60 years

Inclusion criteria
Patients between 18 and 60 years old with flu-type infections.

Exclusion criteria
Patients who had been ill for more than three days from a flu-like infection; not readily cooperative; with additional infections, for instance, of the urological tract; those under treatment with antihistamines, antibiotics, and other relevant medications that influenced the disease profile; those who suffered other autoimmune diseases or immunologically relevant chronic diseases; patients who showed secondary infections such as bronchitis, pneumonia, pleuritis, and septic infections; bacterial illnesses such as pneumoconiosis and fungal infections; pussy angina tonsilleris; a sublingually measured fever of more than 40.5°C; or other serious illnesses.

End points
Subjects were assessed at the beginning of treatment, after three to four days, and after eight to ten days. The target parameter was length of illness and symptom score. The control parameters were clinically objective reports (inflamed nose, swelling of the lymph glands, coated tongue, rhoncus) and flu symptoms reported by the patients (sense of weakness/exhaustion, chills/perspiration, burning eyes, nasal congestion or secretions, sore throat, ear pain, limb or muscle pain, headaches, and cough). Secondary parameters were occurrence of new symptoms, severity of illness (score), comparison of blood workups, and red blood cell sedimentation rate.

Results
Patients treated with 450 mg echinacea extract did not differ significantly from patients treated with placebo in clinically objective scores. However, patients treated with the higher dose of echinacea extract (900 mg) differed significantly from the placebo group for clinically objective scores, and for the patient-reported symptoms, after three to four days. In addition, there was a significant difference in clinical report score between days 3 and 4 and days 8 and 10.

Side effects
None mentioned.

Authors' comments
The therapeutic effectiveness of 900 mg echinacea for patients with flu-type symptoms was good to very good. The therapeutic effect of taking 450 mg of echinacea extract was satisfactory to poor, as was the placebo.

Reviewer's comments
This study was poorly designed and described. The primary end points were duration of illness, symptoms, and results of physical exam; the data regarding duration of illness could not be found in the report. Also, the study title is misleading. No tests of immune function were conducted. There may be improvement at the higher dose, but the SDs overlap and statistics are not adequately described. No adverse events were described, so it is difficult to know if data about adverse events were recorded. (Translation reviewed) (0, 3)

Product Profile: *Echinacea pallida* (Generic)

Manufacturer	None
U.S. distributor	None
Botanical ingredient	**Echinacea root extract**
Extract name	None given

Quantity	No information
Processing	Aqueous alcoholic extract
Standardization	No information
Formulation	Liquid

Source(s) of information: Dorn, Knick, and Lewith, 1997.

Clinical Study: *Echinacea pallida* (Generic)

Extract name	None given
Manufacturer	None
Indication	**Cold; upper respiratory tract infection** (treatment)
Level of evidence	**II**
Therapeutic benefit	**Yes**

Bibliographic reference
Dorn M, Knick E, Lewith G (1997). Placebo-controlled, double-blind study of *Echinacea pallidae* radix in upper respiratory tract infections. *Complementary Therapies in Medicine* 3 (1): 40-42.

Trial design
Parallel.

Study duration	8 to 10 days
Dose	90 drops extract (900 mg root per day)
Route of administration	Oral
Randomized	Yes
Randomization adequate	Yes
Blinding	Double-blind
Blinding adequate	Yes
Placebo	Yes
Drug comparison	No
Site description	Single center
No. of subjects enrolled	160
No. of subjects completed	Not given
Sex	Male and female
Age	Not given

Inclusion criteria
Subjects over 18 years old with an upper respiratory tract infection (infection could be either viral, indicated by a raised differential lymphocyte count, or bacterial, indicated by a raised differential neutrophil count), and with a symptom score of >15 at entry. Patients should not have been sick for more than three days prior to the start of the study. A record of the frequency of infection over the past three years was noted at trial entry.

Exclusion criteria
Subjects with infections involving other organs, being treated with other drugs that might interact with a herbal preparation, suffering from fungal infections or pneumonia, or had other significant diseases such as multiple sclerosis.

End points
Symptoms were recorded at entry into the trial, after day three or four, and again on day eight or ten of the trial. The main end points were the length of the illness and the resolution of cold and cough symptoms.

Results
Compared to placebo, the length of the illness was reduced from 13 days to 9.8 days in putative bacterial infections or 9.1 in putative viral infections ($p < 0.0001$). The lymphocytosis and differentia neutrophil counts also fell at a far faster rate in the treatment group compared to the placebo group. Overall symptom scores and whole clinical scores were significantly improved for the treatment group compared to placebo ($p < 0.0004$ and $p < 0.001$, respectively).

Side effects
None mentioned.

Authors' comments
From these results it is quite clear that *Echinacea pallidae* radix shortens the course in URTI as compared with placebo. The specific clinical signs and symptoms improved and in fact disappeared far more swiftly with real treatment than with placebo treatment. This was correlated with appropriate changes in the lymphocyte and neutrophil count, but past history of recurrent infections had no influence on outcome.

Reviewer's comments
The authors use a lymphocyte versus neutrophil count to allocate causation of the URI as viral or bacterial. I am not sure of the use of this technique or its validity. The authors state that counts declined at a faster rate in the treatment group but do not show data. Also, the symptoms of a URI listed as "weakness" and "pain in arms and legs" are not the usual symptoms of a URI. (4, 2)

Product Profile: *Echinacea angustifolia/E. purpurea* (Generic)

Manufacturer	None
U.S. distributor	None
Botanical ingredient	**Echinacea root extract**
Extract name	None given
Quantity	No information
Processing	Plant to extract ratio 1:11, 30% alcohol. Extracts of either *Echinacea angustifolia* or *Echinacea purpurea*
Standardization	No information
Formulation	Liquid

Source(s) of information: Melchart et al., 1998.

Clinical Study: *Echinacea angustifolia/E. purpurea* (Generic)

Extract name	None given
Manufacturer	None
Indication	**Cold; Upper respiratory tract infection (prevention)**
Level of evidence	**I**
Therapeutic benefit	**No**

Bibliographic reference
Melchart D, Walther E, Linde K, Brandmaier R, Lersch C (1998). Echinacea root extracts for the prevention of upper respiratory tract infections: A double-blind, placebo-controlled randomized trial. *Archives of Family Medicine* 7 (6): 541-545.

Trial design
Parallel. Three-arm study: ethanolic extracts of *Echinacea purpurea* roots, *E. angustifolia* roots, or placebo. Healthy participants took trial preparations from Monday to Friday for 12 weeks.

Study duration	3 months
Dose	50 drops (1ml) twice daily (of either preparation)

Route of administration	Oral
Randomized	Yes
Randomization adequate	Yes
Blinding	Double-blind
Blinding adequate	Yes
Placebo	Yes
Drug comparison	No
Site description	4 military institutions and 1 industrial plant
No. of subjects enrolled	302
No. of subjects completed	289
Sex	Male and female
Age	18-65 years

Inclusion criteria
Persons free of acute illness at time of enrollment.

Exclusion criteria
Acute respiratory tract infection or other infections within the past seven days; serious progressive disease such as tuberculosis, multiple sclerosis, or AIDS; systemic intake of corticosteroids, antibiotics, or immunostimulants in the previous two weeks; allergy to the Asteracea [Compositae] family; and pregnancy.

End points
Main outcome measure was time until first upper respiratory tract infection. Secondary outcome measures were the number of participants with at least one infection, global assessment, and adverse effects.

Results
There was no significant difference between the three groups in the time until first upper respiratory infection. In the *E. angustifolia* group 32 percent had at least one upper respiratory infection, compared with 29 percent in *E. purpurea* group and 37 percent in placebo group. No significant difference between groups in number, severity, or duration of upper respiratory tract infections and quality of life. More subjects in the treatment groups believed they had benefited from taking the medication than those in the placebo group ($p = 0.04$).

Side effects
No adverse effects that were serious or required therapeutic action.

Authors' comments
In this study a prophylactic effect of the investigated echinacea extracts could not be seen. However, based upon the results of this and two other studies, one could speculate that there might be an effect of echinacea products in the order of magnitude of 10 to 20 percent relative risk. Future studies with much larger sample sizes would be needed to prove this effect.

Reviewer's comments
A well-designed, well-described study with clear primary end points. (5, 6)

Product Profile: Esberitox®

Manufacturer	**Schaper & Brümmer GmbH & Co. KG, Germany**
U.S. distributor	**Enzymatic Therapy®**
Botanical ingredient	**White cedar leaf extract**
Extract name	None given
Quantity	2 mg
Processing	Aqueous ethanolic extract
Standardization	No information
Botanical ingredient	**Echinacea root extract**
Extract name	None given
Quantity	7.5 mg
Processing	*Echinacea purpurea* and *Echinacea pallida* plant to extract ratio 1:1, aqueous ethanolic extract
Standardization	No information
Botanical ingredient	**Wild indigo root extract**
Extract name	None given
Quantity	10 mg
Processing	Aqueous ethanolic extract
Standardization	No information
Formulation	Tablet (chewable)

Recommended dose: Adults and children over 12 years, three tablets three times per day; ages 8 to 12, two tablets three times per day; age seven and under, one tablet three times per day.

DSHEA structure/function: Dietary supplement to nutritionally support and stimulate the immune system; unique combination of herbs to promote the body's resistive functions.

Cautions: Not recommended for individuals with autoimmune diseases, HIV infection, or who are allergic to echinacea.

Other ingredients: Lactose, sugar, macrogol, ascorbic acid, magnesium stearate.

Source(s) of information: Product package (Enzymatic Therapy ©1999); information supplied by distributor; Henneicke-von Zepelin et al., 1999.

Clinical Study: Esberitox® N

Extract name	None given
Manufacturer	Schaper & Brümmer GmbH & Co. KG, Germany
Indication	**Common cold** (treatment)
Level of evidence	I
Therapeutic benefit	**Yes**

Bibliographic reference:
Henneicke-von Zepelin HH, Hentschel C, Schnitker J, Kohnen R, Kohler G, Wustenberg P (1999). Efficacy and safety of a fixed combination phytomedicine in the treatment of the common cold (acute viral respiratory tract infection): Results of a randomized, double blind, placebo controlled multicentre study. *Current Medical Research and Opinion* 15 (3): 214-227.

Trial design
Parallel.

Study duration	7 to 9 days
Dose	3 tablets 3 times daily
Route of administration	Oral
Randomized	Yes
Randomization adequate	Yes
Blinding	Double-blind
Blinding adequate	Yes
Placebo	Yes
Drug comparison	No
Site description	15 doctors' practices
No. of subjects enrolled	263
No. of subjects completed	238

Sex	Male and female
Age	18-70 years

Inclusion criteria

Patients were included who were attending their family doctor for an acute common cold.

Exclusion criteria

Acute influenza, the actual cold lasting longer than three days; chronic diseases of the respiratory tract; a fever resulting in a temperature greater than 38.5°C; more than one respiratory tract infection lasting longer than three weeks during the previous year; bacterial respiratory tract infection; progressive systemic diseases; organ transplantation; known impairment of resorption; intake of antibiotics during the study; immunosuppressing, immunostimulating, or immunomodulating medication during four weeks before baseline; allergy tests or vaccination during the study; cytostatic therapy during six months before baseline; severe internal diseases; known clinically relevant abnormalities in laboratory values; pregnancy or lactation; inability to understand the consequences of participation in the study; participation in any other study during this clinical trial of 12 weeks before baseline; and previous participation in this study.

End points

Patients daily documented the intensity of 18 cold symptoms, as well as the cold overall, using a ten-point scale, and estimated their general well-being using the Welzel-Kohnen color scale. In addition, the severity of illness was assessed by the physician using the clinical global impression item 1 (CGI-1) on days 4 and 8. The main outcome measure was a total efficacy measure gauged from the primary end points (rhinitis score, bronchitis score, CGI-1, and general well-being).

Results

Esberitox was effective compared to placebo according to the primary efficacy score ($p < 0.05$). Effect size was 20.6 percent for the "intention to treat" population (ITT) and 23.1 percent for subjects who followed protocol (VC). For general well-being, the effect size was 33.9 percent (VC). The patients who suffered from at least moderate symptoms at baseline showed response rates of 55.3 percent in the Esberitox group and 27.3 percent in the placebo group ($p = 0.017$). In the subgroup of patients who started therapy at an early phase of their cold, the efficacy of the herbal remedy was most prominent ($p = 0.014$ primary efficacy parameter). The therapeutic benefit of Esberitox was observed on day 2, reached significance ($p < 0.05$) on day 4, and continued until the end of the treatment. Improvement was observed three days earlier in the Esberitox group than in the placebo group.

Side effects
Serious adverse events did not occur.

Authors' comments
This study shows that the remedy is effective and safe and that therapeutic benefits consist of a rapid onset of improvement of cold symptoms, particularly if patients are able to start the remedy at the onset of initial symptoms.

Reviewer's comments
Well-designed study. Using the intent-to-treat analysis, the active compound was better than placebo, but only marginally so ($p = 0.0497$). Informed consent was obtained. This is one of the few echinacea studies that actually collected adverse event data and reported them (no significant adverse events occurred). (5, 6)

Clinical Study: Esberitox™

Extract name	None given
Manufacturer	Schaper & Brümmer GmbH & Co. KG, Germany
Indication	**Cold; upper respiratory tract infection** (treatment)
Level of evidence	**III**
Therapeutic benefit	**Undetermined**

Bibliographic reference
Vorberg G (1984). For colds, stimulate the nonspecific immune system; a double-blind study shows: The proven phytotherapeutic Esberitox shortens the duration of symptoms. *Arztliche Praxis* 36 (6): 97-98.

Trial design
Parallel. The control was vitamin C which was called a placebo in the write-up. There was no mention of the quantity of vitamin C.

Study duration	10 days
Dose	2 tablets 3 times daily
Route of administration	Oral
Randomized	Yes
Randomization adequate	No
Blinding	Double-blind
Blinding adequate	No

Placebo	No
Drug comparison	Yes
Drug name	Vitamin C
Site description	Not described
No. of subjects enrolled	100
No. of subjects completed	90
Sex	Male and female
Age	18-60 years

Inclusion criteria
Subjects with acute infections of the upper respiratory tract.

Exclusion criteria
Patients needing primary antibiotic treatment and patients with true viral flu (influenza).

End points
Subjects were assessed prior to the study and after days 3 and 10 of treatment. The parameters used for assessing therapy were subjective and objective pathological symptoms of the cold infection.

Results
After three days, patients taking Esberitox had a significant reduction in fatigue, tiredness, reduced performance, runny nose, sore throat, headache, and subfebrile temperatures compared to placebo ($p < 0.001$). Several symptoms such as purulent secretion, furring, and lymph node swelling remained unaffected by both forms of therapy.

Side effects
None occurred.

Author's comments
The results show a significant superiority of Esberitox over vitamin C in colds. The immunostimulating action of Esberitox leads to an improvement in the endogenous immune response which is relevant to combating an infection in its early phase. The therapeutic use of the drug considerably shortens the duration of illness in most cases and simultaneously contributes to prophylaxis against recurrence.

Reviewer's comments
This study was limited by many flaws. Blinding was inappropriate, as the placebo and active were distinguishable. The statistical analysis is poorly reported: no numbers are supplied; and there are just graphs without standard deviation data. No IRB review was obtained. The study probably would not

allow for replication. Repeated measures would demand a different statistical approach. (1, 0)

Product Profile: Echinacea Plus®

Manufacturer	**Traditional Medicinals, Inc.**
U.S. distributor	**Traditional Medicinals, Inc.**
Formula botanicals	***Echinacea purpurea* (herb)** *E. angustifolia* **(herb)** **Water-soluble dry extract of** *E. purpurea* **(root; ratio 6:1), lemongrass (leaf), spearmint (leaf)**
Quantity	Equivalent
Processing	See Formula botanicals
Standardization	Minimum 20 mg phenolic compounds (cichoric acid, chlorogenic acid, echinacoside) per one tea bag, as determined by HPLC
Formulation	Tea bag

Recommended dose: Three cups or more daily as needed. Pour 8 oz of boiling water over one tea bag and steep, covered, for 10 to 15 minutes.

DSHEA structure/function: Supports the immune system. Induces interferon production if needed by the body.

Cautions: The product should not be used during pregnancy and lactation without medical advice from a practitioner trained in medical herbalism.

Source(s) of information: Product package (Traditional Medicinals ©1999); Echinacea Plus® Herbal Dietary Supplement Technical Paper (©1998).

Clinical Study: Echinacea Plus®

Extract name	None given
Manufacturer	Traditional Medicinals, Inc.
Indication	**Common cold/flu** (treatment)
Level of evidence	**II**
Therapeutic benefit	**Yes**

Bibliographic reference

Lindenmuth GF, Lindenmuth EB (2000). The efficacy of echinacea compound herbal tea preparation on the severity and duration of upper respiratory and flu symptoms: A randomized double-blind placebo-controlled study. *The Journal of Alternative and Complementary Medicine* 6 (4): 327-334.

Trial design

Parallel. The control for Echinacea Plus tea was another tea called Eater's Digest.

Study duration	6 days
Dose	5-6 cups tea the first day of symptoms, titrating down by 1 cup per day over the next 5 days
Route of administration	Oral
Randomized	Yes
Randomization adequate	No
Blinding	Double-blind
Blinding adequate	Yes
Placebo	Yes
Drug comparison	No
Site description	Single center
No. of subjects enrolled	95
No. of subjects completed	95
Sex	Male (7 percent) and female (93 percent)
Age	24-62 years (mean: 39.7)

Inclusion criteria

Employees of a nursing center who reported the earliest symptoms of cold or flu: runny nose, scratchy throat, fever, etc.

Exclusion criteria

Pregnant or nursing mothers; persons who had known allergies to coneflowers, or those who claimed to be allergic to many different flowering plants and pollens; and those who had acute infections and were already placed on antibiotics.

End points

Symptoms were assessed through a questionnaire which asked about the effectiveness of relieving cold or flu symptoms, duration of the cold, and how long it took to notice a change in symptoms.

Results

There was a significant difference between the Echinacea Plus group versus the control group in effectiveness of symptom relief, in number of days of symptoms, and in days of noticeable symptom change (all three $p < 0.001$).

Side effects

No negative effects reported by any subjects.

Authors' comments

Treatment with Echinacea Plus tea at early onset of cold or flu symptoms was effective for relieving these symptoms in a shorter period of time than a placebo.

Reviewer's comments

This study had clearly defined outcome measures and adequate inclusion/exclusion criteria; however, there were several flaws. Alternating assignment was used which does not truly randomize subjects; sample size was relatively small, and no IRB review obtained. Results do suggest shorter duration of symptoms and decrease in severity of symptoms with active treatment. (2, 5)

Elderberry

Other common names: **European elder, black elder**
Latin name: *Sambucus nigra* **L.** [Caprifoliaceae]
Plant part: **Fruit**

Note: Sambucus nigra L. ssp. *canadensis* (L.) R Bolli or
Sambucus canadensis L. is American elder or sweet elder

PREPARATIONS USED
IN REVIEWED CLINICAL STUDIES

European elder or black elder is a common shrub in Europe with
sweet-smelling flowers and shiny black berries. Historically, the
flowers, berries, leaves, and bark have all been used medicinally.
However, the most commonly used plant part is the flower. Preparations of the flowers have been used for their diaphoretic and diuretic
effect in the treatment of colds. In addition, the flowers and berries
are used to make wine, which has been heated until hot and taken for
colds (Wren, Williamson, and Evans, 1988).

The use of an elderberry fruit extract in treatment for flu was borne
out of laboratory testing which found activity against several strains
of influenza virus (Mumcuoglu, 1998). That testing resulted in a
product, Sambucol®, a syrup containing elderberry juice and rasp-
berry extract. Sambucol is manufactured by Razei Bar Industries
Ltd., Israel, and distributed in the United States by Nature's Way
Products Inc.

ELDERBERRY SUMMARY TABLE

Product Name	Manufacturer/ U.S. Distributor	Product Characteristics	Dose in Trials	Indication	No. of Trials	Benefit (Evidence Level-Trial No.)
Sambucol®	Razei Bar Industries Ltd., Israel/Nature's Way Products Inc.	Syrup containing elderberry juice and raspberry extract	Children: 2 tbsp daily, Adults: 4 tbsp daily	Flu	1	Trend (III-1)

SUMMARY OF REVIEWED CLINICAL STUDIES

Sambucol

Flu

Sambucol was tested for the treatment of flu in a small trial with members of a kibbutz. Early symptoms of flu, caused by the influenza virus, are sudden fever, chills, body aches, and eventually a runny nose, headache, and cough. The trial initially included 40 children and adults who had developed flu symptoms within 24 hours before the start of the trial. Participants were given either placebo or Sambucol (two tablespoons per day were given to children, and four tablespoons per day were given to adults) for three days. Only 27 subjects were included in the study evaluation, which reported a significant improvement in symptoms of the flu, including fever, in 93 percent of the treatment group within two days. The placebo group showed such an improvement within six days. The treatment group had a greater increase in antibody titers to influenza B/Panama compared to the control group, but this difference was not significant (Zakay-Rones et al., 1995). According to our reviewer, Dr. Richard O'Connor, evaluation of the clinical effectiveness of Sambucol was limited by the small number of subjects included in the final analysis.

ADVERSE REACTIONS OR SIDE EFFECTS

No side effects were observed in the trial that included 15 subjects in the treatment group, ages 5 to 50 years.

INFORMATION FROM PHARMACOPOEIAL MONOGRAPHS

Sources of Published Therapeutic Monographs

German Commission E
British Herbal Compendium (BHC)

Note: Both the German Commission E and the *British Herbal Compendium* have published monographs on the flower. There is no mention of the fruit in these monographs.

Indications

The German Commission E approves the use of dried, sifted flowers for colds and feverish conditions. The *British Herbal Compendium* also lists these indications. Actions include diaphoretic, diuretic, and increased bronchial secretion (Blumenthal et al., 1998; Bradley, 1992).

Doses

Flower: 10 to 15 g daily (Blumenthal et al., 1998); dried, 3 to 5 g in infusion three times daily (preferably taken hot) (Bradley, 1992).
Fluid extract: 1.5 to 3 g daily (Blumenthal et al., 1998).
Liquid extract: (1:1, 25 percent ethanol), 3 to 5 ml three times daily (Bradley, 1992).
Tincture: 2.5 to 7.5 g daily (Blumenthal et al., 1998); (1:5, 25 percent ethanol), 10 to 25 ml three times daily (Bradley, 1992).

Contraindications

The Commission E and the *BHC* list no known contraindications (Blumenthal et al., 1998; Bradley, 1992).

Adverse Reactions

The Commission E lists no known adverse reactions (Blumenthal et al., 1998).

Drug Interactions

The Commission E lists no known drug interactions (Blumenthal et al., 1998).

REFERENCES

Blumenthal M, Busse W, Hall T, Goldberg A, Gruenwald J, Riggins C, Rister S, eds. (1998). *The Complete German Commission E Monographs: Therapeutic Guide to Herbal Medicines.* Trans. S Klein. Austin, TX: American Botanical Council.

Bradley PR, ed. (1992). *British Herbal Compendium: A Handbook of Scientific Information on Widely Used Plant Drugs,* Volume 1. Dorset, UK: British Herbal Medicine Association.

Mumcuoglu M (1998). *Wonderful Sambucus: The Black Elderberry. How a Tiny Berry Can Defeat Influenza and Protect You.* Jerusalem, Israel: Shmuel Tal Printing Service.

Wren RC, Williamson EM, Evans FJ (1988). *Potter's New Encyclopaedia of Botanical Drugs and Preparations.* Saffron Walden, UK: The SW Daniel Company, Ltd.

Zakay-Rones Z, Varsano N, Zlotnik M, Manor O, Regev L, Schlesinger M, Mumcuoglu M (1995). Inhibition of several strains of influenza virus in vitro and reduction of symptoms by an elderberry extract (*Sambuscus nigra* L.) during an outbreak of influenza B Panama. *Journal of Alternative and Complementary Medicine* 1 (4): 361-369.

DETAILS ON ELDERBERRY PRODUCTS
AND CLINICAL STUDIES

Product and clinical study information is grouped in the same order as in the Summary Table. A profile on an individual product is followed by details of the clinical studies associated with that product. In some instances a clinical study, or studies, supports several products that contain the same principal ingredient(s). In these instances, those products are grouped together.

Clinical studies that follow each product, or group of products, are grouped by therapeutic indication, in accordance with the order in the Summary Table.

Product Profile: Sambucol®

Manufacturer	**Razei Bar Industries, Ltd.**
U.S. distributor	**Nature's Way Products, Inc.**
Botanical ingredient	**Raspberry fruit extract**
Extract name	None given
Quantity	No information
Processing	No information
Standardization	No information
Botanical ingredient	**Elderberry fruit extract**
Extract name	None given
Quantity	3.8 g extract in 2 teaspoons
Processing	No information
Standardization	No information
Formulation	Liquid

Recommended dose: Suggested daily usage: adults take 2 teaspoons daily; children take 1 teaspoon daily. Suggested intensive usage: adults take 2 teaspoons four times daily; children take 1 teaspoon four times daily.

DSHEA structure/function: Popular supplement during the winter season for its health-promoting benefits.

Other ingredients: Glucose syrup, honey, citric acid, natural flavor.

Source(s) of information: Product label.

Clinical Study: Sambucol®

Extract name	None given
Manufacturer	Razei Bar Industries, Ltd.

Indication	**Flu**
Level of evidence	**III**
Therapeutic benefit	**Trend**

Bibliographic reference
Zakay-Rones Z, Varsano N, Zlotnik M, Manor O, Regev L, Schlesinger M, Mumcuoglu M (1995). Inhibition of several strains of influenza virus in vitro and reduction of symptoms by an elderberry extract (*Sambucus nigra* L.) during an outbreak of influenza B Panama. *Journal of Alternative and Complementary Medicine* 1 (4): 361-369.

Trial design
Parallel. Patients received trial medication for three days.

Study duration	6 days
Dose	2 tbsp (children), 4 tbsp (adults) daily
Route of administration	Oral
Randomized	Yes
Randomization adequate	Yes
Blinding	Double-blind
Blinding adequate	Yes
Placebo	Yes
Drug comparison	No
Site description	Dispensary
No. of subjects enrolled	40
No. of subjects completed	27
Sex	Male and female
Age	5-56 years (mean: 22)

Inclusion criteria
Members of a kibbutz with at least three of the following symptoms of less than 24 hours in duration: fever >38°C, myalgia (muscle pain), nasal discharge, and cough.

Exclusion criteria
Patients vaccinated against influenza and those with a sore throat caused by streptococcus A.

End points
Patients were assessed for six days for the following symptoms: fever, rhinitis with flow, headache, pharyngitis, cough, malaise, fatigue, and myalgia. Feelings of improvement or complete cure were also noted. Samples of sera were obtained from patients on their first visit and in the convalescent phase. Sera was tested for antibodies to influenza A and B using the complementation fixation test (CFT) and the hemagglutination inhibition test (HI).

Results
A significant improvement of the symptoms, including fever, was seen in 93.3 percent of the cases in the Sambucol-treated group within two days, whereas in the control group 91.7 percent of the patients showed improvement within six days ($p < 0.001$). A complete cure was achieved within two to three days in nearly 90 percent of the Sambucol group and within at least six days in the placebo group ($p < 0.001$). Differences in antibody titers to influenza B/Panama were higher in the group treated with Sambucol, but these differences were not significant.

Side effects
No side effects observed.

Authors' comments
Considering the efficacy of the extract in vitro on all strains of influenza virus tested, the clinical results, its low cost, and absence of side effects, this preparation could offer a possibility for safe treatment for influenza A and B.

Reviewer's comments
This study is hampered by its small sample size (12 placebo and 15 active treatment patients). The statistics used to calculate odds ratios are not described and are unlikely to have involved regression analysis and log transformed data. The study is not adequately powered. This study needs to be replicated with a larger sample size that is adequately powered and subjected to much more rigorous statistical analysis. Informed consent was obtained, but there was no mention of institutional review board (IRB) approval. (5, 1)

Evening Primrose

Latin name: *Oenothera biennis* **L.** [Onagraceae]
Plant part: **Seed**

PREPARATIONS USED
IN REVIEWED CLINICAL STUDIES

Evening primrose seeds contain up to 25 percent oil. Evening primrose oil (EPO) contains two types of omega-6 fatty acids: linoleic acid (LA) (60 to 80 percent) and gamma-linolenic acid (GLA) (8 to 14 percent) (Schulz, Hänsel, and Tyler, 2001). These acids are considered essential fatty acids (EFAs) because they are required for health and are not synthesized by the body. Linolenic acid deficiency produces visible signs in the skin, including eczema, impetigo, and erythema. Evening primrose oil is used in the formulation of cosmetic products and also as a dietary supplement (Chen, 1999).

Editor's note: Most of the product and manufacturer information supplied as follows comes from the clinical trials themselves, some of which were published as many as twenty years ago. We were unable, after extensive research, to contact any of the companies listed. We suspect that the companies may no longer exist or have been bought out by other companies. Thus the following paragraphs provide information about products that were used in clinical studies but may not exist today.

Efamol® is manufactured in the United Kingdom by Efamol Ltd. Each 500 mg capsule contains 360 mg LA, 50 mg oleic acid, and 45 mg GLA. Efamol is no longer available in the United States.

Epogam® is manufactured by Scotia Pharmaceuticals Ltd. in the United Kingdom. Each 500 mg capsule contains 321 mg LA and 40 mg GLA. One trial used Epogam topically in the form of an emulsion that contained 32 mg GLA/ml. Epogam is not sold in the United States.

EVENING PRIMROSE SUMMARY TABLE

Product Name	Manufacturer/ U.S. Distributor	Product Characteristics	Dose in Trials	Indication	No. of Trials	Benefit (Evidence Level-Trial No.)
Single Ingredient Products						
Efamol®	Efamol Ltd., UK/ None	500 mg EPO capsules including 360 mg LA, 50 mg oleic acid, 45 mg GLA	adults: 2-6 capsules 2 times daily; children: 1-2 capsules 2 times daily	Atopic dermatitis (eczema)	2	Yes (I-1) Undetermined (II-1)
				Uremic skin symptoms in dialysis patients	1	Yes (II-1)
			3 or 4 capsules 2 times daily	Attention deficit/ hyperactivity problems in children	2	No (I-2)
			6 capsules 2 times daily	Rheumatoid arthritis	2*	No (I-2)
			3 capsules 2 times daily	PMS	1	Undetermined (II-1)
Epogam®	Scotia Pharmaceuticals Ltd., UK/ None	500 mg EPO capsules including 321 mg LA, 40 mg GLA	6 capsules 2 times daily	Atopic dermatitis (eczema)	1**	No (I-1)
				Chronic hand dermatitis	1	No (I-1)
				Diabetic neuropathy (nerve degeneration)	1	Yes (I-1)

		Emulsion containing 32 mg GLA/ml	10 ml topical twice daily	Uremic pruritus (itch) in dialysis patients	1	Trend (III-1)
Efamast	Searle, UK/None	500 mg capsules	4 capsules 2 times daily	Fibroadenomas (benign breast lumps)	1	Undetermined (III-1)
Generic	None/None	0.6 ml capsules	4 capsules 2 times daily	Obesity	1	Undetermined (III-1)
Combination Product						
Efamol Marine	Scotia Pharmaceuticals Ltd., UK/None	430 mg EPO plus 107 mg marine fish oil (17 mg eicosapentaenoic acid, 11 mg docosahexaenoic acid)	6 capsules 2 times daily	Rheumatoid arthritis	2*	No (I-2)
				Psoriatic arthritis	1	No (II-1)
				Atopic dermatitis (eczema)	1**	No (I-1)

*One of these studies compared Efamol with Efamol Marine and is listed twice in the table, once with each product.
**This study that compared Epogam with Efamol Marine is listed twice in the table, once with each product.

Efamol Marine is supplied in capsules containing 430 mg EPO plus 107 mg marine fish oil (17 mg eicosapentaenoic acid [EPA], 11 mg docosahexaenoic acid [DHA]). Efamol Marine is manufactured in the United Kingdom by Scotia Pharmaceuticals Ltd. and is not available in the United States.

Efamast capsules, which contain 500 mg EPO, are manufactured by Searle in the United Kingdom. Efamast is not sold in the United States.

One trial used a generic product containing 0.6 ml EPO per capsule.

SUMMARY OF REVIEWED CLINICAL STUDIES

Essential fatty acids, including linoleic acid found in evening primrose oil, cannot be manufactured in the human body, and their supply is dependent on adequate dietary intake. Inadequate intake or compromised conversion to active metabolites can result in symptoms such as hair loss, eczema, disorders in connective tissue, poor wound healing, poor immune and reproductive function, and degeneration of organs, including the liver and kidney (Chen, 1999).

Trials using evening primrose oil preparations have been conducted on subjects with eczema, arthritis, attention-deficit hyperactivity disorder (ADHD, in children), diabetic neuropathy, premenstrual syndrome (PMS), benign fibroadenomas in the breast, and obesity. The majority of trials have focused upon atopic eczema, in which there appears to be a trend toward efficacy. EPO may also help ameliorate the uremic skin symptoms of those undergoing dialysis. In addition, EPO may improve mild diabetic neuropathy. No evidence indicates that it has any effect on ADHD in children, improves symptoms of arthritis or PMS, reduces benign fibroadenomas in the breasts, or helps obese women lose weight.

Atopic eczema or atopic dermatitis is a type of dermatitis in which an inflammation of the skin develops in persons subject to allergic reactions. It is associated with itching, redness, swelling, and blisters that may be weeping and progress to crusted, scaly, and thickened skin. The skin rash can be widespread or limited to a few areas. In teens and young adults, the patches typically occur on the hands and feet (American Academy of Dermatology, 1995).

Efamol and Efamol Marine

Atopic Dermatitis (Eczema)

Two studies explored the use of Efamol in the treatment of atopic eczema. The first study was of good quality, with a crossover design including 80 subjects with moderate to severe atopic eczema, from eight months to 58 years old. The children were given one or two (500 mg) capsules twice daily, and the adults were given two, four, or six (500 mg) capsules twice daily. Each subject was given 12 weeks of EPO and 12 weeks of placebo in random order. An analysis of symptom scores indicated that EPO produced a 30 percent improvement overall in severity of the eczema, while those receiving the higher doses had a 43 percent improvement. At the higher doses for children and adults, EPO was significantly superior to placebo in reducing symptoms of itch, scaling, and patients' general impression of severity. At the lower doses, only itch was significantly reduced compared to placebo (Wright and Burton, 1982).

The second study included 24 adults, with moderate to severe atopic eczema, who were given either placebo or four (500 mg) capsules twice daily for three months. Compared to baseline, patients in the EPO group consumed significantly less topical steroids and had significant improvement in the severity and grade of inflammation, including a reduction in surface area involved. The degree of improvement in clinical parameters in the EPO group was significantly greater compared to the placebo group (Schalin-Karrila et al., 1987). Our reviewer, Dr. John Trimmer Hicks, deemed the study inconclusive due to the small sample size.

Uremic Skin Symptoms in Dialysis Patients

A small study with 16 hemodialysis patients compared the results of Efamol and LA in the treatment of uremic skin symptoms. This good-quality six-week trial compared two capsules twice daily of Efamol (each 500 mg capsule containing 360 mg LA, 50 mg oleic acid, and 45 mg GLA) with pure LA (500 mg capsules). Compared to LA, there was a significant improvement in the combined symptom score (including itch, redness, and dryness) following treatment with

Efamol. There was a trend toward improvement in itch when it was measured independently (Yoshimoto-Furuie et al., 1999).

Attention-Deficit/Hyperactivity Problems in Children

The effect of Efamol on attention-deficit problems or attention-deficit hyperactivity disorder in children was studied in two well-conducted crossover trials. No statistical improvement in overall behavior compared to placebo occurred in either study. The children, with a mean age of nine years, received three or four (500 mg) capsules twice daily for one month. The trials were of good quality but of moderate size; a total of 48 children were included in the two studies (Aman, Mitchell, and Turbott, 1987; Arnold et al., 1989). One study included 10 to 15 mg D-amphetamine as a positive control, and this substance did have a significant effect compared to placebo (Arnold et al., 1989).

Rheumatoid Arthritis

Efamol was tested for efficacy in improving symptoms of rheumatoid arthritis in two good-quality, double-blind, placebo-controlled studies. In both studies the dose was 6 g (12 capsules) per day. Neither study showed an impressive benefit. In the first study, which ran for six months and included 30 subjects, there was no clear benefit in comparison with the placebo (olive oil) (Brzeski, Madhok, and Capell, 1991). The second study compared Efamol with Efamol Marine and placebo. In this study, treatment was given for one year followed by a three-month observation period. Compared to placebo, significantly more patients taking Efamol and Efamol Marine experienced a subjective improvement and were able to reduce their NSAID (nonsteroidal anti-inflammatory drug) therapy. There was no objective improvement in clinical measures, including duration of morning stiffness, grip strength, Ritchie articular index, and pain scale (Belch et al., 1988).

Psoriatic Arthritis

The effect of Efamol Marine on inflammatory arthritis associated with psoriasis (negative for rheumatoid factor) was tested in a well-designed, double-blind, placebo-controlled study involving 32 subjects. The treatment group received 12 capsules per day for nine months. No improvement was seen in either the skin disease or the arthritis. In addition, therapy with Efamol Marine did not decrease the use of NSAIDs to alleviate joint symptoms (Veale et al., 1994).

Premenstrual Syndrome

The effect of Efamol on premenstrual tension was compared to placebo in 30 women over the length of four menstrual cycles. The treatment group was given three (500 mg) capsules twice daily. The PMS symptom scores substantially improved in both the Efamol and placebo groups, and the improvement was slightly greater for the Efamol group. The authors of the study suggested that larger doses and longer treatment length might have shown greater benefit (Puolakka et al., 1985).

Epogam and Efamol Marine

Atopic Dermatitis (Eczema) and Chronic Hand Dermatitis

Two good-quality studies found no benefit from Epogam for dermatitis. The first study was a double-blind, placebo-controlled study including 123 adults and children with atopic dermatitis (eczema), Epogam was compared with Efamol Marine and placebo (paraffin). Subjects were given six capsules twice daily of each treatment. Epogam capsules contained 500 mg EPO, while Efamol Marine capsules contained 430 mg EPO and 107 mg marine fish oil. After 16 weeks, there was no difference in dermatitis symptom scores between either Epogam or Efamol Marine and placebo (Berth-Jones and Graham-Brown, 1993). The second study was a double-blind, placebo-controlled study including 34 subjects with chronic hand dermatitis. In this study, chronic hand dermatitis was defined as dermatitis limited to the hands, excluding eczema. The study ran for four months with continued observation for an additional two months. Improvement was reported in symptoms of dryness, redness, and cracking with Epogam, 12 (500 mg) capsules per day, and placebo (sunflower oil), with no statistical difference between the two (Whitaker, Cilliers, and de Beer, 1996).

Uremic Pruritus (Itch) in Dialysis Patients

A poorly described, double-blind, placebo-controlled study of six months examined the effect of a topical Epogam emulsion on itch (uremic pruritus) experienced by patients undergoing either continuous ambulatory peritoneal dialysis or hemodialysis. Only 16 of the original 33 patients completed the six-month study (five in the placebo group and 11 in the Epogam group). There was no statistically significant difference in the score for itch between the placebo and treatment cream; however, some individuals experienced relief with the Epogam cream, which vanished upon cessation of treatment and was relieved again with use of the cream (Tamimi, Mikhail, and Stevens, 1999).

Diabetic Neuropathy

Epogam was determined to have a positive effect on mild diabetic neuropathy in a well-conducted, double-blind, placebo-controlled study with 84 patients. Treatment with six capsules twice daily, or 6 g per day, for one year improved neurophysiological parameters (motor nerve conduction velocity [MNCV], compound muscle action potential, sensory nerve action potential [SNAP], and warm and cold thresholds) and neurologic parameters (isometric muscle strength and tendon reflexes) compared to baseline, most of them significantly. These parameters mostly deteriorated with placebo (Keen et al., 1993).

Efamast

Fibroadenomas (Benign Breast Lumps)

In a nonrandomized trial including 23 women with benign breast lumps, six months of treatment with four (500 mg) Efamast capsules twice daily was compared to controls who received no treatment. As a result, there was no significant reduction in the size of the lump for women in the treatment group, compared to controls (Kollias et al., 2000).

Generic

Obesity

In a double-blind, placebo-controlled study with 74 obese women (at least 20 percent in excess of ideal body weight), generic EPO was given in a dose of four (0.6 ml) capsules twice daily. Both EPO and placebo groups were given ascorbic acid (250 mg three times daily) and put on a restricted diet. After three months of treatment both the EPO and placebo groups lost some weight, but no indication was found that EPO assisted in weight loss (Haslett et al., 1983)

SYSTEMATIC REVIEWS AND META-ANALYSES

A meta-analysis of nine double-blind, randomized, placebo-controlled studies found Epogam to have highly significant effects on atopic eczema. It appears that the trials, four of parallel design and five of crossover design, were previously unpublished. A total of 311 patients, both children and adults, were included. The majority of adults were given eight (500 mg) capsules per day, but the dose ranged from 4 to 12 capsules. Six trials had a duration of three months, two lasted for two months, and another lasted for one month. Both doctors and patients assessed the severity of the eczema by scoring symptoms at baseline and at several intervals, with an initial assessment after three to four weeks in all studies. Improvements in the Epogam groups in comparison to the placebo groups were often highly significant (two-tail tests, $p < 0.01$), particularly in the case of itch, whereas no improvement, or even a slight deterioration, was seen with placebo. Those treated with Epogam saw progressive improvement, with the effects consistently better at the final assessment point. Higher doses of Epogam produced a greater response, indicating a significant dose-response relationship. In the crossover studies, there was a carryover effect; patients receiving placebo in the second round had little to no deterioration following the earlier benefit from Epogam. When plasma essential fatty acid levels were measured, an improvement in the clinical score for atopic eczema positively correlated with a rise in EFA levels (particularly increased dihomogamma-linolenic acid [DGLA] and arachidonic acid). Finally, improvement with Epogam was in addition to benefits from conventional eczema therapy (Morse et al., 1989).

ADVERSE REACTIONS OR SIDE EFFECTS

Occasional side effects noted in the trials included nausea, diarrhea, and headache.

REFERENCES

Aman MG, Mitchell EA, Turbott SH (1987). The effect of essential fatty acid supplementation by Efamol in hyperactive children. *Journal of Abnormal Child Psychology* 15 (1): 75-90.

American Academy of Dermatology (1995). *Eczema/Atopic Dermatitis*. Schaumburg, IL: American Academy of Dermatology <www.aad.org/pamphlets/eczema/html>.

Arnold LE, Kleykamp D, Votolato NA, Taylor WA, Kontras SB, Tobin K (1989). Gamma-linolenic acid for attention-deficit hyperactivity disorder: Placebo-controlled comparison to D-amphetamine. *Biological Psychiatry* 25 (2): 222-228.

Belch JJF, Ansell D, Madhok R, O'Dowd A, Sturrock RD (1988). Effects of altering dietary essential fatty acids on requirements for non-steroidal anti-inflammatory drugs in patients with rheumatoid arthritis: A double-blind placebo-controlled study. *Annals of the Rheumatic Diseases* 47 (2): 96-104.

Berth-Jones J, Graham-Brown RAC (1993). Placebo-controlled trial of essential fatty acid supplementation in atopic dermatitis. *The Lancet* 341 (8860): 1557-1560.

Brzeski M, Madhok R, Capell HA (1991). Evening primrose oil in patients with rheumatoid arthritis and side-effects of non-steroidal anti-inflammatory drugs. *British Journal of Rheumatology* 30 (5): 370-372.

Chen JK (1999). *Evening Primrose Oil: Continuing Education Module*. Boulder, CO: New Hope Institute of Retailing.

Haslett C, Douglas JG, Chalmers SR, Weighhill A, Munro JF (1983). A double-blind evaluation of evening primrose oil as an antiobesity agent. *International Journal of Obesity* 7 (6): 549-553.

Keen H, Payan J, Allawi J, Walker J, Jamal GA, Weir AI, Henderson LM, Bissessar EA, Watkins PJ, Sampson M, et al. (1993). Treatment of diabetic neuropathy with gamma-linolenic acid. *Diabetes Care* 16 (1): 8-15.

Kollias J, Macmillan RD, Sibbering DM, Burrell H, Robertson JFR (2000). Effect of evening primrose oil on clinically diagnosed fibroadenomas. *The Breast* 9 (1): 35-36.

Morse PF, Horrobin DF, Manku MS, Stewart CM, Allen R, Littlewood S, Wright S, Burton J, Gould DJ, Holt PJ, et al. (1989). Meta-analysis of placebo-controlled studies of the efficacy of Epogam in the treatment of atopic eczema: Relationship between plasma essential fatty acid changes and clinical response. *British Journal of Dermatology* 121 (1): 75-90.

Puolakka J, Makarainen L, Viinikka L, Ylikorkala O (1985). Biochemical and clinical effects of treating the premenstrual syndrome with prostaglandin synthesis precursors. *The Journal of Reproductive Medicine* 30 (3): 149-153.

Schalin-Karrila M, Mattila L, Jansen CT, Uotila P (1987). Evening primrose oil in the treatment of atopic eczema: Effect on clinical status, plasma phospholipid fatty acids and circulating blood prostaglandins. *British Journal of Dermatology* 117 (1): 11-19.

Schulz V, Hänsel R, Tyler VE (2001). *Rational Phytotherapy: A Physicians' Guide to Herbal Medicine,* Fourth Edition. Trans. TC Telgar. Berlin: Springer-Verlag.

Tamimi N, Mikhail A, Stevens P (1999). Role of gamma-linolenic acid in uraemic pruritus. *Nephron* 83 (2): 170-171.

Veale DJ, Torley HI, Richards IM, O'Dowd A, Fitsimons C, Belch JJF, Sturrock RD (1994). A double-blind placebo controlled trial of Efamol Marine on skin and joint symptoms of psoriatic arthritis. *British Journal of Rheumatology* 33 (10): 954-958.

Whitaker DK, Cilliers J, de Beer C (1996). Evening primrose oil (Epogam) in the treatment of chronic hand dermatitis: Disappointing therapeutic results. *Dermatology* 193 (2): 115-120.

Wright S, Burton JL (1982). Oral evening-primrose-seed oil improves atopic eczema. *The Lancet* 2 (8308): 1120-1122.

Yoshimoto-Furuie K, Yoshimoto K, Tanaka T, Saima S, Kikuchi Y, Shay J, Horrobin D, Echizen H (1999). Effects of oral supplementation with evening primrose oil for six weeks on plasma essential fatty acids and uremic skin symptoms in hemodialysis patients. *Nephron* 81 (2): 151-159.

DETAILS ON EVENING PRIMROSE PRODUCTS
AND CLINICAL STUDIES

Product and clinical study information is grouped in the same order as in the Summary Table. A profile on an individual product is followed by details of the clinical studies associated with that product. In some instances a clinical study, or studies, supports several products that contain the same principal ingredient(s). In these instances, those products are grouped together.

Clinical studies that follow each product, or group of products, are grouped by therapeutic indication, in accordance with the order in the Summary Table.

Index to Evening Primrose

Product Profile: Efamol®

Manufacturer	**Efamol Ltd., UK**
U.S. distributor	None
Botanical ingredient	**Evening primrose seed oil**
Extract name	N/A
Quantity	500 mg
Processing	No information
Standardization	360 mg linoleic acid, 50 mg oleic acid, and 45 mg gamma-linolenic acid in each capsule
Formulation	Capsule

Source(s) of information: Schalin-Karrila et al., 1987; Wright and Burton, 1982.

Clinical Study: Efamol®

Extract name	N/A
Manufacturer	Efamol Ltd., UK
Indication	**Atopic eczema**
Level of evidence	**I**
Therapeutic benefit	**Yes**

Bibliographic reference

Wright S, Burton JL (1982). Oral evening-primrose-seed oil improves atopic eczema. *The Lancet* 2 (8308): 1120-1122.

Trial design

Crossover study: 12 weeks of evening primrose oil and 12 weeks of placebo in random order. Patients allowed to continue their normal treatment (mild topical steroid, an emollient, and systemic antihistamines). Adult patients (age 15 to 58) randomly allocated to three dosage groups: A, B, and C received two, four, or six capsules twice daily, respectively. Children (ages 8 months to 14 years) divided into two treatment groups, D and E, and given one or two capsules twice daily. Groups A and D were analyzed separately as low-dose groups.

Study duration	3 months
Dose	Adults: 2 to 6 (500 mg) capsules twice daily; children: 1 to 2 (500 mg) capsules twice daily
Route of administration	Oral
Randomized	Yes
Randomization adequate	Yes
Blinding	Double-blind
Blinding adequate	Yes
Placebo	Yes
Drug comparison	No
Site description	Not described
No. of subjects enrolled	99
No. of subjects completed	80
Sex	Male and female
Age	8 months to 58 years

Inclusion criteria

Clinical diagnosis of moderate or severe atopic eczema, in addition to either a family history of atopy or a personal history of other atopic symptoms.

Exclusion criteria
Patients receiving potent topical steroids or systemic steroid therapy.

End points
Eczema was assessed before the trial and every three weeks during the trial. Degree of scaling, redness, and overall severity were separately assessed on a 10 cm linear scale. Each patient (or parent) also assessed the severity of itching. In the adult patients blood was also taken at 0, 12, and 24 weeks for blood count, urea, electrolytes, and liver-function tests.

Results
In the analysis of the mean symptom scores for all 99 patients, and the impressions of doctors and patients, evening primrose oil produced an improvement of about 30 percent in overall severity of the eczema, and the adults responded better than the children. For patients in the high-dose groups, the overall improvement in severity was about 43 percent, and the patient's self-assessment showed that the EPO was significantly superior to the placebo with regard to itch ($p < .003$), scaling ($p < .002$), and general impression of severity ($p < .01$). In the low-dose groups, itching was the only symptom which responded better to evening primrose oil than placebo ($p < .05$). The doctors' assessments also showed a beneficial effect of EPO on overall severity of the condition ($p < .002$). The other symptom scores showed the same trend but failed to reach statistical significance. No significant effect resulted from the order of the treatment.

Side effects
None mentioned in paper.

Authors' comments
This study has shown that larger doses of linoleic and gamma-linolenic acid in the form of evening primrose seed oil significantly improves the symptoms of atopic eczema, particularly in adults. The relatively poor results with evening primrose seed oil in children may be due to the greater placebo effect in children, or it may be that the doses of evening primrose seed oil used were not adequate.

Reviewer's comments
A good study with pretty convincing efficacy. (5, 6)

Clinical Study: Efamol®

Extract name	N/A
Manufacturer	Efamol Ltd., UK

Indication	**Atopic eczema**
Level of evidence	**II**
Therapeutic benefit	**Undetermined**

Bibliographic reference

Schalin-Karrila M, Mattila L, Jansen CT, Uotila P (1987). Evening primrose oil in the treatment of atopic eczema: Effect on clinical status, plasma phospholipid fatty acids and circulating blood prostaglandins. *British Journal of Dermatology* 117 (1): 11-19.

Trial design

Parallel. Two-week pretrial washout for dermatitis medication.

Study duration	3 months
Dose	4 (500 mg) capsules twice daily
Route of administration	Oral
Randomized	Yes
Randomization adequate	Yes
Blinding	Double-blind
Blinding adequate	Yes
Placebo	Yes
Drug comparison	No
Site description	Not described
No. of subjects enrolled	25
No. of subjects completed	24
Sex	Male and female
Age	19-31 years

Inclusion criteria

Moderate to severe atopic eczema, in addition to either a family history of atopy or atopic respiratory symptoms.

Exclusion criteria

None mentioned.

End points

Patients were monitored for extent and severity of eczema. Blood samples were also taken to monitor effect of treatment on plasma phospholipids. Extent and severity of the eczema was estimated on a linear scale from 0 (no symptoms) to 100 (worst possible). Percentage of body surface involved was estimated, and the degree of inflammation, dryness, and itch graded on a scale of 0: none, 1: mild, 2: moderate, 3: severe. The amount of emollient cream and topical steroids used by patients during the study (as rescue medication) was also recorded.

Results

Patients in the evening primrose oil group consumed significantly less topical steroids over the course of 12 weeks (60 g versus 200 g, $p < .05$). A statistically significant improvement was observed in overall severity and grade of inflammation ($p <. 001$), a significant reduction in surface area involved, as well as in dryness and itching ($p < .01$). Patients in the placebo group also showed a significant reduction in inflammation ($p < .05$). However, in every clinical parameter, the degree of improvement was significantly greater in the EPO group than in the placebo group. The level of DGLA increased significantly in the EPO group.

Side effects

No side effects were observed in the study.

Authors' comments

Although the patients were allocated to the two groups at random, the mean initial status of the eczema was somewhat worse in the EPO group than in the placebo group, which made it difficult to estimate the real effect of EPO. However, significantly greater improvement in every parameter in the EPO group, and the fact that the patients in the placebo group needed about three times as much topical steroids as did those in the EPO group, suggest that EPO was superior to placebo.

Reviewer's comments

The study was well designed and conducted, but the results were weakened by the small sample size. (5, 4)

Clinical Study: Efamol®

Extract name	N/A
Manufacturer	Efamol Ltd., UK
Indication	**Uremic skin symptoms** in hemodialysis patients
Level of evidence	**II**
Therapeutic benefit	**Yes**

Bibliographic reference

Yoshimoto-Furuie K, Yoshimoto K, Tanaka T, Saima S, Kikuchi Y, Shay J, Horrobin D, Echizen H (1999). Effects of oral supplementation with evening primrose oil for six weeks on plasma essential fatty acids and uremic skin symptoms in hemodialysis patients. *Nephron* 81 (2): 151-159.

Trial design
Parallel. Evening primrose oil compared with linoleic acid. Group receiving LA took two (500 mg) capsules twice daily. After six weeks, the group receiving evening primrose oil continued treatment for another six weeks to study the biochemical effects of EPO.

Study duration	6 weeks
Dose	2 (500 mg) capsules twice daily
Route of administration	Oral
Randomized	Yes
Randomization adequate	Yes
Blinding	Double-blind
Blinding adequate	Yes
Placebo	No
Drug comparison	Yes
Drug name	Linoleic acid
Site description	Not described
No. of subjects enrolled	16
No. of subjects completed	16
Sex	Male and female
Age	23-79 years

Inclusion criteria
Patients undergoing hemodialysis who suffered from pruritus and other uremic skin symptoms (i.e., dryness or erythema). Severe dryness of the skin and erythrematous lesions were a prerequisite for participation in the study.

Exclusion criteria
None mentioned.

End points
Assessments of skin symptoms were performed at the beginning of the study and weekly thereafter. Plasma composition of essential fatty acids was analyzed from predialysis blood samples taken at weeks 0 and 6, and for patients on EPO, week 12. Severity of uremic skin symptoms (i.e., pruritus, erythema, and dryness) were measured by a grading-scale system. Dryness of the skin and erythrematous lesions were assessed separately by visual inspection by a single investigator and assessed in severity. The intensity of pruritus was assessed with a self-administered questionnaire.

Results

Statistically significant ($p < 0.05$) overall improvement in the EPO group with regard to the three categories of uremic dermatosis, whereas no significant changes observed in skin symptoms of the LA group. At 6 and 12 weeks, patients given EPO showed significant ($p < 0.01$) increases in the mean plasma concentration of dihomogamma-linolenic acid and gamma-linolenic acid. Patients given LA for six weeks showed a significant increase in the mean plasma concentration of LA, a reduction in docosahexaenoic acid, but no significant changes in DGLA concentrations throughout the study. No significant differences were observed in gross lipid profiles for either group over the duration of the study.

Side effects

EPO was very well tolerated with no adverse clinical symptoms.

Authors' comments

Oral supplementation with EPO significantly improved skin scores during the six-week intervention period, while LA did not. EPO (containing 0.18 g/day of GLA) produced significant elevations in the plasma concentrations of DGLA; supplementation with LA did not. This finding is in good agreement with previous data obtained from healthy subjects and suggests that conversion of LA into GLA is the rate-limiting step in humans. Thus, supplementation with EPO (rich in GLA) rather than LA is an effective means for accelerating the synthesis of DGLA in patients on dialysis.

Reviewer's comments

This is a very detailed and internally consistent set of data, even though the study group was small. The trial is rated Level II due to the small sample size. (5, 5)

Clinical Study: Efamol®

Extract name	N/A
Manufacturer	Efamol Ltd., UK
Indication	**Attention-deficit problems** in children
Level of evidence	**I**
Therapeutic benefit	**No**

Bibliographic reference

Aman MG, Mitchell EA, Turbott SH (1987). The effect of essential fatty acid supplementation by Efamol in hyperactive children. *Journal of Abnormal Child Psychology* 15 (1): 75-90.

Trial design

Crossover. Subjects received either Efamol or placebo for four weeks in randomized order with a one-week washout period between the two phases.

Study duration	1 month
Dose	3 (500 mg) capsules twice daily
Route of administration	Oral
Randomized	Yes
Randomization adequate	Yes
Blinding	Double-blind
Blinding adequate	Yes
Placebo	Yes
Drug comparison	No
Site description	Not described
No. of subjects enrolled	31
No. of subjects completed	30
Sex	Male and female
Age	Mean: 8.86 years

Inclusion criteria

Children were admitted to the study if their scores on both the Attention Problem subscale of the Revised Behavior Problem Checklist and the Inattention scale of the Conners Teacher Rating Scale exceeded the 90th percentile. Most children (26/31) qualified for the study through this criteria. Several children (5/31) had been seen by a child psychiatrist as part of another study and were given a diagnosis of attention deficit disorder (either with or without hyperactivity). Children were perceived to have attention deficits in both the home and the classroom.

Exclusion criteria

Neurological disorders; mental retardedness; less than a year's duration of inattention, impulsivity, or overactivity; children receiving medication at the time of study.

End points

Subjects were assessed prior to the study and twice during each four-week treatment phase on a variety of cognitive, motor, and standardized rating scale measures. Parents rated the children on the Revised Behavior Problem Checklist, and teachers rated the children on the Conners Teacher Rating Scale. Teachers also completed the ADD-H: Comprehensive Teacher's Rating Scale to assess hyperactivity. Subjects were assessed at each visit for side effects using the Dosage Record and Treatment Emergent Symptom Scale (DOTES). At the pretest and after each treatment phase, a blood sample was taken to determine levels of essential fatty acids.

Results

There were some suggestions of therapeutic changes following administration of Efamol, but the large majority of measures failed to show an effect when the rigorous criterion of significance of $p < 0.0012$ was applied. Only two behavioral measures, response time on the distraction task and parent ratings of attention problems, showed significant change. During treatment with Efamol, palmitoleic acids levels decreased significantly and dihomo-gamma-linolenic acid levels increased (14 percent over placebo). The remaining essential fatty acids showed no significant changes, although there was a tendency for alpha-linolenic acid to decrease.

Side effects

No significant side effects in the Efamol group.

Authors' comments

It must be concluded that essential fatty acid supplementation, employed with hyperactive children unselected for baseline EFA concentrations and treated at the present dosage, had relatively few clinical or cognitive effects. However, the rationale for employing essential fatty acid supplementation with hyperactive children appears reasonable on the basis of clinical characteristics and previous work suggesting EFA deficiencies in these children.

Reviewer's comments

Well-designed and well-conducted study. Evening primrose oil does not appear to have any efficacy in hyperactive children. (5, 6)

Clinical Study: Efamol®

Extract name	N/A
Manufacturer	Efamol Ltd., UK
Indication	**Attention-deficit hyperactivity disorder** in children
Level of evidence	**I**
Therapeutic benefit	**No**

Bibliographic reference

Arnold LE, Kleykamp D, Votolato NA, Taylor WA, Kontras SB, Tobin K (1989). Gamma-linolenic acid for attention-deficit hyperactivity disorder: Placebo-controlled comparison to D-amphetamine. *Biological Psychiatry* 25 (2): 222-228.

Trial design
Latin-square, double-crossover study. The three groups were D-amphetamine group (one capsule [10 or 15 mg based on body weight] D-amphetamine + eight capsules placebo); Efamol group (one capsule placebo + eight capsules Efamol); and placebo (nine capsules placebo).

Study duration	1 month
Dose	4 (500 mg) capsules twice daily
Route of administration	Oral
Randomized	Yes
Randomization adequate	Yes
Blinding	Double-blind
Blinding adequate	Yes
Placebo	Yes
Drug comparison	Yes
Drug name	D-amphetamine
Site description	Not described
No. of subjects enrolled	18
No. of subjects completed	18
Sex	Male
Age	6-12 years (mean: 9)

Inclusion criteria
Aged between 6 and 12 years; normal intelligence; diagnosis of attention deficit disorder wth hyperactivity by DSM-III criteria; score of 18 or more on Conners Hyperactivity Index; and a sum of 24 or more on the first six items of the Davids Hyperkinetic Rating Scale.

Exclusion criteria
Use of psychoactive drugs in the week preceding the study; history of seizures.

End points
At screening, at baseline, and every two weeks during the 12 treatment weeks, each subject had blind behavioral ratings by parents and teachers. The teachers used the Conners' Teacher Rating Scale (CTRS).

Results
Behavorial ratings following Efamol treatment were not significantly different from either placebo or D-amphetamine on most measures. Parents' ratings generally showed no difference between Efamol and placebo but a moderate response to D-amphetamine. Teachers' ratings found significant response to D-amphetamine only on the hyperactivity factor of the CTRS, with Efamol response between placebo and D-amphetamine. Post hoc

sample subdivision showed that the six subjects who had D-amphetamine immediately preceding Efamol showed no benefit from Efamol administration, whereas the other 12 subjects showed a response to Efamol closer to D-amphetamine than to placebo.

Side effects
None mentioned in paper.

Authors' comments
Gamma-linolenic acid should be considered to be an experimental treatment for ADHD. The data reported here do not establish its effectiveness. Further studies should use designs that control for a possible sequence interaction and should probably use ten EPO capsules per day.

Reviewer's comments
In this well-conducted study, D-amphetamine was statistically significantly better than placebo, but Efamol (containing GLA) was not. (5, 5)

Clinical Study: Efamol®

Extract name	N/A
Manufacturer	Efamol Ltd., UK
Indication	**Rheumatoid arthritis**
Level of evidence	**I**
Therapeutic benefit	**No**

Bibliographic reference
Brzeski M, Madhok R, Capell HA (1991). Evening primrose oil in patients with rheumatoid arthritis and side-effects of non-steroidal anti-inflammatory drugs. *British Journal of Rheumatology* 30 (5): 370-372.

Trial design
Parallel. Patients were given either evening primrose oil (Efamol) or olive oil (placebo).

Study duration	6 months
Dose	6 g/day (540 mg GLA per day)
Route of administration	Oral
Randomized	Yes
Randomization adequate	Yes
Blinding	Double-blind
Blinding adequate	Yes

Placebo   Yes
Drug comparison   No

Site description   Not described

No. of subjects enrolled 40
No. of subjects completed 30
Sex   Male and female
Age   16-75 years

Inclusion criteria
Patients with rheumatoid arthritis and upper gastrointestinal lesions due to nonsteroidal anti-inflammatory drugs (i.e., peptic ulcer or gastritis at endoscopy or on barium meal, or symptoms strongly suggestive of these diagnoses).

Exclusion criteria
Patients taking systemic corticosteroids were excluded.

End points
Patients were allowed to continue routine medication (NSAIDs, H2 blockers, analgesics). After three months, patients were asked every week to attempt reduction of their NSAIDs and analgesics. At zero, three, and six months, the following assessments were performed: daily use of NSAIDs and analgesia; morning stiffness; 100 mm horizontal visual analog scales for pain and well-being; Ritchie articular index and health assessment questionnaire (HAQ); and Hb, platelets, erythrocyte sedimentation rate (ESR), C-reactive protein (CRP), globulins, and plasma fatty acid analysis.

Results
The evening primrose oil group had significantly reduced morning stiffness at three months with a trend to reduction at six months. In the placebo group, there was a significant reduction in articular index and pain at six months, and a trend to reduced morning stiffness at six months. There was no change in well-being, HAQ scores, or laboratory parameters of inflammation in either group. Of the 13 patients completing treatment in the EPO group, ten showed a significant rise in plasma dihomogamma-linolenic acid (a metabolite of gamma-linolenic acid), suggesting good compliance with the study. No patients stopped NSAIDs, but three in each group reduced the dose of NSAID by one tablet (e.g., t.d.s. to b.i.d.). One patient in the evening primrose group increased NSAID dosage. Four patients taking placebo and one patient taking EPO reduced analgesia dosage, and two in each group increased dosage.

Side effects
No major effects reported in paper. Several patients dropped out of the study due to nausea, which occurred equally in both groups.

Authors' comments
The study found that only 23 percent (3 out of 13) of patients completing treatment with EPO could reduce their NSAID dose and none could stop, similar to placebo. This contrasts with a previous study in which the same dose of EPO enabled 25 percent to stop and an additional 38 percent to reduce NSAID dose after six months without clinical deterioration. In that study, patients had less severe rheumatoid arthritis and none was on second-line therapy. EPO may thus be beneficial only in mild rheumatoid arthritis. We are unable to recommend EPO for severe rheumatoid arthritis. It is disappointing that we have been unable to confirm the possibility of substituting EPO for NSAIDs in patients with NSAID-induced gastrointestinal side effects. It is interesting that olive oil enabled as many patients to reduce NSAIDS as did EPO and produced improvement in more clinical parameters than EPO.

Reviewer's comments
In this well-designed and well-described study, there was no clear benefit of EPO for patients with rheumatoid arthritis. (5, 6)

Clinical Study: Efamol®

Extract name	N/A
Manufacturer	Efamol Ltd., UK
Indication	**Premenstrual syndrome**
Level of evidence	**II**
Therapeutic benefit	**Undetermined**

Bibliographic reference
Puolakka J, Makarainen L, Viinikka L, Ylikorkala O (1985). Biochemical and clinical effects of treating the premenstrual syndrome with prostaglandin synthesis precursors. *The Journal of Reproductive Medicine* 30 (3): 149-153.

Trial design
Crossover.

Study duration   4 menstrual cycles
Dose   3 (500 mg) capsules twice a day, 15th day of the menstrual cycle until the 1st day of the next cycle
Route of administration   Oral

Randomized   Yes
Randomization adequate   Yes
Blinding   Double-blind
Blinding adequate   Yes

Placebo   Yes
Drug comparison   No

Site description   Not described

No. of subjects enrolled   30
No. of subjects completed   Not given
Sex   Female
Age   25-47 years (mean: 38.5)

Inclusion criteria
Severe and incapacitating premenstrual syndrome, with symptoms starting between the fourteenth and nineteenth day of the cycle (mean: fifteenth day).

Exclusion criteria
None mentioned.

End points
Women recorded their premenstrual symptoms at the end of each cycle, before and during the trial. Numerous symptoms were scored, forming the PMS score. Blood samples were obtained from 22 patients during both the Efamol and placebo phases of the trial, as well as from 25 healthy control women. Blood samples were collected between the twelfth to fourteenth days and twentieth to twenty-sixth days and, with the exception of the controls, on the second to fifth days of the next cycle. Blood samples were measured for the stable metabolites of PGI2 (6-keto-PGF1alpha) and TxA2 (TxB2).

Results
The PMS score significantly ($p < 0.001$) decreased following treatment with Efamol and placebo. However, the decrease was greater with Efamol treatment, 62 percent compared to 40 percent with placebo ($p < 0.05$). Depression was alleviated significantly ($p < 0.01$) more frequently by Efamol than by placebo. Irritability was not improved by either. No differences arose in plasma 6-keto-PGF1alpha and serum TxB2 levels in women with or without PMS before the trial. Efamol treatment decreased the formation of TxB2 dur-

ing the luteal phase of the cycle but had no effect on plasma 6-keto-PGF1alpha or on various pituitary or ovarian hormones.

Side effects
None reported in paper.

Authors' comments
Findings are consistent with the idea that essential fatty acids may modulate responses to hormones in PMS. Clinically, both the active and placebo groups improved substantially, but at the dose regime used, the additional effect of Efamol was only small. Larger dosages and longer treatment could improve the therapeutic effect of Efamol in PMS, as has been suggested by an open study on patients who failed to respond to other treatment.

Reviewer's comments
Both Efamol and placebo worked equally well for PMS, but Efamol's efficacy cannot be determined from this trial. (4, 5)

Product Profile: Epogam®

Manufacturer	**Scotia Pharmaceuticals Ltd., UK**
U.S. distributor	None
Botanical ingredient	**Evening primrose seed oil**
Extract name	N/A
Quantity	500 mg
Processing	No information
Standardization	321 mg linoleic acid, 40 mg gamma-linolenic acid in each capsule
Formulation	Capsule

Source(s) of information: Berth-Jones and Graham-Brown, 1993; Whitaker, Cilliers, and de Beer, 1996.

Clinical Study: Epogam®

Extract name	N/A
Manufacturer	Scotia Pharmaceuticals Ltd., UK
Indication	**Atopic dermatitis**
Level of evidence	**I**
Therapeutic benefit	**No**

Bibliographic reference
Berth-Jones J, Graham-Brown RAC (1993). Placebo-controlled trial of essential fatty acid supplementation in atopic dermatitis. *The Lancet* 341 (8860): 1557-1560.

Trial design
Parallel. Three-arm study: patients received six capsules twice daily of Epogam, Efamol Marine (one capsule contained 430 mg EPO and 107 mg marine fish oil), or placebo (liquid paraffin). Subjects participating in this study were divided according to age into two groups: adults and children up to 12 years of age. These two groups were randomized separately to achieve age balance in the three treatment groups. Treatment with sedative antihistamines continued throughout the study if used by patients at entry into the study.

Study duration	4 months
Dose	6 capsules twice daily
Route of administration	Oral
Randomized	Yes
Randomization adequate	Yes
Blinding	Double-blind
Blinding adequate	Yes
Placebo	Yes
Drug comparison	Yes
Drug name	Efamol Marine
Site description	Dermatology department outpatients
No. of subjects enrolled	123
No. of subjects completed	102
Sex	Male and female
Age	2-60 years

Inclusion criteria
Outpatients with atopic dermatitis; equal numbers of adults and children (aged up to 12 years).

Exclusion criteria
None mentioned in paper.

End points
Subjects were examined at 0, 4, 8, and 16 weeks, and again after an eight-week washout phase. Patients were allowed to use topical steroids and emollients as required. Disease activity was monitored by clinical severity scores recorded by the investigator, topical steroid requirements, and symptom scores recorded by subjects. The primary response criterion was mean

change from baseline in Leicester score at 16 weeks. The body was divided into ten zones. Each zone was scored for erythema, excoriation, dryness, cracking, and lichenification. Usage of topical steroids was assessed by weighing the tubes of unused medication. Each week, patients recorded itch, dryness, scaling, redness, and overall impression on separate 10 cm visual analog scales.

Results
At 16 weeks, there was no significant difference in mean Leicester scores between either active treatment or placebo (improvements: 8.48 in Epogam group, 2.45 in Efamol Marine group, and 7.15 in placebo group). The only significant differences for individual components were in favor of placebo over Efamol Marine for erythema ($p = 0.04$) and cracking ($p = 0.05$). Mean percentage of skin affected at 16 weeks fell 3.26 percent in the Epogam group, fell 0.11 percent in the Efamol Marine group, and rose 3.26 percent in the placebo group, with no significant differences between either treatment or placebo. Reduction in topical steroid use occurred in all groups; however, the greatest reduction was recorded for the placebo group. In the patient response diaries, the greatest mean overall reduction in visual analog scales was seen in the placebo group. However, there were no significant differences from placebo at 16 weeks in total score or in any component. In particular, there was no significant difference in pruritus (itch) score.

Side effects
None mentioned in paper.

Authors' comments
This study has demonstrated no response of atopic dermatitis to essential fatty acid supplementation nor any evidence of an additional effect when n3 series EFAs were used in combination with EFAs of the n6 series.

Reviewer's comments
In this well-designed and well-executed study, the authors argue that all prior studies were flawed and that their study is not! They were unable to document any efficacy of evening primrose oil with atopic dermatitis. (5, 6)

Clinical Study: Epogam®

Extract name	N/A
Manufacturer	Scotia Pharmaceuticals Ltd., UK
Indication	**Chronic hand dermatitis**
Level of evidence	**I**
Therapeutic benefit	**No**

Bibliographic reference
Whitaker DK, Cilliers J, de Beer C (1996). Evening primrose oil (Epogam) in the treatment of chronic hand dermatitis: Disappointing therapeutic results. *Dermatology* 193 (2): 115-120.

Trial design
Parallel. Medication or placebo (sunflower oil) was given for 16 weeks and observation continued for another eight weeks. A group of ten healthy age- and sex-matched subjects acted as controls.

Study duration	6 months
Dose	12 (500 mg) capsules per day
Route of administration	Oral
Randomized	Yes
Randomization adequate	Yes
Blinding	Double-blind
Blinding adequate	Yes
Placebo	Yes
Drug comparison	No
Site description	Dermatology department outpatients
No. of subjects enrolled	39
No. of subjects completed	34
Sex	Male and female
Age	19-75 years

Inclusion criteria
Chronic stable hand dermatitis lasting over a year.

Exclusion criteria
Patients with an inflammatory skin disorder other than eczema; allergic contact dermatitis with eczema reactions that resolved after allergen avoidance; patients with severe intercurrent illnesses; or patients currently receiving oral steroids, PUVA therapy (a combination of psoralen and ultraviolet radiation), immune suppressants, phenothiazines, or antidepressants.

End points
Patients were evaluated clinically at baseline and at four-week intervals throughout the twenty-four weeks. Unlimited quantities of standard emollient and a limited amount of a semipotent group III topical steroid cream could be used during the trial. Topical steroid use was monitored by weighing the unused cream at each visit. A 100 mm visual analog scale was used to evaluate dryness, redness, itch, cracking, vesiculation, edema, and overall impression of hand dermatitis. Standard patch test using European standard

of allergens, hematogram, and serum IgE values were determined. Skin biopsies for epidermal lipograms and histology as 5 mm punchbiopsies were taken from the lateral palmar quadrant in the area of greatest activity at 0, 16, and 24 weeks. Plasma, red cells, and separated epidermal lipograms were performed at weeks 0, 16, and 24. Histologically, skin was evaluated for signs of acute, subacute, or chronic hand dermatitis.

Results
After 16 weeks of therapy, both the Epogam and placebo groups had statistical clinical improvement in dryness, redness, and cracking with no statistical difference between the two. After 24 weeks (washout period weeks 16 to 24), the Epogam group additionally had statistically significant improvement in itch, vesiculation, and edema. At baseline, four patients in the Epogam group, three in the placebo group, and all of the control group showed normal histology. During the first 16 weeks of the trial, seven Epogam patients and 15 placebo patients showed histological improvement. During the washout phase of the trial, the histological parameters of both groups were comparable to week 16. No significant difference was found in the change in Odland bodies or intracellular multilamellar lipid sheets or epidermal GLA content. No statistically significant decrease in topical steroid use was found.

Side effects
None mentioned in paper.

Authors' comments
The similarity of favorable results between the two patient groups underlines that hand dermatitis is often characterized by a chronic relapsing course. It is possible that the trial period fell into the natural improvement phase of the disease. Regular follow-up visits made the patients more aware of their condition, and clinical guidance could have enhanced the use of emollients and avoidance of allergens. This study therefore indicates that orally administered GLA for chronic hand dermatitis has no superior therapeutic value to that of placebo. The significant improvement of all clinical parameters at the end of the trial for both study groups emphasizes the necessity of long-term randomized and controlled double-blind studies.

Reviewer's comments
This was a well-designed study showing evening primrose oil is not efficacious in this type of dermatitis. (5, 5)

Clinical Study: EF4 (Epogam)®

Extract name	N/A
Manufacturer	Scotia Pharmaceuticals Ltd., UK

Indication	**Diabetic neuropathy** (nerve degeneration)
Level of evidence	I
Therapeutic benefit	**Yes**

Bibliographic reference
Keen H, Payan J, Allawi J, Walker J, Jamal GA, Weir AI, Henderson LM, Bissessar EA, Watkins PJ, Sampson M, et al. (1993). Treatment of diabetic neuropathy with gamma-linolenic acid. *Diabetes Care* 16 (1): 8-15.

Trial design
Parallel.

Study duration	1 year
Dose	6 capsules twice daily (480 mg/day GLA)
Route of administration	Oral
Randomized	Yes
Randomization adequate	Yes
Blinding	Double-blind
Blinding adequate	Yes
Placebo	Yes
Drug comparison	No
Site description	7 centers
No. of subjects enrolled	111
No. of subjects completed	84
Sex	Male and female
Age	18-70 years (mean: 53)

Inclusion criteria
Mild diabetic neuropathy with clinical evidence such as parasthesia, numbness, weakness, impaired reflexes, or pain; idiopathic diabetes mellitus of either main clinical type; no major changes in diabetes management for at least six months; at least two of the following neurophysiological criteria in the same limb: peroneal MNCV <40 m/s at 34°C, sural MNCV <40 m/s at 34°C, sural SNAP <5μV, and heat threshold or cold threshold outside the 99 percent confidence limit for normal individuals.

Exclusion criteria
Other forms of neuropathy, including carpal tunnel syndrome; or severe neuropathy (immeasurable conduction in common peroneal nerve and/or absent sural sensory potential).

End points
Patients were evaluated at baseline and at 3, 6, and 12 months. The following neurophysiological measurements were performed on limbs: motor nerve conduction velocity (m/s), compound muscle action potential (CMAP) amplitudes (mV), sensory nerve action potential amplitudes (µV), and warm and cold threshold measurements. Neurological examination consisted of isometric muscle strength measurements in wrists, fingers, and toes, and tendon reflexes in upper and lower limbs. Sensation was also assessed for upper and lower limbs. Blood taken at each visit was tested for glucose, hemoglobin A1 (HbA, a measure of blood glucose control), routine hematology, urea, electrolytes, total protein, albumin, fructosamine, alkaline phosphatase, gamma-glutamyl transferase, and aspartate aminotransferase.

Results
All ten neurophysiological parameters improved with evening primrose oil, eight significantly. All ten parameters modestly deteriorated with placebo, four significantly. All six neurological assessments improved with EPO, two significantly. Five of the six assessments deteriorated with placebo, three significantly so. Hemoglobin A1 levels significantly influenced a patient's response to EPO. When the starting level of HbA was less than or equal to 10 percent, improvement with treatment was considerably greater for all 16 parameters than if the HbA starting level was greater than 10 percent.

Side effects
The treatment was well tolerated. No major biochemical or clinical adverse effects were attributable to the treatment.

Authors' comments
Gamma-linolenic acid was found to be superior to placebo. This supports the view that an important factor contributing to the neuropathy of diabetes may be a reduced formation of linoleic acid metabolites. Administration of GLA to patients with mild diabetic polyneuropathy may prevent deterioration and, in some cases, reverse the condition. The treatment is not associated with any important adverse events and may offer an advance in the management of diabetic neuropathy.

Reviewer's comments
The results seem indisputable. EPO has a clear effect on diabetic neuropathy. (5, 6)

Clinical Study: Epogam®

Extract name	N/A
Manufacturer	Scotia Pharmaceuticals Ltd., UK

Indication   **Uremic pruritus** (itch) in dialysis patients
Level of evidence **III**
Therapeutic benefit **Trend**

Bibliographic reference
Tamimi N, Mikhail A, Stevens P (1999). Role of gamma-linolenic acid in uraemic pruritus. *Nephron* 83 (2): 170-171.

Trial design
Parallel.

Study duration	6 months
Dose	Epogam emulsion (10 ml) (32 mg/ml) twice daily
Route of administration	Topical
Randomized	No
Randomization adequate	No
Blinding	Double-blind
Blinding adequate	No
Placebo	Yes
Drug comparison	No
Site description	Not described
No. of subjects enrolled	33
No. of subjects completed	16
Sex	Not given
Age	Not given

Inclusion criteria
Dialysis patients on continuous ambulatory peritoneal dialysis (CAPD) or hemodialysis (HD) with intractable itching (pruritus).

Exclusion criteria
None mentioned.

End points
Severity of pruritus and response to treatment assessed by a questionnaire based on severity, frequency, and distribution of pruritus; scratching; number of sleeping hours; and frequency of waking up during the night for scratching. Renal and liver function tests, full blood count, cholesterol, triglycerides, uric acid levels, ferritin, magnesium, zinc, and parathormone levels were measured at the beginning and end of the study.

Results

Epogam had no effect on hematological and biochemical parameters measured. The difference in itching score between groups failed to reach statistical significance ($p < 0.08$). However, some patients derived marked relief from itching. In two cases, itching recurred after cessation of EPO and was relieved again after EPO was reissued.

Side effects

None mentioned in paper.

Authors' comments

Treatment effects are not instantaneous, as time is needed to reconstitute the normal fatty acid balance in the cutaneous cells. The optimal dose and duration of treatment seems not to be known. This study suggests that evening primrose oil may be beneficial in alleviating the symptoms of dialysis itch, and the mechanism may be through reversal or modulation of the pathological changes alluded to previously, but further studies are needed to confirm this.

Reviewer's comments

This study was briefly described in a letter to the editor. The issue of randomization was not addressed, the sex and age of subjects were not described, the data were summarized in insufficient detail to permit analysis, and there was a large number of dropouts. The placebo was also not described. (1, 2)

Product Profile: Efamast

Manufacturer	**Searle, UK**
U.S. distributor	None
Botanical ingredient	**Evening primrose seed oil**
Extract name	N/A
Quantity	500 mg
Processing	No information
Standardization	No information
Formulation	Capsule

Source(s) of information: Kollias et al., 2000.

Clinical Study: Efamast

Extract name	N/A
Manufacturer	Searle, UK

Indication	**Fibroadenomas** (benign breast lumps)
Level of evidence	**III**
Therapeutic benefit	**Undetermined**

Bibliographic reference

Kollias J, Macmillan RD, Sibbering DM, Burrell H, Robertson JFR (2000). Effect of evening primrose oil on clinically diagnosed fibroadenomas. *The Breast* 9 (1): 35-36.

Trial design

Parallel. Twenty-three women were given the treatment, and 19 women served as controls and received no treatment.

Study duration	6 months
Dose	4 (500 mg) capsules twice daily
Route of administration	Oral
Randomized	No
Randomization adequate	No
Blinding	Open
Blinding adequate	No
Placebo	No
Drug comparison	No
Site description	1 hospital breast unit
No. of subjects enrolled	23
No. of subjects completed	20
Sex	Female
Age	22-49 years (median: 29)

Inclusion criteria

Female patients with breast lumps classified as benign (less than 3 cm and having benign characteristics) who did not wish to have lumps removed surgically.

Exclusion criteria

None mentioned.

End points

Clinical size of breast lumps measured in two dimensions using calipers and ultrasound measurements taken in 3D prior to initial fine needle aspiration. Measurements were repeated at six months.

Results
After six months, change in mean ultrasound size of fibroadenomas in treatment and control groups was not statistically significant ($p = 0.6$). In the Efamast group, 11 out of 21 fibroadenomas reduced in size (52 percent), while in the control group, 8 out of 19 fibroadenomas reduced in size (42 percent), a non-statistically significant comparison between the two groups. No fibroadenomas in either group became impalpable.

Side effects
None mentioned in paper.

Authors' comments
The present study failed to demonstrate that the administration of oil of evening primrose was followed by any appreciable size reduction in women with fibroadenomas compared with a control group. The small number of patients used in this study made statistical evaluation between groups difficult.

Reviewer's comments
This study is flawed by its lack of randomization, blinding, placebo control, and small sample size. (1, 3)

Product Profile: Evening Primrose Oil (generic)

Manufacturer	None
U.S. distributor	None
Botanical ingredient	**Evening primrose seed oil**
Extract name	N/A
Quantity	No information
Processing	No information
Standardization	No information
Formulation	Capsule

Source(s) of information: Haslett et al., 1983.

Clinical Study: Generic

Extract name	N/A
Manufacturer	None

Indication	**Obesity**
Level of evidence	**III**
Therapeutic benefit	**Undetermined**

Bibliographic reference
Haslett C, Douglas JG, Chalmers SR, Weighhill A, Munro JF (1983). A double-blind evaluation of evening primrose oil as an antiobesity agent. *International Journal of Obesity* 7 (6): 549-553.

Trial design
Patients were divided into two groups: (A) 40 subjects suffering from refractory obesity. These subjects had attended the obesity clinic for one year or more and had failed to lose weight in the previous three months (during which they had not received an antiobesity agent). (B) 60 subjects referred to the clinic for the first time. In each group, the subjects were divided into two groups—placebo and active treatment. Subjects were given carbohydrate-restricted dietary advice designed to provide 1,000 calories per day. They were also given a supply of ascorbic acid tablets (250 mg/tablet) and told to take them three times per day.

Study duration	3 months
Dose	4 (0.6 ml) capsules twice daily
Route of administration	Oral
Randomized	No
Randomization adequate	No
Blinding	Double-blind
Blinding adequate	No
Placebo	Yes
Drug comparison	No
Site description	Hospital obesity clinic
No. of subjects enrolled	100
No. of subjects completed	74
Sex	Female
Age	19-61 years (mean: 42)

Inclusion criteria
Women at least 20 percent in excess of ideal body weight.

Exclusion criteria
Subjects outside the age range of 16 to 69; cardiac failure; dependent edema; nonstable endocrine disease such as poorly controlled diabetes or untreated hypothyroidism; subjects taking salicylates or other medications known to interfere with prostaglandin synthesis or action.

End points
Subjects assessed hunger rating on a linear analog scale from 0 to 100. They were weighed and blood was obtained for hematological and biochemical analysis every two weeks.

Results
In group A, mean weight loss achieved after two weeks was 1.1 kg in the placebo group and 0.9 kg in the evening primrose oil group. In group B, mean weight loss after two weeks was 4.1 kg in the placebo group and 3.2 kg in the EPO group. There was no statistical difference with either group. Eighteen reported a reduction in appetite, nine of whom were receiving placebo.

Side effects
Two subjects complained of hair loss (one active, one placebo), and three subjects taking EPO complained of skin changes.

Authors' comments
In this double-blind study, EPO was given in a high-dose regime and ascorbic acid was administered concurrently in order to facilitate the conversion of gamma-linolenic acid to prostaglandin. Overall weight losses achieved in those subjects treated at time of referral to the clinic are comparable to previous experience. Neither in these subjects nor in those with refractory obesity did EPO exert a clinically relevant antiobesity effect. Findings show that EPO is of no practical value in the treatment of the obese female subject.

Reviewer's comments
Despite the methodological flaws, one might have expected some trends if there was any efficacy here. The trial was not randomized, and the statistical methods were not adequately described. (1, 3)

Product Profile: Efamol Marine

Manufacturer	**Scotia Pharmaceuticals Ltd., UK**
U.S. distributor	None
Botanical ingredient	**Evening primrose seed oil**
Extract name	N/A
Quantity	430 mg
Processing	No information
Standardization	No information
Formulation	Capsule

Other ingredients: Marine fish oil (107 mg, contains 17 mg eicosapentaenoic acid and 11 mg docosahexaenoic acid).

Source(s) of information: Veale et al., 1994; Berth-Jones and Graham-Brown, 1993.

Clinical Study: Efamol Marine

Extract name	N/A
Manufacturer	Efamol Ltd., UK
Indication	**Rheumatoid arthritis**
Level of evidence	**I**
Therapeutic benefit	**No**

Bibliographic reference
Belch JJF, Ansell D, Madhok R, O'Dowd A, Sturrock RD (1988). Effects of altering dietary essential fatty acids on requirements for non-steroidal anti-inflammatory drugs in patients with rheumatoid arthritis: A double-blind placebo-controlled study. *Annals of the Rheumatic Diseases* 47 (2): 96-104.

Trial design
Parallel. Three-arm study: Efamol; Efamol Marine; and placebo. Patients taking Efamol were given 12 capsules (540 mg GLA) per day. Each group's capsules also contained 120 mg/day of vitamin E as an antioxidant. During the first three months of treatment, patients were instructed to take the treatment along with their usual NSAIDs. From 3 to 12 months, patients were instructed to decrease or stop taking their NSAIDs if possible without exacerbation of rheumatoid arthritis symptoms. From 12 to 15 months, patients were instructed to maintain, if possible, their current dose of NSAIDs. At 12 months, all patients received placebo capsules without vitamin E in order to assess whether any improvement in condition was due to vitamin E and to monitor relapse. The last phase of the trial was single-blinded.

Study duration	1 year 3 months
Dose	12 capsules (450 mg GLA, 240 mg EPA) per day
Route of administration	Oral
Randomized	Yes
Randomization adequate	Yes
Blinding	Double-blind
Blinding adequate	Yes
Placebo	Yes
Drug comparison	Yes
Drug name	Efamol

Site description   Not described

No. of subjects enrolled 49
No. of subjects completed 34
Sex   Male and female
Age   28-74 years (mean: 49)

Inclusion criteria

Classical or definite rheumatoid arthritis as defined by the American Rheumatism Association. Patients with mild rheumatoid arthritis requiring first-line NSAID therapy for control of symptoms.

Exclusion criteria

Patients with severe rheumatoid arthritis requiring second-line therapy.

End points

Patients were monitored monthly for the first six months, then every three months thereafter. Full metrological assessment was carried out at 0, 3, 6, 12, and 15 months, including duration of morning stiffness in minutes, grip strength of each hand, Ritchie articular index, and a 10 cm visual analog pain scale completed by patients. Side effects were noted. Patients were asked to assess whether they had received any benefit from treatment. Blood was drawn and assessed for erythrocyte sedimentation rate (ESR), C reactive protein levels, and hemoglobin and rheumatoid factor.

Results

The amount of NSAIDs after 12 months was reduced for 11 of 15 patients taking Efamol ($p < 0.003$), 12 of 15 taking Efamol Marine ($p < 0.002$), and 5 of 15 taking placebo ($p < 0.05$). At that time, improvement was reported by 94 percent on Efamol, 93 percent on Efamol Marine, and 30 percent on placebo. However, there were no significant changes in clinical or lab measurements in any of the groups throughout the study. After the three-month run-out placebo phase at the end of the trial, 100 percent of Efamol patients and 80 percent of Efamol Marine patients, compared with only 14 percent of placebo patients, had returned to baseline or become worse. Overall, the only difference between the Efamol and Efamol Marine groups was that the Efamol Marine group had an earlier response to treatment.

Side effects

Two patients in the Efamol group experienced nausea and diarrhea (respectively) and subsequently withdrew from the study. Two patients in the Efamol Marine group experienced nausea and headache (respectively), but neither withdrew from the study.

Authors' comments

It is possible to decrease or stop NSAID treatment in some patients with rheumatoid arthritis by introducing Efamol or Efamol Marine treatment. It should be noted, however, that although patients claimed a subjective improvement, no change was recorded in any of the measures conventionally used to measure disease activity. It would seem that these oils may be best used in clinical situations in which NSAID therapy should be avoided.

Reviewer's comments
This was a well-designed study, but there was no clear benefit of evening primrose oil for rheumatoid arthritis. These results are in contrast to trials in which eicosapentanoic acid in fish oil has shown a consistent trend toward efficacy in rheumatoid arthritis. (5, 6)

Clinical Study: Efamol Marine

Extract name	N/A
Manufacturer	Scotia Pharmaceuticals Ltd., UK
Indication	**Psoriatic arthritis**
Level of evidence	**II**
Therapeutic benefit	**No**

Bibliographic reference
Veale DJ, Torley HI, Richards IM, O'Dowd A, Fitsimons C, Belch JJF, Sturrock RD (1994). A double-blind placebo controlled trial of Efamol Marine on skin and joint symptoms of psoriatic arthritis. *British Journal of Rheumatology* 33 (10): 954-958.

Trial design
Parallel. For nine months, patients took either Efamol Marine (evening primrose oil plus fish oil) or placebo, followed by three months run-out phase in which all took placebo. For the first three months, patients maintained their normal intake of NSAIDs. After that, patients were asked to reduce their intake and maintain that decrease providing that they experienced no worsening of joint symptoms.

Study duration	9 months
Dose	12 capsules (480 mg GLA, 240 mg EPA, 132 mg DHA) per day
Route of administration	Oral
Randomized	Yes
Randomization adequate	Yes
Blinding	Double-blind
Blinding adequate	Yes

Placebo	Yes
Drug comparison	No
Site description	Not described
No. of subjects enrolled	38
No. of subjects completed	32
Sex	Male and female
Age	18-76 years (mean: 40)

Inclusion criteria
Chronic stable plaque psoriasis and inflammatory arthritis; negative for rheumatoid factor (RF) (latex); involvement of at least one peripheral joint with or without sacroiliitis; stable dose of paracetamol and/or NSAID for at least one month prior to study.

Exclusion criteria
Patients suffering from epilepsy, undergoing treatment with systemic steroids, beta-blocking drugs, or phenothiazines.

End points
Clinical assessments of inflammatory joint disease, grip strength, number of active joints, Ritchie articular index, duration of morning stiffness, and NSAID intake were performed at 0, 1, 3, 6, 9, and 12 months. Prostatic skin disease severity was assessed using a 100 mm visual analog scale. The patient recorded changes in skin itch. At each visit, blood tests for hemoglobin, white cell count, platelet count, ESR, CRP, immunoglobulins, urea, electrolytes, and liver enzymes were performed. The effect on arachidonic acid metabolism was determined by measuring levels of TXB_2 in serum and LTB_4 in supernatants following stimulation of polymorphonuclear (PMN) cells.

Results
No significant differences were found between the two groups in clinical or laboratory indices of arthritis disease activity at 6, 9, or 12 months. Three patients in the Efamol group and four patients in the placebo group were able to discontinue use of NSAIDs without worsening their condition. No significant difference was observed in skin disease severity or activity between the two groups. The level of LTB_4 decreased over the study period in the Efamol group and was significantly different at nine months in comparison to baseline ($p < 0.03$). No significant change occurred in the placebo group. TXB_2 levels consistently were lower in the Efamol group than in the placebo group. During the last three months (the placebo phase) of the trial, significant increases in TXB_2 levels in the Efamol group suggested a rebound increase in production. This increase did not occur in the placebo group.

Side effects
Two patients in the active treatment group withdrew due to diarrhea.

Authors' comments
This trial failed to demonstrate that fish oil could substitute for NSAID therapy in psoriatic arthritis. However, it did demonstrate metabolic effects on prostanoid and leukotriene metabolism suggesting that larger doses of fish oil might produce a clinical response.

Reviewer's comments
A well-designed study with appropriate inclusion/exclusion criteria and outcome measures. However, the study was too small to document differences in response rates. (5, 4)

Garlic

Latin name: *Allium sativum* **L.** [Liliaceae]
Plant part: **Bulb**

PREPARATIONS USED
IN REVIEWED CLINICAL STUDIES

Garlic has been used as a medicine for more time and by more cultures than perhaps any other plant. Garlic is unique in its high sulfur content, which is four times greater than that of the other high sulfur-containing vegetables and fruits, such as onion, broccoli, cauliflower, or apricots. The most abundant sulfur compound in garlic is alliin, which is typically present at 10 mg per gram fresh weight. When garlic cloves are cut, crushed, or chewed there is a conversion, within seconds, of alliin to allicin by the enzyme allinase. Allicin is thought to be important to the beneficial effects of garlic and is also responsible for its characteristic odor. Therapeutic effects are also attributed to other sulfur compounds (Lawson, 1996).

Garlic powder is the product most similar to fresh cloves in chemical composition, as it is dehydrated at a low oven temperature and then pulverized. When carefully prepared, the allinase activity is preserved. A very important aspect of the effective quality of garlic powder products is that allicin can be formed after consumption. Therefore, many garlic supplements are standardized to their "allicin potential." Because the enzyme allinase, necessary to produce allicin, is destroyed by the acidic pH of the stomach, many garlic preparations are enteric coated. This coating delays dissolution of the capsule or tablet until it reaches the intestine (Lawson, 1996).

Powdered garlic preparations tested in clinical studies include Kwai®, Pure-Gar®, as well as unbranded or generic dried garlic. Kwai is manufactured by Lichtwer Pharma AG in Germany and distributed in the United States by Lichtwer Pharma US, Inc. The tablets contain a preparation known as LI 111 that is standardized to contain

GARLIC SUMMARY TABLE

Product Name	Manufacturer/ U.S. Distributor	Product Characteristics	Dose in Trials	Indication	No. of Trials	Benefit (Evidence Level-Trial No.)
Kwai®	Lichtwer Pharma AG, Germany/ Lichtwer Pharma U.S., Inc.	Dried garlic, standardized to 1.3 % alliin, 0.6% allicin	300 mg 3 times daily, total 900 mg	Hyperlipid-emia, hyper-cholesterol-emia, hyperlipo-proteinemia (elevated blood lipid levels)	15	Yes (I-2, II-1, III-3) Trend (II-2, III-1) No (I-3, II-2) Undetermined (III-1)
				Lipids and lipoproteins in normal volunteers	1	Undetermined (III-1)
				Atheroscle-rosis	1	Trend (II-1)
				Postmeal lipid levels	1	Undetermined (II-1)
				Increased spontane-ous platelet aggregation	1	Trend (II-1)

Product	Manufacturer/Source	Form	Dose	Indication	No.	Effectiveness
Pure-Gar®	Essentially Pure Ingredients™/ Essentially Pure Ingredients™	Dried garlic, 0.3% allicin	680 mg twice daily, total 1,360 mg	Hypercholesterolemia (elevated cholesterol levels)	1	Yes (II-1)
Generic	None	Dried garlic	594 to 1,350 mg daily	Hyperlipoproteinemia	1	No (III-1)
Generic	Government Pharmaceutical Organization, Thailand/ None	Spray-dried garlic	700 mg daily	Hyperlipoproteinemia	1	Undetermined (III-1)
				Diabetes (NIDDM)	1	Undetermined (III-1)
Kyolic® Aged Garlic Extract™, HI-PO™ Formula 100	Wakunaga of America Co., Ltd./ Wakunaga of America Co., Ltd.	Aged garlic (ethanolic extract)	2.4 to 7.2 g daily	Hypercholesterolemia	2	Yes (I-1) Undetermined (III-1)
				Blood clotting factors	1	MOA (I-1)
				Lipid oxidation	1	MOA (III-1)
Kyolic® Liquid Aged Garlic Extract™	Wakunaga of America Co., Ltd./ Wakunaga of America Co., Ltd.	Aged garlic (ethanolic extract)	4 (1 ml) capsules daily	Hypercholesterolemia	1	Undetermined (III-1)

GARLIC SUMMARY TABLE (continued)

Product Name	Manufacturer/ U.S. Distributor	Product Characteristics	Dose in Trials	Indication	No. of Trials	Benefit (Evidence Level-Trial No.)
Garlic oil	None	Oil, ethyl acetate extracted	Equivalent of 2 g raw garlic daily/0.25 mg oil per kg body weight	Heart disease	2	Yes (II-1, III-1)
Garlic oil	General Nutrition Research Laboratories/None	Oil, cold pressed	18 mg daily	Cardiovascular risk factors	1	Yes (II-1)
Tegra	Hermes Arzneimittel GmbH, Germany/None	Oil, steam distilled, bound to cyclodextrin	10 mg daily	Hypercholesterolemia	1	No (II-1)
Garlic (raw)	None	Raw	10 g daily	Hypercholesterolemia	1	Trend (III-1)
				Cardiovascular risk factors	1	Trend (III-1)

600 mcg allicin in 100 mg garlic powder. Kwai is also sold as Sapec®. Pure-Gar is a brand of garlic powder supplied as raw material to manufacturers that incorporate it into numerous branded products. It is manufactured by Essentially Pure Ingredients™, which is owned by Natrol, Inc.

Aged garlic extract (AGE) is prepared by storing sliced garlic in 15 to 20 percent aqueous ethanol for 18 to 20 months. After this time, the liquid is filtered and concentrated. Most of the sulfur compounds responsible for the characteristic garlic odor are removed during processing. There are few allicin or alliin-derived compounds. The sulfur compound measured for quality purposes is S-allylcysteine. Aged garlic extract is available in both liquid and dry forms. The liquid form contains 10 percent ethanol (Lawson, 1996). Kyolic® Aged Garlic Extract™ is provided by Wakunaga of America Co., Ltd. The trials reviewed used both dry and liquid forms; however, the doses used in the trials were much higher than those suggested in the available product literature.

Garlic contains only a very small amount of oil-soluble compounds. Commercial garlic oil is produced by steam distillation of chopped garlic, a process that converts allicin and other thiosulfinates to oil-soluble allyl sulfides. Garlic oils are also prepared by maceration with organic solvents or common plant oils such as soybean oil. Garlic oils contain mostly alliin-derived compounds. In addition, vinyldithiins and ajoene are present. Garlic oils are not usually characterized by their sulfide content, but tend rather to be promoted as containing a specific amount of "pure garlic oil" (Lawson, 1996).

Three garlic oil preparations have been tested in clinical studies, including ethyl acetate extracted, cold pressed, and steam distilled. The ethyl acetate preparation was made by extracting peeled, crushed garlic cloves with ethyl acetate, evaporating the solvent, and finally dissolving the resultant oil in soy oil. No details were provided for the manufacturer of the "cold-pressed garlic oil" used in the reviewed clinical trial, except that the oil was provided by General Nutrition Research Laboratories. Steamed distilled garlic oil is commonly referred to as the "essential oil of garlic." It is produced by steam distillation of crushed garlic cloves but, as garlic itself contains very little essential oil, the term is a misnomer. Commercial-grade products are often diluted with a vegetable oil. We list one trial that used a proprietary product called Tegra, which contains garlic oil bound to cyclodextrin. Tegra is manufactured by Hermes Arzneimittel GmbH in Germany and is not sold in the United States.

Finally, two trials used fresh garlic that was consumed raw.

SUMMARY OF REVIEWED CLINICAL STUDIES

Clinical trials using garlic preparations have mostly focused on the possible reduction in risk for atherosclerotic heart disease. Elevated plasma (blood) lipids (cholesterol and triglycerides) are considered risk factors for heart disease, and much of preventative treatment has focused on lowering these levels to within parameters considered normal.

Sources for cholesterol are dietary intake of animal fats and production by the liver. Cholesterol is transported in the blood by lipoproteins, and the major categories of lipoproteins are very low-density lipoproteins (VLDL), low-density lipoproteins (LDL), and high-density lipoproteins (HDL). VLDL and LDL transport fats, primarily triglycerides (TG) and cholesterol, from the liver to cells throughout the body. Elevations of either VLDL or LDL are associated with an increase in risk for developing atherosclerosis, a primary cause of heart attack and stroke. The role of HDL is to return fats to the liver. Hence the ratios of total cholesterol (TC) to HDL cholesterol and LDL to HDL indicate whether cholesterol is being deposited into tissues or broken down and excreted. It is recommended that total serum cholesterol be less than 200 mg/dl, LDL be less than 130 mg/dl, HDL cholesterol be greater than 35 mg/dl, and triglyceride levels be less than 150 mg/dl (Pizzorno and Murray, 1999).

Cholesterol levels above 240 mg/dL are generally treated with statin drugs, such as lovastatin (Mevacor) and simvastatin (Zocor). Statins inhibit the activity of 3-hydroxy-3-methylglutaryl coenzyme A (HMG-CoA) reductase, an enzyme involved in the biosynthesis of cholesterol. A reduction in serum cholesterol levels of 25 to 45 percent can be expected with statins (Hardman et al., 1996).

Two other classes of drugs used to reduce cholesterol levels are bile acid sequestrants and nicotinic acid (niacin). Bile acid sequestrants are anion exchange resins that prevent the normal reabsorption of bile salts from the intestine. The reduction in bile reabsorption causes an increase in demand for bile salts to replenish the supply. As bile contains cholesterol, this results in a decrease in plasma levels and a restoration of bile acid production. Treatment often results in reductions in plasma cholesterols levels of 15 to 30 percent. Nicotinic acid (niacin) has diverse actions affecting lipoprotein metabolism. It appears to reduce VLDL levels through transient inhibition of liposis, delivery of free fatty acids to the liver, triglyceride synthesis, and VLDL-triglyceride transport. A reduction of 10 to 20 percent in plasma cholesterol levels is common with this treatment (Hardman et al., 1996).

The garlic preparations studied clinically for reduction in risk for atherosclerotic heart disease include dried garlic, aged garlic, garlic oil, and raw garlic. The end points of those trials include elevated serum cholesterol, hypertension, blood clotting factors, and lipid oxidation. By far, the most extensive number of studies has been conducted on the ability of dried garlic, essentially Kwai, to reduce elevated levels of plasma lipids, especially cholesterol.

Kwai Garlic

A total of 19 controlled studies on Kwai garlic were reviewed. All but two of these studies investigated the potential role of Kwai garlic on serum lipid levels. Six of these studies also reported results on blood pressure testing, and three also examined lipid oxidation. In all but five studies, 900 mg of dried garlic powder was used daily and administered in 300 mg doses three times per day. Most of the trials were conducted for a period of three months or longer.

Hyperlipidemia, Hypercholesterolemia, Hyperlipoproteinemia (Elevated Blood Lipid Levels)

Of the trials which examined the possible beneficial effect of Kwai on plasma lipid profiles, nine studies were positive and eight studies were negative. In the positive trials, statistically significant reductions in serum total cholesterol were reported after one to three months of treatment.

Three studies of good quality reported significant reductions in total cholesterol. A study with 219 subjects reported a reduction in mean serum total cholesterol from 266 to 235 mg/dl after four months of treatment, a reduction of 12 percent. The author stated that the greatest benefit was seen with the subgroup of patients with initial cholesterol levels between 250 and 300 mg/dl, compared to the subgroup with initial levels between 200 and 250 mg/dl (Mader, 1990). Another high-quality trial with 94 subjects with total serum cholesterol levels above 250 mg/dl compared Kwai (900 mg/day) to bezafibrate (600 mg/day). Bezafibrate belongs to a class of drugs that lowers the levels of triglyceride-rich lipoproteins, such as VLDL, and modestly raises HDL levels (Hardman et al., 1996). In this study, garlic reduced mean serum cholesterol from 282 mg/dl to 210 mg/dl after 12 weeks of treatment, a reduction of 25 percent. Bezafibrate reduced total cholesterol to a similar extent, with no significant difference between the two groups. Over the 12 weeks of the study, both groups also had significant decreases in LDL and triglyceride levels as well as a significant increase in HDL levels (Holzgartner, Schmidt, and Kuhn, 1992). In the third good-quality, placebo-controlled trial with 47 subjects with mild hypertension, the total cholesterol in the treatment group fell from 268 mg/dl to 239 mg/dl after eight weeks, and to 230 mg/dl after 12 weeks (Auer et al., 1990). A modest (6 percent) reduction in elevated total cholesterol, from 262 to 247 mg/dl after three months, was reported in a good-quality, placebo-controlled study with 42 subjects. In this study, LDL was also significantly reduced in comparison to placebo (Jain et al., 1993).

Four other placebo-controlled studies, deemed poor quality, reported significant reductions, in the range of 9 to 21 percent, of elevated total cholesterol. The first study included 52 subjects and reported a significant reduction in total cholesterol compared to baseline and placebo after six months. LDL levels also decreased significantly compared to baseline in the treatment group. There was no significant change to triglyceride or HDL levels (De A Santos and Grunwald, 1993). In a small crossover trial with 19 subjects, treated for four months, there was a significant reduction in total cholesterol compared to baseline, an insignificant increase in HDL, and no change in triglyceride levels (Melvin and Chappell, 1996). A parallel study with 40 subjects reported a significant drop in total cholesterol and triglyceride levels compared to placebo after four months (Vorberg and Schneider, 1990). The fourth study included 46 subjects with elevated cholesterol and used a combination of single- and double-blinding to compare the effects of garlic, fish oil (12 g/day), both garlic and fish oil, and placebo on lipid levels following three months of treatment. As a result, those receiving garlic and garlic plus fish oil had a reduction in both total cholesterol and LDL. Fish oil alone did not lower cholesterol and slightly elevated LDL. By contrast, triglycerides were reduced by fish oil as well as the combination of fish oil and garlic, but not by garlic alone (Adler and Holub, 1997).

Seven good-quality, placebo-controlled studies including participants with elevated lipid levels reported no significant effects on cholesterol levels. The most remarkable was a six-month study that included 106 subjects with an initial mean total cholesterol of roughly 270 mg/dl. This very well conducted and designed study showed no significant differences in serum lipids, lipoproteins, apolipoprotein A1 or B, or resistance of LDL to oxidation (Neil et al., 1996). The second trial with 30 children aged eight to 18 with a baseline level of total cholesterol of 265 mg/dl reported no effect on lipid levels after two months (McCrindle, Helden, and Conner, 1998). A third study with 42 subjects with initial cholesterol levels of 262 mg/dl also reported no change in lipid levels after three months (Isaacsohn et al., 1998). A crossover study with 29 subjects with mildly elevated cholesterol (254 mg/dl) found no significant differences in plasma cholesterol or other lipids after three months of treatment. There was also no effect on experimental ex vivo oxidation of LDL (Simons et al., 1995). A placebo-controlled trial with 50 subjects with moderately elevated cholesterol (245 mg/dl) found no effect from three months of treatment with Kwai on levels of triglycerides, total cholesterol, LDL, or HDL (Superko and Krauss, 2000). Another good-quality study with 68 healthy volunteers with slightly elevated cholesterol (223 mg/dl) found no significant reductions in total cholesterol or triglyceride levels at the end of 15 weeks of treatment (Saradeth et al., 1994). A study including 120 subjects with mildly elevated cholesterol levels of 228 mg/dl reported no change after one month of treatment (Kiesewetter et al., 1991).

A poor-quality study, including 60 non-insulin-dependent diabetics (NIDDM) with elevated cholesterol (254 mg/dl), showed a trend toward reduction of serum total cholesterol and LDL that was not significant at the end of three months of treatment. However, HDL cholesterols rose in comparison to the placebo group (Mansell et al., 1996).

There are several possible explanations for the mixed results of Kwai in regard to serum cholesterol levels. One suggestion is that studies must be designed carefully to optimize outcome. In only a few studies was diet carefully controlled, and this aspect may be important in evaluating the potential benefit of garlic. Another consideration is the formulation of the Kwai product. If the release of contents is not timed properly, the full allicin potential may not be reached, rendering the product inactive. A recent paper explored the release of allicin under simulated gastrointestinal conditions (USP method for dissolution testing). The authors were able to test the lots of Kwai used in clinical studies in the dissolution test. They found that the amount of allicin released from garlic powder tablets under simulated gastrointestinal conditions correlated well with the success or failure of such tablets to lower serum cholesterol values in controlled clinical trials. Of interest was a highly significant difference in the effect on serum cholesterol found between trials conducted on Kwai garlic tablets before 1993 and those conducted in 1993 and later. The sharp decline in the effectiveness of the tablets is paralleled by sharp declines in both the acid resistance and the allicin release from the tablets, apparently caused by a change in the coating of the tablet (Lawson, Wang, and Papadimitriou, 2001).

Elevated Blood Pressure

Two of the previously described studies that included patients with hypertension (blood pressure ≥140/90 mmHg, systolic/diastolic) reported decreases in blood pressure, both systolic and diastolic, of 11 to 17 percent (Auer et al., 1990; De A Santos and Grunwald, 1993). Four other studies that measured blood pressure and included subjects without hypertension reported little to no effect (Adler and Holub, 1997; Kiesewetter et al., 1991; McCrindle, Helden, and Conner, 1998; Simons et al., 1995). It appears that garlic may have a normalizing effect, reducing only blood pressure that is already elevated.

Lipids and Lipoproteins in Normal Volunteers

A crossover study included ten subjects with initial normal lipid levels who were given 600 mg LI 111 or placebo for two-week treatment periods with a one-week washout period in between. Kwai garlic did not alter levels of total cholesterol, LDL, or HDL. The authors of the study commented that two weeks was probably too short a time to see any significant changes in lipid levels. However, there was a significant reduction in ex vivo oxidation of apoB-containing lipo-proteins after two weeks compared to baseline (Phelps and Harris, 1993).

Antioxidant Activity

Two studies reviewed previously examined the role of Kwai in re-ducing oxidation of lipoproteins and did not find any benefit. These studies, which included hyperlipidemic subjects, also did not report any cholesterol-lowering activity (Neil et al., 1996; Simons et al., 1995). These results contrast the results of the study reviewed which reported a reduction in ex vivo oxidation of apoB-containing lipo-proteins in subjects with normal lipid levels (Phelps and Harris, 1993). It is possible that the discrepancy between these findings is due to the variability in the bioavailability of allicin in Kwai products, as previously discussed.

Atherosclerosis

A well-conducted study included 152 subjects with advanced atherosclerotic plaques as measured by ultrasound. The subjects were given 900 mg LI 111 or placebo for four years. As a result, the plaque volume in the treatment group decreased by 2.6 percent. The plaque volume in the placebo group increased by 16 percent, and there was a significant difference between the two groups. An analysis of sub-groups found that those subjects aged 50 to 80 years had a larger re-duction in plaque size (6 to 13 percent) compared to placebo. Further subgroup analysis reported that the reductions compared to placebo were 4.4 percent for men and 58 percent for women. The significance of the result with women was questioned, as the predominately youn-ger women in the placebo group (age range 40 to 55 years) had a dras-tic increase in plaque volume (53 percent), while the mainly older women (aged over 55 years) in the garlic group had a plaque reduc-tion of 4.6 percent (Koscielny et al., 1999).

Postmeal Lipid Levels

In a novel approach, lipid levels were measured before and after a high-fat meal in groups of healthy volunteers taking placebo or Kwai garlic (900 mg daily), at baseline, and after three and six weeks. The increase in triglycerides after the meal was less in the garlic group than in the placebo group, but it was not significant due to the small number of participants (24) and the large variation in individual lipid levels. However, after six weeks, the garlic group had a significant decrease in fasting triglyceride levels compared to the placebo group (Rotzsch et al., 1992).

Platelet Aggregation

Authors of a good-quality study, with 120 subjects given 800 mg Kwai garlic for one month, reported a reduction in spontaneous platelet aggregation, from 10 to 56 percent depending upon the test method (Kiesewetter et al., 1991). This study indicated a possible use for Kwai garlic in the inhibition of thrombocyte aggregation in patients unable to tolerate aspirin.

Pure-Gar

Hypercholesterolemia (Elevated Cholesterol Levels)

A fairly well-designed study included 35 renal failure patients with hypercholesterolemia. The subjects were given placebo or Pure-Gar, a preparation standardized to deliver 4 mg allicin per day for three months. Baseline levels of total cholesterol were significantly reduced from 290 to 275 mg/dl and levels of LDL from 193 to 182 mg/dl, while there was no such effect from placebo (Lash et al., 1998).

Generic Dried Garlic Preparations

Hyperlipoproteinemia (Elevated Blood Lipid Levels)

There was no benefit to cardiovascular risk parameters in two poorly described, placebo-controlled, crossover studies including subjects with hyperlipoproteinemia that were reported together. The first study included 34 subjects and used an unnamed commercial dried garlic preparation at a dose of 594 mg per day. The second study included 51 subjects and used a specially prepared supplement at 1350 mg per day. Following six weeks of treatment, there was no effect on total cholesterol, HDL, LDL, or triglycerides in either study. In addition, the second study found no effect on whole blood coagulation time, prothrombin time, or fibrinogen levels (Luley et al., 1986).

Another poorly described study was conducted with a garlic preparation supplied by the Thai government. In the trial of crossover design, 30 subjects with hyperlipoproteinemia did not experience any significant effects on plasma lipid levels. Baseline lipid levels for total cholesterol (280 mg/dl), triglycerides (355 mg/dl), and HDL (38 mg/dl) did not change significantly following a dose of 700 mg dried garlic per day for two months (Plengvidlya et al., 1998).

Diabetes (NIDDM)

Another poorly described study was conducted with the garlic preparation supplied by the Thai government. This was a placebo-controlled study conducted with 33 diabetic patients with mildly elevated serum cholesterol (228 mg/dl). Treatment for one month, with 700 mg dried garlic per day, had no effect on blood glucose, serum insulin, or lipid levels compared to baseline. This study included a highly heterogeneous sample of non-insulin-dependent diabetics, and the sample size may have been too small to show any changes (Sitprija et al., 1987).

Kyolic Aged Garlic Extract

We reviewed five studies with Kyolic Aged Garlic Extract, one using the liquid formulation. Three studies indicated a reduction in lipid levels for those with hyperlipidemia. One study indicated a reduction in platelet aggregation, and two studies indicated reductions in platelet adhesion. Another study demonstrated weak, inconsistent antioxidant activity that was not as powerful as supplementation with vitamin E.

Hypercholesterolemia (Elevated Cholesterol Levels) and Platelet Function

A three-part, six-month pilot study included 51 volunteers, some of whom had elevated cholesterol. The participants were treated with liquid AGE, four (1 ml) capsules daily, or placebo for six months.

Lowering of cholesterol, triglycerides, LDL, and VLDL was reported in the majority of those with elevated baseline levels. The garlic preparation did not affect those whose lipids levels were normal to begin with. In a subgroup with initial cholesterol levels between 220 and 440 mg/dl, 11 of 15 subjects on AGE had a greater than 10 percent lowering of cholesterol (Lau, Lam, and Wang-Cheng, 1987). Our reviewer, Dr. David Heber, concluded that the results of the study were undetermined due to the poor methodology and small sample size.

A study with 34 subjects, with serum cholesterol levels from 220 to 285 mg/dl, reported a 7 percent reduction in serum total cholesterol and a 10 percent reduction in LDL cholesterol compared to baseline after five months of treatment with 7.2 g AGE daily. No change was seen in the placebo group (Yeh et al., 1997). This study was rated as being poor quality.

A good-quality, double-blind, crossover study included 41 moderately hypercholesterolemic men (serum cholesterol levels from 220 to 290 mg/dl). Treatment with a dose of nine (800 mg) capsules (a total of 7.2 g) daily over four to six months led to a 6 to 7 percent reduction in total serum cholesterol compared to placebo. In addition, LDL decreased by 4 percent, blood pressure decreased by 5.5 percent, and there was a 30 percent reduction in platelet adhesion to fibrinogen (Steiner et al., 1996).

Another double-blind, crossover study, with 28 normal healthy adults, studied the effect of 2.4 to 7.2 g AGE per day for six weeks on the function of platelets taken from the subjects' blood. Significant reductions in platelet aggregation with several agonists (epinephrine, adenosine diphosphate [ADP], collagen) were reported, although no consistent increase in response followed an increase in dose. Platelet adhesion to collagen- and fibrinogen-coated surfaces was also reduced by intake of AGE (Steiner and Li, 2001).

Lipid Oxidation

A poor-quality study compared the effects of seven days of administration of either 2.4 g of AGE, 6 g raw garlic, or 0.8 g vitamin E on LDL oxidation in a total of nine subjects. The authors found that AGE provided an inconsistent protection of LDL oxidation which was less than what was observed with vitamin E supplementation (Munday et al., 1999).

Garlic Oil

Four studies on garlic oil are described. Two of these studies used an ethyl acetate extract of crushed garlic, another study used a cold-pressed garlic oil, and the remaining study used a steam-distilled garlic oil preparation bound to cyclodextrin.

Heart Disease

The two studies using the ethyl acetate preparation were double-blind, placebo-controlled studies showing a clear cholesterol-lowering effect in patients with heart disease. The first study, with a dose equivalent to 4 g raw garlic per day for three months, reported a 13 percent decrease in cholesterol (from 253 to 220 mg/dl) and a 15 percent decrease in triglycerides (from 130 to 110 mg/dl) in patients taking garlic oil. High-density lipoprotein cholesterol was increased by 22 percent, and platelet aggregation was also reduced (Bordia, Verma, and Srivastava, 1998). The strength of the evidence in this trial was reduced, as neither the randomization process nor the placebo were described in any detail. The second study, an overall good placebo-controlled study, enrolled subjects with high cholesterol levels (250 to 350 mg/dl). The garlic oil was administered in a dose of 0.25 mg oil per kg body weight (15 g oil, corresponding to 30 g raw garlic, for a 132 lb person) for ten months. After eight months, serum cholesterol was reduced by 18 percent (from a mean of 298 to 244 mg/dl), and this trend continued over the next two months after treatment stopped (dropping to 228 mg/dl) (Bordia, 1981).

Cardiovascular Risk Factors

A study with cold-pressed oil showed a beneficial effect on serum lipid levels in a small, placebo-controlled pilot trial including 20 healthy volunteers. Cholesterol levels dropped from 195 to 180 mg/dl and HDL levels rose from 56 to 69 mg/dl compared to baseline. There was also a reduction in platelet aggregation following a dose of 18 mg of oil, equivalent to 9 g fresh garlic, for four weeks (Barrie, Wright, and Pizzorno, 1987).

Hypercholesterolemia (Elevated Cholesterol Levels)

A study using steam-distilled garlic oil bound to cyclodextrin (Tegra) was widely publicized following publication in the *Journal of the American Medical Association*. This crossover study used a dose of 5 mg twice daily, equivalent to four or five fresh cloves, administered for three months to a total of 25 subjects with moderate hypercholesterolemia. The authors reported no effect on cholesterol metabolism (Berthold, Sudhop, and von Bergmann, 1998a). However, the study was criticized because of the use of steam distillation, which converts allicin to other sulfur compounds, the small dose, and the "prolonged release" formulation that bound the oil to cyclodextrin. In an accompanying letter to the editor, Dr. Lawson reported that the bioavailability of garlic sulfur compounds in this formulation appears to have been limited. Under simulated gastrointestinal conditions (USP methods) only 1.8 mg of the 5 mg present in each tablet was released. In addition, an experiment with two volunteers found only 25 to 40 percent of the expected sulfur on the breath, and whole tablets and large pieces were found in the stool 21 to 24 hours later (Lawson, 1998). The authors of the study replied that the product was specially formulated for slow release, and analysis of 400 stool samples for the trial did not reveal undigested tablets (Berthold, Sudhop, and von Bergmann, 1998b).

Raw Garlic

Hypercholesterolemia (Elevated Cholesterol Levels)
and Cardiovascular Risk Factors

Two studies on raw garlic show changes that can be interpreted as beneficial for cardiovascular risk. In both trials, the garlic groups consumed 10 g raw garlic after breakfast for two months, and the control groups were not given anything. The first study included 25 healthy subjects who had never ingested garlic before, with initial cholesterol levels of 160 to 250 mg/dl. This study reported a 15 percent reduction in cholesterol levels from baseline (Bhushan et al., 1979). The second study included 50 healthy volunteers with a mean initial serum cholesterol level of 213 mg/dl. Significant changes were reported in the garlic group, in cholesterol (16 percent decrease), clotting time (17 percent increase), and fibrinolysis (22 percent decrease). No significant change in these parameters occurred in the placebo group (Gadkari and Joshi, 1991). The main problems with these studies are that they were not blinded, and eating raw garlic after breakfast could have other effects on the diet that were not accounted for in the control groups.

META-ANALYSES AND SYSTEMATIC CLINICAL REVIEWS

The Agency for Healthcare Research and Quality, an agency in the U.S. Department of Health and Human Services, sponsored a systematic review of garlic through one of its evidence-based practice centers (EPC). The evidence report summarized the effects of garlic on cardiovascular-related factors and disease, associations between garlic and cancer, as well as possible adverse effects. Preparations ranging from dehydrated garlic, aged garlic extracts, and garlic oil macerates to distillates, raw garlic, and combination tablets were pooled together.

The review of cardiovascular-related effects was limited to randomized, controlled trials in humans lasting at least four weeks. The report examined 37 randomized, controlled trials, all but one in adults. Compared with placebo, various garlic preparations led to small, statistically significant reductions in total cholesterol after one month (range of average pooled reduction: 1.2 to 17.3 mg/dl) and even greater reductions after three months (range of average pooled reduction: 12.4 to 25.4 mg/dl). However, eight trials with outcomes at six months showed no significant reduction in total cholesterol compared with placebo. The reason for this disparity was not apparent. Changes in LDL levels and triglycerides mirrored total cholesterol results following three months of treatment. No significant changes to HDL levels were seen after three months.

Potential cardiovascular benefits, other than lipid lowering, that were evaluated in the report are summarized as follows. Effects on blood pressure in 27 small, randomized, placebo-controlled studies were mixed, with some studies reporting a small significant decrease in blood pressure and others reporting no effect. There was no effect on blood glucose in subjects with or without diabetes in 12 small, randomized trials. Two small short trials reported no effect on serum insulin or C peptide levels compared with placebo. Ten small trials, all but one in adults, showed positive effects on platelet aggregation and both positive and negative effects on plasma viscosity and fibrinolytic activity. The report stated that insufficient data were available to confirm or refute garlic's effect on clinical outcomes such as heart attack, peripheral vascular occlusive disease, and atherosclerosis.

Reviews of associations between garlic and cancer were limited to controlled studies that reported precancerous or cancerous lesions in humans consuming varying amounts of garlic. Scant data, primarily from case-control studies, suggest that garlic is associated with decreased odds of certain cancers (laryngeal, gastric, colorectal, and endometrial cancer, and adenomatous colorectal polyps) (Mulrow et al., 2000).

Another meta-analysis of randomized, double-blind, placebo-controlled clinical trials for treating hypercholesterolemia (mean total cholesterol of at least 200 mg/dl or 5.17 mM) was published in the same year as the EPC report. In the 13 trials included in the analysis (a total of 796 persons), treatment with garlic reduced total cholesterol significantly more than placebo ($p < 0.01$); the weighted mean difference was 0.41 mmol/l, equivalent to a 5.8 percent reduction in total cholesterol. An analysis of only six diet-controlled studies with the highest scores for methodological quality found no significant difference in comparison with placebo. The authors concluded that although the data suggest garlic is superior to placebo in reducing total cholesterol, the size of the effect is modest and the reliability of the effect is debatable. Therefore, the implication for clinical use is that garlic supplements may not be an effective way to decrease serum total cholesterol (Stevinson, Pittler, and Ernst, 2000). As in the previous analysis, all forms of garlic preparations were evaluated together.

A meta-analysis examining the effect of garlic on blood pressure concluded that a dose of 600 to 900 mg/day of dried garlic (Kwai) appears to lower systolic and diastolic blood pressure over a period from one to three months. However, the authors concluded that insufficient evidence existed at that time to recommend garlic as an effective antihypertensive agent for routine clinical use. Eight randomized controlled trials, which included 415 subjects, were reviewed. Only three of the trials were specifically conducted with hypertensive subjects (Silagy and Neil, 1994).

EPIDEMIOLOGICAL STUDIES

A critical review of the epidemiologic literature on garlic and can-cer found that the evidence from available studies suggests a preven-tive effect of garlic consumption in stomach and colorectal cancers. Site-specific case-controlled studies, for which multiple reports were available, suggest a protective effect of a high intake of raw and/or cooked garlic. Cohort studies confirm this inverse association for colorectal cancer. However, no link was found with garlic supple-ments as analyzed in four cohort studies and one case-controlled re-port (Fleischauer and Arab, 2001).

A case-controlled epidemiological study with 202 adults, from 50 to 80 years old, was included in a study evaluating the possible pro-tective effects of garlic on elasticity of the aorta. The garlic group took at least 300 mg/day of Kwai powdered garlic for at least two years. The elastic properties of the artery were measured using pulse-wave velocity and pressure-standardized elastic vascular resistance. Both measurements were statistically lower in the garlic group ($p < 0.0001$). Aortic elastic properties decreased with increasing age and increased blood pressure in both groups. However, the decrease was significantly lower for the garlic group ($p < 0.0001$). The authors concluded that chronic garlic powder intake reduces age-related in-creases in aortic stiffness (Breithaupt-Grögler et al., 1997).

ADVERSE REACTIONS OR SIDE EFFECTS

Adverse reactions in the 19 controlled studies on Kwai garlic were mild and not observed in all subjects. Bad breath was the most fre-quently noted side effect, followed by body odor and mild gastro-intestinal distress. The adverse reaction noted in some of the studies of other dried garlic preparations and aged garlic was garlic body odor. The studies on garlic oil preparations noted garlic odor. Ab-dominal distension was also noted in the study using the steam-distilled preparation bound to cyclodextrin.

A meta-analysis of 13 trials reported that adverse events most commonly included gastrointestinal symptoms and garlic breath (Stevinson, Pittler, and Ernst, 2000). According to the EPC report, adverse effects of oral ingestion of garlic include "smelly" breath and body odor. In addition, the EPC report cited possible, but unproven, adverse effects of flatulence, esophageal and abdominal pain, small intestinal obstruction, dermatitis, rhinitis, asthma, and bleeding (Mulrow et al., 2000).

INFORMATION FROM PHARMACOPOEIAL MONOGRAPHS

Sources of Published Therapeutic Monographs

British Herbal Compendium (BHC)
European Scientific Cooperative on Phytotherapy (ESCOP)
German Commission E
World Health Organization (WHO)

Indications

The German Commission E, along with the European Scientific Cooperative on Phytotherapy, the World Health Organization, and the *British Herbal Compendium,* state that garlic bulbs are supportive to dietary measures taken when blood lipid levels are elevated and that they can be used as preventative measures for age-dependent vascular changes (atherosclerosis) (Blumenthal et al., 1998; ESCOP, 1997; WHO, 1999; Bradley, 1992). The *BHC* and WHO maintain that garlic can be used to treat hypertension, and these two monographs, in addition to ESCOP, also suggest garlic for respiratory infections (WHO, 1999; Bradley, 1992; ESCOP, 1997). The *BHC* and ESCOP also suggest garlic for catarrhal conditions. Other indications listed include atheroma (Bradley, 1992), urinary tract infections, ringworm and rheumatic conditions, dyspepsia (WHO, 1999), and circulation improvement in peripheral arterial vascular disease (ESCOP, 1997). The actions of garlic listed by the Commission E include antibacterial, antimycotic, lipid-lowering, inhibition of platelet aggregation, prolongation of bleeding and clotting time, and enhancement of fibrinolytic activity (Blumenthal et al., 1998). The *BHC* lists the following actions: lowers blood cholesterol and triglycerides, hypotensive, lowers blood viscosity, activates fibrinolysis, inhibits platelet aggregation, antimicrobial, anti-inflammatory, and anthelmintic (Bradley, 1992).

Doses

Preparations equivalent to: 4 to 12 mg of alliin (approx. 2 to 5 mg of allicin) daily (Bradley, 1992); 6 to 10 mg of alliin (approx. 3 to 5 mg of allicin) daily (ESCOP, 1997)
Fresh: 4 g fresh garlic daily (Blumenthal et al., 1998); 2 to 5 g fresh (air-dried) bulb (Bradley, 1992)
Dried powder: 0.4 to 1.2 g daily (Bradley, 1992); 0.5 to 1 g daily (ESCOP, 1997)
Oil: 2 to 5 mg (Bradley, 1992)
Extract: 300 to 1,000 mg (as solid material) (WHO, 1999)
Tincture: (1:5, 45 percent ethanol) 2 to 4 ml 3 times daily (ESCOP, 1997)
Note: ESCOP suggests specific dosages for certain indications:
- For prophylaxis of atherosclerosis: the equivalent of 6 to 10 mg of alliin (approx. 3 to 5 mg of allicin) daily, typically contained in one clove of garlic or in 0.5 to 1 g of dried garlic powder (ESCOP, 1997)
- For upper respiratory tract infections: 2 to 4 g of dried bulb or 2 to 4 ml of tincture (1:5, 45 percent ethanol), 3 times daily (ESCOP, 1997)

Treatment Period

ESCOP advises long-term treatment in the prevention of atherosclerosis and prophylaxis or treatment of peripheral arterial vascular diseases (ESCOP, 1997).

Contraindications

The Commission E, *BHC,* and ESCOP list no known contraindications (Blumenthal et al., 1998; Bradley, 1992; ESCOP, 1997).

Adverse Reactions

The Commission E, *BHC,* and ESCOP note that gastrointestinal symptoms, changes to the intestinal flora, or allergic reactions rarely occur (Blumenthal et al., 1998; Bradley, 1992; ESCOP, 1997). The WHO lists one reported case of spontaneous spinal epidural hematoma, which was associated with excessive ingestion of fresh garlic cloves (WHO, 1999).

Precautions

The WHO states that consumption of large amounts of garlic may increase the risk of postoperative bleeding and that garlic should be taken with food to prevent gastrointestinal upset (WHO, 1999). ESCOP also advises caution when taking garlic after surgical operations (ESCOP, 1997).

Drug Interactions

ESCOP and the Commission E list no known drug interactions (Blumenthal et al., 1998; ESCOP, 1997). However, the WHO states that patients on warfarin therapy should be warned that garlic supplements may increase bleeding time. Blood clotting times have been reported to double in patients taking warfarin and garlic supplements (WHO, 1999).

REFERENCES

Adler AJ, Holub BJ (1997). Effect of garlic and fish-oil supplementation on serum lipid and lipoprotein concentrations in hypercholesterolemic men. *American Journal of Clinical Nutrition* 65 (2): 445-450.

Auer W, Eiber A, Hertkorn E, Hoehfeld E, Koehrle U, Lorenz A, Mader F, Merx W, Otto G, Schmid-Otto B, et al. (1990). Hypertension and hyperlipidaemia: Garlic helps in mild cases. *The British Journal of Clinical Practice* S69: 3-6.

Barrie S, Wright J, Pizzorno J (1987). Effects of garlic oil on platelet aggregation, serum lipids and blood pressure in humans. *Journal of Orthomolecular Medicine* 2 (1): 15-21.

Berthold H, Sudhop T, von Bergmann K (1998a). Effect of a garlic oil preparation on serum lipoproteins and cholesterol metabolism. *Journal of the American Medical Association* 279 (23): 1900-1902.

Berthold H, Sudhop T, von Bergmann K (1998b). Effect of garlic on serum lipids: In reply to the letter to the editor. *Journal of the American Medical Association* 280 (18): 1568.

Bhushan S, Sharma SP, Singh SP, Agrawal S, Indrayan A, Seth P (1979). Effect of garlic on normal blood cholesterol level. *Indian Journal of Physiology and Pharmacology* 23 (3): 211-214.

Blumenthal M, Busse W, Hall T, Goldberg A, Gruenwald J, Riggins C, Rister S, eds. (1998). *The Complete German Commission E Monographs: Therapeutic Guide to Herbal Medicines.* Trans. S Klein. Austin, TX: American Botanical Council.

Bordia A (1981). Effect of garlic on blood lipids in patients with coronary heart disease. *The American Journal of Clinical Nutrition* 34 (10): 2100-2103.

Bordia A, Verma SK, Srivastava KC (1998). Effect of garlic *(Allium sativum)* on blood lipids, blood sugar, fibrinogen and fibrinolytic activity in patients with coronary artery disease. *Prostaglandins, Leukotrienes, and Essential Fatty Acids* 58 (4): 257-263.

Bradley PR, ed. (1992). *British Herbal Compendium: A Handbook of Scientific Information on Widely Used Plant Drugs,* Volume 1. Dorset, UK: British Herbal Medicine Association.

Breithaupt-Grögler K, Ling M, Boudoulas H, Belz GG (1997). Protective effect of chronic garlic intake on elastic properties of aorta in the elderly. *Circulation* 96 (8): 2649-2655.

De A Santos OS, Grunwald J (1993). Effect of garlic powder tablets on blood lipids and blood pressure—Six month placebo controlled, double blind study. *The British Journal of Clinical Research* 4: 37-44.

European Scientific Cooperative on Phytotherapy (ESCOP) (1997). *Allii sativi* bulbus: Garlic. *Monographs on the Medicinal Uses of Plant Drugs.* Fascicle 3. Exeter, UK: European Scientific Cooperative on Phytotherapy.

Fleischauer AT, Arab L (2001). Garlic and cancer: A critical review of the epidemiologic literature. *The Journal of Nutrition* 131 (3S): 1032S-1040S.

Gadkari, J, Joshi V (1991). Effect of ingestion of raw garlic on serum cholesterol level, clotting time and fibrinolytic activity in normal subjects. *Journal of Postgraduate Medicine* 37 (3): 128-131.

Hardman JG, Limbird LE, Molinoff PB, Ruddon RW, Gilman AG (1996). *Goodman and Gillman's The Pharmacological Basis of Therapeutics,* Ninth Edition. New York: McGraw-Hill.

Holzgartner H, Schmidt U, Kuhn U (1992). Comparison of the efficacy and tolerance of a garlic preparation vs. bezafibrate. *Arzneimittel-Forschung/ Drug Research* 42 (12): 1473-1477.

Isaacsohn JL, Moser M, Stein EA, Dudley K, Davey J, Lishkov E, Black HR (1998). Garlic powder and plasma lipids and lipoproteins. *Archives of Internal Medicine* 158 (11): 1189-1194.

Jain AK, Vargas R, Gotzkowsky S, McMahon FG (1993). Can garlic reduce levels of serum lipids? A controlled clinical study. *The American Journal of Medicine* 94 (6): 632-635.

Kiesewetter H, Jung F, Pindur G, Jung EM, Mrowietz C, Wenzel E (1991). Effect of garlic on thrombocyte aggregation, microcirculation, and other risk factors. *International Journal of Clinical Pharmacology, Therapy and Toxicology* 29 (4): 151-155.

Koscielny J, Klubendorf D, Latza R, Schmitt R, Radtke H, Siegel G, Kiesewetter H (1999). The antiatherosclerotic effect of *Allium sativum*. *Atherosclerosis* 144 (1): 237-249.

Lash JP, Cardoso, LR, Mesler PM, Walczak DA, Pollak R (1998). The effect of garlic on hypercholesterolemia in renal transplant patients. *Transplantation Proceedings* 30 (1): 189-191.

Lau BHS, Lam F, Wang-Cheng R (1987). Effect of an odor-modified garlic preparation on blood lipids. *Nutrition Research* 7: 139-149.

Lawson LD (1996). The composition and chemistry of garlic cloves and processed garlic. In *Garlic, the Science and Therapeutic Application of Allium sativum L. and Related Species*. Eds. HP Koch, LD Lawson. Baltimore, MD: Williams and Wilkins, pp. 37-107.

Lawson LD (1998). Effect of garlic on serum lipids: Letter to the editor. *Journal of the American Medical Association* 280 (18): 1568.

Lawson LD, Wang ZJ, Papadimitriou D (2001). Allicin release under simulated gastrointestinal conditions from garlic powder tablets employed in clinical trials on serum cholesterol. *Planta Medica* 67 (1): 13-18.

Luley C, Lehmann-Leo W, Moeller B, Martin T, Schwartzkopff W (1986). Lack of efficacy of dried garlic in patients with hyperlipoproteinemia. *Arzneimittel-Forschung/Drug Research* 36 (1): 766-768.

Mader FH (1990). Treatment of hyperlipidaemia with garlic powder tablets. *Arzneimittel-Forschung/Drug Research* 40 (10): 1111-1116.

Mansell P, Reckless JPD, Lloyd J, Leatherdale B (1996). The effect of dried garlic powder tablets on serum lipids in non-insulin dependent diabetic patients. *European Journal of Clinical Research* 8: 25-26.

McCrindle BW, Helden E, Conner WT (1998). Garlic extract therapy in children with hypercholesterolemia. *Archives of Pediatric and Adolescent Medicine* 152 (11): 1089-1094.

Melvin KR, Chappell MA (1996). Effects of garlic powder tablets on patients with hyperlipidaemia in Canadian clinical practice. *European Journal of Clinical Research* 8: 15-36.

Mulrow CD, Lawrence V, Ackermann R, Ramirez G, Morbidoni L, Aguilar C, Arterburn J, Block E, Chiquette E, Gardener C, et al. (2000). Garlic: Effects on cardiovascular risks and disease, protective effects against cancer and clinical adverse effects. Evidence Report/Technology Assessment No. 20, AHRQ Publication No. 01-E023, October. Rockville, MD: Agency for Healthcare Research and Quality.

Munday JS, James KA, Fray LM, Kirkwood SW, Thompson KG (1999). Daily supplementation with aged garlic extract, but not raw garlic protects low density lipoprotein against in vitro oxidation. *Atherosclerosis* 143 (2): 399-404.

Neil HAW, Silagy CA, Lancaster T, Hodgeman J, Vos K, Moore JW, Jones L, Cahill J, Fowler GH (1996). Garlic powder in the treatment of moderate hyperlipidemia: A controlled trial and meta-analysis. *Journal of the Royal College of Physicians of London* 30 (4): 329-334. (Further analysis reported in Byrne DJ, Neil HAW, Vallance DT, Winder AF [1999]. *Clinica Chimica Acta: International Journal of Clinical Chemistry* 285 [1-2]: 21-33.)

Phelps S, Harris WS (1993). Garlic supplementation and lipoprotein oxidation susceptibility. *Lipids* 28 (5): 475-477.

Pizzorno JE, Murray MT, eds. (1999). *Textbook of Natural Medicine,* Second Edition, Volume 2. London: Churchill Livingstone.

Plengvidlya C, Sitprija S, Chinayon, S, Pasatrat S, Tunkayoon M (1998). Effects of spray dried garlic preparation on primary hyperlipoproteinemia. *Journal of the Medical Association of Thailand* 71 (5): 248-252.

Rotzsch W, Richter V, Rassoul F, Walper A (1992). Reduction in postprandial lipaemia caused by *Allium sativum:* Controlled double-blind trial involving test persons with low HDL2-cholesterol levels. *Arzneimittel-Forschung/Drug Research* 42 (10): 1223-1227.

Saradeth T, Seidl S, Resch KL, Ernst E (1994). Does garlic alter the lipid pattern in normal volunteers? *Phytomedicine* 1: 183-185.

Schulz V, Hänsel R, Tyler VE (2001). *Rational Phytotherapy: A Physicians' Guide to Herbal Medicine,* Fourth Edition. Trans. TC Telger. Berlin: Springer-Verlag.

Silagy CA, Neil HAW (1994). A meta-analysis of the effect of garlic on blood pressure. *Journal of Hypertension* 12 (4): 463-468.

Simons LA, Balasubramaniam S, von Konigsmark M, Parfitt A, Simons J, Peters W (1995). On the effect of garlic on plasma lipids and lipoproteins in mild hypercholesterolaemia. *Atherosclerosis* 113 (2): 219-225.

Sitprija S, Plengvidlya C, Kangkaya V, Bhuvapanich S, Tunkayoon M (1987). Garlic and diabetes mellitus phase II clinical trial. *Journal of the Medical Association of Thailand* 70 (2): 223-227.

Steiner M, Khan AH, Holbert D, Lin RI (1996). A double-blind crossover study in moderately hypercholesterolemic men that compared the effect of aged garlic extract and placebo administration on blood lipids. *American Journal of Clinical Nutrition* 64 (6): 866-870. (Platelet studies published by Steiner M, Lin RS [1998]. *Journal of Cardiovascular Pharmacology* 31 [6]: 904-908.)

Steiner M, Li W (2001). Aged garlic extract, a modulator of cardiovascular risk factors: A dose-finding study on the effects of AGE on platelet functions. *Journal of Nutrition* 131 (3s): 980S-984S.

Stevinson C, Pittler MH, Ernst E (2000). Garlic for treating hypercholesterolemia, a meta-analysis of randomized clinical trials. *Annals of Internal Medicine* 133 (6): 420-429.

Superko R, Krauss RM (2000). Garlic powder, effect on plasma lipids, postprandial lipemia, low-density lipoprotein particle size, high-density lipoprotein subclass distribution and lipoprotein (a). *Journal of the American College of Cardiology* 35 (2): 321-326.

Vorberg G, Schneider B (1990). Therapy with garlic: Results of a placebo-controlled, double-blind study. *The British Journal of Clinical Practice* S69: 7-11.

World Health Organization (WHO) (1999). *WHO Monographs on Selected Medicinal Plants,* Volume 1. Geneva: World Health Organization.

Yeh YY, Lin RI, Yeh SM, Evans S (1997). Garlic reduces plasma cholesterol in hypercholesterolemic men maintaining habitual diets. In *Food Factors for Cancer Prevention.* Eds. H Ohigashi, T Osawa, J Terao, S Watanabe, T Yoshikawa. Tokyo: Springer-Verlag, pp. 226-230.

DETAILS ON GARLIC PRODUCTS
AND CLINICAL STUDIES

Product and clinical study information is grouped in the same order as in the Summary Table. A profile on an individual product is followed by details of the clinical studies associated with that product. In some instances a clinical study, or studies, supports several products that contain the same principal ingredient(s). In these instances, those products are grouped together.

Clinical studies that follow each product, or group of products, are grouped by therapeutic indication, in accordance with the order in the Summary Table.

Index to Garlic Products

Product Profile: Kwai®

Manufacturer	**Lichtwer Pharma AG, Germany**
U.S. distributor	**Lichtwer Pharma U.S., Inc.**
Botanical ingredient	**Garlic clove powder**
Extract name	**LI III**
Quantity	100 mg concentrated dry garlic, equivalent to 300 mg fresh garlic

Processing	Garlic cloves are cut into slices and carefully dried in 50-60°C air for several hours. The dried slices are ground into powder and sieved
Standardization	600 mcg allicin per tablet
Formulation	Tablet

Recommended dose: Take two tablets three times daily with liquid, ideally with meals. Cholesterol-lowering results observed after 12 weeks of usage.

DSHEA structure/function: Clinically proven to lower cholesterol.

Cautions: If a disease or health-related condition requires the lowering of cholesterol, consult a doctor.

Other ingredients: Lactose, powdered cellulose, silicon dioxide, magnesium stearate, sucrose, magnesium silicate (mineral source), hydroxypropyl methylcellulose, gelatin, beeswax.

Comments: There are two other Kwai products: Kwai® 150 mg and Kwai® Heart Fit™. They have 150 mg and 300 mg garlic powder, respectively. Kwai® Heart Fit™ also contains vitamins A, C, and E. Kwai® is also sold as Sapec®.

Source(s) of information: Product package; Kwai® LI 111: Product Information, Lichtwer Pharma AG, 1999; Auer et al., 1990.

Clinical Study: Kwai®

Extract name	LI 111
Manufacturer	Lichtwer Pharma AG, Germany
Indication	**Hyperlipidemia** (elevated blood lipid levels)
Level of evidence	**I**
Therapeutic benefit	**Yes**

Bibliographic reference
Mader FH (1990). Treatment of hyperlipidaemia with garlic powder tablets. *Arzneimittel-Forschung/Drug Research* 40 (10): 1111-1116.

Trial design
Parallel.

Study duration	4 months
Dose	4 tablets daily (800 mg garlic powder)

Route of administration	Oral
Randomized	Yes
Randomization adequate	Yes
Blinding	Double-blind
Blinding adequate	Yes
Placebo	Yes
Drug comparison	No
Site description	30 general practices
No. of subjects enrolled	261
No. of subjects completed	219
Sex	Male and female
Age	47-71 years (mean: 59)

Inclusion criteria
Total serum cholesterol values of 200 to 300 mg/dl and/or triglyceride values of 200 to 300 mg/dl.

Exclusion criteria
None mentioned.

End points
Total cholesterol and triglyceride levels, as well as supine and diastolic blood pressure, were measured.

Results
After four months, mean cholesterol levels dropped in the garlic group by 12 percent (266 to 235 mg/dl) and triglyceride levels by 17 percent (226 to 188 mg/dl). The difference between the garlic and placebo groups was highly significant ($p < 0.001$). Subgroup analysis showed that patients with initial total cholesterol levels between 250 to 300 mg/dl showed the most improvement compared with placebo. Effects, if any, on blood pressure were not mentioned.

Side effects
Mild garlic smell in 21 percent of garlic and 9 percent of placebo groups. Also minor gastrointestinal upset.

Author's comments
Standardized garlic tablets at a sufficiently high dose can be considered as an alternative for general practitioners in the treatment of mild and medium forms of hyperlipidemia.

Reviewer's comments
This is a good study showing a statistically significant reduction in serum cholesterol and triglycerides with 800 mg garlic powder daily. The length of treatment was appropriate for observing lipid-lowering effects. (5, 6)

Clinical Study: Kwai®

Extract name	LI 111
Manufacturer	Lichtwer Pharma AG, Germany
Indication	**Hyperlipoproteinemia** (elevated blood lipid levels)
Level of evidence	**I**
Therapeutic benefit	**Yes**

Bibliographic reference
Holzgartner H, Schmidt U, Kuhn U (1992). Comparison of the efficacy and tolerance of a garlic preparation vs. bezafibrate. *Arzneimittel-Forschung/ Drug Research* 42 (12): 1473-1477.

Trial design
Parallel. Pretrial period with placebo (six weeks) proceeded drug comparison trial with 600 mg/day bezafibrate. All patients advised to observe a low-fat "step I" diet for the duration of the study.

Study duration	3 months
Dose	1 (300 mg) tablet 3 times daily
Route of administration	Oral
Randomized	Yes
Randomization adequate	Yes
Blinding	Double-blind
Blinding adequate	Yes
Placebo	No
Drug comparison	Yes
Drug name	Bezafibrate
Site description	5 general practices
No. of subjects enrolled	98
No. of subjects completed	94
Sex	Male and female
Age	44-69 years

Inclusion criteria
Primary type IIa, IIb, or IV hyperlipoproteinemia according to Fredrickson. Cholesterol and/or triglycerides higher than 250 mg/dl at the end of the pretrial phase.

Exclusion criteria
Pregnancy, nursing, drug or alcohol abuse, severe renal and hepatic insufficiency, diabetes mellitus, and any therapy with other lipid-lowering agents or with anticoagulants.

End points
Patients were evaluated before the treatment period and after 28, 56, and 84 days. Levels of total cholesterol, high-density lipoprotein cholesterol, low-density lipoprotein cholesterol, triglycerides, and blood pressure and heart rate were determined.

Results
Both medications caused a statistically significant reduction in total cholesterol, LDL cholesterol, and triglycerides, and an increase in HDL cholesterol. Following 12 weeks of treatment, mean cholesterol levels in the garlic group decreased from 282 to 210 mg/dl and in the bezafibrate group from 287 to 208 mg/dl ($p < 0.001$ for both). There was no significant difference between the groups.

Side effects
Side effects were mentioned by five patients in both treatment groups (lack of appetite, fatigue, and myalgia), none of which led to withdrawal of the patients.

Authors' comments
It can be concluded that garlic tablets standardized to 1.3 percent alliin at a sufficient dose are equivalent to other lipid-lowering agents in therapeutic administration.

Reviewer's comments
This was a well-run and well-designed study showing garlic to have effects equivalent to those of bezafibrate. The treatment length was appropriate. (5, 6)

Clinical Study: Kwai®

Extract name	LI 111
Manufacturer	Lichtwer Pharma AG, Germany

Indication	**Hyperlipidemia and hypertension**
	(elevated blood lipids and blood pressure)
Level of evidence	**II**
Therapeutic benefit	**Yes**

Bibliographic reference

Auer W, Eiber A, Hertkorn E, Hoehfeld E, Koehrle U, Lorenz A, Mader F, Merx W, Otto G, Schmid-Otto B, et al. (1990). Hypertension and hyperlipidaemia: Garlic helps in mild cases. *The British Journal of Clinical Practice* S69: 3-6.

Trial design

Parallel. Pretrial run-in period of two weeks.

Study duration	3 months
Dose	2 (100 mg) capsules 3 times daily
Route of administration	Oral
Randomized	Yes
Randomization adequate	No
Blinding	Double-blind
Blinding adequate	Yes
Placebo	Yes
Drug comparison	No
Site description	11 general practices
No. of subjects enrolled	47
No. of subjects completed	Not given
Sex	Male and female
Age	51-65 years

Inclusion criteria

Patients with mild hypertension (WHO stages I and II) and diastolic blood pressure between 95 and 104 mmHg on two measurements two weeks apart.

Exclusion criteria

Patients being treated with other antihypertensive agents or lipid-lowering agents, cases with severe forms of hypertension and hyperlipidemia, and patients who were seriously ill and might be expected to deteriorate or suffer complications suddenly during the period of the trial.

End points

Supine and standing blood pressure, pulse rates, serum cholesterol, and triglycerides were measured before admission to the trial, after the two-week pretrial period, and 4, 8, and 12 weeks after start of treatment. At the start and the end of the trial, serum glutamate-pyruvate transaminase (SGPT), serum glutamate oxaloacetate transaminase (SGOT), gamma-glutamyl transferase (GT), and blood sugar were measured.

Results
Supine diastolic blood pressure in the garlic group fell from 102 to 91 mmHg after eight weeks ($p < 0.05$) and to 89 mmHg after 12 weeks ($p < 0.01$). Supine systolic blood pressure fell after 12 weeks from 171 to 152 mmHg ($p < 0.05$). There was no significant change in blood pressure in the placebo group. The serum cholesterol and triglycerides were also significantly reduced after 8 and 12 weeks of treatment. Total serum cholesterol fell from 268 mg/dl after eight weeks ($p < 0.05$) and to 230 mg/dl after 12 weeks ($p < 0.05$), a decrease of 14 percent. In the placebo group, on the other hand, no significant differences occurred. No significant changes were found in pulse rate, SGPT, SGOT, gamma GT, or blood sugar levels.

Side effects
No serious side effects were reported. In three cases a slight smell of garlic was noted.

Authors' comments
This trial demonstrated that a preparation of garlic powder, which was free of side effects, significantly reduced blood pressure, total cholesterol, and triglycerides. Doctors now have a medication at their disposal which can be used adjunctively with diet and behavior alterations to reduce raised blood pressure and raised lipid levels, and thus contribute to a reduction in cardiovascular risk.

Reviewer's comments
This was a well-run and well-designed study with an appropriate length. The randomization process and the withdrawals were not described. (2, 6)

Clinical Study: Kwai®

Extract name	LI 111
Manufacturer	Lichtwer Pharma AG, Germany
Indication	**Hyperlipidemia** (elevated blood lipid levels)
Level of evidence	**II**
Therapeutic benefit	**Trend**

Bibliographic reference

Jain AK, Vargas R, Gotzkowsky S, McMahon FG (1993). Can garlic reduce levels of serum lipids? A controlled clinical study. *The American Journal of Medicine* 94 (6): 632-635.

Trial design

Parallel. Pretrial two-week washout period.

Study duration	3 months
Dose	1 (300 mg) tablet 3 times daily
Route of administration	Oral
Randomized	Yes
Randomization adequate	No
Blinding	Double-blind
Blinding adequate	Yes
Placebo	Yes
Drug comparison	No
Site description	Single center
No. of subjects enrolled	42
No. of subjects completed	42
Sex	Male and female
Age	Mean: 52 years

Inclusion criteria

Serum total cholesterol levels greater than or equal to 220mg/dl at two consecutive visits two weeks apart.

Exclusion criteria

Older than 70 years; history of drug or alcohol abuse; impaired hepatic function test results greater than 20 percent above normal; unstable angina; myocardial infarction or coronary bypass surgery within six months; diabetes mellitus; known secondary hypercholesterolemia due to nephrotic syndrome or hyperthyroidism; serum creatinine level greater than 2.0 mg/dl; or use of lipid-lowering agents within one month prior to enrollment.

End points

Lipid profiles from fasting blood samples were determined before and after the two-week washout period, as well as after 6 and 12 weeks of treatment. Total cholesterol, triglycerides, high-density lipoprotein cholesterol (HDL-C), low-density lipoprotein cholesterol (LDL-C), and serum glucose were determined.

Results

The baseline serum TC level of 262 +/– 34 mg/dl was reduced to 247 +/– 40 mg/dl ($p < 0.001$) after 12 weeks of standardized garlic treatment, a reduction of 6 percent. This reduction was significant compared with a 1 percent reduction with placebo ($p < 0.01$). LDL-C was reduced by 11 percent by garlic treatment and 3 percent by placebo ($p < 0.05$). No significant changes were recorded in HDL-C, TG, serum glucose, blood pressure, and other monitored parameters.

Side effects

In general, garlic tablets were well tolerated without any significant odor problems. One patient complained of belching and bad taste.

Authors' comments

Treatment with standardized garlic, 900 mg/day, produced a significantly greater reduction in serum TC and LDL-C than placebo.

Reviewer's comments

This is a relatively well-designed and well-run study. The reduction in serum cholesterol and LDL cholesterol in the treatment group was actually quite modest compared to control. The treatment length was appropriate. The two groups were comparable, but the randomization process was not described. (3, 5)

Clinical Study: Kwai®

Extract name	LI 111
Manufacturer	Lichtwer Pharma AG, Germany
Indication	**Hypercholesterolemia** (elevated cholesterol levels)
Level of evidence	**III**
Therapeutic benefit	**Yes**

Bibliographic reference

De A Santos OS, Grunwald J (1993). Effect of garlic powder tablets on blood lipids and blood pressure—Six month placebo controlled, double blind study. *The British Journal of Clinical Research* 4: 37-44.

Trial design

Parallel. Patients were instructed to follow a low-fat/low-cholesterol diet.

Study duration	6 months
Dose	1 (900 mg powder) tablet daily

Route of administration	Oral
Randomized	Yes
Randomization adequate	No
Blinding	Double-blind
Blinding adequate	No
Placebo	Yes
Drug comparison	No
Site description	1 general practice
No. of subjects enrolled	60
No. of subjects completed	52
Sex	Male and female
Age	43-60 years

Inclusion criteria
Patients with total cholesterol values over 6.5 mmol/l.

Exclusion criteria
Patients treated with other antihypertensive agents or lipid-lowering agents, severe forms of hypertension and hyperlipidemia, and serious illness.

End points
Blood pressure was measured at baseline and then monthly. Serum cholesterol, triglycerides, low-density lipoprotein cholesterol, and high-density lipoprotein cholesterol were measured at baseline and after three and six months. General well-being was assessed monthly.

Results
Serum cholesterol in the garlic group was statistically reduced after six months compared to placebo ($p < 0.05$). Initial serum cholesterol in the garlic group was reduced from 6.92 to 6.31 mmol/l, a 9 percent reduction. Values for LDL were reduced by nearly 10 percent by garlic and 6 percent by placebo. Mean systolic blood pressure was reduced in the garlic group by 17 percent, from 145 to 120 mmHg ($p < 0.001$). Mean diastolic blood pressure was also reduced, from 90 to 80 mmHg ($p < 0.01$). Blood pressure remained unchanged in the placebo group. Well-being was improved in the active group by 20 percent ($p < 0.001$).

Side effects
No significant side effects.

Authors' comments
Patients given dietary advice and treatment with standarized garlic tablets

produced a significantly greater reaction of total cholesterol and blood pressure than that of placebo.

Reviewer's comments
This study was flawed by the inadequately described statistical methods, blinding, and randomization. The treatment length was appropriate. (1, 5)

Clinical Study: Kwai®

Extract name	LI 111
Manufacturer	Lichtwer Pharma AG, Germany
Indication	**Hyperlipidemia** (elevated blood lipid levels)
Level of evidence	**III**
Therapeutic benefit	**Trend**

Bibliographic reference
Melvin KR, Chappell MA (1996). Effects of garlic powder tablets on patients with hyperlipidaemia in Canadian clinical practice. *European Journal of Clinical Research* 8: 15-36.

Trial design
Crossover. At beginning of trial subjects were randomized to placebo or garlic; on day 30 both groups were given garlic; and on day 60 subjects were again blinded to the original placebo or garlic groups.

Study duration	4 months
Dose	1 (300 mg) tablet 3 times daily
Route of administration	Oral
Randomized	Yes
Randomization adequate	No
Blinding	Double-blind
Blinding adequate	No
Placebo	Yes
Drug comparison	No
Site description	1 clinical practice
No. of subjects enrolled	34
No. of subjects completed	19
Sex	Male and female
Age	41-77 years (mean: 54)

Inclusion criteria
Elevated cholesterol and off all other drug therapy.

Exclusion criteria
None mentioned.

End points
Physical exam (clinical history, pill compliance, weight, blood pressure, and diet status) and biochemical lipid profiles in fasting state were taken at baseline and at each 30-day visit.

Results
Total serum cholesterol levels decreased by 12 percent ($p < 0.03$) on average by day 120 in the active treatment group, from an average of 6.99 mmol/l at baseline to 6.09 mmol/l. The placebo group did not show a significant decrease in cholesterol. No significant effect on serum triglycerides was seen in either group. High-density lipoprotein levels increased with garlic but did not reach statistical significance.

Side effects
None listed.

Authors' comments
Garlic powder tablets have a role in cholesterol management as an adjunctive therapy in most cases of significant hyperlipidemia.

Reviewer's comments
This study had a small sample size with a wide age range, and a very moderate reduction in serum cholesterol was observed in these patients. Also, 30 days minimum active treatment (e.g., placebo group from days 30 to 60) may not be long enough to notice effects. The randomization and blinding were not adequately described. (1, 3)

Clinical Study: Kwai®

Extract name	LI 111
Manufacturer	Lichtwer Pharma AG, Germany
Indication	**Hypercholesterolemia** (elevated cholesterol levels)
Level of evidence	**III**
Therapeutic benefit	**Yes**

Bibliographic reference
Vorberg G, Schneider B (1990). Therapy with garlic: Results of a placebo-controlled, double-blind study. *The British Journal of Clinical Practice* S69: 7-11.

Trial design
Parallel. Pretrial washout period of 14 days.

Study duration	4 months
Dose	900 mg daily
Route of administration	Oral
Randomized	Yes
Randomization adequate	No
Blinding	Double-blind
Blinding adequate	No
Placebo	Yes
Drug comparison	No
Site description	1 general practice
No. of subjects enrolled	40
No. of subjects completed	40
Sex	Male and female
Age	Mean: 50 years

Inclusion criteria
Serum cholesterol between 230 and 350 mg/dl after 14-day washout period.

Exclusion criteria
Patients receiving therapy for diabetes mellitus, advanced renal insufficiency, or for lipid lowering.

End points
Cholesterol, triglycerides, and blood pressure were measured before the study, at the end of the washout period, and at 4, 8, 12, and 16 weeks after beginning of therapy.

Results
Total cholesterol in the garlic group dropped by week 8 and continued through week 16, from 294 to 232 mg/dl, 21 percent of the starting value; this change was significant ($p < 0.001$). Reductions in triglyceride levels were also significantly different from placebo at week 16 ($p < 0.05$). Blood pressure also dropped significantly. In addition, results of a self-evaluation questionnaire indicated that patients in the drug group had a greater feeling of well-being.

Side effects
None reported.

Authors' comments
The main finding of our study was the reduction in serum cholesterol by the garlic preparation. Blood pressure and triglyceride reductions were also significantly different between garlic and placebo groups, particularly with respect to change from baseline values. All these effects increased continuously during the 16-week treatment period.

Reviewer's comments
The garlic reduced cholesterol and triglycerides compared to placebo. The length of the trial was appropriate, but the randomization and blinding were not described in sufficient detail. (1, 5)

Clinical Study: Kwai®

Extract name	LI 111
Manufacturer	Lichtwer Pharma AG, Germany
Indication	**Hypercholesterolemia** (elevated cholesterol levels)
Level of evidence	**III**
Therapeutic benefit	**Yes**

Bibliographic reference
Adler AJ, Holub BJ (1997). Effect of garlic and fish-oil supplementation on serum lipid and lipoprotein concentrations in hypercholesterolemic men. *American Journal of Clinical Nutrition* 65 (2): 445-450.

Trial design
Parallel. Four-arm, double-placebo trial: (1) placebo, (2) garlic, (3) fish oil (12 g/day providing 3.6 g n-3 fatty acids), and (4) both garlic and fish oil. Three-week run-in phase.

Study duration	3 months
Dose	1 (300 mg) capsule 3 times daily
Route of administration	Oral
Randomized	Yes
Randomization adequate	No
Blinding	Double/single-blind
Blinding adequate	No

Placebo	Yes
Drug comparison	Yes
Drug name	Fish oil
Site description	Single center
No. of subjects enrolled	50
No. of subjects completed	46
Sex	Male
Age	Mean: 45.9 years

Inclusion criteria

Total cholesterol concentration >5.2 mmol/l; medications were allowed as long as they were not initiated within four weeks of the beginning of the study.

Exclusion criteria

Subjects taking lipid-altering or blood pressure-altering medications or supplements within four weeks of study start, with diabetes mellitus, or with cardiovascular disease.

End points

Fasting blood samples were taken at weeks 0, 3, 6, 9, and 12, and were analyzed for total cholesterol, low-density lipoprotein cholesterol, high-density lipoprotein cholesterol, and triglycerides. Blood pressure and heart rate were measured. Fatty acid composition of total serum phospholipid was analyzed at weeks 0 and 12. Two three-day dietary records were kept.

Results

In the placebo group, mean serum total cholesterol, LDL-C, and triacylglycerols were not significantly changed in relation to baseline. Mean group total cholesterol concentrations were significantly lower with garlic + fish oil (−12.2 percent) and with garlic (−11.5 percent) after 12 weeks but not with fish oil alone. Mean LDL-C concentrations were reduced with garlic + fish oil (−9.5 percent) and with garlic (−14.2 percent) but were raised with fish oil (+8.5 percent). Mean triacylglycerol concentrations were reduced with garlic + fish oil (−34.3 percent) and fish oil alone (−37.3 percent). The garlic groups (with and without fish oil) had significantly lower ratios of total cholesterol to HDL-C and LDL-C to HDL-C. Mean systolic, diastolic, and arterial blood pressures for all subjects at entry were 120.1, 80.0, and 94.0 mmHg, respectively. By week 12, reductions of 2.4 to 4.2 percent ($p < 0.05$ or $p < 0.005$, respectively) in mean systolic, diastolic, and arterial pressures were found for all three treatment groups (garlic alone, fish oil alone, and garlic + fish oil) relative to the placebo group.

Side effects
Odor due to garlic was reported in 20 percent of the subjects taking garlic pills. One subject reported a slight feeling of nausea with fish oil.

Authors' comments
Garlic supplementation significantly decreased both total cholesterol and LDL-C, whereas fish oil supplementation significantly decreased triacyl-glycerol concentrations and increased LDL-C concentrations in hyper-cholesterolemic men. The combination of garlic and fish oil reversed the moderate fish oil-induced rise in LDL-C.

Reviewer's comments
In this study, the garlic supplement alone reduced total cholesterol and LDL cholesterol. Garlic pills and placebo pills were administered in a double-blinded manner, but fish oil capsules and oil placebo capsules were only single-blinded. There was no description of the randomization process. (1, 6)

Clinical Study: Kwai®

Extract name	LI 111
Manufacturer	Lichtwer Pharma AG, Germany
Indication	**Hyperlipidemia** (elevated blood lipid levels)
Level of evidence	I
Therapeutic benefit	**No**

Bibliographic reference
Neil HAW, Silagy CA, Lancaster T, Hodgeman J, Vos K, Moore JW, Jones L, Cahill J, Fowler GH (1996). Garlic powder in the treatment of moderate hyperlipidemia: A controlled trial and meta-analysis. *Journal of the Royal College of Physicians of London* 30 (4): 329-334. (Further analysis reported in Byrne DJ, Neil HAW, Vallance DT, Winder AF [1999]. *Clinica Chimica Acta: International Journal of Clinical Chemistry* 285 [1-2]: 21-33.)

Trial design
Parallel. During a preliminary six-week screening period, dietary guidelines were given: a daily intake of less than 300 mg cholesterol and about 35 g of fiber was recommended.

Study duration	6 months
Dose	1 (300 mg powder) capsule 3 times daily

Route of administration	Oral
Randomized	Yes
Randomization adequate	Yes
Blinding	Double-blind
Blinding adequate	Yes
Placebo	Yes
Drug comparison	No
Site description	1 general practice
No. of subjects enrolled	115
No. of subjects completed	106
Sex	Male and female
Age	35-64 years

Inclusion criteria
Total cholesterol concentration of 6.5 to 9.0 mmol/L on screening and a repeat fasting concentration of 6.0 to 8.5 mmol/L, with a low-density lipoprotein cholesterol of 3.5 mmol/L or above.

Exclusion criteria
Fasting triglyceride concentration of 5.6 mmol/L or above; high-density lipoprotein cholesterol concentration of 2.0 mmol/L or above; hyperlipidemia secondary to any recognized cause; treatment with a lipid-lowering drug; hospitalization for severe illness within the previous three months; and pregnancy or breast-feeding.

End points
Concentrations of total cholesterol, low-density lipoprotein cholesterol, high-density lipoprotein cholesterol, apolipoprotein (apo) A1 and B, and triglycerides were determined. Blood samples were analyzed six weeks before the trial, at the beginning, and at the end of the trial. The second report analyzed resistance of LDL to oxidation, LDL subfraction composition, and levels of circulating antibody to oxidized LDL.

Results
There were no significant differences between the groups receiving garlic and placebo in the mean concentrations of serum lipids, lipoproteins, or apo A1 or B, by analysis either on intention-to-treat or treatment received. An analysis limited to those subjects with better than 75 percent compliance again found no significant differences. The second report showed no significant difference in oxidative resistance lag time, LDL composition, or levels of antibodies to oxidized LDL.

Side effects
Garlic odor was noted.

Authors' comments
In this trial, garlic was less effective in reducing total cholesterol than suggested by previous meta-analysis. The results do not support the hypothesis that dietary garlic supplementation decreases the susceptibility of isolated LDL to oxidation and that patterns of LDL fractions in plasma might be involved. Levels of lipoprotein in plasma were also not changed. Other mechanisms of cardiovascular benefit are, however, not excluded.

Reviewer's comments
This is a very well conducted and designed study with an appropriate length. There were no significant effects on plasma total cholesterol, HDL or LDL cholesterol, triglycerides, or apolipoproteins compared with the placebo. (5, 6)

Clinical Study: Kwai®

Extract name	LI 111
Manufacturer	Lichtwer Pharma AG, Germany
Indication	**Hyperlipidemia** (elevated blood lipid levels)
Level of evidence	**I**
Therapeutic benefit	**No**

Bibliographic reference
McCrindle BW, Helden E, Conner WT (1998). Garlic extract therapy in children with hypercholesterolemia. *Archives of Pediatric and Adolescent Medicine* 152 (11): 1089-1094.

Trial design
Parallel. Patients were instructed to stop taking lipid-lowering medications for at least eight weeks before the study.

Study duration	2 months
Dose	1 (300 mg) capsule 3 times daily
Route of administration	Oral
Randomized	Yes
Randomization adequate	Yes

Blinding	Double-blind
Blinding adequate	Yes
Placebo	Yes
Drug comparison	No
Site description	Single center
No. of subjects enrolled	30
No. of subjects completed	30
Sex	Male and female
Age	Mean: 14.0 years

Inclusion criteria

Eight to eighteen years old, a positive family history of hypercholesterolemia or premature atherosclerotic cardiovascular disease in first-degree relatives, a minimum fasting total cholesterol level at enrollment higher than 4.8 mmol/l (>185 mg/dl), participation in a dietary counseling program, and compliance with a National Cholesterol Education Program Step II diet for at least six months.

Exclusion criteria

Presence of secondary causes of hyperlipidemia, a history of major surgery, or serious illness three months or less prior to enrollment.

End points

Fasting blood samples were taken at baseline and at trial end point. Total cholesterol, triglycerides, high-density lipoprotein cholesterol, low-density lipoprotein cholesterol, lipoprotein(a), apolipoprotein B-100 and A-1, homocysteine, and fibrogen were determined. Blood pressure was monitored along with diet via a food frequency questionnaire.

Results

Baseline lipid values were as follows: total cholesterol 265 mg/dl; LDL cholesterol 206 mg/dl; HDL cholesterol 37 mg/dl; and triglycerides 112 mg/dl. There was no significant relative attributable effect of garlic extract on fasting total cholesterol or LDL cholesterol. Likewise, no significant effect was seen on the levels of HDL cholesterol, triglycerides, apolipoprotein B-100, lipoprotein(a), fibrinogen, homocysteine, or blood pressure (no patients had hypertension at baseline). There was a small effect on apolipoprotein A-1.

Side effects

Minor effects noted: headache, upset stomach, and garlic odor on breath. There were no differences in adverse effects between groups.

Authors' comments
Garlic extract therapy has no significant effect on cardiovascular risk factors in pediatric patients with familial hyperlipidemia.

Reviewer's comments
This is an excellent study that showed no significant reduction in serum lipids or blood pressure compared to placebo. The treatment length was appropriate. (5, 6)

Clinical Study: Kwai®

Extract name	LI 111
Manufacturer	Lichtwer Pharma AG, Germany
Indication	**Hypercholesterolemia** (elevated cholesterol levels)
Level of evidence	**I**
Therapeutic benefit	**No**

Bibliographic reference
Isaacsohn JL, Moser M, Stein EA, Dudley K, Davey J, Lishkov E, Black HR (1998). Garlic powder and plasma lipids and lipoproteins. *Archives of Internal Medicine* 158 (11): 1189-1194.

Trial design
Parallel. Entry into the study following eight weeks of diet stabilization.

Study duration	3 months
Dose	1 (300 mg) tablet 3 times daily
Route of administration	Oral
Randomized	Yes
Randomization adequate	Yes
Blinding	Double-blind
Blinding adequate	Yes
Placebo	Yes
Drug comparison	No
Site description	2 outpatient clinics
No. of subjects enrolled	50
No. of subjects completed	42
Sex	Male and female
Age	44-70 years

Inclusion criteria

Mean plasma LDL-C level, determined at two visits (four and two weeks before randomization), of 4.1 mmol/l (160 mg/dl) or higher (with no single value <4.0 mmol/l [155 mg/dl]), and a mean plasma triglyceride level lower than 4.0 mmol/l (350 mg/dl).

Exclusion criteria

Secondary cause of hypercholesterolemia including hypothyroidism, nephrotic syndrome (treatment with hormones known to affect lipids, uncontrolled diabetes), unstable angina, or myocardial infarction occurring within two months of entry into the study, active liver disease, chronic renal disease (creatinine level >265 µmol/l [>3mg/dl]), or severe metabolic or endocrine disorders. All lipid-lowering drugs were discontinued six weeks before entry into the study.

End points

Dietary assessment using a three-day diet diary and food rating record was made after four and eight weeks of diet stabilization, and after 12 weeks of treatment. Fasting blood samples were drawn to determine plasma lipid and lipoproteins, apolipoproteins, chemistry profiles, and complete blood counts. Heart rate and blood pressure were also measured.

Results

Baseline levels for total cholesterol were 250 mg/dl and 274 mg/dl for the placebo and garlic groups, respectively. An adjusted percentage of change was calculated and compared between the two groups as the baseline numbers were statistically different. At the conclusion of the trial there were no significant lipid or lipoprotein changes in either placebo or garlic-treated groups and no significant difference between the two groups.

Side effects

Three patients complained of garlic breath, two of body odor. Three patients in both groups complained of gastrointestinal problems.

Authors' comments

Garlic powder (900 mg/d) treatment for 12 weeks was ineffective in lowering cholesterol levels in patients with hypercholesterolemia.

Reviewer's comments

This was a well-conducted study. A small but statistically significant increase in diastolic blood pressure was observed in the placebo group. Otherwise, no significant differences observed between groups. The treatment length was appropriate. (5, 6)

Clinical Study: Kwai®

Extract name	LI 111
Manufacturer	Lichtwer Pharma AG, Germany
Indication	**Hypercholesterolemia** (elevated cholesterol levels)
Level of evidence	**II**
Therapeutic benefit	**No**

Bibliographic reference
Simons LA, Balasubramaniam S, von Konigsmark M, Parfitt A, Simons J, Peters W (1995). On the effect of garlic on plasma lipids and lipoproteins in mild hypercholesterolaemia. *Atherosclerosis* 113 (2): 219-225.

Trial design
Crossover. After a baseline dietary period of 28 days, subjects were assigned to garlic or placebo for 12 weeks followed by 28 days washout, followed by 12 weeks with alternate treatment. All subjects were placed on an isocaloric, fat-restricted diet.

Study duration	3 months
Dose	1 (300 mg) tablet 3 times daily
Route of administration	Oral
Randomized	Yes
Randomization adequate	No
Blinding	Double-blind
Blinding adequate	Yes
Placebo	Yes
Drug comparison	No
Site description	Single center
No. of subjects enrolled	31
No. of subjects completed	29
Sex	Male and female
Age	42-69 years

Inclusion criteria
Mild hypercholesterolemia in the range 6.0 to 7.8 mol/l after 28 days on standard dietary advice; plasma triglyceride below 3.0 mmol/l; not using lipid-regulating, antihypertensive, or antioxidant drugs.

Exclusion criteria
No active renal or liver disease, diabetes, or unstable coronary artery dis-

ease. No intake of garlic or other nutritional supplements throughout the study.

End points
At point of recruitment and continuing throughout the study, each subject received dietary instruction in an isocaloric, fat-restricted diet. Clinical observations and blood sampling were performed every 28 days, for a total of nine visits. Blood pressure was measured, as well as plasma cholesterol and triglycerides.

Results
Comparing the period on garlic with that on placebo, there were no significant differences in plasma cholesterol, low-density lipoprotein cholesterol, high-density lipoprotein cholesterol, plasma triglycerides, lipoprotein(a) concentrations, or blood pressure (baseline 120/80 +/– 14/8 mmHg). Garlic showed no demonstrable effect on oxidizability of LDL, on the ratio of plasma lathosterol to cholesterol (a measure of cholesterol synthesis), or on LDL receptor expression in lymphocytes.

Side effects
Minor gastrointestinal disturbances such as abdominal bloating, nausea, or flatulence; body odor; garlic taste.

Authors' comments
We conclude from the present study in subjects with mild to moderate hypercholesterolemia that garlic powder tablets at a dose of 900 mg/day appeared to have no significant effect on plasma cholesterol or other lipid and lipoprotein parameters.

Reviewer's comments
The garlic supplementation showed no beneficial effect on plasma lipids. The trial had a good crossover/washout design. (3, 6)

Clinical Study: Kwai®

Extract name	LI 111
Manufacturer	Lichtwer Pharma AG, Germany
Indication	**Hypercholesterolemia** (elevated cholesterol levels)
Level of evidence	**II**
Therapeutic benefit	**No**

Bibliographic reference
Superko R, Krauss RM (2000). Garlic powder, effect on plasma lipids, post-prandial lipemia, low-density lipoprotein particle size, high-density lipopro-tein subclass distribution and lipoprotein(a). *Journal of the American College of Cardiology* 35 (2): 321-326.

Trial design
Parallel. Patients followed the American Heart Association Step I diet for at least two weeks before entry into the trial. Before the laboratory tests, sub-jects fasted for 16 hours and avoided alcohol for 48 hours.

Study duration	3 months
Dose	1 (300 mg) tablets 3 times daily
Route of administration	Oral
Randomized	Yes
Randomization adequate	Yes
Blinding	Double-blind
Blinding adequate	Yes
Placebo	Yes
Drug comparison	No
Site description	Lipid research clinic
No. of subjects enrolled	50
No. of subjects completed	50
Sex	Not given
Age	Mean: 53 years

Inclusion criteria
Subjects with moderate hypercholesterolemia: low-density lipoprotein cho-lesterol between 150 and 200 mg/dl and triglycerides <300 mg/dl.

Exclusion criteria
Subjects with heterozygous familial hypercholesterolemia, a systemic dis-ease that could affect blood lipids, body weight greater than 30 percent of ideal, use of lipid-lowering drugs in the preceding two months, or other medi-cations known to change blood lipids.

End points
LDLC, HDLC, very-low-density lipoproteins, low-density lipoproteins, total cholesterol, and triglyceride levels were measured. Apolipoprotein (apo) B and lipoprotein(a) [Lp(a)] levels were also measured, as well as post-priandial triglyceride response.

Results
At the end of the trial, Kwai garlic tablets had no significant effect on levels of fasting triglycerides, postprandial triglycerides, LDL cholesterol, LDL subclass distribution, LDL peak particle diameter, HDL subclass distribution, HDL cholesterol, total cholesterol, Lp(a), or apo B. There were also no changes compared to the placebo group with respect to body mass index, diastolic or systolic blood pressure, or diet variables.

Side effects
None mentioned.

Authors' comments
The double-blind, randomized clinical trial we report confirms this lack of effect of garlic on routine measures of triglycerides, total, LDL, and HDL cholesterol. However, it contributes new information to the field by further revealing no significant effect of 300 mg t.i.d. of Kwai garlic on LDL peak particle diameter, LDL subclass distribution, apo B, Lp(a), HDL subclass distribution, and postprandial lipemia.

Reviewer's comments
This is a good-quality study. (5, 6)

Clinical Study: Kwai®

Extract name	LI 111
Manufacturer	Lichtwer Pharma AG, Germany
Indication	**Hypercholesterolemia** (elevated cholesterol levels)
Level of evidence	**II**
Therapeutic benefit	**Trend**

Bibliographic reference
Saradeth T, Seidl S, Resch KL, Ernst E (1994). Does garlic alter the lipid pattern in normal volunteers? *Phytomedicine* 1: 183-185.

Trial design
Parallel. Pretrial two-week washout period.

Study duration	15 weeks
Dose	600 mg daily
Route of administration	Oral
Randomized	Yes

Randomization adequate	Yes
Blinding	Double-blind
Blinding adequate	Yes
Placebo	Yes
Drug comparison	No
Site description	Single center
No. of subjects enrolled	72
No. of subjects completed	68
Sex	Male and female
Age	Mean: 39.2 years

Inclusion criteria
Between 18 and 50 years, and healthy with constant blood baseline measurements before and after two-week pretrial washout period.

Exclusion criteria
Pregnant women, and individuals taking fresh garlic or garlic medication prior to the trial, showing clinical signs of atherosclerotic diseases, impaired liver function, or inflammatory diseases were excluded. Persons taking fibrinolytic agents, anticoagulants, or fibrates were also not admitted.

End points
Baseline measurements were taken at the beginning and end of the two-week washout period, and trial measurements were taken after 5, 10, and 15 weeks of treatment. Total cholesterol, triglycerides, and blood pressure were monitored.

Results
There was a drop in total cholesterol in the garlic group which was significant after ten weeks but insignificant at the 15 weeks measurement (223 to 210 and 214 mg/dl). Triglycerides decreased numerically (124 to 118 mg/dl) without reaching the level of significance. Blood pressure remained constant throughout. No changes occurred in the placebo group.

Side effects
Not mentioned.

Authors' comments
The medication of garlic induces changes in blood lipids, even if these variables had been normal to start with.

Reviewer's comments
This study demonstrated that 600 mg dried garlic per day led to a slight decrease in total cholesterol compared with placebo in volunteers with normal

lipid levels at baseline. In this well-designed and well-conducted study, a level of evidence point was lost because of inappropriate inclusion/exclusion criteria. (5, 5)

Clinical Study: Kwai®

Extract name	LI 111
Manufacturer	Lichtwer Pharma AG, Germany
Indication	**Hypercholesterolemia** (elevated cholesterol levels) in diabetics
Level of evidence	**III**
Therapeutic benefit	**Undetermined**

Bibliographic reference
Mansell P, Reckless JPD, Lloyd J, Leatherdale B (1996). The effect of dried garlic powder tablets on serum lipids in non-insulin dependent diabetic patients. *European Journal of Clinical Research* 8: 25-26.

Trial design
Parallel.

Study duration	3 months
Dose	1 (300 mg of dried garlic) tablet 3 times daily
Route of administration	Oral
Randomized	Yes
Randomization adequate	No
Blinding	Not described
Blinding adequate	No
Placebo	Yes
Drug comparison	No
Site description	1 general practice
No. of subjects enrolled	60
No. of subjects completed	60
Sex	Male and female
Age	42-75 years (median: 63)

Inclusion criteria
Non-insulin-dependent diabetics with well-controlled diabetes, on diet or tablets, with a serum total cholesterol between 6.0 and 8.0 mmol/l.

Exclusion criteria
None mentioned.

End points
Blood samples and blood pressure measurements were taken at baseline and after 6 and 12 weeks.

Results
Serum total cholesterol and serum low-density lipoprotein cholesterol in garlic group were reduced ($p < 0.07$ and $p < 0.05$, respectively) at week 6, but not at week 12. High-density lipoprotein cholesterol in the garlic group rose compared to placebo ($p < 0.05$). LDL-C/HDL-C ratio fell at 6 and 12 weeks ($p < 0.05$). There were no differences in very low density lipoprotein cholesterol, HDL-C2 and HDL-C3, triglycerides or in apolipoprotein A1 or B compared with placebo. Garlic tablets also had no effect on fasting blood glucose, HbA1c, serum insulin, or c peptide. It was not mentioned whether there was an effect on blood pressure.

Side effects
Odor noted at least once weekly.

Authors' comments
Dried garlic tablets had a beneficial effect on LDL-C/HDL-C ratio in moderately hypercholesterolemic non-insulin-dependent diabetic patients—a potential reduction in cardiovascular risk. No significant effect on blood pressure or diabetic control.

Reviewer's comments
Although the placebo was identical to treatment, the degree of blinding was not mentioned. The randomization process was not clearly described. Insufficient detail was given for the inclusion and exclusion criteria. However, the outcome measures were clearly defined, and the treatment length was appropriate. (0, 3)

Clinical Study: Kwai®

Extract name	LI 111
Manufacturer	Lichtwer Pharma AG, Germany
Indication	**Lipids and lipoproteins** in normal volunteers
Level of evidence	**III**
Therapeutic benefit	**Undetermined**

Bibliographic reference
Phelps S, Harris WS (1993). Garlic supplementation and lipoprotein oxidation susceptibility. *Lipids* 28 (5): 475-477.

Trial design
Crossover. Two-week treatment periods with a one-week washout period between treatment periods. Subjects' diets were monitored.

Study duration	2 weeks
Dose	6 (100 mg of powdered garlic) tablets daily
Route of administration	Oral
Randomized	Yes
Randomization adequate	No
Blinding	Double-blind
Blinding adequate	No
Placebo	Yes
Drug comparison	No
Site description	1 general practice
No. of subjects enrolled	10
No. of subjects completed	Not given
Sex	Male and female
Age	Mean: 32 years

Inclusion criteria
Healthy, normolipidemics. Smoking and exercise patterns were kept constant throughout the study.

Exclusion criteria
Subjects could not be taking medications that may affect the serum lipids, garlic, or have a significant amount of antioxidants in diet.

End points
Blood samples were drawn at the beginning and end of each test period. Lipids and lipoproteins were analyzed. Diets were monitored with three-day diaries, one per treatment period.

Results
Garlic supplementation did not alter plasma total cholesterol, low-density lipoprotein or high-density lipoprotein cholesterol, or triglyceride levels. Garlic significantly reduced the susceptibility of the apoB-containing lipoproteins to copper-induced oxidation ($p < 0.05$). Only half of the group experienced

this change, with two patients showing remarkable changes. Values with placebo were unchanged.

Side effects
None listed.

Authors' comments
We conclude that 600 mg of Kwai taken for only two weeks significantly decreased the lipoprotein oxidation susceptibility without altering serum cholesterol levels in normal adults.

Reviewer's comments
This was a very brief study with a small sample size. Garlic supplementation reduced apo-B lipoprotein fraction susceptibility to oxidation, but because the sample size was very small, the value of this finding is undetermined in a "real life" setting. Also, randomization, blinding, and dropouts were not adequately described. (0, 5)

Clinical Study: LI 111

Extract name	LI 111
Manufacturer	Lichtwer Pharma AG, Germany
Indication	**Atherosclerosis**
Level of evidence	**II**
Therapeutic benefit	**Trend**

Bibliographic reference
Koscielny J, Klubendorf D, Latza R, Schmitt R, Radtke H, Siegel G, Kiesewetter H (1999). The antiatherosclerotic effect of *Allium sativum. Atherosclerosis* 144 (1): 237-249.

Trial design
Parallel.

Study duration	4 years
Dose	900 mg powder daily
Route of administration	Oral
Randomized	Yes
Randomization adequate	No
Blinding	Double-blind
Blinding adequate	Yes

Placebo	Yes
Drug comparison	No
Site description	Single center
No. of subjects enrolled	280
No. of subjects completed	152
Sex	Male and female
Age	40-80 years

Inclusion criteria

Advanced atherosclerosis plaques as measured by ultrasound in the carotid bifurcation and/or the femoral arteries; at least one of the established risk factors such as high systolic blood pressure, hypercholesterolemia, diabetes mellitus, and smoking.

Exclusion criteria

Severe internal diseases such as functional disorders of the heart, circulation, liver, kidney, and lung, decompensated heart failure, severe arrythmias, acute myocardial infarction (<6 months ago), lung emphysema, asthma bronchiale, systolic blood pressure >180 mmHg, hypotension <110 mmHg, renal failure (creatinine >2.0 mg/dl); pregnancy; simultaneous treatment with aspirin, naftidrofuryl, pentoxifylline, omega-3-fatty acid, calcium antagonists, and oral antithrombotic agents; and hemodynamically relevant stenotic lesions in the examined arteries.

End points

Change of plaque volume in the common carotid and femoral artery and changes in the combined intimal-medial thickness (IMT). Plasma viscosity, platelet aggregation, total blood cholesterol, low-density lipoprotein cholesterol, high-density lipoprotein cholesterol, triglycerides, and glucose were also measured. Doppler pressure assessments of the brachial, dorsal pedal, and posterior artery, of blood pressure, and of heart rate were obtained.

Results

The arteriosclerotic plaque volume increased by 15.6 percent over four years in the placebo group. In the garlic group a decrease of 2.6 percent was observed. There was a significant difference of 18.3 percent between placebo and garlic groups. Breaking the groups down by sex and age showed differences in results. The age-dependent representation of the plaque volume shows an increase between 50 to 80 years that is diminished with garlic treatment by 6 to 13 percent. Further subgroup analysis found that the reductions compared to placebo were 4.4 percent for men and 58 percent for women. However, there was an unequal age distribution of women in the placebo and garlic groups. The predominately younger women in the placebo group (aged 40 to 55 years) had a drastic increase in plaque volume (53 percent), while the mainly older women (aged over 55 years) in the garlic group had a plaque reduction of 4.6 percent. Plasma lipid levels and blood pressure measurements were not mentioned.

Side effects
Annoyance with odor.

Authors' comments
These results substantiate that not only a preventative but also possibly a curative role in artherosclerosis therapy (plaque regression) may be ascribed to garlic remedies.

Reviewer's comments
This is a well-conducted and well-designed study with an appropriate treatment length. There was no description of the randomization process. (3, 6)

Clinical Study: Kwai®

Extract name	LI 111
Manufacturer	Lichtwer Pharma AG, Germany
Indication	**Effect on postmeal lipid levels**
Level of evidence	**II**
Therapeutic benefit	**Undetermined**

Bibliographic reference
Rotzsch W, Richter V, Rassoul F, Walper A (1992). Reduction in postprandial lipaemia caused by *Allium sativum:* Controlled double-blind trial involving test persons with low HDL2-cholesterol levels. *Arzneimittel-Forschung/Drug Research* 42 (10): 1223-1227.

Trial design
Parallel. Lipid levels were measured before and after a high-fat meal. Pretrial washout period of one week.

Study duration	1 dose and 6 weeks
Dose	1 (300 mg) tablet 3 times daily
Route of administration	Oral
Randomized	Yes
Randomization adequate	No
Blinding	Double-blind
Blinding adequate	Yes

Placebo	Yes
Drug comparison	No
Site description	Single center
No. of subjects enrolled	24
No. of subjects completed	24
Sex	Male and female
Age	23-53 years

Inclusion criteria
Volunteers with low initial high-density lipoprotein 2-cholesterol concentrations in the plasma, below 10 mg/dl in men and 15 mg/dl in women.

Exclusion criteria
None mentioned.

End points
Lipid concentrations in the serum were measured three times each day on the first, twenty-second, and forty-third day of treatment; measurements were taken both before as well as three and five hours after intake of 100 g butter.

Results
The postprandial increase in triglyceride levels was much lower in the garlic group than the placebo group, but it was not statistically significant. However, after six weeks, garlic caused a significant decrease in fasting triglyceride levels compared to placebo. There was an increase in HDL2-cholesterol in the garlic group, but this was not statistically different from placebo.

Side effects
None discussed.

Authors' comments
In everyday life, this would mean that the single administration of garlic together with a high-fat meal will slightly improve triglyceride values, but a major preventive effect will be obtained only by regular administration over longer periods of time.

Reviewer's comments
The single-day treatment to observe postprandial changes in plasma lipids is of limited value. The six weeks of continuous administration led to a reduction in fasting triglycerides. The trial was limited by the small sample size (12 in each group), as well as inadequately described randomization. (2, 5)

Clinical Study: LI 111

Extract name	LI 111
Manufacturer	Lichtwer Pharma AG, Germany
Indication	**Increased spontaneous platelet aggregation**
Level of evidence	**II**
Therapeutic benefit	**Trend**

Bibliographic reference

Kiesewetter H, Jung F, Pindur G, Jung EM, Mrowietz C, Wenzel E (1991). Effect of garlic on thrombocyte aggregation, microcirculation, and other risk factors. *International Journal of Clinical Pharmacology, Therapy and Toxicology* 29 (4): 151-155.

Trial design

Parallel. Trial preceded by a one-week washout period.

Study duration	1 month
Dose	4 (200 mg powdered garlic) tablets daily
Route of administration	Oral
Randomized	Yes
Randomization adequate	No
Blinding	Double-blind
Blinding adequate	Yes
Placebo	Yes
Drug comparison	No
Site description	Single general practice
No. of subjects enrolled	120
No. of subjects completed	Not given
Sex	Male and female
Age	19-26 years

Inclusion criteria

Subjects with constantly increased spontaneous thrombocyte (platelet) aggregation. Measurements were made three times during the washout phase (days 0, 3, and 7) and the values measured on days 3 and 7 had to be pathological.

Exclusion criteria

None mentioned.

End points

Spontaneous thrombocyte aggregation was measured during washout phase (days 0, 3, and 7) and on days 14, 21, 28, and 35. Blood pressure, blood glucose, cholesterol, triglycerides, fibrinogen, thrombocyte, and leukocyte count were also determined.

Results

Spontaneous thrombocyte aggregation in the garlic group decreased significantly, by 56.3 percent by the Breddin method and 10.3 percent by the Grotemeyer method. The microcirculation of the skin increased by 47.6 percent, plasma viscosity in garlic group decreased by 3.2 percent, diastolic blood pressure decreased by 9.5 percent (from 74 +/− 9 to 67 +/− 5 mmHg), and blood glucose concentration decreased by 11.6 percent. There was no change in systolic blood pressure, total cholesterol levels, or triglyceride levels. The mean total cholesterol level at baseline for the garlic group was 228 mg/dl.

Side effects

None mentioned.

Authors' comments

The vascular protective effect of garlic, by influencing the mentioned risk parameters for cardiovascular diseases, must be pointed out. Especially interesting is the thrombocyte aggregation inhibiting effect. Thus, garlic may be useful in cases of acetylsalicyclic acid intolerance.

Reviewer's comments

This is a well-designed and well-conducted study showing that garlic powder may be useful for inhibition of thrombocyte aggregation in patients unable to use aspirin. The treatment length was appropriate and the blinding was adequately described. (2, 6)

Product Profile: Pure-Gar®

Manufacturer	**Essentially Pure Ingredients™**
U.S. distributor	**Essentially Pure Ingredients™**
Botanical ingredient	**Garlic clove dried**
Extract name	N/A
Quantity	No information
Processing	Proprietary quick "cool dry" process
Standardization	0.3% allicin
Formulation	Tablet

Source(s) of information: Essentially Pure Ingredients™ Web page (www.essentiallypure.com/products.htm); Lash et al., 1998.

Clinical Study: Pure-Gar®

Extract name	N/A
Manufacturer	Essentially Pure Ingredients™
Indication	**Hypercholesterolemia** (elevated cholesterol levels) in renal transplant patients
Level of evidence	**II**
Therapeutic benefit	**Yes**

Bibliographic reference
Lash JP, Cardoso, LR, Mesler PM, Walczak DA, Pollak R (1998). The effect of garlic on hypercholesterolemia in renal transplant patients. *Transplantation Proceedings* 30 (1): 189-191.

Trial design
Parallel. Patients were on National Cholesterol Education Program Step One restriction diet.

Study duration	3 months
Dose	1 tablet (680 mg dried garlic) twice daily
Route of administration	Oral
Randomized	Yes
Randomization adequate	No
Blinding	Double-blind
Blinding adequate	Yes
Placebo	Yes
Drug comparison	No
Site description	1 general practice
No. of subjects enrolled	35
No. of subjects completed	35
Sex	Male and female
Age	41-51 years

Inclusion criteria
Renal transplanted patients with total serum cholesterol greater than 240 mg/dL and LDL cholesterol greater than 160 mg/dL by two consecutive fast-

ing determinations, with stable renal allograft function for more than six months.

Exclusion criteria
Triglycerides >500 mg/dL, nephritic syndrome, and use of other hypolipemic medications within a six-month period.

End points
Lipid profile, such as cholesterol, triglycerides, LDL, and HDL, were measured.

Results
Garlic was effective in decreasing both total and LDL cholesterol levels (290 to 275 mg/dl; 193 to 182 mg/dl). This benefit was apparent after six weeks and maintained at 12 weeks. No change was observed in the placebo group in total or LDL cholesterol.

Side effects
One case each of diarrhea and epigastric pain.

Authors' comments
Although garlic had significant beneficial effects, treated patients still had hyperlipidemia which was severe enough to consider the addition of standard pharmacotherapy. There may be a role for garlic in combination therapy with a HMG-CoA reductase inhibitor. It is possible that garlic supplementation could decrease the dosage of the HMG-CoA reductase inhibitor required and thereby minimize the chance for drug toxicity.

Reviewer's comments
In this study, garlic clearly shows cholesterol-lowering effect in renal failure patients. It is a well-designed and well-executed study; however, the randomization process was not described in any detail. (3, 5)

Product Profile: Dried Garlic

Manufacturer	None
U.S. distributor	None
Botanical ingredient	**Garlic clove dried**
Extract name	N/A
Quantity	No information
Processing	No information
Standardization	No information
Formulation	Tablet

Source(s) of information: Luley et al., 1986.

Clinical Study: Garlic (Dried)

Extract name	N/A
Manufacturer	None
Indication	**Hyperlipoproteinemia** (elevated blood lipid levels)
Level of evidence	**III**
Therapeutic benefit	**No**

Bibliographic reference
Luley C, Lehmann-Leo W, Moeller B, Martin T, Schwartzkopff W (1986). Lack of efficacy of dried garlic in patients with hyperlipoproteinemia. *Arzneimittel-Forschung/Drug Research* 36 (1): 766-768.

Trial design
Crossover after six weeks. Two studies are reported here. Study 1 had 34 subjects who were given 594 mg/day of an unnamed commercial preparation of dried garlic. Study 2 had 51 subjects who were given 1350 mg/day of a preparation especially prepared for the study.

Study duration	6 weeks
Dose	(1) 3 (66 mg) three times daily;
	(2) 1 (450 mg) three times daily
Route of administration	Oral
Randomized	Yes
Randomization adequate	No
Blinding	Double-blind
Blinding adequate	No
Placebo	Yes
Drug comparison	No
Site description	1 general practice
No. of subjects enrolled	34, 51
No. of subjects completed	34, 51
Sex	Not given
Age	Not given

Inclusion criteria
Patients with hyperlipoproteinemia types IIa, IIb, and IV.

Exclusion criteria
None mentioned.

End points
Total cholesterol, HDL cholesterol, LDL cholesterol, triglycerides, and several safety parameters were measured every three weeks in both studies. Study 2 had additional tests, including apolipoprotein A and B levels, euglobulin, lysis time, fibrin split products, prothrombin time, whole blood coagulation time, and fibrinogen levels.

Results
Neither dosage of dried garlic showed any significant effect on any of the parameters measured.

Side effects
Bad smell reported in study 2.

Authors' comments
The administration of pills containing dried garlic in the concentration studied should not be recommended as an antiatherosclerotic agent.

Reviewer's comments
No benefit to cardiovascular risk was found from dried garlic pills. The randomization and blinding were not described in any detail. (1, 5)

Product Profile: Spray-Dried Garlic

Manufacturer	**Government Pharmaceutical Organization, Thailand**
U.S. distributor	None
Botanical ingredient	**Garlic clove dried**
Extract name	N/A
Quantity	350 mg
Processing	Spray-dried garlic
Standardization	No information
Formulation	Capsule

Source(s) of information: Plengvidlya et al., 1998.

Clinical Study: Garlic (Dried)

Extract name	N/A
Manufacturer	Government Pharmaceutical Organization, Thailand

Indication	**Hyperlipoproteinemia** (elevated blood lipid levels)
Level of evidence	**III**
Therapeutic benefit	**Undetermined**

Bibliographic reference

Plengvidlya C, Sitprija S, Chinayon, S, Pasatrat S, Tunkayoon M (1998). Effects of spray dried garlic preparation on primary hyperlipoproteinemia. *Journal of the Medical Association of Thailand* 71 (5): 248-252.

Trial design

Crossover after two months.

Study duration	2 months
Dose	1 (350 mg) capsule twice daily
Route of administration	Oral
Randomized	Yes
Randomization adequate	No
Blinding	Double-blind
Blinding adequate	No
Placebo	Yes
Drug comparison	No
Site description	1 general practice
No. of subjects enrolled	30
No. of subjects completed	30
Sex	Male and female
Age	42-60 years

Inclusion criteria

Patients with primary hyperlipoproteinemia, with moderately increased serum triglycerides and cholesterol.

Exclusion criteria

Patients with complicated diseases, or diseases causing secondary hyperlipoproteinemia, and those previously receiving any lipid-lowering drugs.

End points

Blood samples were taken at baseline and after one, two, three, and four months. Serum lipid profiles, total cholesterol, triglycerides, and HDL-C were determined.

Results

The results showed some trends for reduction of serum cholesterol and se-rum triglycerides, and elevation of serum high-density lipoprotein choles-terol. However, no statistical significance was demonstrated by analysis of variance for comparison with the baseline and placebo. Baseline lipid levels were as follows: total cholesterol 280 mg/dl; triglycerides 355 mg/dl; and HDL cholesterol 38 mg/dl.

Side effects
None mentioned.

Authors' comments
The lipid-lowering effects of this garlic preparation were not confirmed.

Reviewer's comments
No statistical lowering of serum lipid levels was observed. The sample size was too small, and the randomization and blinding processes were not ade-quately described. (1, 4)

Clinical Study: Garlic (Dried)

Extract name	N/A
Manufacturer	Government Pharmaceutical Organization, Thailand

Indication	**Diabetes** (NIDDM)
Level of evidence	**III**
Therapeutic benefit	**Undetermined**

Bibliographic reference
Sitprija S, Plengvidlya C, Kangkaya V, Bhuvapanich S, Tunkayoon M (1987). Garlic and diabetes mellitus phase II clinical trial. *Journal of the Medical As-sociation of Thailand* 70 (2): 223-227.

Trial design
Parallel. Subjects were instructed to have dietary control for the month pre-ceding the experiment and to continue this dietary control during the study.

Study duration	1 month
Dose	350 mg twice daily
Route of administration	Oral

Randomized	Yes
Randomization adequate	No

Blinding	Double-blind
Blinding adequate	No
Placebo	Yes
Drug comparison	No
Site description	Outpatient clinic
No. of subjects enrolled	40
No. of subjects completed	33
Sex	Male and female
Age	42-60 years

Inclusion criteria
Subjects with non-insulin-dependent diabetes without complication and who had no prior treatment.

Exclusion criteria
None mentioned.

End points
Glucose tolerance test performed after overnight fast (12 hours). Blood glucose and serum insulin were determined at fasting and at 30, 60, 120, and 180 minutes via venous blood. Blood total cholesterol, triglycerides, high-density lipoprotein, and liver function were determined. The tests were measured before and one month after treatment.

Results
Garlic produced an insignificant change in blood glucose and serum insulin levels compared to baseline. There was also no significant change in total cholesterol, triglycerides, or in high-density lipoprotein. The baseline levels were as follows: total cholesterol 228 mg/dl; triglycerides 203 mg/dl; and HDL 42 mg/dl.

Side effects
No significant effects observed.

Authors' comments
Garlic produced no significant change to blood glucose, serum insulin, and lipid profile. Toxic effects to the liver were not observed.

Reviewer's comments
This study was conducted on a small, heterogeneous group of 40 diabetics. Neither the randomization nor blinding processes were adequately described. (1, 5)

Product Profile: Kyolic® Aged Garlic Extract™, HI-PO™ Formula 100

Manufacturer	**Wakunaga of America Co., Ltd.**
U.S. distributor	**Wakunaga of America Co., Ltd.**
Botanical ingredient	**Garlic bulb extract**
Extract name	None given
Quantity	300 mg
Processing	Aqueous ethanol extract of fresh bulb
Standardization	*S*-allylcysteine
Formulation	Capsule

Recommended dose: Take two capsules with a meal twice daily.

DSHEA structure/function: Supports cardiovascular health; supports a healthy heart and overall circulatory function.

Other ingredients: Whey, magnesium stearate (vegetable source).

Comments: Kyolic Aged Garlic Extract also comes in tablet, caplet, and liquid forms. Kyolic Aged Garlic Extract can also be found in combination with various other herbs and vitamins.

Source(s) of information: Product label; information from manufacturer.

Clinical Study: Aged Garlic Extract

Extract name	None given
Manufacturer	Wakunaga of America Co., Ltd.
Indication	**Hypercholesterolemia** (elevated cholesterol levels)
Level of evidence	**III**
Therapeutic benefit	**Undetermined**

Bibliographic reference
Yeh YY, Lin RI, Yeh SM, Evans S (1997). Garlic reduces plasma cholesterol in hypercholesterolemic men maintaining habitual diets. In *Food Factors for Cancer Prevention*. Eds. H Ohigashi, T Osawa, J Terao, S Watanabe, T Yoshikawa. Tokyo: Springer-Verlag, pp. 226-230.

Trial design
Parallel. Pretreatment baseline period of four weeks.

Study duration	5 months
Dose	3 (800 mg) capsules 3 times daily
Route of administration	Oral
Randomized	Yes
Randomization adequate	No
Blinding	Double-blind
Blinding adequate	No
Placebo	Yes
Drug comparison	No
Site description	Single center
No. of subjects enrolled	34
No. of subjects completed	34
Sex	Male
Age	35-55 years

Inclusion criteria
Plasma total cholesterol between 220 mg/dl and 285 mg/dl.

Exclusion criteria
Acute or chronic disease of the liver, kidney, skin, digestive system, thyroid, and blood as evaluated from a medical questionnaire and a clinical blood test.

End points
Fasting blood samples drawn at baseline (average of three measurements at one, two, and four weeks of pretreatment), and at two, four, and five months, were analyzed for plasma cholesterol. Three-day food records were taken at baseline and after two and four months of treatment.

Results
After five months of treatment with garlic, the mean plasma level of total cholesterol was reduced by 7 percent (18 mg/dl) and LDL cholesterol was decreased by 10 percent (17 mg/dl) from the baseline values. Levels remained unchanged in the placebo group. Neither garlic nor placebo altered the plasma levels of high-density lipoprotein cholesterol and tricylglycerol. Garlic treatment did not affect body weight, body mass index, or blood pressure.

Side effects
No major side effects were observed. Two subjects complained of mild unpleasant breath, and one reported occasional heartburn.

Authors' comments
We conclude that daily supplementation of aged garlic extract for five months without diet modifications has a mild cholesterol-lowering effect in hypercholesterolemic men.

Reviewer's comments
This study was limited by the small sample size (17 men in each group). The placebo capsules contained a common food ingredient, but there was no mention as to whether their appearance was identical to that of garlic capsules. There was no description of the randomization process either. (1, 5)

Clinical Study: Aged Garlic Extract

Extract name	None given
Manufacturer	Wakunaga of America Co., Ltd.
Indication	**Hypercholesterolemia** (elevated cholesterol levels)
Level of evidence	**I**
Therapeutic benefit	**Yes**

Bibliographic reference
Steiner M, Khan AH, Holbert D, Lin RI (1996). A double-blind crossover study in moderately hypercholesterolemic men that compared the effect of aged garlic extract and placebo administration on blood lipids. *American Journal of Clinical Nutrition* 64 (6): 866-870. (Platelet studies published by Steiner M, Lin RS [1998] *Journal of Cardiovascular Pharmacology* 31 [6]: 904-908.)

Trial design
Crossover. Four-week baseline period, followed by six-month treatment period of garlic or placebo, and then a four-month period with switched treatments. Participants were advised to follow the National Cholesterol Education Program Step 1 diet for the length of the study.

Study duration	10 months
Dose	9 (800 mg) capsules per day
Route of administration	Oral
Randomized	Yes
Randomization adequate	Yes
Blinding	Double-blind
Blinding adequate	Yes

Placebo   Yes
Drug comparison   No

Site description   Single center

No. of subjects enrolled   52
No. of subjects completed   41
Sex   Male
Age   32-68 years

Inclusion criteria
Plasma total cholesterol between 220 mg/dl and 290 mg/dl; normal results on a physical examination.

Exclusion criteria
None mentioned.

End points
During the baseline and treatment periods, lipid profiles (total, HDL, and LDL cholesterol, and triglycerols) were analyzed at weekly intervals. Blood pressure was also measured. In a subgroup of ten compliant subjects divided between the garlic and placebo groups, platelet adhesion and aggregation studies were performed at three and six months during the first intervention period, at three months during the second intervention period, and two to three months after termination of the study.

Results
Maximal reduction in total serum cholesterol of 6.1 percent or 7.0 percent in comparison with the average concentration during the placebo administration and baseline evaluation period, respectively. Low-density lipoprotein cholesterol was also decreased by aged garlic extract, 4 percent in comparison with placebo period concentrations. In addition, there was a 5.5 percent decrease in systolic blood pressure and a modest reduction of diastolic blood pressure in response to garlic. Platelet adhesion to fibrogen was reduced by >30 percent during garlic administration. Platelets also required higher concentrations of epinephrine and collagen, but not ADP, to aggregate.

Side effects
Allergy to coating material of the capsules, gastrointestinal complaints, and perception of unusual body odor.

Authors' comments
Dietary supplementation with aged garlic extract has beneficial effects on the lipid profile and blood pressure of moderately hypercholesterolemic subjects. AGE administration can produce an inhibition of some of the platelet functions important for initiating thromboembolic events in the arterial circu-

lation. Together, AGE provides a combination of therapeutic effects directed against the major pathogenic factors of atherosclerosis and associated thrombotic events.

Reviewer's comments
This is a well-designed and well-conducted peer-reviewed study showing a modest decrease in both cholesterol and blood pressure. (5, 6)

Clinical Study: Aged Garlic Extract

Extract name	None given
Manufacturer	Wakunaga of America Co., Ltd.
Indication	**Blood clotting factors** in normal volunteers
Level of evidence	I
Therapeutic benefit	**MOA**

Bibliographic reference
Steiner M, Li W (2001). Aged garlic extract, a modulator of cardiovascular risk factors: A dose-finding study on the effects of AGE on platelet functions. *Journal of Nutrition* 131 (3s): 980S-984S.

Trial design
Crossover. There was an initial six-week baseline period during which no treatment was given. Patients were then randomized to receive placebo or AGE three (800 mg) capsules per day for six weeks; the dosage was then raised to six (800 mg) capsules per day for six weeks; and finally the dosage was raised to nine (800 mg) capsules per day for another six weeks. After a two-week washout period, patients were switched to the other treatment for a repeat of the same dosing regimen.

Study duration	18 weeks
Dose	3, 6, or 9 (800 mg) capsules daily (2.4 to 7.2 g daily)
Route of administration	Oral
Randomized	Yes
Randomization adequate	Yes
Blinding	Double-blind
Blinding adequate	Yes
Placebo	Yes
Drug comparison	No

Site description   Not described

No. of subjects enrolled   34
No. of subjects completed   28
Sex   Male and female
Age   Not given

Inclusion criteria
Normal individuals in good physical health.

Exclusion criteria
None mentioned.

End points
Every two weeks blood was sampled and processed for adhesion and platelet aggregation studies. Aggregation tests were carried out with the following agonists: arachidonic acid, adenosine diphosphate (ADP), epinephrine, and collagen. Platelet adhesion was tested for all subjects on surfaces coated with collagen, and for a subgroup of subjects on surfaces coated with fibrinogen and von Willebrand factor.

Results
Platelet aggregation using the agonist ADP resulted in a significant increase in the threshold for individuals consuming AGE, compared to baseline and placebo only at the highest dose (7.2 g AGE daily, $p < 0.05$). With the collagen-induced aggregation, all doses of AGE saw a significant increase in the threshold compared to baseline and placebo. For epinephrine-induced aggregation, AGE significantly inhibited aggregation (increased threshold) only at the lower doses (2.4 and 4.8 g) compared to placebo and baseline. At low shear rates (~1/30 s), there were significant, but small, reductions in platelet aggregation to collagen-coated surfaces for the two higher doses (4.8 to 7.2 g AGE). For high shear rates (~1/1200 s) there was a dose response for reduction in platelet adhesion to collagen-coated surfaces; 7.2 g AGE produced the highest reduction. For the subgroup tested for platelet adhesion to fibrinogen- and von Willebrand factor-coated surfaces, adhesion to the former was significantly inhibited by all doses of AGE, with greater inhibition at the two higher doses. Adhesion to von Willebrand factor-coated surfaces was inhibited only at doses of 7.2 g AGE.

Side effects
Side effects included body odor, allergy, and gastrointestinal complaints such as flatulence and heartburn.

Authors' comments
The inhibition of several risk factors achieved by AGE should make it a very useful dietary supplement in the prevention of cardiovascular disease.

Reviewer's comments
This is a good study. (5, 6)

Clinical Study: High Potency Kyolic®

Extract name	None given
Manufacturer	Wagner Probiotics (Wakunaga of America Co., Ltd.)
Indication	**Lipid oxidation** in normal volunteers
Level of evidence	**III**
Therapeutic benefit	**MOA**

Bibliographic reference

Munday JS, James KA, Fray LM, Kirkwood SW, Thompson KG (1999). Daily supplementation with aged garlic extract, but not raw garlic protects low density lipoprotein against in vitro oxidation. *Atherosclerosis* 143 (2): 399-404.

Trial design

Three-arm Latin-square design study: 6 g raw garlic, 2.4 g aged garlic extract, or 0.8 g DL-alpha-tocopherol. Subjects took each supplement for seven days, interrupted by a seven-day washout period with no supplements.

Study duration	7 days
Dose	2 capsules (total of 2.4 g) aged garlic extract daily
Route of administration	Oral
Randomized	Yes
Randomization adequate	No
Blinding	Double-blind
Blinding adequate	No
Placebo	No
Drug comparison	Yes
Drug name	DL-alpha-tocopherol and raw garlic
Site description	Single center
No. of subjects enrolled	9
No. of subjects completed	9
Sex	Male and female
Age	24-49 years

Inclusion criteria

Nonsmoking volunteers.

Exclusion citeria
Person who had consumed significant quantities of garlic or taken any medication, including dietary supplements, during the month preceding the study.

End points
At the beginning and the end of each seven-day supplement period, a fasting blood sample was taken and the concentration of plasma lipoproteins and the oxidizability of LDL determined.

Results
Alpha-tocopherol (vitamin E) supplementation produced LDL which was significantly ($p < 0.05$) more resistant to oxidation than LDL isolated from subjects receiving AGE. LDL from subjects receiving AGE was more resistant ($p < 0.01$) to oxidation than LDL from nonsupplemented subjects (i.e., when subjects were on washout periods between treatments). The oxidation resistance of LDL from subjects receiving raw garlic was not significantly different to LDL from subjects receiving no supplements or subjects receiving AGE. The decrease in LDL oxidation resulting from alpha-tocopherol supplementation was consistent. In contrast, that resulting from supplementation of AGE or raw garlic was variable. No significant changes in plasma lipoprotein or triglyceride concentrations were observed.

Side effects
No adverse effects with AGE or alpha-tocopherol; body odor with raw garlic.

Authors' comments
These results suggest that if antioxidants are proven to be antiatherogenic, the combined antioxidant and serum cholesterol-lowering actions of AGE may make it useful in reducing the progression of atherosclerosis.

Reviewer's comments
This study was flawed by the small sample size and short treatment period. Both AGE and raw garlic had unimpressive effects on LDL oxidation compared to vitamin E. There was no placebo due to the inclusion of raw garlic. (1, 5)

Product Profile: Kyolic® Liquid Aged Garlic Extract™

Manufacturer	**Wakunaga of America Co., Ltd.**
U.S. distributor	**Wakunaga of America Co., Ltd.**
Botanical ingredient	**Garlic bulb extract**
Extract name	None given

Quantity	No information
Processing	Aqueous ethanolic extract of the bulb (aged 20 months) and produced without heat
Standardization	*S*-allylcysteine
Formulation	Liquid

Recommended dose: As a dietary supplement, take one-quarter to one-half teaspoon, or 30 to 60 drops (one or two filled 00 size capsules) with a meal twice daily.

Other ingredients: Water, residual alcohol from extraction.

Source(s) of information: Product package; information from manufacturer.

Clinical Study: Kyolic® Liquid Aged Garlic Extract™

Extract name	None given
Manufacturer	Wakunaga of America Co., Ltd.
Indication	**Hypercholesterolemia** (elevated cholesterol levels)
Level of evidence	**III**
Therapeutic benefit	**Undetermined**

Bibliographic reference
Lau BHS, Lam F, Wang-Cheng R (1987). Effect of an odor-modified garlic preparation on blood lipids. *Nutrition Research* 7: 139-149.

Trial design
Three-part study. Part 1 (hyperlipidemic group): 32 patients (ages 45 to 68; 27 finished study) with elevated serum cholesterol and triglycerides. Part 2 (normolipidemic group): 14 patients (ages 18 to 32) with serum cholesterol and triglycerides in normal range. Part 3 (hyperlipidemics): 10 patients (ages 56 to 67), uncontrolled study.

Study duration	6 months
Dose	4 (1 ml, 250 mg active garlic components per ml) capsules daily
Route of administration	Oral
Randomized	Yes
Randomization adequate	No

Blinding	Single-blind
Blinding adequate	No
Placebo	Yes
Drug comparison	No
Site description	Single center
No. of subjects enrolled	56
No. of subjects completed	51
Sex	Male and female
Age	3 different age groups

Inclusion criteria

Healthy volunteers with no obvious medical problems at the time of the study. First study: initial cholesterol in the range of 220 to 440 mg/dl; second study: initial cholesterol in the range of 150 to 200 mg/dl; third study: initial cholesterol in the range of 240 to 380 mg/dl.

Exclusion criteria

Those taking medications, on special diets, smokers, or alcohol users.

End points

Fasting blood measurements of serum cholesterol, triglycerides, and lipoproteins taken at baseline and at monthly intervals.

Results

Lowering of cholesterol, triglycerides, and low density and very low density lipoproteins with a rise of high-density lipoprotein was observed in the majority of hyperlipidemic subjects who took garlic. Part 1 reported that 11 out of 15 subjects had a decrease in serum cholesterol of greater than 10 percent. The effect was significant compared to placebo. Garlic did not significantly influence cholesterol and triglyceride levels of those whose baseline levels were in the normal range. The lowering of lipid levels was not observed during the first and second month of treatment. In fact, the majority showed a rise in lipid values during that period.

Side effects

No serious side effects reported.

Authors' comments

This study conforms previous reports of lowering cholesterol and triglycerides using various garlic preparations. Furthermore, it suggests that odor-modified garlic extract may be used in conjunction with dietary modification for control of hyperlipidemia. Of special interest was the initial rise in cholesterol, triglycerides, and LDL/VLDL with garlic supplementation, suggesting possible mobilization of tissue lipids into the circulation during this phase of garlic ingestion.

Reviewer's comments
This was a three-part study, each with an inadequate number of participants. Although parts 1 and 2 were placebo controlled, part 3 was not. Blinding appeared to be single, and the randomization process was not described. (1, 5)

Product Profile: Garlic Oil, Ethyl Acetate Extracted

Manufacturer	None
U.S. distributor	None
Botanical ingredient	**Garlic clove extract**
Extract name	None given
Quantity	Equivalent of 1 g raw garlic
Processing	Peeled garlic cloves were crushed, extracted in ethyl acetate, the solvent evaporated, and the resultant oil dissolved in soy oil
Standardization	No information
Formulation	Capsule

Source(s) of information: Bordia, Verma, and Srivastava, 1998.

Clinical Study: Garlic Oil, Ethyl Acetate Extraction

Extract name	None given
Manufacturer	None
Indication	**Heart disease; coronary artery disease**
Level of evidence	**III**
Therapeutic benefit	**Yes**

Bibliographic reference
Bordia A, Verma SK, Srivastava KC (1998). Effect of garlic *(Allium sativum)* on blood lipids, blood sugar, fibrinogen and fibrinolytic activity in patients with coronary artery disease. *Prostaglandins, Leukotrienes, and Essential Fatty Acids* 58 (4): 257-263.

Trial design

Parallel. Two-week pretrial baseline period.

Study duration	3 months
Dose	2 capsules (each equivalent to 1 g raw garlic) twice daily
Route of administration	Oral
Randomized	No
Randomization adequate	No
Blinding	Not described
Blinding adequate	No
Placebo	Yes
Drug comparison	No
Site description	1 general practice
No. of subjects enrolled	60
No. of subjects completed	60
Sex	Not given
Age	51-66 years

Inclusion criteria

Patients who had myocardial infarctions more than six months ago, with or without angina. Those with angina were stable with drugs. All patients stopped intake of nitrates and aspirin two weeks prior to study.

Exclusion criteria

None mentioned.

End points

Two pretrial fasting blood samples were collected at an interval of two weeks to examine baseline parameters. Patients were then evaluated every month for clinical symptoms and side effects. At intervals of one and one-half months and three months of administration, fasting blood samples were obtained and examined for lipid profile, fibrinogen, fibrinolytic activity, and blood sugar levels.

Results

Patients taking garlic showed a significant reduction in total cholesterol (from 252.9 to 220.5 mg/dl, 12.8 percent) and triglycerides (15.2 percent) compared to baseline (both $p < 0.01$) after three months of treatment. Their HDL-C and fibrinolytic activity increased significantly (22.3 percent and 55.1 percent, respectively) compared to baseline ($p < 0.05$ and $p < 0.01$, respectively). There was no change in fibrinogen levels. Those on placebo had no significant changes to any of the parameters compared to baseline. Neither group showed any change to blood glucose levels.

Side effects
None listed.

Authors' comments
In the light of these data and those of others on the lipid-regulating effects of garlic coupled with its enhanced fibrinolytic activity and anticoagulant, eicosanoid modulatory, and antioxidant effects, garlic might find a place among the arsenal of dietary agents showing protection against the diseases of the cardiovascular system and possibly other diseases as well.

Reviewer's comments
This study had clear and statistically positive results: cholesterol was lowered by 13 percent at three months; triglycerides were lowered by 15.2 percent; HDL increased by 22.3 percent; and platelet aggregation was inhibited. Neither the randomization process nor the placebo were described in any detail. It is unclear if this trial was blinded or open. (1, 6)

Clinical Study: Garlic Oil, Ethyl Acetate Extraction

Extract name	None given
Manufacturer	None
Indication	**Coronary heart disease patients with hypercholesterolemia** (elevated cholesterol levels)
Level of evidence	**II**
Therapeutic benefit	**Yes**

Bibliographic reference
Bordia A (1981). Effect of garlic on blood lipids in patients with coronary heart disease. *The American Journal of Clinical Nutrition* 34 (10): 2100-2103.

Trial design
Parallel. Two-part study. Part 1 included 20 healthy individuals given garlic for six months followed by two months without garlic. Part 2 included 68 coronary heart disease patients who were divided into two groups and given either garlic or placebo for ten months.

Study duration	10 months
Dose	0.25 mg oil per kg body weight in 2 divided doses; e.g., 15 mg/60 kg person
Route of administration	Oral
Randomized	Yes
Randomization adequate	No
Blinding	Double-blind
Blinding adequate	Yes
Placebo	Yes
Drug comparison	No
Site description	Not described
No. of subjects enrolled	68
No. of subjects completed	62
Sex	Not given
Age	42-62 years

Inclusion criteria
Patients with coronary heart disease with serum cholesterol levels from 250 to 350 mg/dl.

Exclusion criteria
Patients with hyperlipidemia secondary to other conditions such as nephrotic syndrome, liver, pancreas or biliary tract disease, or uncontrolled diabetes and other endocrinological diseases; patients with serious complications or severe hyperlipidemia requiring specific therapy and strict dietary restriction.

End points
Fasting blood samples were collected initially (mean of two samples at a one-week interval) and then after every month. Samples were analyzed for serum cholesterol, triglycerides, phospholipids, and lipoproteins.

Results
In the first part of the study, serum cholesterol dropped (233 to 200 mg/dl, $p < 0.05$), serum triglycerides dropped (110 to 92 mg/dl, $p < 0.05$), and high-density lipoprotein increased (29 to 41 mg/dl, $p < 0.001$) after six months. In part 2, garlic administration raised serum cholesterol in the first month but decreased it by 18 percent after eight months (298 to 244 mg/dl, $p < 0.05$). Serum cholesterol continued to decrease for two months after treatment had stopped (to 228 mg/dl). Serum triglycerides also decreased significantly ($p < 0.05$). There was no change in these levels in the control group. By the end of 8 months, the HDL levels increased ($p < 0.001$) while the LDL levels

decreased ($p < 0.05$). The cholesterol/phospholipid ratio reduced following garlic administration but not with placebo.

Side effects
Epigastric discomfort, diarrhea.

Author's comments
The essential oil of garlic has shown a distinct hypolipidemic action in patients of coronary heart disease.

Reviewer's comments
Overall, this is a good study showing a reduction in cholesterol with ethylacetate extract of garlic oil over eight months. (3, 6)

Product Profile: Garlic Oil, Cold Pressed

Manufacturer	**General Nutrition Research Laboratories**
U.S. distributor	None
Botanical ingredient	**Garlic clove extract**
Extract name	None given
Quantity	18 mg oil is equivalent to 9 g raw garlic
Processing	Cold-pressed garlic oil extracted from fresh garlic
Standardization	No information
Formulation	Perle

Other ingredients: Coconut oil (158 mg), glycerin (30 mg), gelatin (54 mg).

Source(s) of information: Barrie, Wright, and Pizzorno, 1987.

Clinical Study: Garlic Oil, Cold Pressed

Extract name	None given
Manufacturer	General Nutrition Research Laboratories
Indication	**Cardiovascular risk factors** in normal volunteers
Level of evidence	**II**
Therapeutic benefit	**Yes**

Bibliographic reference
Barrie S, Wright J, Pizzorno J (1987). Effects of garlic oil on platelet aggregation, serum lipids and blood pressure in humans. *Journal of Orthomolecular Medicine* 2 (1): 15-21.

Trial design
Crossover after four weeks. Three-week washout between treatment periods.

Study duration	4 weeks
Dose	18 mg of garlic oil (extracted from 9 g of fresh garlic)
Route of administration	Oral
Randomized	Yes
Randomization adequate	No
Blinding	Double-blind
Blinding adequate	Yes
Placebo	Yes
Drug comparison	No
Site description	1 general practice
No. of subjects enrolled	20
No. of subjects completed	20
Sex	Not given
Age	Mean: 26 years

Inclusion criteria
Good health.

Exclusion criteria
Signs of degenerative cardiovascular disease.

End points
Platelet aggregation percentages, serum lipid levels, and blood pressure readings measured before and after each supplementation period.

Results
During garlic administration, there was a significant reduction (16.4 percent) in platelet aggregation ($p < 0.005$), in serum cholesterol (from 195 to 180 mg/dl, $p < 0.001$), and the mean blood pressure (94 to 88 mmHg, $p < 0.009$), as well as a rise in the mean HDL levels (from 56 to 69 mg/dl, $p < 0.001$). In addition, there was a rise in arachidonic acid in red cell phospholipids following garlic administration.

Side effects
None noted.

Authors' comments
The results of this study suggest that garlic has therapeutic potential as an antiatherosclerotic, antithrombotic, and antihypertensive agent in normal healthy adults.

Reviewer's comments
This is a well-designed study overall; however, 20 subjects is too small to judge in a crossover design. (3, 5)

Product Profile: Tegra

Manufacturer	**Hermes Arzneimittel GmbH, Germany**
U.S. distributor	None
Botanical ingredient	**Garlic clove extract**
Extract name	None given
Quantity	5 mg, equivalent to 4 to 5 g fresh garlic
Processing	Steam-distilled garlic oil preparation
Standardization	No information
Formulation	Enteric coated

Other ingredients: Beta cyclodextrin.

Source(s) of information: Berthold, Sudhop, and von Bergmann, 1998a.

Clinical Study: Tegra

Extract name	None given
Manufacturer	Hermes Arzneimittel GmbH, Germany
Indication	**Hypercholesterolemia** (elevated cholesterol levels)
Level of evidence	**II**
Therapeutic benefit	**No**

Bibliographic reference
Berthold H, Sudhop T, von Bergmann, K (1998a). Effect of a garlic oil prepa-

ration on serum lipoproteins and cholesterol metabolism. *Journal of the American Medical Association* 279 (23): 1900-1902.

Trial design
Crossover study after 12 weeks. Pretrial single-blind washout period for four weeks, and a four-week single-blind washout between treatment periods.

Study duration	3 months
Dose	5 mg garlic oil twice daily, equivalent to 4 to 5 fresh garlic cloves
Route of administration	Oral
Randomized	Yes
Randomization adequate	Yes
Blinding	Double-blind
Blinding adequate	Yes
Placebo	Yes
Drug comparison	No
Site description	Single outpatient clinic
No. of subjects enrolled	26
No. of subjects completed	25
Sex	Male and female
Age	51-66 years

Inclusion criteria
Moderate hypercholesterolemia (total cholesterol 240 to 348 mg/dl and triglycerides <265 mg/dl). Any lipid-lowering drugs or drugs which would interfere with lipid metabolism were not allowed for eight weeks prior to start. No additional intake of garlic or other food supplements allowed.

Exclusion criteria
Active liver or renal diseases, diabetes, thyroid dysfunction, history of coronary heart disease, pathological values in clinical chemistry or routine hematological parameters, and alcohol or drug abuse.

End points
Serum lipoprotein concentrations, cholesterol absorption, and cholesterol synthesis measured at beginning of study and ends of both treatment periods. Food intake was assessed at the end of the treatment periods using seven-day food records. During the last week of each treatment period, cholesterol absorption and endogenous cholesterol synthesis were measured by double isotope feeding using deuterated $[D_6]$cholesterol and $[D_4]$sitosterol.

Results
Lipoprotein levels were virtually unchanged at the end of both treatment periods. Cholesterol absorption, cholesterol synthesis, mavalonic acid excretion, and changes in the ratio of lathosterol to cholesterol were not different in garlic and placebo treatment.

Side effects
Garlic odor; slight abdominal discomfort in a few cases caused by garlic and placebo.

Authors' comments
The commercial garlic oil preparation had no influence on serum lipoproteins, cholesterol absorption, or cholesterol synthesis. Garlic therapy for treatment of hypercholesterolemia cannot be recommended on the basis of this study.

Reviewer's comments
Tegra garlic oil is steam distilled and bound to cyclodextrin. The use of this special preparation may affect the bioavailable dose compared to other garlic oil. Otherwise, this is a well-conducted study. (5, 5)

Product Profile: Garlic (Raw)

Manufacturer	None
U.S. distributor	None
Botanical ingredient	**Garlic clove**
Extract name	N/A
Quantity	No information
Processing	Raw
Standardization	No information

Source(s) of information: Bhushan et al., 1979; Gadkari and Joshi, 1991.

Clinical Study: Garlic (Raw)

Extract name	N/A
Manufacturer	None

Indication	**Hypercholesterolemia** (elevated cholesterol levels)
Level of evidence	**III**
Therapeutic benefit	**Trend**

Bibliographic reference

Bhushan S, Sharma SP, Singh SP, Agrawal S, Indrayan A, Seth P (1979). Effect of garlic on normal blood cholesterol level. *Indian Journal of Physiology and Pharmacology* 23 (3): 211-214.

Trial design

Parallel. Treatment group was compared to a control group taking nothing.

Study duration	2 months
Dose	10 g of raw garlic daily
Route of administration	Oral
Randomized	Yes
Randomization adequate	No
Blinding	Open
Blinding adequate	No
Placebo	No
Drug comparison	No
Site description	1 general practice
No. of subjects enrolled	25
No. of subjects completed	25
Sex	Male
Age	18-35 years

Inclusion criteria

Healthy subjects who had never ingested garlic before with initial cholesterol levels of 160 to 250 mg/dl.

Exclusion criteria

During test period, no intake of any drug, onion, smoking, or tobacco chewing was allowed. Physical activity was restricted.

End points

Fasting blood samples collected and serum cholesterol tested before study and after two months.

Results

There was a significant decrease in serum cholesterol (33.2 mg/dl) in the raw garlic group compared to baseline (15 percent reduction, *p* < 0.00001);

whereas serum cholesterol in the control group did not change significantly. A comparison of the two groups revealed a significant difference ($p < 0.05$).

Side effects
None noted.

Authors' comments
Raw garlic can be advocated for daily ingestion in order to lower one's blood cholesterol level even if it is within normal limits.

Reviewer's comments
This study was flawed by its small sample size and lack of blinding. The randomization process was also not described. (0, 5)

Clinical Study: Garlic (Raw)

Extract name	N/A
Manufacturer	None
Indication	**Cardiovascular risk factors** in normal volunteers
Level of evidence	**III**
Therapeutic benefit	**Trend**

Bibliographic reference
Gadkari, J, Joshi V (1991). Effect of ingestion of raw garlic on serum cholesterol level, clotting time and fibrinolytic activity in normal subjects. *Journal of Postgraduate Medicine* 37 (3): 128-131.

Trial design
Parallel. Treatment group compared was to a control group taking nothing.

Study duration	2 months
Dose	10 g of raw garlic daily
Route of administration	Oral
Randomized	Yes
Randomization adequate	No
Blinding	Open
Blinding adequate	No
Placebo	No
Drug comparison	No
Site description	1 general practice

No. of subjects enrolled   50
No. of subjects completed   50
Sex   Not given
Age   17-22 years

Inclusion criteria
Healthy subjects who had never ingested garlic before.

Exclusion criteria
None mentioned.

End points
Fasting blood samples were taken before the study and after two months of treatment. Serum cholesterol, fibrinolytic activity, and clotting time were measured.

Results
After two months of treatment, there was a significant decrease in serum cholesterol (from 213.3 to 180.0 mg/dl), an increase in clotting time (from 4.14 to 5.02 min), and an increase in fibrinolytic activity in the raw garlic group (all $p < 0.001$), whereas there was no significant change in the control group.

Side effects
None noted.

Authors' comments
Garlic may be useful for prevention of thromboembolic phenomenon.

Reviewer's comments
The outcome measures and inclusion/exclusion criteria were clearly defined and appropriate. However, the study was not blinded, the randomization process was not described, and the effects of garlic on fibrinolysis, cholesterol, and clotting time could be due to other factors. (0, 6)

Ginger

Latin name: ***Zingiber officinale*** **Roscoe** [Zingiberaceae]
Plant parts: **Root, rhizome**

PREPARATIONS USED IN REVIEWED CLINICAL STUDIES

Ginger root (rhizome) is a common spice that has long been esteemed as an appetite stimulant and an aid to digestion. It has been
used in China for roughly 2,500 years and is a common ingredient in
traditional Chinese herbal formulas. Ginger has a distinct aroma due
to its essential oil, which contains approximately 60 components, including geranial and neral. Ginger's flavor is due to its pungent prin-
cipals, which include gingerols and products formed from gingerols,
the shogaols and zingerone. Shogaols and gingerols, especially 6-
gingerol, have demonstrated antiemetic activity in animal studies
(Awang, 1992; ESCOP, 1996).

Zintona® contains a standardized dried ginger root powder. It is a
registered trademark of Dalidar Pharma Ltd. and is registered as an
OTC pharmaceutical in several European countries. Dalidar has been
acquired by Makhteshim-Agan Industries, Ltd., Israel, a subsidiary
of Koor Industries. Several trials were conducted on Zintona supplied
by Pharmaton S.A., Switzerland. Zintona is no longer sold in the
United States.

WS 1540 is an extract of ginger rhizome. It is manufactured by Dr.
Willmar Schwabe GmbH & Co. in Germany. This extract is not available in the United States.

Eurovita Extract 33 (EV ext-33) is a ginger extract with a standardized amount of hydroxy-methoxy-phenyl compounds. It is manufactured by Eurovita A/S and is not available in the United States.

Several studies used generic preparations of powdered ginger root
and rhizome. Few details were provided to characterize these ginger
preparations. Most studies just described the product as powdered

GINGER SUMMARY TABLE

Product Name	Manufacturer/ U.S. Distributor	Product Characteristics	Dose in Trials	Indication	No. of Trials	Benefit (Evidence Level-Trial No.)
Zintona®	Dalidar Pharma Ltd., Israel/ None	Dried root powder	Ages 3-6: 250 mg; over 6 yrs: 500 mg before departing and then every 4 h	Motion sickness	4	Yes (I-1, II-1) Trend (III-1) MOA (III-1)
WS 1540	Dr. Willmar Schwabe GmbH & Co., Germany/ None	Extract of rhizome (WS 1540)	2 × 2 (10 mg) capsules	Gastrointestinal motility	1	MOA (II-1)
Eurovita Extract 33	Eurovita A/S, Denmark/None	Standardized to content of hydroxymethoxy-phenyl compounds	170 mg 3 times daily	Osteoarthritis	1	No (I-1)
Generic	None/None	Powdered ginger	0.94-1 g daily	Motion sickness	3	Trend (III-2) MOA (III-1)
			0.5-2 g daily	Nausea	7	Yes (I-1, II-1) Undetermined (II-1, III-3) No (I-1)
			1 g	Gastric motility	1	MOA (I-1)
			4 g daily	Cardiovascular risk factors	1	MOA (III-1)
Generic (raw and stem)	None/None	Chopped ginger root or stem ginger	15 g raw or 40 g stem ginger daily	Cardiovascular risk factors	1	MOA (III-1)

ginger and gave the dose. None of the studies mentioned profiling the ginger for quantities of gingerols, nor were any other chemical analyses mentioned. Bordia, Verma, and Srivastava (1997) remark in their discussion that the sample used in their study was almost 50 percent lower in measured constituents than two other samples which they also obtained. However, they did not specify the constituents they measured or give any values. One study used ginger that complied with the British Pharmacopoeia monograph of 1988 and was supplied by Blackmores Ltd. (Sydney, Australia) (Arfeen et al., 1995). Two studies used powdered ginger specially prepared for the trial by Martindale Pharmaceuticals Pty. Ltd. in England (Phillips, Ruggier, and Hutchinson, 1993; Phillips, Hutchinson, and Ruggier, 1993). Again, however, characterization of the product was not mentioned.

One trial used raw Brazilian ginger root supplied by Toko Rinus, Nijmegen, and stem ginger supplied by Ambition, Polak Import, Rotterdam, both of the Netherlands. No further description was provided (Janssen et al., 1996).

SUMMARY OF REVIEWED CLINICAL STUDIES

Ginger products have been tested in clinical studies for effectiveness in reducing nausea and vomiting due to administration of chemotherapy, emergence from general anesthesia following surgery, morning sickness associated with pregnancy, and, most commonly, for motion sickness. Vertigo, nausea, vomiting, cold sweat, and pallor are typical signs of motion sickness. Motion sickness is often caused by the perception of movement by the inner ear, especially when it conflicts with information from the eyes and other senses. The inner ear contains sensors for motion in the vestibular system. The vomiting reflex is mediated via the vagal and sympathetic pathways of the nervous system and can be stimulated by pain, smell, sight, motion, cytotoxic drugs, and irritants in the stomach.

Agents commonly used to prevent nausea and vomiting include serotonin inhibitors (e.g., ondansetron), dopamine antagonists (metoclopramide, chlorpromazine, promenthazine, etc.), antihistamines (dimenhydrinate, diphenhydramine, meclizine, etc.), corticosteroids, cannabinoids, and benzodiazepines. Scopolamine, given orally, parenterally, or transdermally, is regarded as the most potent drug for the prophylaxis and treatment of motion sickness. However, the antihistamines, especially dimenhydrinate, are also commonly used (Hardman et al., 1996).

The ability of ginger to inhibit the formation of inflammatory mediators and its antioxidant activity in vitro led to testing an extract for a possible clinical application for osteoarthritis (deterioration of the joints characterized by pain, inflammation, and reduced function). Common first-line treatments for relief of symptoms of rheumatic diseases are the nonsteroidal anti-inflammatory drugs (NSAIDs), which include aspirin, acetaminophen, indomethacin, ibuprofen, and diclofenac (Hardman et al., 1996).

Zintona

Motion Sickness

Three studies with Zintona demonstrated a benefit for this ginger product on motion sickness. A fourth study indicated that the mode of action of Zintona is gastrointestinal, rather than through the central nervous system.

The first of two good-quality studies compared the ability of Zintona and six other agents (standard pharmaceuticals) to prevent seasickness on a six-hour sea voyage. The trial included 1,475 volunteers who filled out a questionnaire regarding their degree of discomfort, nausea, and vomiting. Zintona was given in a dose of 500 mg (two tablets) two hours prior to departure and again four hours later. Completed questionnaires indicated that all treatments offered some benefit, with no statistical difference between them (Schmid et al., 1994). The other good-quality study included 60 cruise ship passengers, with a history of motion sickness, who received either Zintona (500 mg before sailing and every four hours afterward) or dimenhydrinate (100 mg before sailing and every fours hours afterward) for two days. Both treatments were equally effective in preventing seasickness (Riebenfeld and Borzone, 1999).

In one study, 28 children, four to eight years old, were treated to prevent motion sickness on a two-day trip that included journeying by car, boat, and/or airplane. They were given either Zintona (250 mg for those aged three to six or 500 mg for those older than six, 30 minutes before the trip and every four hours as needed) or dimenhydrinate (12.5 or 25 mg 30 minutes before the trip and every four hours as needed). As rated by pediatric physicians, Zintona was more effective and had fewer side effects (Cereddu, 1999). The trial was rated as having a trend toward therapeutic benefit by our reviewers, Drs. Karriem Ali and Richard Aranda, due to a lack of detail in the study report.

A three-arm, crossover, mode-of-action study with 38 participants determined that ginger did not prevent motion sickness with the same central nervous system mechanism as dimenhydrinate. The study measured the nystagmus response (involuntary eye movements) to optokinetic stimuli (a moving stripe pattern), vestibular stimuli (water irrigation of the ears), and to being spun in a rotary chair. Ginger, 1g Zintona given 90 minutes before stimuli, had no influence on experimentally induced nystagmus, compared to baseline and placebo. In contrast, dimenhydrinate, 100 mg, reduced the nystagmus response to all stimuli. The authors concluded that ginger most likely acts through a mechanism involving the gastrointestinal tract, in contrast to dimenhydrinate which acts through the central nervous system (Holtmann et al., 1989).

WS 1540

Gastrointestinal Motility

A crossover trial measured the effect of 200 mg ginger extract WS 1540 (corresponding to 2 g ginger root) on gastrointestinal motility in 12 healthy volunteers. Ginger or placebo was given in the morning after fasting and at noon before lunch. Gastroduodenal motility was tested in the morning and for an hour after lunch. In comparison to placebo, ginger increased the number, frequency, and amplitude of gastric contractions in the fasting state and to a lesser degree following a meal (Micklefield et al., 1999).

Eurovita Extract 33

Osteoarthritis

Eurovita Extract 33 (EV ext-33), a ginger extract, was compared to ibuprofen (a NSAID) and placebo in a well-conducted crossover study with 56 participants with osteoarthritis. Each treatment arm, with daily administration of 510 mg ginger extract, 1200 mg ibuprofen, or placebo, was three weeks in duration with a one-week washout period in between. As a result, ibuprofen was more effective than ginger and placebo in reducing pain, improving range of motion, and reducing consumption of acetaminophen (another NSAID). Benefit from ibuprofen was significantly better than placebo. Ginger was more effective than placebo, but not significantly (Bliddal et al., 2000).

Generic

Motion Sickness

The effect of powdered ginger on experimentally induced motion sickness was tested in two studies, both given low ratings. In the first study, prevention of experimentally induced motion sickness was measured in a one-dose crossover experiment. Motion sickness was induced by stimulation of the vestibular system (inner ear) through irrigating the left ear with water. Ginger, 1 g powdered root given one hour before the procedure, was effective in reducing vertigo but not nystagmus in comparison with placebo. As no statistically significant change in nystagmus was demonstrated, the author suggested that ginger does not directly affect the vestibular system (Grøntved and Hentzer, 1986). The second study was a three-arm, open, experimental study with motion sickness induced by a tilted rotating chair. The study compared the benefit of powdered ginger root (940 mg), dimenhydrinate (100 mg), and placebo (powdered chickweed herb). Administration of ginger allowed the subjects to stay in the chair longer and diminished feelings in their stomachs compared to those in the other two groups (Mowrey and Clayson, 1982).

Another study explored the effects of ginger on motion sickness experienced by Navy cadets. Seventy-nine men were given either ginger (1 g powered root) or placebo (lactose) on their first trip on the high seas. Ginger significantly reduced the tendency to vomit and experience cold sweats. The symptoms of nausea and vertigo were also reduced, but not significantly (Grøntved et al., 1988).

Nausea

A small study included 11 subjects undergoing chemotherapy with 8-methoxy psoralen (8-MOP). The subjects monitored their nausea following 8-MOP treatments with or without the addition of ginger (1.6 g powdered root). As a result, treatment with ginger reduced the nausea score (Meyer et al., 1995). The level of evidence of this trial was low due to poor experimental design.

The ability of ginger to treat postoperative nausea and vomiting was tested in four trials. One trial rated as good quality failed to show a benefit. The other three studies were rated as having undetermined benefit due to poor methodology. The good-quality study was a three-arm study in which females undergoing gynecological laparoscopic surgery received either 500 mg ginger, 1000 mg ginger, or placebo one hour before induction of anesthesia. Three hours after the operation patients were questioned as to whether they had experienced any nausea or vomiting after gaining consciousness. No significant benefit was derived from the ginger (Arfeen et al., 1995).

A larger study with 111 women undergoing gynecological laparoscopic surgery compared ginger and droperidol with placebo in a double-dummy protocol with four arms. All treatments were administered one hour before surgery (ginger 1 g orally; droperidol 1.25 mg intravenously), and the ginger treatment was repeated after surgery. As a result, there were no significant differences in the incidences of postoperative nausea with either treatment alone or with both treatments together (Visalyaputra et al., 1998). Our reviewers, Drs. Ali and Aranda, commented that the sample size was inadequate and the differences in surgical techniques might have affected the results of this study.

In another study, 120 women undergoing laparoscopic surgery were given metoclopramide (10 mg), ginger (1 g), or placebo one hour before induction of anesthesia. In this study the incidence of nausea and vomiting following surgery for both treatment groups was less than with placebo (Phillips, Ruggier, and Hutchinson, 1993). However, Drs. Ali and Aranda rated the benefit as undetermined, as measuring the number of nausea complaints per patients does not have a clear correlation with severity or antiemetic effect.

In a study with 60 women undergoing major gynecological surgery, ginger (1 g) was compared to metoclopramide (10 mg IV) and placebo in a double-dummy design. The ginger capsules were given one and one-half hours before surgery, and the metoclopramide was given at the induction of anesthesia. As a result of treatment, the ginger and metoclopramide groups both experienced significantly less nausea after surgery compared to the placebo group. There was also less need for additional treatment with metoclopramide after surgery in the active treatment groups (Bone et al., 1990). The level of evidence was rated low due to limitations of the methodology.

Ginger was reported to significantly reduce nausea and vomiting associated with pregnancy in two good-quality studies using a dose of 250 mg powdered ginger four times daily for four days. The first trial included 27 women in a crossover design, in which the women were given either placebo or powdered ginger for four days with a two-day washout period in between. Subjective assessments by the women revealed that 70 percent felt greater relief from ginger (Fischer-Rasmussen et al., 1990). The second study was a larger, parallel, placebo-controlled study with 67 pregnant women that measured nausea and vomiting using a visual analog scale and the five-item Likert scale. Using the Likert scale, 28 out of 32 subjects in the ginger group had relief from nausea compared to 10 out of 35 in the placebo group. Ginger did not have an adverse effect on pregnancy outcome (Vutyavanich, Kraisarin, and Ruangsri, 2001).

Gastric Motility

A crossover trial with 16 healthy volunteers examined the effect of powdered ginger (1 g) or placebo on gastric emptying rates. Paracetamol was administered at the same time as either ginger or placebo, and the mean, peak, and time of peak plasma concentrations of the drug were used as a marker for gastric emptying rates. Ginger did not affect gastric emptying rates, as the paracetamol pharmacokinetics were the same for both groups (Phillips, Hutchinson, and Ruggier, 1993).

Cardiovascular Risk Factors

A placebo-controlled trial explored the benefit of ginger for 60 patients with stable cardiovascular disease. The subjects had a history of heart attack and were taking nitrates and aspirin. The aspirin was stopped two weeks before the study. A dose of 4 g powdered ginger root for three months did not affect experimentally induced platelet aggregation, fibrinogen levels, blood lipid levels, or blood sugar levels. Only a higher, single dose of 10 g powdered ginger reduced experimentally induced platelet aggregation (Bordia, Verma, and Srivastava, 1997). Omissions in descriptions of trial methodology made this trial difficult to evaluate.

A crossover study examined the possible effect of ginger on platelet activity. Platelets were removed from 18 healthy volunteers following two weeks' administration of either 15 g raw ginger, 40 g cooked stem ginger, or placebo. There was no effect by either form of ginger on platelet activity as measured by stimulated release of thromboxane B2 (Janssen et al., 1996). The description of the preparations used in this trial was insufficient, and the study would have been stronger if a comparison with powdered ginger, the more common form of ginger, was included.

SYSTEMATIC REVIEWS AND META-ANALYSES

A systematic review of randomized controlled trials was conducted on six studies exploring the possible efficacy of ginger for nausea and vomiting. The studies addressed four different clinical conditions: seasickness (one study), morning sickness (one study), chemotherapy-induced nausea (one study), and postoperative nausea (three studies). Only the data from the three studies on postoperative nausea were pooled for statistical analysis (Bone et al., 1990; Phillips, Ruggier, and Hutchinson, 1993; Arfeen et al., 1995). The pooled absolute risk reduction for the incidence of postoperative nausea indicated that 1 g ginger taken before surgery gave no benefit over placebo (Ernst and Pittler, 2000).

ADVERSE REACTIONS OR SIDE EFFECTS

No serious side effects associated with powdered ginger or ginger extracts were reported in the trials reviewed. Occasionally participants reported headache and abdominal discomfort. A comparison trial with adults reported fewer side effects with Zintona (13 percent) compared with dimenhydrinate (40 percent). The doses were 500 mg and 100 mg, respectively, every four hours for two days (Riebenfeld and Borzone, 1999).

A trial with 28 children reported no side effects for those given ginger, whereas for those taking dimenhydrinate, 69 percent complained of dry mouth. In that trial, children aged three to six years received 250 mg Zintona every four hours for two days and those aged six to eight years received 500 mg every four hours for two days; those taking dimenhydrinate received either 12.5 or 25 mg in the same dosing regimen (Cereddu, 1999).

In two trials including a total to 100 pregnant women given 250 mg powdered ginger four times daily for four days, there were no reports of major adverse events or effects on the outcome of pregnancy (Fischer-Rasmussen et al., 1990; Vutyavanich, Kraisarin, and Ruangsri, 2001). Only minor side effects, including headache and abdominal discomfort, were reported.

INFORMATION FROM PHARMACOPOEIAL MONOGRAPHS

Sources of Published Therapeutic Monographs

German Commission E
British Herbal Compendium (BHC)
World Health Organization (WHO)
European Scientific Cooperative on Phytotherapy (ESCOP)
United States Pharmacopoeia—Drug Information (USP-DI)

Indications

Ginger root is widely recommended for the treatment of dyspepsia and the prevention or prophylaxis of motion sickness (Blumenthal et al., 1998; Bradley, 1992; WHO, 1999; ESCOP, 1996). The *British Herbal Compendium,* the WHO, and ESCOP state that ginger can be used to treat vomiting in pregnancy, while the latter two also suggest ginger for postoperative nausea and vomiting (Bradley, 1992; WHO, 1999; ESCOP, 1996). Other indications listed by the *BHC* include colic, anorexia, bronchitis, and rheumatic complaints (Bradley, 1992). The WHO also lists the following indications: flatulence, colic, vomiting, diarrhea, spasm, colds, flu, appetite stimulation, narcotic antagonist, and inflammation in migraine headache and rheumatic and muscular disorders (WHO, 1999). The *United States Pharmacopoeia—Drug Information* botanical monograph series lists the following reported uses of ginger rhizome: the prevention of nausea and vomiting after operations and the prevention and treatment of vomiting and nausea associated with motion sickness (*USP-DI*, 1998).

Actions stated by the Commission E are antiemetic, positively inotropic, promoting secretion of saliva and gastric juices, cholagogue, and increases tonus and peristalsis in the intestines (Blumenthal et al., 1998). The *BHC* also lists several actions, including carminative, antiemetic, spasmolytic, peripheral circulatory stimulant, and anti-inflammatory (Bradley, 1992).

Doses

Rhizome: 2 to 4 g rhizome daily or equivalent preparations (Blumenthal et al., 1998; WHO, 1999)
- Powdered rhizome: single doses of powdered rhizome, 1 to 2 g, or 0.25 to 1 g three times daily (Bradley, 1992); 0.5 to 2 g of the powdered drug daily or divided doses (adults and children over six years) (ESCOP, 1996)

Tincture:
- Weak ginger tincture BP: (1:5, 90 percent ethanol) 1.5 to 3 ml three times daily (Bradley, 1992)
- Strong ginger tincture BP: (1:2, 90 percent ethanol), 0.25 to 0.5 ml three times daily (Bradley, 1992)

Note: The *BHC*, WHO, and *USP-DI* suggest specific dosages for certain indications:

As an antiemetic: single doses of powdered rhizome, 1 to 2 g (Bradley, 1992)

For motion sickness: (adults and children over six years) 0.5 g, 2 to 4 times daily (WHO, 1999); 1 g ginger 30 to 60 minutes before travel (*USP-DI*, 1998)

For dyspepsia: 2 to 4 g daily, as powdered plant material or extracts (WHO, 1999)

For postoperative nausea or vomiting: 1 g ginger taken 30 to 60 minutes before surgery (*USP-DI*, 1998)

Treatment Period

No restrictions are listed by ESCOP (1996).

Contraindications

The Commission E and WHO suggest that ginger should be used only after consultation with a physician when the patient has gallstones (Blumenthal et al., 1998; WHO, 1999). The WHO also states that patients taking anticoagulant drugs or those with blood coagulation disorders should consult their physicians before self-medicating with ginger (WHO, 1999). The *USP-DI* suggests that pharmacologic doses of ginger are not recommended for children and pregnant or breastfeeding women (*USP-DI*, 1998). The *BHC* and ESCOP list no known contraindications (Bradley, 1992; ESCOP, 1996).

Adverse Reactions

ESCOP lists heartburn as a possible adverse reaction, while the Commission E states that ginger has no known adverse reactions (ESCOP, 1996; Blumenthal et al., 1998). The *USP-DI* also lists minor heartburn as the only reported adverse reaction to ginger (*USP-DI*, 1998).

Precautions

ESCOP has no reported precautions for ginger, while the WHO suggests that it is not recommended for children less than six years of age (ESCOP, 1996; WHO, 1999). The *USP-DI* suggests that patients with an increased risk of hemorrhage or those taking anticoagulants should use ginger with caution (*USP-DI*, 1998).

Drug Interactions

Although the Commission E states no known drug interactions, the WHO states that ginger may affect bleeding times and immunological parameters owing to its ability to inhibit thromboxane synthase and to act as a prostacyclin agonist; the ESCOP claims that ginger may enhance absorption of sulfaguanidine (Blumenthal et al., 1998; WHO, 1999; ESCOP, 1996).

REFERENCES

Arfeen Z, Owen H, Plummer, JL, Ilsley AH, Sorby-Adams RAC, Doecke CJ (1995). A double-blind randomized controlled trial of ginger for the prevention of postoperative nausea and vomiting. *Anaesthesia and Intensive Care* 23 (4): 449-452.

Awang DVC (1992). Ginger. *Canadian Pharmaceutical Journal, Revue Pharmaceutique Canadienne (CPJ RPC):* 309-311.

Bliddal H, Rosetzsky A, Schlichting P, Weidner MS, Andersen LA, Ibfelt H-H, Christensen K, Jensen ON, Barslev J (2000). A randomized, placebo-controlled, cross-over study of ginger extracts and ibuprofen in osteoarthritis. *Osteoarthritis and Cartilage* 8 (1): 9-12.

Blumenthal M, Busse W, Hall T, Goldberg A, Gruenwald J, Riggins C, Rister S, eds. (1998). *The Complete German Commission E Monographs: Therapeutic Guide to Herbal Medicines.* Trans. S Klein. Austin, TX: American Botanical Council.

Bone ME, Wilkinson DJ, Young JR, McNeil J, Charlton S (1990). Ginger root—A new antiemetic: The effect of ginger root on postoperative nausea and vomiting after major gynecological surgery. *Anaesthesia* 45 (8): 669-671.

Bordia A, Verma SK, Srivastava KC (1997). Effect of ginger (*Zingiber officinale* Rosc.) and fenugreek (*Trigonella foenumgraceum* L.) on blood lipids, blood sugar and platelet aggregation in patients with coronary artery disease. *Prostaglandins, Leukotrienes, and Essential Fatty Acids* 56 (5): 379-384.

Bradley PR, ed. (1992). *British Herbal Compendium: A Handbook of Scientific Information on Widely Used Plant Drugs,* Volume 1. Dorset, UK: British Herbal Medicine Association.

Cereddu P (1999). Motion sickness in children: Results of a double-blind study with ginger (Zintona®) and dimenhydrinate. Reviewed and edited by Fulder S and Brown D. *Healthnotes Review of Complementary and Integrative Medicine* 6 (2): 102-107.

Ernst E, Pittler MH (2000). Efficacy of ginger and vomiting: A systematic review of randomized clinical trials. *British Journal of Anaesthesia* 84 (3): 367-371.

European Scientific Cooperative on Phytotherapy (ESCOP) (1996). Zingiberis rhizoma: Ginger. *Monographs on the Medicinal Uses of Plant Drugs.* Fascicle 1. Exeter, UK: European Scientific Cooperative on Phytotherapy.

Fischer-Rasmussen W, Kjaer SK, Dahl C, Asping U (1990). Ginger treatment of hyperemesis gravidarum. *European Journal of Obstetrics and Gynecology and Reproductive Biology* 38 (1): 19-24.

Grøntved A, Brask T, Kambskard J, Hentzer E (1988). Ginger root against seasickness, a controlled trial on the open sea. *Acta Otolaryngologica* 105 (1-2): 45-49.

Grøntved A, Hentzer E (1986). Vertigo-reducing effect of ginger root, a controlled clinical study. *ORL; Journal for Oto-rhino-laryngology and Its Related Specialties* 48 (5): 282-286.

Hardman JG, Limbird LE, Molinoff PB, Ruddon RW, Gillman AG (1996). *Goodman and Gillman's The Pharmacological Basis of Therapeutics,* Ninth Edition. New York: McGraw-Hill.

Holtmann S, Clarke AH, Scherer H, Hohn M (1989). The anti-motion sickness mechanism of ginger, a comparative study with placebo and dimenhydrinate. *Acta Otolaryngologica* 108 (3-4): 168-174.

Janssen PLTMK, Meyboom S, van Staveren WA, de Vegt F, Katan MB (1996). Consumption of ginger (*Zingiber officinale* Roscoe) does not affect ex vivo platelet thromboxane production in humans. *European Journal of Clinical Nutrition* 50 (11): 772-774.

Meyer K, Schwartz J, Crater D, Keyes B (1995). *Zingiber officinale* (ginger) used to prevent 8-MOP-associated nausea. *Dermatology Nursing* 7 (4): 242-244.

Micklefield GH, Redeker Y, Meister V, Jung O, Greving I, May B (1999). Effect of ginger on gastroduodenal motility. *International Journal of Clinical Pharmacology and Therapeutics* 37 (7): 341-346.

Mowrey D, Clayson D (1982). Motion sickness, ginger and psychophysics. *The Lancet* 1 (8273): 655-657.

Phillips S, Hutchinson S, Ruggier R (1993). *Zingiber officinale* does not affect gastric emptying rate: A randomized, placebo-controlled, crossover trial. *Anaesthesia* 48 (5): 393-395.

Phillips S, Ruggier R, Hutchinson SE (1993). *Zingiber officinale* (Ginger)—An antiemetic for day case surgery. *Anaesthesia* 48 (8): 715-717.

Riebenfeld D, Borzone L (1999). Randomized double-blind study comparing ginger (Zintona®) and dimenhydrinate in motion sickness. Reviewed and edited by S Fulder and D Brown. *Healthnotes Review of Complementary and Integrative Medicine* 6 (2): 98-101.

Schmid R, Schick T, Steffen R, Tschopp A, Wilk T (1994). Comparison of seven commonly used agents for prophylaxis of seasickness. *Journal of Travel Medicine* 1 (4): 203-206.

United States Pharmacopoeia—Drug Information (1998). Botanical monograph series: Ginger. Rockville, MD: The United States Pharmacopoeial Convention, Inc.

Visalyaputra S, Petchpaisit N, Somcharoen K, Choavaratana R (1998). The efficacy of ginger root in the prevention of postoperative nausea and vomiting after outpatient gynaecological laparoscopy. *Anaesthesia* 53 (5): 506-510.

Vutyavanich T, Kraisarin T, Ruangsri R-A (2001). Ginger for nausea and vomiting in pregnancy: Randomized, double-masked, placebo-controlled trial. *Obstetrics and Gynecology* 97 (4): 577-582.

World Health Organization (WHO) (1999). *WHO Monographs on Selected Medicinal Plants*, Volume 1. Geneva, Switzerland: World Health Organization.

DETAILS ON GINGER PRODUCTS
AND CLINICAL STUDIES

Product and clinical study information is grouped in the same order as in the Summary Table. A profile on an individual product is followed by details of the clinical studies associated with that product. In some instances a clinical study, or studies, supports several products that contain the same principal ingredient(s). In these instances, those products are grouped together.

Clinical studies that follow each product, or group of products, are grouped by therapeutic indication, in accordance with the order in the Summary Table.

Index to Ginger

Product Profile: Zintona®

Manufacturer	**Dalidar Pharma Ltd., Israel**
U.S. distributor	None
Botanical ingredient	**Ginger root**
Extract name	**Zintona**
Quantity	250 mg
Processing	Dried root powder
Standardization	Pungent phenolic compounds
Formulation	Capsule

Recommended dose: Take two capsules one-half hour prior to travel or meals. Up to two capsules may be taken every four hours during travel.

DSHEA structure/function: Maintains a calm stomach, especially during travel.

Cautions: As with any supplement, contact a doctor if currently taking prescription medicine, or if pregnant or nursing a baby.

Other ingredients: Gelatin, colloidal anhydrous silica, sodium lauryl sulfate.

Source(s) of information: Quanterra™ Stomach Comfort product package (©1999 Warner-Lambert Co.); Riebenfeld and Borzone, 1999.

Clinical Study: Zintona®

Extract name	Zintona
Manufacturer	Pharmaton S.A., Switzerland (Dalidar Pharma Ltd., Israel)
Indication	**Motion sickness; seasickness**
Level of evidence	**II**
Therapeutic benefit	**Yes**

Bibliographic reference
Schmid R, Schick T, Steffen R, Tschopp A, Wilk T (1994). Comparison of seven commonly used agents for prophylaxis of seasickness. *Journal of Travel Medicine* 1 (4): 203-206.

Trial design
Parallel. Subjects received one of seven substances frequently used to prevent seasickness and matching placebo of another substance in a double-dummy method. Nobody received only placebo. The comparison medications were Touristil (cinnarizine 20 mg, domperidone 15 mg), Marzine (cyclizine 50 mg), Dramamine (dimenhydrinate 50 mg, caffeine 50 mg), Peremesin (meclozine 25 mg, caffeine 20 mg), Stugeron (cinnarizine 25 mg), and Scopoderm TTS (scopolamine 0.5 mg). In most cases, subjects took the medication two hours prior to departure. For Touristil and Zintona an additional dose was administered four hours later. Stugeron and Scopoderm TTS were administered the previous evening. A second dose of Stugeron was given the following morning. The whale-watching tour lasted six hours and went out on high seas.

Study duration	1 day
Dose	500 mg 2 hours prior to departure and after 4 hours
Route of administration	Oral

Randomized	Yes
Randomization adequate	Yes
Blinding	Double-blind
Blinding adequate	No
Placebo	No
Drug comparison	Yes
Drug name	Touristil, Marzine, Dramamine, Peremesin, Stugeron, Scopoderm TTS
Site description	Ship
No. of subjects enrolled	1741
No. of subjects completed	1475
Sex	Male and female
Age	16-65 years

Inclusion criteria
Tourists participating in a whale-watching tour in Norway between the ages of 16 and 65 years old.

Exclusion criteria
Pregnant or nursing women, persons who had used antiemetic or anti-allergic drugs within the past 48 hours, patients with glaucoma, and persons with a history of adverse reactions to any of the substances to be tested.

End points
The outcome measures were vomiting, malaise (modified Graybiel criteria), and subjective reports of adverse events. The information was collected via a questionnaire gathered at the end of the trip.

Results
Questionnaires were completed by 85.5 percent of volunteers ($n = 1489$). Those who tried to avoid seasickness by fixing their eyes on the horizon, by putting cotton in their ears, or by wearing a "sea band" on the wrist were excluded from analysis. None of the study medications offered complete protection from seasickness. All had similar rates of efficacy compared to an earlier trip without prophylaxis when 80 percent got sick. No statistical difference was seen between treatments. In each treatment group, 4.1 to 10.2 percent experienced vomiting and 16.4 to 23.5 percent experienced malaise (nausea and discomfort).

Side effects
No serious adverse reactions reported. Sleepiness and tiredness were reported generally for all seven agents.

Authors' comments
Six of the seven medications may be recommended for prevention of sea-sickness; Scopolamine TTS seems the least attractive. Ginger was as potent as the others.

Reviewers' comments
The ginger root product (Zintona) demonstrated similar efficacy to the pharmaceutical agents tested. The experimental design did not include a baseline measurement of nausea/vomiting sensitivity. This study is of a type similar to a phase II clinical development trial; however, no conclusive phase I type (effective and toxic dose ranges) data were presented or referenced. (3, 5)

Clinical Study: Zintona®

Extract name	Zintona
Manufacturer	Dalidar Pharma Ltd., Israel
Indication	**Motion sickness; seasickness**
Level of evidence	I
Therapeutic benefit	**Yes**

Bibliographic reference
Riebenfeld D, Borzone L (1999). Randomized double-blind study comparing ginger (Zintona®) and dimenhydrinate in motion sickness. Reviewed and edited by Fulder S and Brown D. *Healthnotes Review of Complementary and Integrative Medicine* 6 (2): 98-101.

Trial design
Parallel. Cruise ship passengers received either Zintona or dimenhydrinate (100 mg one-half hour before sailing and 100 mg every four hours) for two days.

Study duration	2 days
Dose	500 mg one-half hour before sailing and every 4 hours thereafter
Route of administration	Oral
Randomized	Yes
Randomization adequate	Yes
Blinding	Double-blind
Blinding adequate	Yes
Placebo	No
Drug comparison	Yes

Drug name   Dimenhydrinate (Dramamine)

Site description   Cruise ship

No. of subjects enrolled   60
No. of subjects completed 60
Sex   Male and female
Age   10-77 years (mean: 37)

Inclusion criteria
Cruise ship passengers with a history of motion sickness.

Exclusion criteria
Not mentioned.

End points
Therapeutic effectiveness was evaluated by the following parameters: a physician's examination of general condition, especially central nervous system and gastrointestinal function; severity of motion sickness symptoms rated according to a point system by physicians; and subjects' self-reported assessment of severity of motion sickness.

Results
Twenty-one patients taking Zintona reported very good results compared to 15 in the dimenhydrinate group. The ship's physician reported equal results (primarily good or very good) for both Zintona and dimenhydrinate (statistical improvement for both $p < 0.05$). General conditions, such as malaise, appetite, and vomiting, improved equally well in both groups. Change in degree of motion sickness was slightly (nonsignificant) better for dimenhydrinate for treatment of motion sickness.

Side effects
Side effects in the Zintona group (13.3 percent) were significantly less than in the dimenhydrinate group (40 percent) ($p < 0.001$). Drowsiness and headache were reported with Zintona, while dimenhydrinate was associated with drowsiness, gastric distress, and cold sweats.

Authors' comments
Zintona is as effective as dimenhydrinate for treatment of motion sickness and has a lower incidence of side effects.

Reviewers' comments
The study, as designed, allowed for noninferiority comparison to the existing treatment, but the analysis of treatment based upon primarily subjective assessment methods would have benefited from a placebo arm. The study did not include a general gastrointestinal history or otherwise rule out comorbid conditions. The sample size was probably appropriate, given the significant

results; however, no power calculation was presented. The trial length was adequate. It is unclear if the adverse events were intrinsic to the clinical syndrome of motion sickness. (Edited version of the paper reviewed) (5, 6)

Clinical Study: Zintona®

Extract name	Zintona
Manufacturer	Dalidar Pharma Ltd., Israel
Indication	**Motion sickness**
Level of evidence	**III**
Therapeutic benefit	**Trend**

Bibliographic reference
Cereddu P (1999). Motion sickness in children: Results of a double-blind study with ginger (Zintona®) and dimenhydrinate. Reviewed and edited by Fulder S and Brown D. *Healthnotes Review of Complementary and Integrative Medicine* 6 (2): 102-107.

Trial design
Parallel. Subjects received either Zintona (ages three to six years: 250 mg 30 minutes before beginning a two-day trip [by car, boat, and/or airplane], then 250 mg every four hours as needed; ages six and above: 500 mg in the same pattern) or dimenhydrinate (12.5 mg or 25 mg 30 minutes before beginning the trip and 12.5 or 25 mg every four hours as necessary). There was a one-week washout period before the trial, and no drugs similar to those being tested were given during this time.

Study duration	2 days
Dose	3 to 6 years, 250 mg every 4 hours; 6+ years, 500 mg every four hours
Route of administration	Oral
Randomized	Yes
Randomization adequate	No
Blinding	Double-blind
Blinding adequate	No
Placebo	No
Drug comparison	Yes
Drug name	Dimenhydrinate (Dramamine)
Site description	Travel in car, boat, or airplane
No. of subjects enrolled	28

No. of subjects completed   28
Sex   Male and female
Age   4-8 years

Inclusion criteria
Children with previous history of motion sickness which was determined by a questionnaire.

Exclusion criteria
Children younger than three years of age, concomitant illnesses, anemic, or could not cooperate with the study design.

End points
The severity of motion sickness was determined by the pediatric physician and included subjective symptoms (vertigo, body temperature, headache, increased salivation, stomachache, nausea, dryness of mouth) and objective symptoms (pallor, cold sweat).

Results
In the physicians' ratings, Zintona was reported as having good results in 100 percent of the subjects while dimenhydrinate rated good in only 31 percent and modest results in 69 percent. Therapeutic effect was noted within 30 minutes in the Zintona group compared with 60 minutes for the dimenhydrinate ($p < 0.00001$).

Side effects
No subject taking Zintona reported any side effects, while 69.23 percent of cases in the dimenhydrinate group complained of dry mouth and 23.07 percent had vertigo.

Author's comments
This small study provides some indication that a safe traditional medicinal food is quite effective in decreasing vertigo, nausea, sweating, pallor, and, in general, the symptoms of motion sickness.

Reviewers' comments
It is unclear whether each subject experienced the same mode(s) and duration of travel. Given the day-to-day variance in the study population, the described and applied statistical methods are inadequate. The randomization method used did not create well-matched groups with respect to history and severity of motion sickness. Because the data collected were relative-subjective, this difference could serve as a confounder both toward overestimating and underestimating efficacy (i.e., a subject with severe symptoms could either be more refractory to treatment effects or could experience, and so report, a greater relative sense of symptomatic relief). The washout period was an interesting idea, but not of any apparent value in this trial. The refer-

ences presented regarding the dosage range involved studies of significantly older patients. This is concerning, as pediatric dosing—especially in patients under six years of age—warrants thorough study and consideration for any agent. The circumstance of unsubstantiated dosage choices in vulnerable subjects in this study demands mention here again, that this study is of a type most similar to a phase II clinical development trial, yet no conclusive phase I type data (effective and toxic dose ranges) were presented or referenced. The trial length was likely adequate. (Edited version of the paper reviewed) (1, 3)

Clinical Study: Zintona®

Extract name	Zintona
Manufacturer	Pharmaton S.A., Switzerland (Dalidar Pharma Ltd., Israel)
Indication	**Motion sickness; induced nystagmic activity**
Level of evidence	**III**
Therapeutic benefit	**MOA**

Bibliographic reference
Holtmann S, Clarke AH, Scherer H, Hohn M (1989). The anti-motion sickness mechanism of ginger, a comparative study with placebo and dimenhydrinate. *Acta Otolaryngologica* 108 (3-4): 168-174.

Trial design
Crossover. Three-arm study: subjects were given either ginger, dimenhydrinate (100 mg), or placebo (lactose). Preparations were administered 90 minutes before stimulus routines. There were washout periods of 48 hours between sessions.

Study duration	1 day
Dose	1000 mg single dose
Route of administration	Oral
Randomized	Yes
Randomization adequate	No
Blinding	Double-blind
Blinding adequate	No
Placebo	Yes
Drug comparison	Yes
Drug name	Dimenhydrinate (Dramamine)

Site description   Single center

No. of subjects enrolled   38
No. of subjects completed   38
Sex   Male and female
Age   22-34 years (mean 26.3)

Inclusion criteria
Subjects with a distinct, symmetrical response to caloric and rotatory vestibular stimuli and normal gain in the optokinetic test.

Exclusion criteria
Subjects exhibiting a spontaneous nystagmus in their electronystagmography (ENG) recording with an intensity of more than 1 degree per second were also excluded from the study.

End points
The extent to which nystagmic activity (involuntary movements of the eye), induced by vestibular stimuli (water irrigation of the ears), optokinetic stimuli (a moving strip pattern), and being spun in a rotary chair, was affected was measured in a model for testing motion sickness. Eye movements were recorded using standard ENG equipment, and the evaluation was performed by automatic nystagmus analysis.

Results
Ginger root had no influence on the experimentally induced nystagmus, compared with baseline and placebo. Dimenhydrinate was found to cause a reduction in the nystagmus response to caloric, rotatory, and optokinetic stimuli. It can be concluded that neither the vestibular nor the oculomotor system, both of which are of decisive importance in the occurrence of motion sickness, are influenced by ginger.

Side effects
None mentioned.

Authors' comments
The mechanism of action of ginger is of a different nature than the CNS mechanism of action of the commonly used anti-motion sickness drugs. These reports and findings lend support to the thesis that the antiemetic mechanism of action of powdered ginger root is of gastrointestinal nature.

Reviewers' comments
The sample size may have been appropriate; however, no power calculation was presented. The trial had a very poor presentation of data. The data were not clearly presented in one bar graph, and other graphs and charts did not allow for assessment of statistical significance between groups. It is unclear

whether lactose is sufficiently gastrointestinally inactive to serve as a placebo in this study. The treatment length was adequate. (1, 4)

Product Profile: WS 1540

Manufacturer	**Dr. Willmar Schwabe GmbH & Co., Germany**
U.S. distributor	None
Botanical ingredient	**Ginger rhizome extract**
Extract name	**WS 1540**
Quantity	100 mg, corresponding to 1 g ginger root
Processing	No information
Standardization	No information
Formulation	Capsule

Source(s) of information: Micklefield et al., 1999.

Clinical Study: WS 1540

Extract name	WS 1540
Manufacturer	Dr. Willmar Schwabe GmbH & Co., Germany
Indication	**Gastroduodenal motility**
Level of evidence	**II**
Therapeutic benefit	**MOA**

Bibliographic reference
Micklefield GH, Redeker Y, Meister V, Jung O, Greving I, May B (1999). Effect of ginger on gastroduodenal motility. *International Journal of Clinical Pharmacology and Therapeutics* 37 (7): 341-346.

Trial design
Two-period crossover trial. Ginger or placebo were given at 8 a.m. after fasting and at 12 noon before a meal. Seven days elapsed between experiments.

Study duration	1 day
Dose	2 (100 mg extract) capsules twice daily
Route of administration	Oral

Randomized	Yes
Randomization adequate	No
Blinding	Double-blind
Blinding adequate	No
Placebo	Yes
Drug comparison	No
Site description	Laboratory
No. of subjects enrolled	12
No. of subjects completed	12
Sex	Male
Age	24-44 years

Inclusion criteria
Male volunteers aged 18 to 50 years.

Exclusion criteria
Symptoms or anamnestic indications of gastrointestinal disorders or serious abdominal surgeries (except appendectomies), other severe disorders, and any concomitant medication.

End points
Fasting and postprandial (up to one hour after a meal) gastroduodenal motility was recorded using a manometric catheter. The motility parameters, including the number, the frequency, and the amplitude of contractions, were measured in the gastric corpus, antrum, and duodenum. The phases of the migrating motor complex (MMC) were as follows: phase I motor quiescence; phase II pressure waves >10 mmHg at a rate higher than two per ten minutes; and phase III rhythmic contractile activity at maximum frequency (two per minute in the antrum for at least one minute, 10 to 12 per minute in the duodenum for at least two minutes).

Results
In the fasting state, ginger significantly increased the number and frequency of contractions during phase II in the corpus and phase III in the antrum. The only significant effect on the duodenum was the frequency of contractions during phase II. Postprandially, ginger significantly increased the number and frequency of contractions in the corpus and amplitude in the antrum but otherwise showed only a trend toward activity compared to placebo. Ginger had no effect on the postprandial motility index compared to placebo.

Side effects
None observed.

Authors' comments
Oral ginger improves gastroduodenal motility in the fasting state and after a standard test meal.

Reviewers' comments
The small sample size was acceptable for this physiologic study (mechanism of action). The trial length was adequate. (3, 4)

Product Profile: Eurovita Extract 33

Manufacturer	**Eurovita A/S, Denmark**
U.S. distributor	None
Botanical ingredient	**Ginger root extract**
Extract name	**EV ext-33**
Quantity	No information
Processing	No information
Standardization	Hydroxy-methyl-phenyl compounds
Formulation	Capsule

Source(s) of information: Bliddal et al., 2000.

Clinical Study: Eurovita Extract 33

Extract name	EV ext-33
Manufacturer	Eurovita A/S, Denmark
Indication	**Osteoarthritis**
Level of evidence	**I**
Therapeutic benefit	**No**

Bibliographic reference
Bliddal H, Rosetzsky A, Schlichting P, Weidner MS, Andersen LA, Ibfelt H-H, Christensen K, Jensen ON, Barslev J (2000). A randomized, placebo-controlled, cross-over study of ginger extracts and ibuprofen in osteoarthritis. *Osteoarthritis and Cartilage* 8 (1): 9-12.

Trial design
Crossover. One-week washout period preceded three three-week treatment periods. Patients received either ginger extract, ibuprofen (400 mg three times daily), or placebo. Acetaminophen was given as a rescue drug during

the washout period and during the rest of the study in a maximum dose of 3 g daily.

Study duration	3 weeks
Dose	170 mg three times daily
Route of administration	Oral
Randomized	Yes
Randomization adequate	Yes
Blinding	Double-blind
Blinding adequate	Yes
Placebo	Yes
Drug comparison	Yes
Drug name	Ibuprofen
Site description	Multicenter
No. of subjects enrolled	75
No. of subjects completed	56
Sex	Male and female
Age	24-87 years (mean: 66)

Inclusion criteria
Outpatients fluent in Danish, over the age of 18, with clinical dysfunction and pain due to osteoarthritis of the hip or knee. Mean duration of osteoarthritis was 7.7 years, and mean Lequesne index was 11.8 at entry.

Exclusion criteria
Exclusion criteria included rheumatoid arthritis, neurological disorders, severe medical diseases, and dementia. No injections in joints were accepted within six months before the study start.

End points
The primary outcome measure was a 100 mm visual analog scale (VAS) for pain assessment. Other end points included the Lequesne index for either hip or knee, range of motion, consumption of acetaminophen, and the investigator's preference of medication in the different treatment periods. Measurements were taken at baseline (after the washout period) and at the end of each treatment period. Patients also kept a diary with a four-point Likert pain scale during each treatment period.

Results
For the VAS, a ranking of efficacy was found for the three treatment periods: ibuprofen > ginger extract > placebo ($p < 0.0001$). The same ranking trend was found for the rescue medication (acetaminophen) consumption ($p < 0.01$). The Lesquesne index changed positively during treatment, also with

the same ranking of treatment efficacy. For these tests, there were significant differences between ibuprofen and ginger extract and between ibuprofen and placebo, but there was no significant difference between ginger extract and placebo. The patients' diaries were not assessable, as many were not filled out properly. No differences in range of motion were noted in any of the treatment periods. Investigators had a 66 percent preference in favor of ibuprofen for all periods.

Side effects
Four patients withdrew due to side effects: intestinal strangulation (placebo); restless legs (placebo); bad taste (ginger); and nausea (ibuprofen). Other adverse events were mostly gastrointestinal: bad taste; dyspepsia; changes in stools/intestinal trouble; or nausea. Three patients had allergic reactions (one in each treatment group).

Authors' comments
This study demonstrates a ranking of efficacy on pain level and function in patients with osteoarthritis of the hip or knee with ibuprofen being more effective than ginger extract (E.ext-33) and placebo. However, a carryover effect may blur possible effects of the later treatment periods, and based on the present results, caution should be observed in the interpretation of a crossover study of ginger extract.

Reviewers' comments
This study is of a type most similar to a phase II or IV clinical development trial; however, no conclusive phase I type (effective and toxic dose ranges) data were presented or referenced. In such an experimental circumstance, only a positive result can be considered definitive, as a negative result may occur simply due to an ineffective dosing regimen. Therefore, the results presented apply only to the particular standardized ginger extract (Eurovita 33). Lack of therapeutic benefit cannot be assumed categorically for all ginger preparations. The trial length was potentially inadequate, given that the dose-response pharmacokinetics of ginger are unknown. (5, 6)

Product Profile: Ginger (Powdered)

Manufacturer	None
U.S. distributor	None
Botanical ingredient	**Ginger root**
Extract name	N/A
Quantity	No information
Processing	Powdered plant material
Standardization	No information
Formulation	Capsule

Clinical Study: Ginger (Powdered)

Extract name	N/A
Manufacturer	None
Indication	**Motion sickness; vertigo and nystagmus**
Level of evidence	**III**
Therapeutic benefit	**MOA**

Bibliographic reference

Grøntved A, Hentzer E (1986). Vertigo-reducing effect of ginger root, a controlled clinical study. ORL; *Journal for Oto-rhino-laryngology and Its Related Specialties* 48 (5): 282-286.

Trial design

Crossover study. At least 48 hours between one-day sessions in which either ginger or placebo was administered one hour before testing.

Study duration	1 day
Dose	1 g of powdered ginger root
Route of administration	Oral
Randomized	Yes
Randomization adequate	No
Blinding	Double-blind
Blinding adequate	Yes
Placebo	Yes
Drug comparison	No
Site description	Single center
No. of subjects enrolled	8
No. of subjects completed	8
Sex	Not given
Age	16-56 years (median: 33.5)

Inclusion criteria

Healthy volunteers.

Exclusion criteria

Persons having spontaneous nystagmus, food allergy, or abnormal otomicroscopy were excluded.

End points

Subjects were adapted to darkness and placed supine with their head bent

30 degrees forward. The vestibular system was stimulated by irrigating the left ear with water. The provoked nystagmus was recorded by electronystagmography. The subject evaluated the degree of vertigo on a scale of 0 to 5. Recording of vertigo and nystagmus was carried out three times at 20-minute intervals after intake of treatment.

Results
Ginger root reduced the induced vertigo significantly compared to placebo ($p < 0.05$). There was no statistically significant action upon the duration or the maximum slow-phase velocity of nystagmus.

Side effects
None reported by the subjects.

Authors' comments
Ginger root reduced the induced vertigo significantly better than placebo. Investigations indicate that ginger root, similar to sympathomimetics and parasympatholytics, dampens the induced vestibular impulses to the autonomic centers of the central nervous system and possibly the cerebral cortex. Ginger root does not appear to affect the vestibular system directly, as no statistically significant change in nystagmus was demonstrable.

Reviewers' comments
The sample size may not have been appropriate; no power calculation was presented. The washout period was brief and not of fixed duration, but likely adequate if ginger's mechanism is direct (versus centrally mediated). (3, 3)

Clinical Study: Ginger (Powdered)

Extract name	N/A
Manufacturer	None
Indication	**Motion sickness**
Level of evidence	**III**
Therapeutic benefit	**Trend**

Bibliographic reference
Mowrey D, Clayson D (1982). Motion sickness, ginger and psychophysics. *The Lancet* 1 (8273): 655-657.

Trial design
Parallel. Three-arm study. Subjects were told that they were to be given either dimenhydrinate or harmless herbs. Subjects were given either dimenhydrinate

(100 mg), powdered ginger (940 mg), or placebo (powdered chickweed herb) 20 to 25 minutes before testing.

Study duration	1 day
Dose	2 capsules (total of 940 mg of powdered ginger)
Route of administration	Oral
Randomized	No
Randomization adequate	No
Blinding	Open
Blinding adequate	No
Placebo	Yes
Drug comparison	Yes
Drug name	Dimenhydrinate (Dramamine)
Site description	Laboratory
No. of subjects enrolled	36
No. of subjects completed	36
Sex	Male and female
Age	18-20 years

Inclusion criteria

Subjects were selected based on self-rated extreme or very high susceptibility to motion sickness.

Exclusion criteria

None mentioned.

End points

Subjects were blindfolded and placed on a tilted, rotating chair for up to six minutes. They were asked to quantify the feelings in their stomachs every 15 seconds. The experiment was stopped if the subject vomited.

Results

None of the subjects in the placebo and dimenhydrinate groups was able to stay in the chair for six minutes, whereas half of the subjects in the ginger group stayed for the full time ($p < 0.001$). The magnitude of gastrointestinal sensations was greatest with placebo, intermediate with dimenhydrinate, and lowest with ginger.

Side effects

None noted.

Authors' comments
Powdered ginger was superior to dimenhydrinate in preventing gastrointestinal symptoms of testing motion sickness.

Reviewers' comments
The "time in chair" measurements imply superiority of ginger over placebo.
The validity of chickweed as a placebo in this study is a concern. Subjects
were also not evaluated for other medications, gastrointestinal and central
nervous system disorders, or other relevant medical history. The experimental design did not sufficiently control the variables involved in the unknown
nature of the physiologic mechanism, analytic method, and pharmacokinetics. The experimental and analytical methods did not produce a convincing picture from the data. Indeed, the analytical methodology was as
much of an experimental variable as the tested agents. Power function analysis should have been established first without treatment, then with an effective agent versus a valid placebo. It is not clear whether the pharmacokinetics of ginger are amenable to a study of ±30 minutes duration. (1, 3)

Clinical Study: Ginger (Powdered)

Extract name	N/A
Manufacturer	Dispensary at Odense University Hospital, Denmark
Indication	**Motion sickness; seasickness**
Level of evidence	**III**
Therapeutic benefit	**Trend**

Bibliographic reference
Grøntved A, Brask T, Kambskard J, Hentzer E (1988). Ginger root against
seasickness, a controlled trial on the open sea. *Acta Otolaryngologica* 105
(1-2): 45-49.

Trial design
Parallel. Conditions of heavy seas, a few days from port.

Study duration	4 hours
Dose	1 g of powdered ginger root
Route of administration	Oral
Randomized	Yes
Randomization adequate	No
Blinding	Double-blind
Blinding adequate	Yes

Placebo	Yes
Drug comparison	No
Site description	Fully rigged training ship
No. of subjects enrolled	80
No. of subjects completed	79
Sex	Male
Age	16-19 years (median: 17)

Inclusion criteria
Subjects not accustomed to high seas and not especially susceptible to motion sickness.

Exclusion criteria
None mentioned.

End points
Every hour for four hours, subjects noted a score for each of the following seasickness symptoms: nausea, vertigo, vomiting, and cold sweats.

Results
Ginger root significantly reduced the tendency to vomit and cold sweat compared to placebo ($p < 0.05$). Ginger root also reduced the symptoms of nausea and vertigo but not significantly.

Side effects
None reported.

Authors' comments
Powdered ginger has at least some effect on symptoms of motion sickness. Contrary to all conventionally used anti-motion sickness drugs, no side effects were reported.

Reviewers' comments
The sample size may not have been appropriate; no power calculation was presented. A larger sample size may have provided greater data resolution. (3, 3)

Clinical Study: Ginger (Powdered)

Extract name	N/A
Manufacturer	None

Indication   **Nausea due to chemotherapy agent**
Level of evidence   **III**
Therapeutic benefit   **Undetermined**

Bibliographic reference
Meyer K, Schwartz J, Crater D, Keyes B (1995). *Zingiber officinale* (ginger) used to prevent 8-MOP-associated nausea. *Dermatology Nursing* 7 (4): 242-244.

Trial design
Linear comparison. Nausea due to chemotherapy agent 8-MOP alone was noted before the trial and then compared to nausea felt after administration of both 8-MOP and ginger. Ginger was administered 30 minutes prior to 8-MOP ingestion.

Study duration	Not given
Dose	3 capsules of 530 mg each (1.6 g total)
Route of administration	Oral
Randomized	No
Randomization adequate	No
Blinding	Open
Blinding adequate	No
Placebo	No
Drug comparison	No
Site description	Hospital
No. of subjects enrolled	11
No. of subjects completed	11
Sex	Male and female
Age	23-80 years (median: 54)

Inclusion criteria
Patients undergoing monthly photopheresis therapy (psoralen, 8-MOP) and who regularly complained of nausea as a result.

Exclusion criteria
None mentioned.

End points
Patients completed a survey, rating their nausea on scale of 0 to 4 (no nausea to severe nausea). Serum was drawn to assess 8-MOP levels.

Results
Total score for nausea decreased from 22.5 (individual average 2.045) prior

to the trial, to 8.0 (individual average 0.727) after administration of ginger. Serum levels of 8-MOP remained therapeutic in 10 out of 11 patients (the one patient with subtherapeutic levels had connective tissue disease with gastrointestinal involvement).

Side effects
Three patients described heartburn symptoms.

Authors' comments
As a nonprescription item with minimal side effects, ginger is worth a trial as an antiemetic in both photopheresis and other therapies involving psoralen.

Reviewers' comments
This trial had an exceptionally poor experimental design and discussion. The trial used a subjective assessment of a subjective condition without blinding or placebo. Comparing experimental results to memory of prior experiences is not sound methodology. The MOP levels were not compared to a baseline level for this patient group. No justification or explanation was given for administering ginger 30 minutes prior to administering 8-MOP; the pharmacokinetics of this agent are not well established. (1, 3)

Clinical Study: Ginger (Powdered)

Extract name	N/A
Manufacturer	Blackmores Ltd., Australia
Indication	**Nausea and vomiting** (postoperative)
Level of evidence	**I**
Therapeutic benefit	**No**

Bibliographic reference
Arfeen Z, Owen H, Plummer, JL, Ilsley AH, Sorby-Adams RAC, Doecke CJ (1995). A double-blind randomized controlled trial of ginger for the prevention of postoperative nausea and vomiting. *Anaesthesia and Intensive Care* 23 (4): 449-452.

Trial design
Parallel. Patients received diazepam (10 mg) as oral presurgery medication plus two study medication capsules, one hour before induction of anesthesia. There were three groups of patients. They received either two placebo capsules, one capsule of 500 mg ginger plus one placebo capsule, or two capsules containing 500 mg ginger. Anesthesia was induced using thio-

pentone 4 to 5 mg/kg followed by vecuronium 0.1 mg/kg. Intraoperative and postoperative analgesia was provided by intravenous morphine.

Study duration	1 day
Dose	1 or 2 capsules of 500 mg ginger powder
Route of administration	Oral
Randomized	Yes
Randomization adequate	No
Blinding	Double-blind
Blinding adequate	Yes
Placebo	Yes
Drug comparison	No
Site description	Single center
No. of subjects enrolled	108
No. of subjects completed	108
Sex	Female
Age	19-70 years (mean: 32.3 years)

Inclusion criteria
Patients between 18 and 75 years undergoing gynecological laparoscopic surgery, American Society of Anesthesiology (ASA) physical status 1 or 2, under general anesthesia.

Exclusion criteria
Patients with known allergy to ginger or intolerance to spicy foods, who were pregnant or lactating, or receiving other antiemetic treatment.

End points
Three hours after the operation, patients were questioned as to whether they had experienced any nausea or vomiting since regaining consciousness. Nausea was graded as either present with one of three categories of severity or as absent, and vomiting was categorized as present or absent.

Results
The incidence of nausea and vomiting increased slightly but nonsignificantly with increasing dose of ginger. The incidence of moderate or severe nausea was 22 percent for placebo, 23 percent for 500 mg ginger, and 36 percent for 1000 mg ginger. The incidence of vomiting was 17 percent, 14 percent, and 31 percent in groups receiving 0, 500, and 1000 mg ginger, respectively.

Side effects
Flatulence, bloated feeling, and heartburn were reported in the ginger group.

Authors' comments
Powdered ginger (British Pharmacopoeia grade, 1988) is ineffective in reducing the incidence of postoperative nausea and vomiting.

Reviewers' comments
This is an excellent study. The subjects were limited to ASA 1 and 2 females. The inclusion of morphine in the anesthetic regimen and variations in surgical technique are covariables. The results may have been different for different surgeons or anesthetic techniques. The trial length was adequate. (3, 6)

Clinical Study: Ginger (Powdered)

Extract name	N/A
Manufacturer	Pharmacy Department of Mahidol University, Thailand
Indication	**Nausea and vomiting** (postoperative)
Level of evidence	**II**
Therapeutic benefit	**Undetermined**

Bibliographic reference
Visalyaputra S, Petchpaisit N, Somcharoen K, Choavaratana R (1998). The efficacy of ginger root in the prevention of postoperative nausea and vomiting after outpatient gynaecological laparoscopy. *Anaesthesia* 53 (5): 506-510.

Trial design
Parallel. Ginger and/or droperidol were given using a double-placebo method yielding 4 groups. Group 1: placebo capsules and 0.5 ml IV saline; group 2: placebo capsules plus 1.25 mg droperidol IV; group 3: two capsules of 0.5 g powdered ginger root plus saline IV; group 4: two capsules of 0.5 powdered ginger plus 1.25 mg droperidol IV. Study medications were taken one hour before induction of anesthesia induced with thiopentone (5 mg/kg) and fentanyl (1 µg/kg). One-half hour before discharge, every patient received another two capsules of either ginger root (0.5 g per capsule) or placebo. Paracetamol tablets were given for postoperative pain.

Study duration	1 day
Dose	2 (0.5 g) capsules before and after surgery
Route of administration	Oral
Randomized	Yes
Randomization adequate	No

Blinding	Double-blind
Blinding adequate	Yes
Placebo	Yes
Drug comparison	Yes
Drug name	Droperidol
Site description	Single center
No. of subjects enrolled	120
No. of subjects completed	111
Sex	Female
Age	Mean: 32.75 years

Inclusion criteria
Women age 20 to 40 years with ASA grade 1 or 2 who were scheduled for elective gynecological diagnostic laparoscopy.

Exclusion criteria
Patients who had received opioids or antiemetic drugs within 24 hours of the operation.

End points
The incidence and severity of nausea as well as the frequency of vomiting were recorded during the period in the recovery room and for 24 hours afterward. The degree of dizziness and sedation upon arrival into the recovery room were also recorded.

Results
There were no significant differences in the incidences of postoperative nausea, which were 32 percent, 20 percent, 22 percent, and 33 percent, and vomiting which were 35 percent, 15 percent, 25 percent, and 25 percent in the placebo, droperidol, ginger, and ginger plus droperidol groups, respectively.

Side effects
Not addressed.

Authors' comments
Ginger powder in the dose of 2 g, droperidol 1.25 mg, or both are ineffective in reducing the incidence of postoperative nausea and vomiting after gynecological laparoscopy.

Reviewers' comments
This trial had an insufficient sample size, and the variations in surgical technique may have affected the ability of this study to produce statistically sig-

nificant results. The subjects were limited to ASA 1 and 2, middle-aged females. The trial length was adequate. (3, 5)

Clinical Study: Ginger (Powdered)

Extract name	N/A
Manufacturer	Martindale Pharmaceuticals Pty Ltd., UK
Indication	**Nausea and vomiting** (postoperative)
Level of evidence	**III**
Therapeutic benefit	**Undetermined**

Bibliographic reference
Phillips S, Ruggier R, Hutchinson SE (1993). *Zingiber officinale* (ginger)—An antiemetic for day case surgery. *Anaesthesia* 48 (8): 715-717.

Trial design
Parallel. Three study groups: group A given two capsules of metoclopramide (10 mg total); group B given two capsules of powdered ginger root (1 g total); and group C given placebo. Study medications were administered one hour before induction of anesthesia. Anesthesia was induced with propofol 2.5 mg/kg and fentanyl 1 to 2 µg/g followed by atracurium 0.3 mg/kg.

Study duration	1 day
Dose	2 (500 mg) capsules of powdered ginger root
Route of administration	Oral
Randomized	Yes
Randomization adequate	No
Blinding	Double-blind
Blinding adequate	Yes
Placebo	Yes
Drug comparison	Yes
Drug name	Metoclopramide
Site description	Single center
No. of subjects enrolled	120
No. of subjects completed	120
Sex	Female
Age	Mean: 33.6 years

Inclusion criteria

Gynecological patients, ASA grades 1 to 3, scheduled for elective laparoscopic surgery as day patients.

Exclusion criteria

Patients who were pregnant or had ingested alcohol, opioids, or antiemetics in the 24 hours before surgery.

End points

Nausea and vomiting were observed at discharge from recovery room, at hospital discharge, and 24 hours postoperatively. The presence of pain and possible side effects were also recorded.

Results

The incidence of nausea and vomiting was similar in patients given metoclopramide and ginger (27 percent and 21 percent, respectively) and less than those who received placebo (41 percent).The requirement for postoperative antiemetics was lower in those patients receiving ginger. The requirements for postoperative analgesia recovery time and time until discharge were the same in all groups.

Side effects

There was no difference in the incidence of side effects between the three groups.

Authors' comments

Ginger is an effective and promising antiemetic suitable for day case patients with no documented side effects.

Reviewers' comments

The sample size may have been appropriate, given the significant results; however, no power calculation was presented. The standard/threshold for administering antiemetic treatment was not presented. Postoperative antiemetic regimen variation is a confounding covariable. Measuring the number of nausea complaints per patient does not have a clear correlation with severity or antiemetic efficacy. The anesthetic agent used, propofol, has known antiemetic effects. Perhaps the most relevant statements were that the mean time from induction to discharge was the same in all groups. Therefore there was no demonstrated impact on the parameter of primary motivation for the study—"delayed hospital discharge." "Antiemetics required more often" sounds convincing; however, it is meaningless without an established standard/threshold for treatment. Even then, it says more about the efficacy of the postoperative antiemetic regimen than it does the preoperative prophylaxis. The trial length was adequate. (3, 4)

Clinical Study: Ginger (Powdered)

Extract name	N/A
Manufacturer	Pharmacy Department at St. Bartholomew's Hospital, England

Indication	**Nausea and vomiting** (postoperative)
Level of evidence	**III**
Therapeutic benefit	**Undetermined**

Bibliographic reference
Bone ME, Wilkinson DJ, Young JR, McNeil J, Charlton S (1990). Ginger root—A new antiemetic: The effect of ginger root on postoperative nausea and vomiting after major gynecological surgery. *Anaesthesia* 45 (8): 669-671.

Trial design
Parallel. Ginger was compared to placebo and metoclopramide. Group 1 was given two capsules powdered ginger root (total 1 g) and placebo injection. Group 2 was given placebo capsules and metoclopramide (10mg) IV. Group 3 was given a double placebo. Capsules were given at the time of premedication and 1.5 hours before surgery, and intravenous medication was given at the induction of anesthesia. Patients were premedicated intramuscularly with papaveretum and scopolamine (hyoscine). Anesthesia was induced with a sleep dose of thiopentone, followed by alcuronium or vecuronium. Both ginger and placebo capsules were flavored with a "nonactive chemical essence of ginger." Nausea and vomiting after surgery were treated with metoclopramide, 10 mg intramuscularly, as required. Papaveretum or paracetamol was administered upon request for pain.

Study duration	1 day
Dose	2 capsules (500 mg) powdered ginger
Route of administration	Oral
Randomized	Yes
Randomization adequate	No
Blinding	Double-blind
Blinding adequate	Yes
Placebo	Yes
Drug comparison	Yes
Drug name	Metoclopramide
Site description	Hospital
No. of subjects enrolled	60
No. of subjects completed	60

| Sex | Female |
| Age | 16-65 years (mean: 40.6) |

Inclusion criteria
Patients with ASA grades 1 or 2, scheduled for major gynecological surgery.

Exclusion criteria
Patients who received opioid analgesia or antiemetics in the 24 hours before surgery.

End points
Patients were observed for symptoms of nausea and vomiting after recovery from anesthesia in recovery room, and at 4, 12, and 24 hours after the operation.

Results
Significantly fewer incidences of nausea were recorded in the group that received ginger root compared with placebo ($p < 0.05$). The number of incidences of nausea in the groups that received either ginger root or metoclopramide were similar. The administration of an antiemetic after the operation was significantly greater in the placebo group compared to the other two groups ($p < 0.05$).

Side effects
Very low and did not differ between treatments.

Authors' comments
Ginger root significantly reduced the incidence of postoperative emetic sequelae compared to placebo and had the same effect as metoclopramide.

Reviewers' comments
The nausea/vomiting data (N/V) were grouped rather than presented as individual numbers for each period. No prior history of predisposition to N/V was mentioned, e.g., CNS (vestibular) or GI disorders, or emetogenic medications taken. The sample size may not have been appropriate, as no power calculation was presented. The placebo group was older with a lower incidence of postoperative N/V and motion sickness and had shorter surgical times. The ginger group received more papaveretum intraoperatively. The nonuniform administration of papaveretum and paracetamol for postoperative analgesia creates a potentially confounding covariable. The administration of scopolamine (hyoscine) as an antiemetic creates a covariable which is a potential cofounder; unrecognized synergetic or other interactions are possible given that the mechanism of action of ginger is unknown. No reference was presented to demonstrate that the ginger flavoring used for the ginger and placebo pills lacks antiemetic or other potentially confounding bioactivity. The trial length was adequate. (3, 3)

Clinical Study: Ginger (Powdered)

Extract name	N/A
Manufacturer	None
Indication	**Severe nausea and vomiting in pregnancy** (hyperemesis gravidarum)
Level of evidence	**II**
Therapeutic benefit	**Yes**

Bibliographic reference
Fischer-Rasmussen W, Kjaer SK, Dahl C, Asping U (1990). Ginger treatment of hyperemesis gravidarum. *European Journal of Obstetrics and Gynecology and Reproductive Biology* 38 (1): 19-24

Trial design
Crossover. Four-day treatment periods with a two-day washout period in between.

Study duration	4 days
Dose	250 mg 4 times daily
Route of administration	Oral
Randomized	Yes
Randomization adequate	No
Blinding	Double-blind
Blinding adequate	No
Placebo	Yes
Drug comparison	No
Site description	Hospital (OB/GYN department)
No. of subjects enrolled	30
No. of subjects completed	27
Sex	Female
Age	18-39 years (mean: 26.4)

Inclusion criteria
Pregnant women admitted to the hospital with hyperemesis (nausea and vomiting) before the twentieth week of gestation and with symptoms lasting more than two days.

Exclusion criteria
Inability to take capsules. Subjects with gastrointestinal symptoms with probable origin in gallbladder or liver disease, duodenal ulcer, pancreatitis, etc.

End points

The severity and relief of symptoms were assessed using scoring systems. The severity score, conducted before the trial, noted the degree of nausea, vomiting, and weight loss. The relief score, evaluated on days 5 and 11 (after treatment) included a subjective assessment by the patient. Subjects were also observed for acetonuria and disturbance of hematocrit values.

Results

Subjective assessments by the women revealed that 70.4 percent stated preference to the period in which they received the ginger capsules, 14.8 percent preferred the placebo, and the remainder were unable to state a preference. The relief scores showed a significantly greater relief for ginger, especially in reducing the number of attacks of vomiting and the degree of nausea.

Side effects

No side effects were reported. No deformed infants were born. One spontaneous abortion occurred.

Authors' comments

Powdered root of ginger in daily doses of 1 g during four days was better than placebo in diminishing or eliminating vomiting during pregnancy.

Reviewers' comments

This is a good-quality study. No justification was given for the length of the washout period (two days). The subjective scale is not balanced between exacerbation and amelioration. The trial length was adequate. (5, 4)

Clinical Study: Ginger (Powdered)

Extract name	N/A
Manufacturer	None
Indication	**Nausea and/or vomiting in pregnancy**
Level of evidence	I
Therapeutic benefit	**Yes**

Bibliographic reference

Vutyavanich T, Kraisarin T, Ruangsri R-A (2001). Ginger for nausea and vomiting in pregnancy: Randomized, double-masked, placebo-controlled trial. *Obstetrics and Gynecology* 97 (4): 577-582.

Trial design

Parallel. Subjects were advised to divide their meals into frequent small ones low in fat and rich in carbohydrates.

Study duration	4 days
Dose	1 (250 mg) capsule 4 times daily
Route of administration	Oral
Randomized	Yes
Randomization adequate	No
Blinding	Double-blind
Blinding adequate	No
Placebo	Yes
Drug comparison	No
Site description	University hospital
No. of subjects enrolled	70
No. of subjects completed	67
Sex	Female
Age	Mean: 28.5 years

Inclusion criteria

Women who had attended an antenatal clinic before 17 weeks gestation and had nausea of pregnancy, with or without vomiting.

Exclusion criteria

Subjects were excluded if they had other medical disorders such as gastrointestinal diseases or hepatitis that may manifest with vomiting or nausea; were mentally retarded; had geographic or language barriers; had taken other medication in the previous week that might alleviate or aggravate nausea or vomiting; were unable to take the medication as prescribed; or were otherwise unable to participate in the trial.

End points

The primary outcome was improvement in symptoms of nausea. A visual analog scale and a Likert scale were used to measure nausea. Subjects completed a visual analog scale at their first visit and twice daily for the four days of treatment (at noon and bedtime). The five-item Likert scale was used at the one-week follow-up visit to assess the patients' response to ginger or placebo. Patients also recorded the number of vomiting episodes in the 24 hours prior to treatment and on each of the treatment days. Other secondary end points included side effects and adverse effects on pregnancy such as preterm birth, abortion, perinatal death, congenital anomaly, and delivery mode.

Results

The visual analog scores (after therapy minus baseline) of the subjects taking ginger decreased significantly as compared to the placebo group scores ($p = 0.014$). The number of vomiting episodes was also significantly decreased in the ginger group compared to the placebo group ($p < 0.001$). Using the Likert scale, 28 out of 32 subjects in the ginger group had improvement in symptoms of nausea compared to 10 of 35 in the placebo group ($p < 0.001$).

Side effects

Minor side effects occurred in both groups. Effects reported in the ginger group included headache, abdominal discomfort, heartburn, and diarrhea. Ginger did not have an adverse effect on pregnancy outcome.

Authors' comments

A significant improvement in nausea scores was found in subjects who received ginger compared with those who received placebo. Ginger also significantly reduced the mean number of vomiting episodes during the four days of treatment.

Reviewers' comments

Dietary modification to small, low-fat, carbohydrate-rich meals is a potential confounding variable. Compliance with prescribed diet was not assessed/reported. The ginger preparation used was well described but not chemically characterized (i.e., fresh Thai ginger, dried at 60°C for 24 hours, and ground into powder). The treatment length was adequate. (5, 6)

Clinical Study: Ginger (Powdered)

Extract name	N/A
Manufacturer	Martindale Pharmaceuticals Pty Ltd., UK
Indication	**Gastric motility; gastric emptying rate**
Level of evidence	**I**
Therapeutic benefit	**MOA**

Bibliographic reference

Phillips S, Hutchinson S, Ruggier R (1993). *Zingiber officinale* does not affect gastric emptying rate: A randomized, placebo-controlled, crossover trial. *Anaesthesia* 48 (5): 393-395.

Trial design

Crossover study. Patients received two capsules of either ginger or placebo in each study period. After at least a week they switched treatments. Before each study period, subjects abstained from alcohol and paracetamol for 24 hours and fasted for at least two hours.

Study duration	1 day
Dose	2 capsules (500 mg) powdered ginger root
Route of administration	Oral
Randomized	Yes
Randomization adequate	Yes
Blinding	Double-blind
Blinding adequate	Yes
Placebo	Yes
Drug comparison	No
Site description	Hospital
No. of subjects enrolled	16
No. of subjects completed	16
Sex	Male and female
Age	Not given

Inclusion criteria
Healthy volunteers at least 18 years old.

Exclusion criteria
Patients who were pregnant, had a gastrointestinal disease, or were taking any medication that affected gastric emptying.

End points
Gastric emptying was measured using a paracetamol absorption technique. The rate of gastric emptying was assessed by comparing the mean, peak, and time of peak plasma paracetamol concentrations, time to first detection of paracetamol in plasma, and the area under the paracetamol concentration time curve. Venous blood was taken at the same time as capsule administration and every 15 minutes for two hours.

Results
Ingestion of ginger did not affect gastric emptying. The mean and peak plasma paracetamol concentrations were similar in both groups.

Side effects
None reported by subjects.

Authors' comments
The antiemetic effect of ginger is not associated with an effect on gastric emptying.

Reviewers' comments
No documentation is given to support the assumption that ginger smell and taste additives have no gastrointestinal or pharmacologic effect. It is unclear whether lactose is suitably gastrointestinally inactive to serve as a placebo. The trial length was adequate. (5, 5)

Clinical Study: Ginger (Powdered)

Extract name	N/A
Manufacturer	None
Indication	**Cardiovascular risk factors; coronary artery disease**
Level of evidence	**III**
Therapeutic benefit	**MOA**

Bibliographic reference
Bordia A, Verma SK, Srivastava KC (1997). Effect of ginger (*Zingiber officinale* Rosc.) and fenugreek (*Trigonella foenumgraceum* L.) on blood lipids, blood sugar and platelet aggregation in patients with coronary artery disease. *Prostaglandins, Leukotrienes, and Essential Fatty Acids* 56 (5): 379-384.

Trial design
Parallel. Ginger was administered in two different doses: 4 g daily for three months and 10 g as a single dose. *Note:* Fenugreek was tested separately and that information is not included in this summary.

Study duration	3 months
Dose	4 g powdered ginger daily, or 10 g single dose
Route of administration	Oral
Randomized	No
Randomization adequate	No
Blinding	Not described
Blinding adequate	No
Placebo	Yes
Drug comparison	No

Site description   Not described

No. of subjects enrolled   60
No. of subjects completed   Not given
Sex   Not given
Age   Not given

Inclusion criteria
Patients with healed myocardial infarction (>6 months) with or without angina, all stable in their symptoms. All subjects were taking nitrates and aspirin; the aspirin was stopped two weeks before the study.

Exclusion criteria
Not mentioned.

End points
Two blood samples were collected before the trial at an interval of two weeks. During the three-month trial, patients were evaluated every month for clinical symptoms. Blood samples were collected after one and one-half months and three months. Blood samples were examined for lipid profile (total serum cholesterol, triglycerides, and HDL-C), blood sugar, plasma fibrinogen, fibrinolytic activity, and platelet aggregation.

Results
Ginger given at 4 g daily did not affect adenosine diphosphate (ADP)- and epinephrine-induced platelet aggregation, or fibrinolytic activity, fibrinogen levels, blood lipids, or blood sugar. However, a single dose of 10 g powdered ginger produced a significant reduction in platelet aggregation after four hours. Both ADP- and epinephrine-induced platelet aggregation were reduced significantly ($p < 0.05$).

Side effects
None noted.

Authors' comments
Ginger's antiartherosclerotic effect could be related to its antioxidant property and/or eicosanoid metabolism, since it did not affect the blood lipids, fibrinolytic activity, and fibrinogen level.

Reviewers' comments
No data were given concerning subjects' medications, medical history (comorbid conditions), or demographics. The sample size may not have been appropriate; no power calculation was presented. This study is of a type more similar to a phase IV clinical development trial; however, no conclusive phase I type (effective and toxic dose ranges) data were presented or referenced. Stopping aspirin in these patients carries a risk which is unwarranted

given the lack of any preliminary data demonstrating clear therapeutic efficacy. The dosage choices of 4 and 10 g were beyond the standard range for other trials. The trial length was apparently adequate. (0, 3)

Product Profile: Ginger (Raw), Stem Ginger

Manufacturer	**Toko Rinus, the Netherlands (root), Ambition, Polak Import, the Netherlands (stem)**
U.S. distributor	None
Botanical ingredient	**Ginger root and stem**
Extract name	N/A
Quantity	No information
Processing	Raw root or stem were cut up and put into custard
Standardization	No information

Source(s) of information: Janssen et al., 1996.

Clinical Study: Ginger (Raw), Stem Ginger

Extract name	N/A
Manufacturer	Toko Rinus, the Netherlands (root); Ambition, Polak Import, the Netherlands (stem)
Indication	**Cardiovascular risk factors; antiplatelet effect**
Level of evidence	**III**
Therapeutic benefit	**MOA**

Bibliographic reference
Janssen PLTMK, Meyboom S, van Staveren WA, de Vegt F, Katan MB (1996). Consumption of ginger (*Zingiber officinale* Roscoe) does not affect ex vivo platelet thromboxane production in humans. *European Journal of Clinical Nutrition* 50 (11): 772-774.

Trial design
Crossover study. Three consecutive two-week periods. Three treatments:

15 g of raw ginger root daily, 40 g of cooked stem ginger daily, or placebo; all supplied in vanilla custard.

Study duration	2 weeks
Dose	15 g of raw ginger root; 40 g stem ginger
Route of administration	Oral
Randomized	Yes
Randomization adequate	No
Blinding	Single-blind
Blinding adequate	No
Placebo	Yes
Drug comparison	No
Site description	Not described
No. of subjects enrolled	18
No. of subjects completed	18
Sex	Male and female
Age	Mean: 22 years

Inclusion criteria
Healthy subjects, nonsmokers, with normal values in routine lab tests.

Exclusion criteria
Subjects with urinary protein or glucose or high blood pressures.

End points
Fasting venous blood was drawn to measure thromboxane B2 production in maximally stimulated platelet-rich plasma at day 12 and day 14 of each treatment period.

Results
Daily treatment of ginger root or stem ginger for 14 days did not affect maximum ex vivo platelet thromboxane B2 production ($p = 0.616$). There was no significant effect on thromboxane production relative to placebo for raw ginger or stem ginger, and no effect of treatment order.

Side effects
None reported.

Authors' comments
The putative antithrombotic activity of ginger in humans cannot be confirmed.

Reviewers' comments
In the "Design and Treatments" section, it is evident that the trial was not conducted in a blinded fashion. The subjects were given their treatment materials to take home on the weekends to mix on their own. It is difficult to imagine how this could have been accomplished without the treatment groups being unblinded. The "cooked stem ginger" preparation was unusual enough that it should have been clearly described botanically, as well as its cooking protocol. The power calculation for this study was presented only by reference to a previous paper written by this author. The number of samples drawn per subject per treatment period was small. For some reason the effects of dry ginger root powder—the most common dosage form—were not evaluated in this study. Due to the broad variation in what could be considered "fresh" Brazilian ginger root or "cooked stem," the results of this study cannot be generally extrapolated to other ginger products/preparations. The trial length was adequate. (1, 4)

Ginkgo

Other common names: **Maidenhair tree**
Latin name: *Ginkgo biloba* **L.** [Ginkgoaceae]
Plant part: **Leaf**

PREPARATIONS USED
IN REVIEWED CLINICAL STUDIES

The ginkgo tree is native to China. It is the last surviving member of its family (Ginkgoaceae) and more closely resembles ancient ferns than deciduous trees. Ginkgo is extremely hardy, and specimens over one thousand years old have been reported in China, Korea, and Japan. The seeds have been used therapeutically in China and eastern Asia for over 2,000 years. Therapeutic use of the leaves has gained popularity in the past 40 years (Schulz, Hänsel, and Tyler, 2001).

Most of the ginkgo leaf products on the market are concentrated extracts with a ratio of roughly 50 parts leaf to 1 part extract. This means that the manufacturing procedure, which uses an acetone-water extraction and several purification steps, yields one kilogram of final product from 50 kilograms of dried ginkgo leaves. Standardized leaf extracts generally contain 22 to 27 percent flavonol glycosides, 5 to 7 percent terpene lactones (2.8 to 3.4 percent ginkgolides A, B, and C, and 2.6 to 3.2 percent bilobalide), and less than 5 ppm ginkolic acids. While many ginkgo constituents are purported to contribute to the herb's therapeutic effect, some of the constituents have been linked to specific pharmacological actions. The ginkgo flavonol glycosides are efficient free-radical scavengers, the ginkgolides inhibit platelet-activating factor, and the ginkgolides and bilobalide have demonstrated neuroprotective properties (Schulz, Hänsel, and Tyler, 2001; Foster and Tyler, 1999).

Ginkgold® and Ginkoba® are manufactured by Dr. Willmar Schwabe GmbH & Co. in Germany and are marketed in the United States by Nature's Way Products, Inc., and Pharmaton Natural Health

GINKGO SUMMARY TABLE

Product Name	Manufacturer/ U.S. Distributor	Product Characteristics	Dose in Trials	Indication	No. of Trials	Benefit (Evidence Level-Trial No.)
Single Ingredient Products						
Ginkgold®; Ginkoba®	Dr. Willmar Schwabe GmbH & Co., Germany/ Nature's Way Products, Inc.	Leaf extract (EGb 761®)	120-240 mg per day, up to 600 mg per day	Normal cognitive functioning	4	Yes (I-1, II-1), Trend (II-1), No (II-1)
				Age-related cognitive impairment	6	Yes (I-3, II-2), No (I-1)
	Pharmaton Natural Health Products			Dementia/ Alzheimer's disease	4	Yes (I-3, III-1)
			120-240 mg per day	Cerebro-vascular insufficiency	6	Yes (I-2, II-1, III-2), Trend (III-1)
			120 or 240 mg per day	Peripheral vascular disease	5	Yes (I-1, II-1, III-3)
			120 or 240 mg per day	Tinnitus (ringing in the ears)	1	Yes (I-1)
			120 or 240 mg per day	Sudden hearing loss	1	Trend (II-1)

Product	Manufacturer	Extract	Dose	Indication	No.	Evidence
Ginkai™* (US), Kaveri® (EU), Ginkyo® (EU)	Indena S.p.A., Italy; Lichtwer Pharma AG, Germany/ Lichtwer Pharma U.S., Inc.	Leaf extract (LI 1370; GinkgoSelect™)	160 or 320 mg per day	Protection against hypoxia	1	Yes (III-1)
				Antioxidant effects	1	Yes (III-1)
			40-240 mg per day	Electrophysiological effects	3	MOA (II-1, III-2)
			150 mg per day	Age-related cognitive impairment	4	Yes (I-1, III-2) Undetermined (III-1)
				Cognitive functioning after brain aneurysm operation	1	Yes (II-1)
				Normal cognitive functioning	1	Yes (II-1)
				Tinnitus (ringing in the ears)	1	No (I-1)
			112.5 or 300 mg per day	Micro-circulation	2	Yes (III-2)
			240 mg	Sleep quality (REM latency)	1	MOA (I-1)

GINKGO SUMMARY TABLE *(continued)*

Product Name	Manufacturer/ U.S. Distributor	Product Characteristics	Dose in Trials	Indication	No. of Trials	Benefit (Evidence Level-Trial No.)
GK501™	Pharmaton S.A., Switzerland/None	Leaf extract (GK 501™)	120-360 mg per day	Normal cognitive functioning	2	Yes (I-2)
Ginkgoforce	Bioforce AG, Switzerland/Bioforce USA	Alcoholic tincture of fresh leaves	60-120 drops per day	Age-related memory impairment	1	Trend (II-1)
Combination Product						
Ginkoba M/E™ (US), Gincosan ® (EU)	Pharmaton S.A., Switzerland/ Pharmaton Natural Health Products	Ginkgo leaf extract (GK501™) and ginseng root extract (G115®)**	80-960 mg daily	Cognitive functioning	3	Yes (I-1, II-1, III-1)

*Products that contain the Indena S.p.A GinkgoSelect extract as a single ingredient are listed below. The extract has been tested clinically but the final formulation has not.

Product Name	Manufacturer/Distributor
Ginkgo Biloba 24%	Enzymatic Therapy
GB24™	Thorne Research
Ginkgo Biloba	Swanson Health Products

**See the ginseng profile for information on the ginseng root extract G115.

Products, respectively. These products contain a patented ginkgo leaf extract called EGb 761® (50:1), which is characterized as containing 24 percent flavonol glycosides and 6 percent terpene lactones. EGb 761 is sold in Europe in products named Tanakan®, Rökan®, and Tebonin® forte.

Ginkai™ contains the ginkgo leaf extract LI 1370 which is standardized to contain 25 percent ginkgo flavonol glycosides and 6 percent terpenoids (ginkgolides and bilobalide). LI 1370 is manufactured by Lichtwer Pharma AG in Germany and contains the GinkgoSelect™ extract manufactured by Indena S.p.A., Italy. Ginkai is sold in the United States by Lichtwer Pharma U.S., Inc. LI 1370 is sold in Europe as Ginkyo® and Kaveri®. GinkgoSelect is also sold in the United States under the names Ginkgo Biloba-24% (Enzymatic Therapy®), GB24™ (Thorne Research), and Ginkgo Biloba (Swanson Health Products).

GK501™ is manufactured in Switzerland by Pharmaton S.A. It is characterized as containing 24 percent ginkgo flavonol glycosides and 6 percent terpene lactones. GK501 is not sold in the United States as a single-ingredient product.

Ginkoba M/E™ is a combination product that contains extracts of ginkgo leaves (GK501) and ginseng root (G115®). GK501 is characterized as containing 24 percent ginkgo flavonol glycosides and 6 percent terpene lactones, and G115 contains 4 percent ginsenosides. Ginkoba M/E is manufactured by Pharmaton S.A. in Switzerland and sold in the United States by Pharmaton Natural Health Products. This product is sold in Europe as Gincosan®.

Ginkgoforce, sold as Geriaforce in Europe, is a liquid tincture of fresh ginkgo leaves. Ginkgoforce has a plant-to-extract ratio of 1:9 and is made with 62 percent alcohol. Ginkgoforce is produced by Bioforce AG in Switzerland and sold by Bioforce USA in the United States.

SUMMARY OF REVIEWED CLINICAL STUDIES

Ginkgo products have been tested in clinical studies for their ability to improve cognitive function in a range of subjects, from normal healthy adults and those with age-related impairment to those with early-stage dementia and Alzheimer's disease. Ginkgo products have also been tested for treatment of cognitive dysfunction attributed to insufficient blood flow to the brain, termed cerebrovascular insufficiency or vascular dementia.

Dementia is a clinical syndrome characterized by losses of cognitive and emotional abilities that are sufficient to interfere with daily functioning and quality of life. The American Psychiatric Association, in its *Diagnostic and Statistical Manual of Mental Disorders* (DSM-IV-TR) (2000), defines the diagnostic features of dementia as memory impairment, deterioration of language function (aphasia), impaired ability to execute activities despite intact muscles, senses, and comprehension of the task (apraxia), and disturbances in executive functioning (the ability to think abstractly and to plan, initiate, sequence, monitor, and conclude complex behavior). Dementia can be mild (work and social activities are impaired but the capacity for independent living remains), moderate (independent living is hazardous and some supervision is required), or severe (daily living activities are impaired, continuous supervision is required, and the person is largely incoherent or mute). Dementia can be caused by Alzheimer's disease, vascular disease, human immunodeficiency virus (HIV), head trauma, Parkinson's disease, Huntington's disease, Pick's disease, Creutzfeldt-Jakob disease, substance abuse, and other medical conditions.

Alzheimer's disease is observed as a gradual and progressive cognitive decline. Diagnosis of Alzheimer's disease is often made once other causes of dementia have been ruled out, due to a lack of laboratory markers. Cerebrovascular disease can cause vascular dementia diagnosed by characteristic neurological signs or laboratory evidence. Symptoms include transient ischemic attacks (ministrokes), hemipareses, tinnitus (ringing in the ears), dizziness, headache, and anxiety (Schulz, Halama, and Hoerr, 2000).

Ginkgo has also been tested in treatment of cramping and pain in the legs while walking, a condition termed intermittent claudication. This condition is due to mild to moderate peripheral arterial disease (peripheral arterial occlusive disease), in which narrowing of the arteries limits the blood supply to the legs. Early stages of the disease are without symptoms, but later stages are associated with leg pain and muscle cramps upon walking and, ultimately, ischemic ulceration, gangrene, and tissue loss. The stages have been classified in a system according to Fontaine: stage I represents those who are asymptomatic with isolated arterial stenosis of the lower limbs; stage II is mild to moderately severe leg pain and muscle cramps upon walking; stage III are those with pain while resting; and stage IV are those with ulcerations and gangrene. Ginkgo has been tested in the treatment of stage IIb, in which subjects have a pain-free walking distance of 200 meters or less (Peters, Kieser, and Holscher, 1998).

EGb 761

By far, the majority of clinical trials on ginkgo have been conducted on products containing the EGb 761 extract. We include here a total of 32 controlled clinical studies covering indications of cognitive function (normal and age-related impairment), dementia (including Alzheimer's disease), insufficient blood flow to the brain or extremities, tinnitus, and antioxidant effects.

Normal Cognitive Functioning

Four trials that looked at the effect of EGb 761 on cognitive function in normal volunteers reported mixed results. The largest study, including 203 adults over 60 years old without cognitive impairment, did not report any benefit from Ginkoba, 40 mg three times daily for six weeks, compared to placebo. The study used a battery of tests to measure cognitive function as well as a self-reported memory function questionnaire and a global rating by a companion (Solomon et al., 2002). Another trial included 40 volunteers (55 to 88 years old) who took 120 mg extract or placebo for six weeks and reported improvements in speed of mental processing following treatment. Participants receiving treatment judged their memory as improved, but objective memory tests did not reveal any statistical improvement (Mix and Crews, 2000). Two small crossover trials examined the effect of one dose of ginkgo on reaction time and memory. In both trials, memory improved one hour after administration of 600 mg extract. One of the trials, with eight women aged 25 to 40 years, reported a selective but marked improvement in working memory (Hindmarch, 1986). The other trial, with 12 females, mean age 22 years, failed to replicate the benefit to working memory but did find evidence of improved secondary memory (Warot et al., 1991). Other measurements of reaction time or the activity of the central nervous system in general did not change in either trial.

Age-Related Cognitive Impairment

Five good-quality trials looked at elderly people with cognitive impairment attributed to aging. All trials used cognitive test batteries, four of them computerized. The patients in these trials all satisfied the criteria of age-associated memory impairment and, in the more extreme trials, mild cognitive impairment. All trials showed statistically significant benefits to one or more aspects of cognitive function, including attention, information processing, and both short- and long-term memory. Four trials ranged in length from three months to one year and used a dose of 120 or 160 mg extract per day. Improvement was observed after one month (Rai, Shovlin, and Wesnes, 1991; Wesnes et al., 1987; Israel et al., 1987; Taillandier et al., 1986). The largest trial (122 subjects) and longest running (one year) reported an increase in the Geriatric Clinical Evaluation score after three months of treatment with continued improvement for the remainder of the year (Taillandier et al., 1986). The fifth trial, which included a series of one-day experiments, showed improvement in a computerized test of information processing completed one hour after taking doses of 320 or 600 mg extract (Allain et al., 1993).

Age-Related Cognitive Impairment/Dementia and Alzheimer's Disease

A study included elderly adults with either dementia or non-demented age-associated memory impairment. A total of 214 participants with a mean age of 83 years included 63 with dementia due to Alzheimer's disease or vascular origins and 151 with age-related memory loss. The majority of the Mini-Mental State Examination (MMSE) scores were in the range of 12 to 24, signaling moderate impairment. The participants were divided into three groups for the initial three months and given 160 or 240 mg EGb 761 or placebo. The groups taking EGb 761 were randomized again to either continue with ginkgo or to take placebo for the rest of the six-month study. The initial placebo group continued to take placebo. An intention-to-treat analysis showed no effect on neuropsychological testing, clinical assessment of symptoms, depressive mood, self-perceived memory, health, or behavior in either the relatively small group that took ginkgo (79) or the placebo group (44) for the entire six months. In addition, no beneficial effects were observed due to the higher ginkgo dose or longer duration of treatment. In short, none of the subgroups benefited from ginkgo compared to placebo (van Dongen et al., 2000).

Dementia and Alzheimer's Disease

Four good-quality trials, two large and two small, found a benefit from treatment with ginkgo on dementia. The two large well-conducted positive trials included a combined total of 293 patients with either Alzheimer's disease or vascular (multiple infarct) dementia. One study used a dose of 240 mg per day and continued for six months (Kanowski et al., 1997). The other used a dose of 120 mg per day and lasted for one year (Le Bars et al., 1997). In both studies, the treatment groups showed improvement after six months of dosing according to the following scales: Sundrom-Kurztest (SKT) (a brief test of cognitive function, memory, and attention), Clinical Global Impressions (CGI) (clinicians' interview-based quantified judgment of the amount of change in overall impairment), Alzheimer's Disease Assessment Scale (ADAS-cog) (a performance-based cognitive test that objectively evaluates memory, language, praxis, and orientation), and Geriatric Evaluation by Relatives Rating Instrument (GERRI) (an inventory completed by the caregiver) (Kanowski et al., 1997; Le Bars et al., 1997). According to our reviewer, Dr. Keith Wesnes, this well-known ginkgo study shows a benefit from ginkgo comparable to current pharmacological therapies of choice, e.g., Aricept. A reanalysis of the Le Bars and colleagues (1997) study included a stratification of Alzheimer's patients according to severity of cognitive impairment. The relative changes from baseline depended upon the severity of the disease. Significant improvement compared to baseline according to the ADAS-cog and GERRI was observed in those with mild cognitive impairment (MMSE more than 23). While in patients with moderate to severe dementia (MMSE less than 23), there was less deterioration in the EGb 761 group compared to baseline than that observed in the placebo group (Le Bars et al., 2002). The two small trials had a combined total of 58 patients with Alzheimer's disease who were given 240 mg per day for three months. The studies demonstrated improvement with treatment, compared with placebo, according to the SKT test (Maurer et al., 1997; Hofferberth, 1994).

Cerebrovascular Insufficiency

Six trials looked at cognitive function in elderly people with dysfunction attributed to insufficient blood flow to the brain. Symptoms of this disorder, called cerebrovascular insufficiency or cerebroorganic psychosyndrome, include transient ischemic attacks, hemipareses, tinnitus, dizziness, headache, and anxiety. Five of the six studies used doses of 120 or 160 mg per day for seven weeks to six months and reported clear and significant benefits in cognitive function that were based upon either performance or subjective ratings. Two of these studies, with a total of 92 subjects, were deemed to be of excellent quality and reported improvement in short-term memory, awareness, and rate of learning (Grassel, 1992; Halama, Bartsch, and Meng, 1988). In the third good-quality, but small, study with 24 subjects, changes in electroencephalogram (EEG) patterns in the treatment group correlated with a reduction in abnormally elevated venous microembolism (a laboratory indicator of blood platelet aggregation). This result indicated an improvement in blood flow may play a role in the clinically observed cognitive improvement (Hofferberth, 1991b). Two other studies had clearly defined positive end points in cognitive function, saccadic eye movement, and EEG changes (Hofferberth, 1989), as well as symptoms of tinnitus, anxiety, attention, higher function, and memory (Arrigo, 1986), but failed to describe the blinding and randomization processes. The sixth study of this group included 20 patients who were depressed, in addition to having cerebrovascular insufficiency. Following a dose of 240 mg per day for two months, there were patterns of improvement in reaction times and depression symptoms in the treatment group in comparison with the placebo group (Halama, 1990).

Peripheral Vascular Disease

Five trials looked at effects of ginkgo on peripheral vascular disease stage IIb according to Fontaine. Subjects had intermittent claudication (leg pain and cramps) and a pain-free walking distance of less than 200 meters. Four of the five trials were placebo controlled and showed important improvements in pain-free walking distances for patients following treatment of 120 mg extract per day for six months. None of the studies indicated any gross improvement in blood flow of the ischemic leg as measured in Doppler studies comparing blood pressure in the ankle to blood pressure in the arm. One excellent-quality, parallel, placebo-controlled trial that included a total of 54 patients reported an increase in pain-free walking distance from 94.5 m to 147 m following treatment. There was also a 42 percent increase in total walking distance for the treatment group, compared to an 8 percent increase in the placebo group (Blume, Kieser, and Holscher, 1996). Three other studies, with a total of 225 subjects, reported similar findings (Bauer, 1984; Thomson et al., 1990; Peters, Kieser, and Holscher, 1998). A six-month dose-response study reported significantly greater increases in pain-free walking distance and maximum walking distance with a doubling of the standard dose; the trial compared the usual 120 mg per day to 240 mg per day (Schweizer and Hautmann, 1999).

Tinnitus

A well-conducted trial focusing on tinnitus (the perception of sound in the absence of external stimuli or "ringing in the ears") reported a clear clinical benefit for those taking ginkgo. In this trial which included 78 patients with tinnitus for at least the previous two months, a dose of 120 mg extract per day produced a statistical reduction in sound volume after ten weeks compared to baseline. No significant change was noted in the placebo group (Morgenstern, 1997).

Sudden Hearing Loss

A trial with 78 adults with sudden hearing loss (of at least 15 dB, within ten days before entry into the study) compared a dose of 24 mg to 240 mg daily for two months. A large majority of subjects in both groups recovered their hearing. The higher dose showed an advantage over the lower dose for those without tinnitus, but not for those with tinnitus (Burschka et al., 2001).

Protection Against Hypoxia

A poorly described placebo-controlled pilot trial using eight healthy male volunteers showed that 160 mg extract per day for two weeks helped reduce the deficits in both attention and saccadic eye movements produced by hypoxia (lack of oxygen to the brain) (Schaffler and Reeh, 1985).

Antioxidant Effects

Another placebo-controlled pilot study demonstrated that taking EGb 761 before surgery limited oxidative stress in plasma and showed signs of improving patient recovery. The study included 15 patients undergoing coronary bypass surgery who were given 320 mg extract per day or placebo for five days before surgery (Pietri et al., 1997).

Electrophysiological Effects

Three studies explored the effect of EGb 761 on brain electroencephalogram recordings. Two of the studies suggested an increase in alpha activity that was consistent with a nootropic or cognitive enhancing action (Itil and Martorano, 1995; Luthringer, d'Arbigny, and Macher, 1995). The third study did not report any clear effect on the EEG profile (Kunkel, 1993). The studies used doses ranging from 40 to 160 mg extract and were all short term with testing following either one treatment or at most five days of treatment.

LI 1370

We reviewed ten studies conducted on ginkgo extract LI 1370. Three of four trials showed a benefit for age-related cognitive impairment. A benefit was also observed for subjects recovering from a brain aneurysm and subsequent operation, as well as normal volunteers. LI 1370 appeared to benefit microcirculation in two studies but showed no benefit for tinnitus in another. A sleep study indicated that LI 1370 does not have cholinergic activity.

Age-Related Cognitive Impairment

The largest trial, which included a total of 209 outpatients, mean age 69, with cerebral insufficiency, reported a significant improvement after six weeks in forgetfulness, depression, and headache with treatment of 150 mg extract per day in comparison to placebo. After 12 weeks, there was significant improvement in additional symptoms of memory gaps, difficulty concentrating, tendency to fatigue, lack of drive, and tinnitus in comparison to placebo (Bruchert, Heinrich, and Ruf-Kohler, 1991). Another good-quality three-month trial with 86 subjects with cerebral insufficiency due to old age reported similar findings. Significant improvement was seen in short-term memory, attention to tasks, and subjective performance from the sixth week onward with a dose of 150 mg extract per day in comparison to placebo (Vesper and Hansgen, 1994).

A trial studied 50 elderly people with failing mental performance. Significant benefits to cognitive function according to both psychometric and neurophysiologic tests were observed after three weeks of treatment compared with placebo. LI 1370 was given in a dose of 50 mg three times daily for six weeks (Hofferberth, 1991a). However, the methodology of the trial was considered poor.

A pilot study with 15 subjects measured EEG changes in mildly impaired subjects with age-related signs of cerebral insufficiency. Treatment with 150 mg LI 1370 for three months did not cause a general change in EEG activity. However, when the subjects were stressed by sleep deprivation, causing a reversible decrease in mental performance, there were significant changes in theta waves and the alpha slow-wave sleep index in the ginkgo group compared to the placebo group. The authors concluded that ginkgo causes EEG changes that are situation and stimulus dependent (Schulz, Jobert, and Breuel, 1991).

Brain Aneurysm

A good-quality trial included 42 people recovering from brain aneurysms and subsequent operations. After 12 weeks of treatment with 150 mg LI 1370 per day, a statistically significant improvement was seen in reaction times, the number of errors, and short-term verbal memory in comparison to baseline and to the placebo group (Maier-Hauff, 1991).

Normal Cognitive Functioning

A dose-comparison trial included 31 healthy volunteers who showed improved performance in short-term memory tasks after two days' dosing with quantities of 50 and 100 mg extract three times daily or 120 mg and 240 mg once daily compared to placebo. More improvement occurred in a subset of older volunteers, but there was no indication of a dose-response relationship for the group as a whole (Rigney, Kimber, and Hindmarch, 1999). Our reviewer, Dr. Wesnes, commented that the authors did not state their method of blinding the five different treatments, nor did they give the rationale for the different dosage regimens.

Tinnitus

A large study included 909 healthy volunteers who had had tinnitus for over a year. They were treated with 50 mg three times daily or placebo for three months. As a result, there was no significant benefit for ginkgo over placebo (Drew and Davies, 2001).

Microcirculation

Two trials demonstrated improvements to microcirculation; one of them also showed improvements in retinal circulation, while the other also showed improvements in blood flow in nail fold capillaries. The first study included a group of 24 hypertensive individuals, with fundus hypertonicus who were treated with 300 mg per day LI 1370 or placebo for six weeks. Retinal blood flow increased, circulation time decreased, and blood viscosity decreased compared to the placebo group (Koza, Ernst, and Sporl, 1991). The second study was a small crossover study with single doses (45 ml solution) containing either 112.5 mg dry extract or a placebo (composed of inactive excipients in the formulation) given to ten healthy subjects. The result was a 15.6 percent decrease in erythrocyte aggregation and a 57 percent increase in blood flow in nail fold capillaries in the ginkgo group (Jung et al., 1990).

Sleep Quality (REM Latency)

A small mode-of-action study explored whether LI 1370 had cholinergic activity, as measured by its effect on latency to rapid eye movement (REM) in sleep. Ten healthy volunteers were given placebo or 240 mg ginkgo two hours before going to bed in a sleep lab. No comparative effect on sleep was measured. However, the authors did not rule out a cholinergic mechanism for LI 1370, as REM sleep can be affected by other factors such as noradrenaline or serotonin function (Murray, Cowen, and Sharpley, 2001).

GK501, Ginkoba M/E

Cognitive Functioning

Cognitive function and attention speed scores improved in a good-quality pilot trial with 20 young volunteers given single doses of 120, 240, or 360 mg GK501 extract. Dose-dependent improvements in attention appeared two and one-half hours after dosing with 240 and 360 mg and were still present after six hours. Changes in speed of memory and accuracy of information did not follow a pattern (Kennedy, Scholey, and Wesnes, 2000).

Another study examined the effects of ginkgo extract GK501, ginseng extract G115, the combination of the two (Ginkoba M/E), and placebo on cognitive functioning up to six hours after dosing in 20 young volunteers. There was a dose-dependent improvement in speed in an arithmetic task (serial threes) with doses of 120, 240, and 360 mg of ginkgo extract. Ginseng improved accuracy and slowed responses in the serial sevens arithmetic task with doses of 200, 400, and 600 mg. Ginkoba M/E produced a sustained increase in the number of serial sevens responses with a dose of 320 mg. Higher doses of 640 and 960 mg also improved accuracy in both serial threes and serial sevens tests (Scholey and Kennedy, 2002).

The product combining extracts GK501 and G115 (Ginkoba M/E) was tested for its effect on cognitive function in three additional trials. Improvements in quality of memory were demonstrated in all three studies, reflecting selective improvement in the ability to store and retrieve information from short- and long-term memory. Other cognitive aspects such as attention were not improved. The first study compared the effects of three doses (80, 160, and 320 mg) for three months on healthy volunteers with neurasthenia (fatigue, lack of motivation, and feelings of inadequacy) (Wesnes et al., 1997). The second study included a large number (256) of healthy, middle-aged volunteers given either 320 mg or placebo daily for three and one-half months. In this trial, benefits persisted 14 days after termination of treatment (Wesnes et al., 2000). The third study compared single doses of 320, 640, or 960 mg of the combination in a small study with healthy young volunteers (Kennedy, Scholey, and Wesnes, 2001).

Geriaforce (Ginkgoforce)

Age-Related Memory Impairment

A large trial (197 subjects) conducted on people with age-induced memory disorders compared two doses of Ginkgoforce (60 or 120 drops per day) with placebo in a six-month trial. The results of the trial were partly compromised by not training the subjects on tests prior to the study, with the result that training effects appeared on all assessments. Nonetheless, improvements were greater with ginkgo on the Benton test measuring visual short-term memory (Degenring and Brautigam, 1999).

META-ANALYSES AND SYSTEMATIC REVIEWS

Several meta-analyses and systematic reviews of the clinical literature on ginkgo have been published. A summary of analyses of trials treating Alzheimer's disease, dementia, cerebral insufficiency, intermittent claudication (a symptom of peripheral arterial disease), and tinnitus is given in this section.

An objective measure of the effect of ginkgo (products not differentiated) on cognitive function in patients with Alzheimer's disease was attempted in a meta-analysis of randomized, placebo-controlled, double-blind studies. The four studies that met the inclusion criteria contained a total of 212 subjects treated with ginkgo and 212 with placebo. The authors found a small but significant effect after three to six months of treatment with 120 to 240 mg ginkgo extract, EGb 761, compared to placebo. The modest effect size (0.40, $p < 0.0001$), calculated from reported p-values for cognitive measures and sample sizes, translated into a 3 percent difference in the Alzheimer's Disease Assessment Scale-cognitive subset (Oken, Storzbach, and Kaye, 1998). Published one year later, a systematic review of the treatment of dementia with ginkgo (EGb 761) included nine double-blind, randomized, placebo-controlled trials. The authors concluded that the majority of trials support the notion that ginkgo is efficacious in delaying the clinical deterioration of patients with dementia, or in bringing about symptomatic improvement. However, the authors also commented that none of the trials were flawless or completely convincing (Ernst and Pittler, 1999).

An evaluation of the treatment of age-related cognitive impairment or dementia of any type with any ginkgo extract compared to placebo was undertaken in a meta-analysis including 33 randomized, double-blind studies. The authors concluded that, compared to placebo, ginkgo showed significant benefit for cognition at doses less than 200 mg/day and more so with doses more than 200 mg/day, both for 12 weeks (95 percent CI $-1.09, -0.05$, $p = 0.03$; 95 percent CI -1.12 to 0.0, $p = 0.008$). Benefits in cognition were also found following 24 weeks with any ginkgo dose (95 percent CI -0.32 to -0.02, $p = 0.03$). Activities of daily living also showed a benefit with doses less than 200 mg/day for 12 weeks. Measures of mood and emotional function showed benefit compared to placebo with doses less than 200 mg/day in treatment lasting 12 weeks and in shorter durations. The authors concluded that overall there is promising evidence of improvement in cognition and function associated with ginkgo. However, they also commented that many of the earlier trials used unsatisfactory methods and were small in size. They could also not rule out publication bias and expressed the need for a large trial using modern methodology and intention-to-treat analysis (Birks et al., 2002).

A meta-analysis of studies exploring the efficacy of the ginkgo preparation LI 1370 (Kaveri® forte) in aged patients with cerebral insufficiency included 11 randomized, placebo-controlled, double-blind trials. In most studies the dose was 150 mg extract per day. The parameters examined were single symptoms, total score of clinical symptoms, and global effectiveness. All single-symptom scores that were analyzed demonstrated superiority compared to placebo. In eight studies, upon which analysis of the total score of clinical symptoms could be conducted, seven of the studies confirmed LI 1370's effectiveness compared to placebo, and one study found no difference between the two. Global effectiveness, as evaluated by physicians and patients, was confirmed in five of six studies that allowed this analysis (Hopfenmuller, 1994).

Significant increases in pain-free walking distance compared to placebo for patients with intermittent claudication was reported in a meta-analysis of eight randomized, placebo-controlled, double-blind studies. Overall, the increase was 34 meters (37 yards). The dose was either 120 mg or 160 mg of various ginkgo extracts, and the length of treatment for the majority of the trials was 24 weeks, with one trial lasting six weeks and another for 12 weeks (Pittler and Ernst, 2000).

A systematic review summarized randomized, controlled trials using ginkgo for tinnitus. Five studies fulfilled the entry criteria, and the results of these studies suggest that ginkgo is effective in treating tinnitus. One study produced a negative result, but the dose used in the study was much lower (29 mg extract daily) than the usual 120 to 160 mg extract per day used in the other studies. The studies used several different products with either liquid or solid formulations, different routes of administration (one trial used injections), and different lengths of treatment (two weeks to three months). The variability in methodology, end point measurement, dose, and patient classification made a firm conclusion about efficacy difficult (Ernst and Stevinson, 1999).

Alzheimer's disease is associated with a deficiency of the neurotransmitter acetylcholinesterase. A relatively new class of drugs that delays the decomposition of the neurotransmitter has been shown to enhance the cognitive performance of persons with that disease. A comparison of efficacy studies of acetylcholinesterase inhibitors with efficacy studies of ginkgo extract EGb 761 was published. The study results were compared using intent-to-treat analyses of the Alzheimer's Disease Assessment Scale (ADAS-Cog) scores. Two ginkgo studies were compared with one study each for the following acetylcholinesterase inhibitors: rivastigmine, tacrine, metrifonate, and donepezil. The authors reported finding a similar delay in disease progression over a six-month period with both types of treatment (Wettstein, 1999/2000).

ADVERSE REACTIONS OR SIDE EFFECTS

Adverse effects noted in the reviewed trials included abdominal complaints, nausea, and dyspepsia. A meta-analysis published in 1998 noted that the incidence of adverse effects was not different from placebo in the four studies reviewed. In these studies the dose was either 120 to 240 mg per day for three to six months and a total of 424 subjects were included (Oken, Storzbach, and Kaye, 1998). A large postmarketing surveillance study including 1,357 doctors who treated 10,815 patients with dementia with ginkgo extract (LI 1370) reported only mild adverse events in 1.7 percent of patients. The main adverse symptoms observed were nausea (0.34 percent), headache (0.22 percent), stomach complaints (0.14 percent), and allergic reactions (0.09 percent) (Burkard and Lehrl, 1991).

Five case reports of bleeding that may be linked to ginkgo were reported between 1996 and 1998. Three of the patients were reported to have been in good health, one 33 years old and the others aged 61 and 72 years (Rowin and Lewis, 1996; Gilbert, 1997; Vale, 1998). Two had cardiovascular disease and were already taking anticoagulants (aspirin, warfarin) (Matthews, 1998; Rosenblatt and Mindel, 1997).

These reports raised concerns regarding ginkgo and its possible effects on blood thinning and/or interactions with other blood thinners. Five clinical studies that have explored this topic are summarized here. Two studies indicate that ginkgo might inhibit platelet aggregation, but none indicate any alteration in bleeding times. One study indicates a lack of interaction with the blood thinner warfarin.

A study reported inhibition of ex vivo platelet aggregation in 12 volunteers administered 240 mg EGb 761 extract for seven days (Klein, 1988). In another study with six healthy males, administration of a single dose of 600 mg EGb 761 extract reduced ex vivo platelet aggregation but did not alter prothrombin bleeding time or skin bleeding time (Guinot et al., 1989). A trial with 50 healthy male volunteers given 240 mg EGb 761 per day or placebo for seven days in a crossover design reported no alteration of bleeding time, coagulation parameters, or platelet activation (Kohler, Funk, and Kieser, in press). Another crossover study which also included 50 healthy males reported no additional effect on bleeding times or platelet aggregation (agonists included adenosine diphosphate, epinephrine, platelet activating factor, and collagen) when 120 mg EGb 761 was administered along with 500 mg aspirin (Wolf, in press). A double-blind, crossover study with 21 middle-aged patients on stable long-term warfarin treatment found that the addition of 100 mg ginkgo extract (Bio-Biloba®, Pharma Nord ApS, Denmark) over four weeks did not alter International Normalized Ratio (INR) values, a standardized measurement of clotting time (Engelsen, Nielsen, and Winter, 2002).

Some indications from animal studies suggest that ginkgo extract may inhibit monoamine oxidase (MAO). MAO inhibitors are used to elevate mood in depressed individuals, but their use as antidepressants has been limited due to concerns over interactions with foods high in tyamine content (e.g., cheese) and many drugs. A small pilot study with ten subjects determined that 129 mg EGb 761 extract per day for one month had no effect on MAO in the brain, neither MAO_A or MAO_B. The authors point out that this study does not rule out MAO inhibition in peripheral organs. However, no reports of adverse events suggest significant MAO inhibition (Fowler et al., 2000).

INFORMATION FROM PHARMACOPOEIAL MONOGRAPHS

Sources of Published Therapeutic Monographs

German Commission E
World Health Organization (WHO)

Indications

The German Commission E approves of the use of a dry extract of the dried leaf that is manufactured using acetone/water with subsequent purification steps, without addition of concentrates or isolated ingredients, and with a drug/extract ratio of 35 to 67:1, on average 50:1. The Commission E and World Health Organization further stipulate that the preparation contain 22 to 27 percent flavone glycosides and 5 to 7 percent terpene lactones, of which approximately 2.8 to 3.4 percent consists of ginkgolides A, B, and C and 2.6 to 3.2 percent bilobalide. The level of ginkgolic acids is below 5 mg/kg. Both organizations indicate use in cases of demential syndromes (in primary degenerative dementia, vascular dementia, and mixed forms of both) with symptoms including memory deficits, disturbances in concentration, depressive emotional condition, dizziness, tinnitus, and headache; improvement of pain-free walking distance in peripheral arterial occlusive disease in stage II of Fontaine (intermittent claudication); and vertigo and tinnitus of vascular and involutional origin (Blumenthal et al., 1998; WHO, 1999).

Doses

Extract:
- Dry: 120 to 240 mg daily in two or three divided doses (WHO, 1999)
- Fluid: (1:1), 0.5 ml three times daily (WHO, 1999)

Note: The Commission E suggests specific dosages for certain indications:
- For demential syndromes: 120 to 240 mg native dry extract in two or three doses daily (Blumenthal et al., 1998)
- For walking improvement, vertigo, and tinnitus: 120-160 mg native dry extract in two or three doses daily (Blumenthal et al., 1998)

Treatment Period

The Commission E suggests these treatment lengths for the following indications: for demential syndromes, treatment length depends on severity of symptoms but should last at least eight weeks for chronic illnesses; for walking improvement, treatment should be at least six weeks; and for vertigo and tinnitus, administration for more than six to eight weeks has no therapeutic benefit (Blumenthal et al., 1998).

Contraindications

The Commission E and the WHO list the following contraindication: hypersensitivity to *Ginkgo biloba* preparations (Blumenthal et al., 1998; WHO, 1999).

Adverse Reactions

The following adverse reactions are listed as occurring infrequently by the Commission E and the WHO: stomach or intestinal upsets, headaches, or allergic skin reaction (Blumenthal et al., 1998; WHO, 1999).

Precautions

The Commission E and the WHO list no known precautions (Blumenthal et al., 1998; WHO, 1999).

Drug Interactions

The Commission E lists no known drug interactions (Blumenthal et al., 1998).

REFERENCES

Allain H, Raoul P, Lieury A, LeCoz F, Gandon JM, d'Arbigny P (1993). Effect of two doses of *Ginkgo biloba* extract (EGb 761) on the dual-coding test in elderly subjects. *Clinical Therapeutics* 15 (3): 549-558.

Arrigo A (1986). Treatment of chronic cerebrovascular insufficiency with *Ginkgo biloba* extract. *Therapiewoche* 36: 5208-5218.

Bauer U (1984). 6-month double-blind randomized clinical trial of *Ginkgo biloba* extract versus placebo in two parallel groups in patients suffering from peripheral arterial insufficiency. *Arzneimittel-Forschung/Drug Research* 34 (6): 716-720.

Birks J, Grimley Evans J, Van Dongen M (2002). *Ginkgo biloba* for cognitive impairment and dementia (Cochrane Review). In *The Cochrane Library*, Issue 4. Oxford: Update Software.

Blume J, Kieser M, Holscher U (1996). Placebo-controlled double-blind study on the efficacy of *Ginkgo biloba* special extract EGb 761 in the maximum-level trained patients with intermittent claudication. *Zeitschrift fur Gefasskrankheiten/Journal for Vascular Diseases* 25 (3): 265-274.

Blumenthal M, Busse W, Hall T, Goldberg A, Gruenwald J, Riggins C, Rister S, eds. (1998). *The Complete German Commission E Monographs: Therapeutic Guide to Herbal Medicines*. Trans. S Klein. Austin, TX: American Botanical Council.

Bruchert E, Heinrich SE, Ruf-Kohler P (1991). Wirksamkeit von LI 1370 bei alteren patienten mit hirnleistungsschwache. *Munchener Medizinische Wochenschrift* 133 (Suppl 1): S9-S14.

Burkard G, Lehrl S (1991). Verhaltnis von Demenzen vom Multi-infarkt-und Alzheimertyp in arzlichen Praxen: Diagnostische und therapeutische Konsequenzen am Beispiel eines *Ginkgo-biloba*-Praparates. *Münchener Medizinische Wochenschrift* 133 (Suppl. 1): S38-S43.

Burschka MA, Hassan HAH, Reineke T, van Bebber L, Caird DM, Mösges R (2001). Effect of treatment with *Ginkgo biloba* extract EGb 761 (oral) on unilateral idiopathic sudden hearing loss in a prospective randomized double-blind study of 106 outpatients. *European Archives of Oto-Rhino-Laryngology* 258 (5): 213-219.

Degenring FH, Brautigam MRH (1999). Geriaforce for the treatment of age-induced memory disorders: A placebo-controlled double-blind study with two dosages. *Schweizerische Zeitschrift fur GanzheitsMedizin* 11 (5): 252-257.

Diagnostic and Statistical Manual of Mental Disorders, Fourth Edition, Text Revision (DSM-IV-TR). Washington, DC: American Psychiatric Association.

Drew S, Davies E (2001). Effectiveness of *Ginkgo biloba* in treating tinnitus: Double blind, placebo controlled trial. *British Medical Journal* 322 (7278): 1-6.

Engelsen J, Nielsen JD, Winter K (2002). Effect of coenzyme Q10 and *Ginkgo biloba* on warfarin dosage in stable, long-term warfarin treated outpatients: A randomized, double blind, placebo-crossover trial. *Thrombosis and Haemostasis* 87 (6): 1075-1076.

Ernst E, Pittler MH (1999). *Ginkgo biloba* for dementia, a systematic review of double-blind, placebo-controlled trials. *Clinical Drug Investigations* 17 (4): 301-308.

Ernst E, Stevinson C (1999). *Ginkgo biloba* for tinnitus: A review. *Clinical Otolaryngology and Allied Sciences* 24 (3): 164-167.

Foster S, Tyler VE (1999). *Tyler's Honest Herbal.* Binghamton, NY: The Haworth Press.

Fowler JS, Wang GJ, Volkow ND, Logan J, Franceschi D, Franceschi M, MacGregor R, Shea C, Garza V, Liu N, Ding YS (2000). Evidence that *Ginkgo biloba* extract does not inhibit MAO A and B in living human brain. *Life Sciences* 66 (9): 141-146.

Gilbert GJ (1997). *Ginkgo biloba. Neurology* 48 (4):1137.

Grassel E (1992). The effect of *Ginkgo biloba* extract on mental performance: Double-blind study conducted under computerized measurement conditions in patients with cerebral insufficiency. *Fortschritte der Medizin* 110 (5): 73-76.

Guinot P, Caffrey E, Lambe R, Darragh A (1989). Tanakan inhibits platelet-activating-factor-induced platelet aggregation in healthy male volunteers. *Haemostasis* 19 (4): 219-223.

Halama P (1990). Treatment with *Ginkgo biloba* in patients with cerebro-vascular insufficiency and refractory depressive symptoms: Results of a placebo-controlled, randomized double-blind pilot study. *Therapiewoche* 40 (51/52): 3760-3765.

Halama P, Bartsch G, Meng G (1988). Randomized, double-blind study on the efficacy of *Ginkgo biloba* extract. *Fortschritte der Medizin* 106 (19): 408-412.

Hindmarch I (1986). Effect of *Ginkgo biloba* extract on short-term memory. *Presse Medicale* 15 (31): 1592-1594.

Hofferberth B (1989). Effect of *Ginkgo biloba* extract on neurophysiological and psychometric findings in patients with cerebro-organic syndrome. *Arzneimittel-Forschung/Drug Research* 39 (8): 918-922.

Hofferberth B (1991a). *Ginkgo biloba* special extract in patients with organic brain syndrome. *Munchener Medizinische Wochenschrift* 133 (Suppl. 1): S30-S33.

Hofferberth B (1991b). Simultaneous determination of electrophysiological, psychometric, and rheological parameters in patients with cerebro-organic psychosyndrome and increased vascular risk—A placebo-controlled double-blind study with *Ginkgo biloba* extract EGb 761. In *Mikrozirkulation in Gehirn und Sinnesorganen.* Eds. R Stodtmeister R, LE Pillunat LE. Stuttgart: Ferdinand Enke Verlag, pp. 64-74.

Hofferberth B (1994). The efficacy of EGb 761 in patients with senile dementia of the Alzheimer type, a double-blind, placebo-controlled study on different levels of investigation. *Human Psychopharmacology* 9: 215-222.

Hopfenmuller W (1994). Nachweis der therapeutischen Wirksamkeit einer ginkgo biloba-spezialextraktes; meta-analysis von 11 klinischen studien bei patienten mit hirnleistungsstorungen im alter. *Arzneimittel-Forschung/Drug Research* 44 (9): 1005-1013.

Israel L, Dell Accio E, Martin G, Hugonot R (1987). *Ginkgo biloba* extract and memory training programs comparative assessment on elderly out-patients. *Psychologie Medicale* 19 (8): 1431-1439.

Itil T, Martorano D (1995). Natural substances in psychiatry (*Ginkgo biloba* in dementia). *Psychopharmacology Bulletin* 31 (1): 147-158.

Jung F, Mrowietz C, Kiesewetter H, Wenzel E (1990). Effect of *Ginkgo biloba* on fluidity of blood and peripheral microcirculation in volunteers. *Arzneimittel-Forschung/Drug Research* 40 (1) 5: 589-593.

Kanowski S, Herrmann WM, Stephan K, Wierich W, Horr R (1997). Proof of efficacy of the *Ginkgo biloba* special extract EGb 761 in outpatients suffering from mild to moderate primary degenerative dementia of the Alzheimer type or multi-infarct dementia. *Phytomedicine* 4 (1): 3-13. (Also published in Kanowski S, Herrmann WM, Stephan K, Wierich W, Horr R [1996] *Pharmacopsychiatry* 29 [2]: 47-56.)

Kennedy DO, Scholey AB, Wesnes KA (2000). The dose-dependent cognitive effects of acute administration of *Ginkgo biloba* to healthy young volunteers. *Psychopharmacology* 151 (4): 416-423.

Kennedy DO, Scholey AB, Wesnes KA (2001). Differential, dose dependent changes in cognitive performance following acute administration of a *Ginkgo biloba/Panax ginseng* combination to healthy young volunteers. *Nutritional Neuroscience* 4 (5): 399-412.

Klein P (1988). Untersuchung uber die Hemmwirkung von *Ginkgo biloba* extract. *Therapiewoche* 38: 2379-2383. Cited in DeFeudis FV (1998). *Ginkgo biloba Extract (EGb 761), from Chemistry to the Clinic.* Wiesbaden: Ullstein Medical.

Kohler S, Funk P, Kieser M (In press). Influence of *Ginkgo biloba* special extract EGb 761® on bleeding time and coagulation: A placebo-controlled, double-blind study in healthy volunteers.

Koza KD, Ernst FD, Sporl E (1991). Retinal blood flow after *Ginkgo biloba* therapy in fundus hypertonicus. *Munchener Medizinische Wochenschrift* 133 (Suppl. 1): S47-S50.

Kunkel H (1993). EEG profile of three different extractions of *Ginkgo biloba. Neuropsychobiology* 27 (1): 40-45.

Le Bars PL, Katz MM, Berman N, Itil TM, Freedman AM, Schatzberg AF (1997). A placebo-controlled, double-blind, randomized trial of an extract of *Ginkgo biloba* for dementia. *The Journal of the American Medical Association* 278 (16): 1327-1332. (This study was reanalyzed and published in Le Bars PL, Kieser M, Itil KZ [2000]. *Dementia and Geriatric Cognitive Disorders* 11 [4]: 230-237.)

Le Bars PL, Velasco FM, Ferguson JM, Dessain EC, Kieser M, Hoerr R (2002). Influence of the severity of cognitive impairment on the effect of the *Ginkgo biloba* extract EGb 761® in Alzheimer's disease. *Nueropsychiobiology* 45 (1): 19-26.

Luthringer R, d'Arbigny P, Macher JP (1995). *Ginkgo biloba* extract (EGb 761), EEG and event-related potentials mapping profile. In *Advances in Ginkgo biloba Extract Research*, Volume 4: *Effects of* Ginkgo biloba *Extract (EGb 761) on Aging and Age-Related Disorders*. Eds. Y Christen, Y Courtois, M-T Droy-Lefaix. Paris: Elsevier, pp. 107-118.

Maier-Hauff K (1991). LI 1370 after cerebral aneurysm operation; efficacy in outpatients with disorders of cerebral functional capacity. *Munchener Medizinische Wochenschrift* 133 (Suppl. 1): S34-S37.

Matthews MK, Jr (1998). Association of *Ginkgo biloba* with intracerebral hemorrhage. *Neurology* 50 (6):1933-1934.

Maurer K, Ihl R, Dierks T, Frolich L (1997). Clinical efficacy of *Ginkgo biloba* special extract EGb 761 in dementia of the Alzheimer type. *Journal of Psychiatry Research* 31 (6): 645-655.

Mix JA, Crews WD (2000). An examination of the efficacy of *Ginkgo biloba* extract EGb 761 on the neuropsychologic functioning of cognitively intact older adults. *The Journal of Alternative and Complementary Medicine* 6 (3): 219-229.

Morgenstern C (1997). *Ginkgo biloba* extract EGb 761 in the treatment of tinnitus aurium. *Fortschritte der Medizin* 115: 7-11.

Murray BJ, Cowen PJ, Sharpley AL (2001). The effect of Li 1370, extract of *Ginkgo biloba*, on REM sleep in humans. *Pharmacopsychiatry* 34 (4): 155-157.

Oken BS, Storzbach DM, Kaye JA (1998). The efficacy of *Ginkgo biloba* on cognitive function in Alzheimer's disease. *Archives of Neurology* 55 (11):1409-1415.

Peters H, Kieser M, Holscher U (1998). Demonstration of the efficacy of *Ginkgo biloba* special extract EGb 761 on the intermittent claudication: A placebo-controlled, double-blind multicenter trial. *Zeitschrift fur Gefasskrankheiten/Journal for Vascular Diseases* 27 (2): 106-110.

Pietri S, Seguin J, d'Argigny P, Drieu K, Culcasi M (1997). *Ginkgo biloba* extract (EGb 761) pretreatment limits free radical-induced oxidative stress inpatients undergoing coronary bypass surgery. *Cardiovascular Drugs and Therapy* 11 (2): 121-131.

Pittler MH, Ernst E (2000). *Ginkgo biloba* extract for the treatment of intermittent claudication: A meta-analysis of randomized trials. *The American Journal of Medicine* 108 (4): 276-281.

Rai GS, Shovlin C, Wesnes KA (1991). A double-blind placebo-controlled study of *Ginkgo biloba* extract (Tanakan) in elderly outpatients with mild to moderate memory impairment. *Current Medical Research and Opinion* 12 (6): 350-355.

Rigney U, Kimber S, Hindmarch I (1999). The effects of acute doses of standardized *Ginkgo biloba* extract on memory and psychomotor performance in volunteers. *Phytotherapy Research* 13 (5): 408-415.

Rosenblatt M, Mindel J (1997). Spontaneous hyphema associated with ingestion of *Ginkgo biloba* extract. *The New England Journal of Medicine* 3336 (15): 1108.

Rowin J, Lewis SL (1996). Spontaneous bilateral subdural hematomas associated with chronic *Ginkgo biloba* ingestion. *Neurology* 46 (6):1775-1776.

Schaffler K, Reeh PW (1985). Double-blind study on the protective effect against hypoxia of a standardized *Ginkgo-biloba* preparation following repeated administration to normal subjects. *Arzneimittel-Forschung/ Drug Research* 35 (2): 1283-1286.

Scholey AB, Kennedy DO (2002). Acute, dose-dependent cognitive effects of *Ginkgo biloba, Panax ginseng* and their combination in healthy young volunteers: Differential interactions with cognitive demand. *Human Psychopharmacology* 17 (1): 35-44.

Schulz H, Jobert M, Breuel HP (1991). Wirkung von spezialextrakt LI 1370 auf das EEG alterer patienten im schlafentzugsmodell. *Munchener Medizinische Wochenschrift* 133 (Suppl. 1): S26-S29.

Schulz J, Hamala P, Hoerr R (2000). *Ginkgo biloba* extracts for the treatment of cerebral insufficiency and dementia. In *Ginkgo biloba*. Ed. TA van Beek. Amsterdam, the Netherlands: Harwood Academic Publishers, pp. 345-370.

Schulz V, Hänsel R, Tyler VE (2001). *Rational Phytotherapy: A Physicians' Guide to Herbal Medicine,* Fourth Edition. Trans. TC Telgar. Berlin: Springer-Verlag.

Schweizer J, Hautmann C (1999). Comparison of two dosages of *Ginkgo biloba* extract Egb 761 in patients with peripheral arterial occlusive disease Fontaine's stage IIb. *Arzneimittel-Forschung/Drug Research* 49 (11): 900-904.

Solomon PR, Adams F, Silver A, Zimmer J, DeVeaux R (2002). Ginkgo for memory enhancement: A randomized controlled trial. *Journal of the American Medical Association* 288 (7): 835-840.

Taillandier J, Ammar A, Rabourdin JP, Ribeyre JP, Pichon J, Niddam S, Pierart H (1986). *Ginkgo biloba* extract in the treatment of cerebral disorders due to aging: A longitudinal multicenter double-blind placebo-controlled drug trial. *La Presse Medicale* 25 (31): 1576-1583.

Thomson GJL, Vohra RK, Carr MH, Walker MG (1990). A clinical trial of *Ginkgo biloba* extract in patients with intermittent claudication. *International Angiology* 9 (2): 75-78.

Vale S (1998). Subarachnoid haemorrhage associated with *Ginkgo biloba*. *The Lancet* 352 (9121): 36.

van Dongen MCJM, van Rossum E, Kessels AGH, Sielhorst HJG, Knipschild PG (2000). The efficacy of ginkgo for elderly people with dementia and age-associated memory impairment: New results of a randomized clinical trial. *Journal of the American Geriatrics Society* 48 (10): 1183-1194.

Vesper J, Hansgen KD (1994). Efficacy of *Ginkgo biloba* in 90 outpatients with cerebral insufficiency caused by old age. *Phytomedicine* 1: 9-16.

Warot D, Lacomblez L, Danjou P, Weiller E, Payan C, Puech AJ (1991). Comparative effects of *Ginkgo biloba* extracts on psychomotor performance and memory in healthy volunteers. *Therapie* 46 (1): 33-36.

Wesnes K, Simmons D, Rook M, Simpson P (1987). A double-blind placebo-controlled trial of Tanakan in the treatment of idiopathic cognitive impairment in the elderly. *Human Psychopharmacology* 2: 159-169.

Wesnes K, Ward T, McGinty A, Petrini O (2000). The memory enhancing effects of a *Ginkgo biloba/Panax ginseng* combination in healthy middle-aged volunteers. *Psychopharmacology* 152 (4): 353-361.

Wesnes KA, Faleni RA, Hefting NR, Hoogsteen G, Houben JJG, Jenkins E, Jonkman JHG, Leonard J, Petrini O, van Lier JJ (1997). The cognitive, subjective and physical effects of a *Ginkgo biloba/Panax ginseng* combination in healthy volunteers with neurasthenic complaints. *Psychopharmacology Bulletin* 33 (4): 677-683.

Wettstein, A (1999/2000). Cholinesterase inhibitors and ginkgo extracts—Are they comparable in the treatment of dementia? *Phytomedicine* 6 (6): 393-401.

Wolf HRD (In press). Effect of *Ginkgo biloba* special extract EGb 761® and acetylsalicyclic acid on coagulation: A randomized, double-blind, crossover study in healthy subjects.

World Health Organization (WHO) (1999). *WHO Monographs on Selected Medicinal Plants*, Volume 1. Geneva, Switzerland: World Health Organization.

DETAILS ON GINKGO PRODUCTS AND CLINICAL STUDIES

Product and clinical study information is grouped in the same order as in the Summary Table. A profile on an individual product is followed by details of the clinical studies associated with that product. In some instances a clinical study, or studies, supports several products that contain the same principal ingredient(s). In these instances, those products are grouped together.

Clinical studies that follow each product, or group of products, are grouped by therapeutic indication, in accordance with the order in the Summary Table.

Index to Ginkgo Products

Product Profile: Ginkgold®

Manufacturer	**Dr. Willmar Schwabe GmbH & Co., Germany**
U.S. distributor	**Nature's Way Products, Inc.**
Botanical ingredient	**Ginkgo leaf extract**
Extract name	**Egb 761®**
Quantity	60 mg
Processing	Plant to extract ratio 50:1, acetone 60% m/m
Standardization	24% flavone glycosides, 6% terpene lactones
Formulation	Tablet

Recommended dose: One tablet two times daily with water at meals. For intensive use, take up to two tablets two times daily with water.

DSHEA structure/function: For improved mental sharpness, concentration, memory, cognitive activity. Supports healthy circulation to the brain as well as the extremities. Maintains healthy blood vessel tone and reduces blood viscosity.

Other ingredients: Cellulose, starch, modified cellulose, silica, magnesium stearate, titanium dioxide, caramel.

Comments: EGb 761 is sold in Europe as Tanakan®, Rökan®, and Tebonin® forte.

Source(s) of information: Product package and label; information provided by distributor.

Product Profile: Ginkoba®

Manufacturer	**Dr. Willmar Schwabe GmbH & Co., Germany**
U.S. distributor	**Pharmaton Natural Health Products**
Botanical ingredient	**Ginkgo leaf extract**
Extract name	**EGb 761®**
Quantity	40 mg
Processing	Plant to extract ratio 50:1
Standardization	24% ginkgo flavone glycosides and 6% terpene lactones
Formulation	Tablet

Recommended dose: One tablet three times daily with water at mealtimes. Optimal effectiveness has been shown after four weeks with continuous uninterrupted use.

DSHEA structure/function: Improves memory and concentration and enhances mental focus by safely increasing the flow of oxygen to the brain. Sharpens mental focus, enhances memory and concentration, and helps contribute to an overall sense of healthy well-being by increasing the natural blood flow of oxygen to the brain.

Cautions: In case of accidental overdose, seek the advice of a professional immediately. If taking a prescription medicine, pregnant or lactating, please contact a doctor before taking Ginkoba. No information is available on the use of ginkgo biloba extract in children under the age of 12.

Other ingredients: Hydroxypropyl methyl cellulose, lactose, talc, polyethylene glycol, magnesium stearate, titanium dioxide, synthetic iron oxides.

Comments: EGb 761 is sold in Europe as Tanakan®, Rökan®, and Tebonin® forte.

Source(s) of information: Product package and insert (© Boehringer Ingelheim Pharmaceuticals Inc., 2000).

Clinical Study: Ginkoba®

Extract name	EGb 761
Manufacturer	Dr. Willmar Schwabe GmbH & Co., Germany
Indication	**Cognitive functioning** in normal elderly volunteers
Level of evidence	**II**
Therapeutic benefit	**No**

Bibliographic reference
Solomon PR, Adams F, Silver A, Zimmer J, DeVeaux R (2002). Ginkgo for memory enhancement: A randomized controlled trial. *Journal of the American Medical Association* 288 (7): 835-840.

Trial design
Parallel.

Study duration	6 weeks
Dose	1 (40 mg) tablet 3 times daily
Route of administration	Oral
Randomized	Yes
Randomization adequate	Yes
Blinding	Double-blind
Blinding adequate	No
Placebo	Yes
Drug comparison	No
Site description	Single center
No. of subjects enrolled	230
No. of subjects completed	203
Sex	Male and female
Age	60-82 years (Mean: 69.3)

Inclusion criteria

Community-dwelling subjects over 60 years old without cognitive impairment (Mini-Mental State Examination scores greater than 26), and generally in good health, with a companion with whom they came in contact regularly (>four times per week for at least one hour) and who was willing to complete a questionnaire. All subjects were independent in daily living tasks such as shopping, managing finances, and transportation.

Exclusion criteria

Subjects were excluded if they had a history of neurologic or psychiatric disorder, had taken antidepressants or other psychoactive medications in the past 60 days, or had a life-threatening illness in the past five years.

End points

The outcome measures, except the companion's questionnaire, were assessed at the beginning and end of the study. These included tests of memory and learning (California Verbal Learning Test, the Logical Memory subscale of the Wechsler Memory Scale-Revised [WMS-R], and the Visual Reproduction subscale); tests of concentration and attention (Stroop Test, Digit Span [WMS-R], Mental Control [WMS-R], Digit Symbol subscale of the Wechsler Adult Intelligence Scale-Revised [WAIS-R]); expressive language tests (Controlled Category Fluency test, Boston Naming Test). The subjects also completed a memory questionnaire. The subjects' companions completed a global evaluation (based on the Caregiver Global Impression of Change [CGIC] rating scale) only at the end of the study.

Results

Compared to the placebo group, the subjects in the ginkgo group did not perform significantly better on any of the outcome measures.

Side effects

Not evaluated.

Authors' comments

These data suggest that when taken following the manufacturer's instructions, this compound provides no measurable benefit in cognitive function to elderly adults with intact cognitive function.

Reviewer's comments

This trial was compromised by learning effects on most tests, due to the absence of prestudy training and use of tests that are known to have training effects. Also, memory was assessed at only one time point and effects might have been seen at other times. The main author was not blinded, a very unusual practice that would have prevented publication in some scientific journals. (3, 6)

Clinical Study: Ginkgold®

Extract name	EGb 761
Manufacturer	Dr. Willmar Schwabe GmbH & Co., Germany
Indication	**Cognitive functioning** in normal volunteers
Level of evidence	I
Therapeutic benefit	**Yes**

Bibliographic reference
Mix JA, Crews WD (2000). An examination of the efficacy of *Ginkgo biloba* extract EGb 761 on the neuropsychologic functioning of cognitively intact older adults. *The Journal of Alternative and Complementary Medicine* 6 (3): 219-229.

Trial design
Parallel.

Study duration	6 weeks
Dose	3 (60 mg capsules) daily
Route of administration	Oral
Randomized	Yes
Randomization adequate	Yes
Blinding	Double-blind
Blinding adequate	Yes
Placebo	Yes
Drug comparison	No
Site description	Single center
No. of subjects enrolled	48
No. of subjects completed	40
Sex	Male and female
Age	55-88 years

Inclusion criteria
No history of significant neurocognitive impairment and a total score of 24 or more on the Mini-Mental State Examination (MMSE).

Exclusion criteria
Histories of active or clinically significant cardiovascular, neurologic, pulmonary, endocrine, renal, hepatic, gastrointestinal, hematologic, or oncologic diseases/disorders; uncontrolled hypertension; learning disabilities; psychi-

atric or substance abuse disorders; treatment with anticoagulant or psychotropic medications; histories of bleeding disorders or hemorrhagic stroke; uncorrected vision; or hearing or motor difficulties that could have possibly precluded their participation and/or compliance with all of the neuropsychologic procedures.

End points
A series of neuropsychologic tests designed to measure cognitive and behavioral functioning were administered prior to treatment and after six weeks. Tests included the MMSE, Stroop Color and Word Test, Trail Making Test, and the Wechsler Memory Scale—Revised Logical Memory I and II and Visual Reproduction I and II subsets. A self-report questionnaire was administered during the second assessment.

Results
Participants who received EGb 761 exhibited significantly more improvement on a task assessing speed of processing abilities by the end of the treatment as compared to placebo. Trends favoring improved performances in EGb 761 group were also demonstrated in three of the four remaining tasks that involved a timed, speed of processing component, although they did not reach statistical significance. Significantly more participants in the EGb 761 group rated their overall abilities to remember by the end of the treatment as "improved," as compared to the placebo group. In contrast, no significant differences were found between the EGb 761 and placebo groups on any of the four objective memory measures.

Side effects
No notable adverse reactions were reported.

Authors' comments
Ginkgo biloba extract EGb 761 may prove efficacious in enhancing certain neurocognitive functions/processes of cognitively intact older adults.

Reviewer's comments
Soundly conducted and excellently reported study. This is one of the few trials on cognitive function in normal, healthy volunteers. The only possible caveat is that the statistical outcome is dependent on one-tailed testing. (5, 6)

Clinical Study: EGb 761®

Extract name	EGb 761
Manufacturer	Dr. Willmar Schwabe GmbH & Co., Germany

Indication   **Cognitive functioning** in normal volunteers
Level of evidence   **II**
Therapeutic benefit   **Trend**

Bibliographic reference
Hindmarch I (1986). Effect of *Ginkgo biloba* extract on short-term memory. *Presse Medicale* 15 (31): 1592-1594.

Trial design
Crossover. Two Latin squares, treatment with one of three doses of EGb 761 (120 mg, 240 mg, and 600 mg extract) or placebo, administered one hour prior to testing. The four treatments were separated by one-week washout intervals.

Study duration	1 day
Dose	120, 240, and 600 mg of EGb 761 extract
Route of administration	Oral
Randomized	Yes
Randomization adequate	No
Blinding	Double-blind
Blinding adequate	Yes
Placebo	Yes
Drug comparison	No
Site description	Not described
No. of subjects enrolled	8
No. of subjects completed	8
Sex	Female
Age	25-40 years (mean: 32)

Inclusion criteria
Healthy female volunteers in good physical condition with no history of disease (cardiovascular, gastric, hepatic, renal, psychiatric).

Exclusion criteria
Any drug therapy (except contraceptives) and confirmed or suspected pregnancy.

End points
Tests consisted of Critical Flicker Fusion Test (CFF) to measure the activity of the central nervous system (CNS) as a whole; Choice Reaction Time (CRT) to measure sensorimotor performance; memory test to measure

short-term memory and rapid discriminant memory; and a 10 cm visual analog scale to evaluate subjective effects.

Results
Short-term memory as assessed by the Sternberg technique was significantly improved one hour after administration of 600 mg ginkgo ($p < 0.0001$). Analysis of mean reaction times from the pooled data of the positive and negative tests shows a significant difference ($p < 0.05$) between placebo and EGb 761. No significant differences were seen in either the Flicker Fusion or Choice Reaction Time Tests.

Side effects
None mentioned in paper.

Author's comments
Only the Sternberg test was modified to a significant degree by administration of EGb 761, suggesting a specific action of the product on central cognitive processes. These findings point to a potential for use of *Ginkgo biloba* extract in the treatment of patients suffering from senile or presenile dementia in whom memory disorders are among the principal clinical symptoms.

Reviewer's comments
This is the first volunteer study of ginkgo with automated cognitive function tests. The sample was small, and the effect was restricted to 1 dose (600 mg) and one of three tests (Sternberg), but the significance of the effect was high. This finding was not replicated in another trial with 12 females using the same dose and tests (Warot et al., 1991). The randomization process was not adequately described and withdrawals and dropouts were not described. (Translation reviewed) (2, 5)

Clinical Study: Tanakan®

Extract name	EGb 761
Manufacturer	Dr. Willmar Schwabe GmbH & Co., Germany
Indication	**Cognitive functioning** in normal volunteers
Level of evidence	**II**
Therapeutic benefit	**Yes**

Bibliographic reference
Warot D, Lacomblez L, Danjou P, Weiller E, Payan C, Puech AJ (1991).

Comparative effects of *Ginkgo biloba* extracts on psychomotor performance and memory in healthy volunteers. *Therapie* 46 (1): 33-36.

Trial design
Crossover. Latin square, with two different ginkgo preparations and matching placebos. Three courses of treatment (600 mg unidentified ginkgo preparation, 600 mg Tanakan and placebo) were separated by one-week intervals. The treatments were given as one acute dose preceding evaluations. Consumption of alcohol and caffeinated beverages was prohibited on the evening before and on the day of evaluation visits.

Study duration	1 day
Dose	600 mg extract
Route of administration	Oral
Randomized	No
Randomization adequate	No
Blinding	Double-blind
Blinding adequate	Yes
Placebo	Yes
Drug comparison	Yes
Drug name	Unidentified ginkgo preparation
Site description	Not described
No. of subjects enrolled	12
No. of subjects completed	12
Sex	Female
Age	19-30 years (mean: 22.3)

Inclusion criteria
Healthy female volunteers with normal scores on Cattell's self-analysis scale, the Eysenck Personality Inventory, and the Mini-Mult test.

Exclusion criteria
None mentioned.

End points
Psychomotor performance and memory were evaluated before and one hour after oral administration of the drugs. Four psychometric tests were employed for analysis: Critical Flicker Frequency (CFF), Choice Reaction Time, memory test (number recognition or Sternberg test), and images (used to explore free recall and recognition of images). Self-evaluation scales in the form of 11 visual analog scales were completed by the subjects to evaluate mood and wakefulness.

Results

No significant change was observed in the CFF threshold, the choice reaction time, and the subjective evaluation measured by the visual analog scales. In the memory test, significant differences were found between placebo and Tanakan ($p < 0.01$) and between Tanakan and the unidentified ginkgo product ($p = 0.05$). Memory performances were maintained one hour after taking Tanakan, while scores obtained after the administration of the unidentified ginkgo or placebo were reduced.

Side effects

None mentioned in paper.

Authors' comments

In order to verify the clinical relevance of these results, the tests need to be repeated in older, healthy volunteers with age-associated memory impairment.

Reviewer's comments

This study with 50 percent more volunteers failed to replicate working memory benefit seen in Hindmarch (1986), but it did find evidence of improved secondary memory (clear benefit of ginkgo on recall scores). Though authors suggest proactive interference may account for effects, this is unlikely. The study participants were not allocated to groups in a randomized manner. (Translation reviewed) (3, 5)

Clinical Study: Tanakan®

Extract name	EGb 761
Manufacturer	Ipsen, France (Dr. Willmar Schwabe Gmbh & Co., Germany)
Indication	**Age-related memory impairment**
Level of evidence	**I**
Therapeutic benefit	**Yes**

Bibliographic reference

Rai GS, Shovlin C, Wesnes KA (1991). A double-blind placebo-controlled study of *Ginkgo biloba* extract (Tanakan) in elderly outpatients with mild to moderate memory impairment. *Current Medical Research and Opinion* 12 (6): 350-355.

Trial design
Parallel. Two weeks prior to the trial patients underwent training on the test procedures.

Study duration	6 months
Dose	1 (40 mg) tablet 3 times daily
Route of administration	Oral
Randomized	Yes
Randomization adequate	Yes
Blinding	Double-blind
Blinding adequate	Yes
Placebo	Yes
Drug comparison	No
Site description	1 hospital geriatric department
No. of subjects enrolled	31
No. of subjects completed	27
Sex	Male and female
Age	54-89 years (mean: 76)

Inclusion criteria
Patients over the age of 50 showing signs of mild to moderate memory impairment of organic origin as classified by the National Institute of Neurological and Communicative Disorders and Stroke (NINCDS, now the NINDS) and the Alzheimer's Disease and Related Disorders Association (ADRDA, now the Alzheimer's Association) for a minimum of three months prior to screening.

Exclusion criteria
Patients presenting with memory problems due to physical illness, metabolic, endocrine, nutritional, neurological, or cardiac disease; functional disorders such as depression; evidence of renal or hepatic failure; presence of severe cardiac disease; myocardial infarction within the preceding six months; poorly controlled diabetes; epilepsy or malignant disease; those on drugs acting on cerebral metabolism or cerebral blood flow; uncooperative patients; and those with a history of drug or alcohol abuse.

End points
Patients were assessed two weeks before the trial, at baseline, and after 12 and 24 weeks of treatment using the following psychometric tests: the Folstein Mini-Mental State Examination; the Kendrick Battery for the detection of dementia in the elderly; a computerized version of the digit recall task; a computerized version of a classification task; latency of auditory event-related potential (ERP), i.e., P300; and an EEG. Change in performance

over time was assessed by subtracting the initial score from the test score at week 12 or week 24.

Results
The results in patients receiving ginkgo extract were significantly superior to placebo on the digit copying subtest of the Kendrick Battery at both week 12 ($p = 0.022$) and week 24 ($p = 0.017$), and on the median reaction time of the classification task at 24 weeks ($p = 0.026$). The EEG between 1 and 3 Hz also showed a statistically significant decrease in the active treatment group for this frequency compared to placebo.

Side effects
None mentioned in paper.

Authors' comments
The findings of an improvement on the digit copying subtest and an improvement in speed on the classification task, both at week 24, confirm that ginkgo extract EGb 761 has a beneficial effect on mental efficiency in elderly patients showing mild to moderate impairment of organic origin.

Reviewer's comments
This is a replication in a different site with differing tests of Wesnes and colleagues (1987) showing that ginkgo improves cognitive function in what is today termed mild cognitive impairment. The trial is small but supportive of beneficial effects. (5, 5)

Clinical Study: Tanakan®

Extract name	EGb 761
Manufacturer	Ipsen, France (Dr. Willmar Schwabe GmbH & Co., Germany)
Indication	**Age-related cognitive impairment**
Level of evidence	**I**
Therapeutic benefit	**Yes**

Bibliographic reference
Wesnes K, Simmons D, Rook M, Simpson P (1987). A double-blind placebo-controlled trial of Tanakan in the treatment of idiopathic cognitive impairment in the elderly. *Human Psychopharmacology* 2: 159-169.

Trial design
Parallel. Pretrial washout period of one to three weeks. Patients were trained on the experimental tasks before the trial began.

Study duration	3 months
Dose	1 (40 mg) tablet 3 times daily
Route of administration	Oral
Randomized	Yes
Randomization adequate	Yes
Blinding	Double-blind
Blinding adequate	Yes
Placebo	Yes
Drug comparison	No
Site description	Not described
No. of subjects enrolled	58
No. of subjects completed	54
Sex	Male and female
Age	62-85 years

Inclusion criteria
Patients who showed mild impairment of everyday functioning using the Crichton Geriatric Behavioral Scale for diagnosis of dementia (a score of 14 or more on the scale, without scoring more than 3 on any individual item).

Exclusion criteria
Patients were excluded if there was a predisposing cause for their symptoms, such as infection, drug toxicity, metabolic, endocrine, or nutritional disease; or if they had a neurological disorder, such as chronic subdural hematoma or cerebral neoplasia. Patients with a possible psychiatric cause for their condition, such as depression, were also excluded, as were those with renal, hepatic, or cardiac insufficiency, with diabetes mellitus, or with malignant disease. Medication with psychotropic drugs was not permitted during the trial.

End points
Cognitive efficiency was measured prior to the trial start, and then at monthly intervals, using a battery of tests of mental ability comprising both computerized and pencil-and-paper tasks. Quality of life was assessed using a behavioral questionnaire both before and after the study.

Results
Results of the tests were combined using two different methods. Both groups improved in accuracy during weeks 8 and 12 compared to baseline. The ginkgo group's reaction times were significantly faster during week 4 and showed trends toward maintaining this level during weeks 8 and 12. No improvement was seen in the placebo group. There was a notable increase

in interest taken in everyday activities for the ginkgo group ($p = 0.015$) but not for the placebo group.

Side effects
Tolerance was very good. One ginkgo patient complained of constipation that resolved itself without interruption of treatment.

Authors' comments
Overall the findings from this study, that ginkgo has a favorable effect on mental efficiency in this population, suggest that the drug could prove effective in the treatment of the early stages of primary degenerative dementia.

Reviewer's comments
This is the first study using computerized tests of cognitive function in elderly impaired patients. It showed clear benefits to accuracy and speed of cognitive function plus improvements to quality of life. The authors used one-tailed testing, but the results would have been significant with two-tailed testing. The sample size was fair but probably at the lower end required to detect an effect in this population. (5, 6)

Clinical Study: Tanakan®

Extract name	EGb 761
Manufacturer	Ipsen, France (Dr. Willmar Schwabe Gmbh & Co., Germany)

Indication	**Age-related cognitive impairment**
Level of evidence	**II**
Therapeutic benefit	**Yes**

Bibliographic reference
Israel L, Dell Accio E, Martin G, Hugonot R (1987). *Ginkgo biloba* extract and memory training programs comparative assessment on elderly out-patients. *Psychologie Medicale* 19 (8): 1431-1439.

Trial design
Parallel. Four treatment arms: treatment with either ginkgo or placebo, and with or without memory training. Patients assigned to the memory training program met with a psychologist once a week for three months.

Study duration	3 months
Dose	2 ml twice daily (160 mg extract per day)

Route of administration	Oral
Randomized	Yes
Randomization adequate	No
Blinding	Double-blind
Blinding adequate	Yes
Placebo	Yes
Drug comparison	No
Site description	Not described
No. of subjects enrolled	80
No. of subjects completed	75
Sex	Male and female
Age	56-83 years (mean: 68.4)

Inclusion criteria
Subjects over 55 years of age who complained about beginning disorders of their cognitive functions (score of 20 to 26 on the Folstein MMSE) and without a depressive syndrome (score <18 on the Yesavage Geriatric Depression Scale [GDS]).

Exclusion criteria
Patients with an acute or chronic associated disease of relative severity; manifest depressions in their case history; patients who were not able to discontinue for the duration of the study a treatment concerning vasoregulation or cerebral metabolism.

End points
Patients were assessed at baseline and after three months using three assessments: the psychologist conducted a series of memory tests; the physician rated the scale of mental dynamics and repercussions of the symptoms on the patient's daily life; and the patient rated himself or herself using the Geriatric Depression Scale, the scale of difficulties of daily living, and questions judging his or her satisfaction with the treatment.

Results
Ginkgo treatment significantly improved immediate memory ($p < 0.01$) and training sessions also improved this factor ($p < 0.01$), though the effects were not additive. Improvement was not seen in patients receiving placebo alone. General evocation memory was significantly improved by training sessions ($p < 0.01$) but not by ginkgo. Neither ginkgo nor training improved learning. Mental fluidity and control was improved in both ginkgo groups ($p < 0.005$), but not by memory training.

Side effects
One ginkgo patient complained of nausea and dyspepsia.

Authors' comments
Whenever possible, a therapeutic combination of ginkgo and memory training has to be recommended since its conjugate action allows patients to obtain a better adaptation to everyday life.

Reviewer's comments
Well-conducted trial in elderly mildly impaired volunteers showing benefits of ginkgo on memory and giving probable evidence that training plus ginkgo is the best overall combination for "immediate memory." The randomization process was not adequately described and the data summary was insufficient (does not permit an alternative analysis or replication). (Translation reviewed) (3, 5)

Clinical Study: Tanakan®

Extract name	EGb 761
Manufacturer	Ipsen, France (Dr. Willmar Schwabe GmbH & Co., Germany)
Indication	**Age-related cognitive impairment**
Level of evidence	**II**
Therapeutic benefit	**Yes**

Bibliographic reference
Taillandier J, Ammar A, Rabourdin JP, Ribeyre JP, Pichon J, Niddam S, Pierart H (1986). *Ginkgo biloba* extract in the treatment of cerebral disorders due to aging: A longitudinal multicenter double-blind placebo-controlled drug trial. *La Presse Medicale* 25 (31): 1576-1583.

Trial design
Parallel.

Study duration	1 year
Dose	2 (2 ml) doses daily (equivalent to 160 mg/day ginkgo extract)
Route of administration	Oral
Randomized	Yes
Randomization adequate	No
Blinding	Double-blind
Blinding adequate	Yes

Placebo	Yes
Drug comparison	No
Site description	4 centers
No. of subjects enrolled	166
No. of subjects completed	122
Sex	Male and female
Age	60-97 years (mean: 82)

Inclusion criteria

Patients over 60 years of age with disorders related to cerebral aging (or signs of chronic cerebral insufficiency), Geriatric Clinical Evaluation Scale (GCES) total score between 21 and 113. Patients also had to be living in the retirement home for at least two months.

Exclusion criteria

Patients were excluded if they had any serious chronic disease or associated pathological disorders: psychosis (chronic delirium, mania, depression); severe neurosis (hysterical, obsessive); neoplasms regardless of the site; chronic alcoholism, etc.

End points

Effectiveness was judged according to the GCES. The examining physician also judged the general clinical state of the patient according to the following classifications: disease absent, mild, moderate, moderately severe, significant, or severe. Assessments were carried out at baseline and at 3, 6, 9, and 12 months.

Results

The ginkgo group showed a significant improvement in the GCES after three months. Improvement continued and after one year reached 17 percent. In comparison, improvement in the placebo group became significant only after one year, reaching 7 percent. The two groups were significantly different after three months ($p = 0.01$). Disease severity was significantly different after six months, when the percentage of patients whose condition was "mild" increased from 25 percent to 37 percent in the ginkgo group and decreased from 23 percent to 16 percent in the placebo group. The clinician judged that 58 percent of patients in the ginkgo group had improved compared to 43 percent of patients in the placebo group.

Side effects

Three patients (one in the ginkgo group) complained of digestive disorders and had to stop treatment.

Authors' comments
The use of the GCES permitted the conclusion at the end of this study that *Ginkgo biloba* extract is effective in disorders due to cerebral aging.

Reviewer's comments
Large and early study of ginkgo in "cerebral disorders due to aging" showing significant benefit in the GCES from three months on. The study was flawed, however, by the inadequate description of both the randomization and the statistical analysis. (Translation reviewed) (3, 5)

Clinical Study: Tanakan®

Extract name	EGb 761
Manufacturer	Ipsen, France (Dr. Willmar Schwabe Gmbh & Co., Germany)
Indication	**Age-related memory impairment**
Level of evidence	I
Therapeutic benefit	**Yes**

Bibliographic reference
Allain H, Raoul P, Lieury A, LeCoz F, Gandon JM, d'Arbigny P (1993). Effect of two doses of *Ginkgo biloba* extract (EGb 761) on the dual-coding test in elderly subjects. *Clinical Therapeutics* 15 (3): 549-558.

Trial design
Crossover. Latin-square study design with three treatments, each separated by six-day intervals. The treatments were 320 mg extract, 600 mg extract, and placebo. Each was given one hour before psychometric testing.

Study duration	1 day
Dose	320 mg or 600 mg extract
Route of administration	Oral
Randomized	Yes
Randomization adequate	Yes
Blinding	Double-blind
Blinding adequate	Yes
Placebo	Yes
Drug comparison	No
Site description	Single center
No. of subjects enrolled	18

No. of subjects completed   Not given
Sex   Male and female
Age   60-80 years (mean: 69.3)

Inclusion criteria
Elderly patients with slight age-related memory impairment, nondemented, reporting a cognitive impairment reflected objectively by a difference of more than one standard deviation in comparison with a group of young subjects on an inclusion memory test. Subjects were receiving no treatment for their cognitive impairment.

Exclusion criteria
None mentioned.

End points
Psychometric testing used a dual-coding technique which evaluates the memory coding of verbal material and images in relation to variable presentation times (1920, 960, 480, 240, and 120 ms). The presentation of each series was followed by an immediate recall test. The point at which the presentation time is too short to allow for verbal coding and storage was considered the breaking point.

Results
Overall analyses showed no significant differences between the three treatments on word recall, drawing recall, or the drawings versus words recalled ($p = 0.06$). In the groups treated with ginkgo extract compared to the placebo group, the breaking point was significantly shifted ($p < 0.05$) toward a shorter presentation time (480 ms for ginkgo versus 960 ms for placebo), and dual coding was observed at 960 ms (versus 1920 ms for placebo).

Side effects
No adverse effects were reported by any of the subjects.

Authors' comments
In comparison with placebo, 320 or 600 mg of ginkgo extract improved the performance on the dual-coding test one hour after administration in elderly subjects with slight memory impairment. The values obtained after treatment with ginkgo extract were closer to the values observed in young healthy subjects.

Reviewer's comments
Well-run acute-dose, three-way crossover study in elderly patients satisfying age-associated memory impairment criteria showing the benefit of ginkgo in a computerized test of information processing. This is an interesting study with novel technique, and good design plus analysis. (4, 6)

Clinical Study: EGb 761®

Extract name	EGb 761
Manufacturer	Dr. Willmar Schwabe GmbH & Co., Germany
Indication	**Age-related memory impairment; Alzheimer's disease; vascular dementia**
Level of evidence	I
Therapeutic benefit	**No**

Bibliographic reference

van Dongen MCJM, van Rossum E, Kessels AGH, Sielhorst HJG, Knips-child PG (2000). The efficacy of ginkgo for elderly people with dementia and age-associated memory impairment: New results of a randomized clinical trial. *Journal of the American Geriatrics Society* 48 (10): 1183-1194.

Trial design

Parallel. Initially a three-arm study, becoming a five-arm study. After a three-week run-in period with placebo, subjects were randomized to receive one of three treatments: 160 mg/day ginkgo extract; 240 mg/day ginkgo extract; or placebo. After three months, the subjects taking ginkgo were randomized again to either continue taking ginkgo with the same dose or to take placebo for another three months. Those in the initial placebo group continued to take placebo throughout the study.

Study duration	6 months
Dose	2 tablets per day (either 160 or 240 mg per day)
Route of administration	Oral
Randomized	Yes
Randomization adequate	Yes
Blinding	Double-blind
Blinding adequate	Yes
Placebo	Yes
Drug comparison	No
Site description	Multicenter
No. of subjects enrolled	256
No. of subjects completed	196
Sex	Male and female
Age	Mean: 82.9 years

Inclusion criteria
Patients at least 50 years old with dementia, including those with Alzheimer's disease and vascular dementia, according to ICD-10 and DSM-III-R, and nondemented patients with age-associated memory impairment.

Exclusion criteria
Exclusion criteria included the following: severe depression; inadequate level of premorbid intelligence; insufficient compliance; a placebo response during three-week washout period; expectation of premature withdrawal; serious comorbidity (particularly pathological conditions considered as nontreatable underlying causes of dementia and cognitive disorders or sources of interference with the trial conduct: brain traumata, tumors, various neurological disorders, severe infectious diseases, or absorption disorders); or taking impermissible cointerventions (e.g., antiparkinson medication, antipsychotic drugs, neuroleptics, antidepressants, cholinergic therapy, or vasoactive drugs).

End points
Outcome measures were assessed at baseline and after 4, 8, 12, 18, and 24 weeks of treatment. The outcome measures included the Zahlennachsprechen Test G (ZN-G, digit span test to test short-term memory); the Wortliste (WL, tests verbal learning); the Zahlen-Verbindungs-Test G (ZVT-G, version of trail-making test that measures planning and organization and cognitive speed); the Sandoz Clinical Assessment-Geriatric Scale (SCAG, rating scale for geriatric symptoms); the Geriatric Depression Scale; self-perceived health status; self-perceived memory status; and the Nürnberger Alters Alltagsaktivitäten Skala (NAA; Nuremberg Gerontopsychological Rating Scale for Activities of Daily Living). The ZVT-G, ZN-G, WL, and NAA are all components of the Nürnberger Alters Inventar (NAI; Nuremberg Gerontopsychological Inventory).

Results
Sixty-three demented and 151 nondemented patients were randomized into the study. The MMSE baseline scores of 80 percent of the population were between 12 and 24, signaling moderate impairment. In general, there was not a dramatic shift in the scores for most of the outcome measures during the treatment with either ginkgo (both doses) or placebo. Intention-to-treat analysis showed no effect on any outcome measure for those given ginkgo ($n = 79$) compared with placebo ($n = 44$) for the entire six-month period.

Side effects
The most common side effects were dizziness, nervousness, and headache. Incidence of side effects was similar in all groups.

Authors' comments
The authors conclude that the trial has failed to reproduce the beneficial effects of ginkgo in older patients with dementia and age-associated memory impairment demonstrated by many previous trials.

Reviewer's comments
This trial was conducted with great care and expertise. My only concern is that there were so many subgroups of patients that this added much variability to the analysis. Nevertheless, a clear negative finding. (5, 6)

Clinical Study: EGb 761®

Extract name	EGb 761
Manufacturer	Dr. Willmar Schwabe GmbH & Co., Germany
Indication	**Alzheimer-type or multi-infarct dementia**
Level of evidence	**I**
Therapeutic benefit	**Yes**

Bibliographic reference
Kanowski S, Herrmann WM, Stephan K, Wierich W, Horr R (1997). Proof of efficacy of the *Ginkgo biloba* special extract EGb 761 in outpatients suffering from mild to moderate primary degenerative dementia of the Alzheimer type or multi-infarct dementia. *Phytomedicine* 4 (1): 3-13. (Also published in Kanowski S, Herrmann WM, Stephan K, Wierich W, Horr R [1996] *Pharmacopsychiatry* 29 [2]: 47-56.)

Trial design
Parallel. Single-blind placebo run-in period of four weeks.

Study duration	6 months
Dose	2 (120 mg) capsules daily
Route of administration	Oral
Randomized	Yes
Randomization adequate	Yes
Blinding	Double-blind
Blinding adequate	Yes
Placebo	Yes
Drug comparison	No
Site description	41 practices
No. of subjects enrolled	216
No. of subjects completed	156
Sex	Male and female
Age	55-82 years

Inclusion criteria
Outpatients, at least 55 years of age with presenile and senile primary degenerative dementia of the Alzheimer's type (DAT) and multi-infarct dementia (MID) according to DSM-III-R; between 6 and 18 points in the Syndrom-Kurztest; between 13 and 25 points in the MMSE (Mini-Mental State Examination); no pronounced cerebral atrophy; and in whom the necessity for full-time care can probably be avoided or postponed.

Exclusion criteria
Patients with disturbances of consciousness, suffering from other cerebral diseases, depression, psychosis, disorders due to cerebral ischemia of hemorrhage, epilepsy, and dementia of an origin other than those defined in the inclusion criteria; unstable metabolism due to severe cardiovascular insufficiency; noncompensated arrhythmia; severe chronic pulmonary diseases; hepatic and renal disorders; hyper- or dehydration; malign hypertension; gastrointestinal disorders leading to uncertain resorption of the investigational drug; diseases that prevented adequate test performance (e.g., noncompensated dysopia and defective hearing), lack of cooperation; the inability to comprehend the instructions; and intake of drugs which might have interfered with the assessment of efficacy (such as psychostimulants, nootropics, centrally acting vasoactive substances, psychotropic substances, and reserpine).

End points
Evaluations at baseline and after 12 and 24 weeks. Adverse events were additionally recorded after 6 and 18 weeks. Three primary parameters were measured: psychopathological assessment using the Clinical Global Impressions scale (CGI), syndrome-relevant cognitive performance according to the Syndrom-Kurztest (SKT), and behavior according to the Nurnberger Alters-Beobachtungsskala (NAB).

Results
The 156 patients who completed the study in accordance to protocol were evaluated according to the following response criteria: changes in the CGI to "much improved" or "very much improved"; a decrease in the SKT score by 4 points; and a decrease in NAB score of 2 points. The frequency of therapy responders in the two treatment groups differed significantly in favor of EGb 761, with $p < 0.005$ in Fisher's Exact Test. The intent-to-treat analysis of 205 patients led to similar efficacy results.

Side effects
A relationship between the study drug and adverse events was considered possible in only five patients. These were allergic skin reactions, gastrointestinal complaints, and headache.

Authors' comments
The results of this clinical study lead to the conclusion that the ginkgo biloba extract EGb 761 is of clinical efficacy in the treatment of outpatients with dementia of the Alzheimer's type and multi-infarct dementia.

Reviewer's comments
Probably the best study conducted on ginkgo and dementia. Clear benefits on SKT and CGI and excellent reporting. (5, 6)

Clinical Study: Tebonin® forte

Extract name	EGb 761
Manufacturer	Dr. Willmar Schwabe GmbH & Co., Germany
Indication	**Alzheimer-type or multi-infarct dementia**
Level of evidence	**I**
Therapeutic benefit	**Yes**

Bibliographic reference
Le Bars PL, Katz MM, Berman N, Itil TM, Freedman AM, Schatzberg AF (1997). A placebo-controlled, double-blind, randomized trial of an extract of *Ginkgo biloba* for dementia. *The Journal of the American Medical Association* 278 (16): 1327-1332. (This study was reanalyzed and published in Le Bars PL, Kieser M, Itil KZ [2000]. *Dementia and Geriatric Cognitive Disorders* 11 [4]: 230-237; and reanalyzed again in Le Bars PL, Velasco FM, Ferguson JM, Dessain EC, Kieser M, Hoerr R [2002] *Neuropsychobiology* 45 [1]: 19-26.)

Trial design
Parallel. Trial was preceded by a two-week, single-blind placebo run-in phase.

Study duration	1 year
Dose	3 (40 mg) tablets daily
Route of administration	Oral
Randomized	Yes
Randomization adequate	Yes
Blinding	Double-blind
Blinding adequate	Yes
Placebo	Yes
Drug comparison	No

Site description   6 centers

No. of subjects enrolled   327
No. of subjects completed 137
Sex   Male and female
Age   45-90 years (mean: 69)

Inclusion criteria
Forty-five years of age or older, diagnosis of uncomplicated dementia according to *Diagnostic and Statistical Manual of Mental Disorders* and *International Statistical Classification of Diseases* criteria, either Alzheimer-type or multi-infarct dementia, a Mini-Mental State Examination (MMSE) score of 9 to 26 (inclusive), and a Global Deterioration Scale score of 3 to 6 (inclusive).

Exclusion criteria
Significant medical conditions including cardiac disease, insulin-dependent diabetes, liver disease, chronic renal insufficiency, another psychiatric disorder as a primary diagnosis, and brain mass or intracranial hemorrhage determined by computed tomography (CT) or magnetic resonance imaging (MRI).

End points
Primary outcome measures were assessed at baseline and at 12, 26, and 52 weeks. They were cognitive impairment according to the cognitive subscale of the Alzheimer's Disease Assessment Scale (ADAS-Cog); daily living and social behavior according to the Geriatric Evaluation by Relatives Rating Instrument (GERRI); and general psychopathology according to the Clinical Global Impression of Change (CGIC). Safety assessments were performed after 4, 12, 26, 39, and 52 weeks.

Results
After six months, the placebo group showed a worsening and the ginkgo group showed minimal improvement resulting in statistically significant differences in favor for ginkgo for the ADAS-cog (1.3 points, $p = 0.04$) and the GERRI (0.12 points, $p = 0.02$). In the one-year intent-to-treat analysis, the ginkgo group had an ADAS-cog score 1.4 points better than the placebo group ($p = 0.04$) and a GERRI score 0.14 points better than the placebo group ($p = 0.0004$). On the ADAS-cog, 27 percent of patients treated with ginkgo achieved at least a four-point improvement, compared with 14 percent taking placebo ($p = 0.005$); on the GERRI, 37 percent were considered improved with ginkgo, compared with 23 percent taking placebo ($p = 0.003$). No difference was seen in the CGIC. The results were reanalyzed following application of a stratification based on the severity of the cognitive impairment in a population of 263 intent-to-treat cases with Alzheimer's disease. In stratum 1, with 122 subjects with MMSE > 23, there was no significant change in ADAS-cog or GERRI for the placebo group. The EGb 761 group

showed significant improvement compared to baseline (ADAS-cog 1.7 points; GERRI 0.09 points). There was no significant difference between the two groups. In stratum 2, with 114 subjects with MMSE < 14, the placebo group deteriorated compared to baseline (ADAS-cog 4.1 points; GERRI 0.18 points). The EGb 761 group showed an insignificant impairment from baseline. However, there was a significant difference between the two treatment groups. A small group of 35 subjects with an MMSE < 15 showed significant decline in the placebo group and an insignificant decline in the EGb 761 group. The difference between the two groups was similar to that in stratum 2.

Side effects
No significant differences compared with placebo were observed in the number of patients reporting adverse events or in the incidence and severity of these events.

Authors' comments
EGb 761 was safe and appears capable of stabilizing and, in a substantial number of cases, improving the cognitive functioning of demented patients for six months to one year. Although modest, the changes induced by EGb were objectively measured by the ADAS-cog and were of sufficient magnitude to be recognized by caregivers in the GERRI. The six-month analysis, unlike the one-year analysis, was obtained with a high rate of patient participation (79 percent of intent-to-treat population). The retrospective stratification analysis showed that the relative changes from baseline depended heavily on the severity at baseline. Improvement was observed in the group of patients with very mild to moderate cognitive impairment, while in more severe dementia, the mean EGb 761 effect should be considered more in terms of stabilization or slowing down of worsening, as compared to the greater deterioration observed with placebo.

Reviewer's comments
This is the most famous ginkgo study. It is well conducted and written up and shows a benefit comparable to current pharmacological therapies of choice, e.g., Aricept. The third analysis of this study shows the ADAS-cog effect is best in the MMSE <24 group compared to the effect in the MMSE >23 group. This information is worthy of comment. (5, 6)

Clinical Study: Tebonin® forte

Extract name	EGb 761
Manufacturer	Dr. Willmar Schwabe GmbH & Co., Germany
Indication	**Alzheimer-type dementia**

Level of evidence   **I**
Therapeutic benefit   **Yes**

Bibliographic reference
Maurer K, Ihl R, Dierks T, Frolich L (1997). Clinical efficacy of *Ginkgo biloba* special extract EGb 761 in dementia of the Alzheimer type. *Journal of Psychiatry Research* 31 (6): 645-655.

Trial design
Parallel. Trial preceded by a seven-day run-in phase.

Study duration	3 months
Dose	6 (40 mg) tablets daily
Route of administration	Oral
Randomized	Yes
Randomization adequate	Yes
Blinding	Double-blind
Blinding adequate	Yes
Placebo	Yes
Drug comparison	No
Site description	Single center
No. of subjects enrolled	20
No. of subjects completed	18
Sex	Male and female
Age	51-75 years

Inclusion criteria
Age 50-80; Hachinski Ischemic Score less than or equal to 4; mild to moderate Alzheimer-type senile dementia (mean Brief Cognitive Rating Scale [BCRS] score 3 to 5); and normal CT finding or a diffuse, possibly asymmetric, atrophy.

Exclusion criteria
Advanced Alzheimer's dementia (inpatient care or constant nursing by another person for daily tasks); intellectual degeneration, states of confusion, or dementia syndromes of another origin, e.g., multi-infarct dementia (Hachinski Ischemic Score > 7); pseudodementia; nonorganic depressive illness or schizophrenic decompensation; aphasia or sensory, motor, and/or visual disturbances that could interfere with psychometric tests; severe organic diseases; neoplasia of any localization; epilepsy; cerebrovascular malformation; alcohol or drug abuse; vasoactive drugs, nootropics, and/or long-term treatment with other drugs proscribed during the study; and lack of patient cooperation already during the run-in phase.

End points

The primary outcome measure was the sum score in the Syndrom-Kurztest. Other psychometric tests, including the trailmaking test (Zahlen Verbindungs Test [ZVT]), Alzheimer's Disease Assessment Scale (ADAS), Clinical Global Impression, and EEG topography, were evaluated descriptively. Patients were assessed at baseline and after one, two, and three months.

Results

Although the EGb 761 group, with a mean sum score of 19.67 points in the SKT, had a poorer baseline level than the placebo group (18.11 points), it improved to 16.78 points with treatment, whereas the placebo group deteriorated to 18.89 points. The differences between the baseline and final values formed the basis for a statistical group comparison, which gave a result favorable to EGb 761, at a significance level of $p < 0.013$. In addition, certain favorable trends were found at the psychopathological (CGI) and dynamic functional (EEG findings) levels. Intergroup differences in the ADAS cognitive and noncognitive subscales did not reach statistical significance, probably because of the small sample size.

Side effects

None reported.

Authors' comments

The results of this trial can be interpreted as evidence of effectiveness of *Ginkgo biloba* special extract EGb 761 in mild to moderate dementia, and of local effects in the central nervous system.

Reviewer's comments

This trial had a small sample but was well conducted and reported with a clear benefit on a good cognitive end point, SKT, in patients with mild/moderate Alzheimer's disease. Some support in CGI and EEG as well. (5, 5)

Clinical Study: Tebonin® forte

Extract name	EGb 761
Manufacturer	Dr. Willmar Schwabe GmbH & Co., Germany
Indication	**Alzheimer-type dementia**
Level of evidence	**III**
Therapeutic benefit	**Yes**

Bibliographic reference

Hofferberth B (1994). The efficacy of EGb 761 in patients with senile dementia of the Alzheimer type, a double-blind, placebo-controlled study on different levels of investigation. *Human Psychopharmacology* 9: 215-222.

Trial design

Parallel.

Study duration	3 months
Dose	6 (40 mg) tablets daily
Route of administration	Oral
Randomized	Yes
Randomization adequate	No
Blinding	Double-blind
Blinding adequate	Yes
Placebo	Yes
Drug comparison	No
Site description	Single center
No. of subjects enrolled	42
No. of subjects completed	40
Sex	Male and female
Age	50-75 years

Inclusion criteria

Hospitalized patients with the clinical diagnosis of incipient senile dementia of the Alzheimer type, aged between 50 and 75 years, Blessed Dementia Scale: sum part A: 0-16, sum part B: 9.5 to 30.5; Hachinski Ischemic Score < 4; normal or diffuse and possible asymmetrically atrophic CT findings.

Exclusion criteria

Those with advanced Alzheimer's dementia; those suffering from intellectual deterioration of confusedness and/or dementia syndrome of other origin including multi-infarctional dementia, Pick's disease, alcoholic dementia, Parkinson's disease, Huntington's disease, lateral amyotrophic sclerosis, chronic subdural hematoma, brain tumors, and dementias based on infectious, toxic, or metabolic/endocrinological factors; those with pseudodementia; those subject to a severe depressive condition; pronounced sensory or motor disturbances; those suffering from severe organic conditions, neoplasias, epilepsy, cerebrovascular malformation, alcohol or drug abuse; patients who were pregnant or not willing to cooperate; or receiving therapy with vasoactive agents, nootropics, psychotonics, tranquilizers, and/or depressants.

End points
The Syndrom-Kurztest (SKT) was the target parameter. Secondary parameters included the saccade test, reaction performance, the Sandoz Clinical Assessment Geriatric Scale (SCAG), and electroencephalography (EEG). Subjects were evaluated at baseline and then at monthly intervals.

Results
Baseline mean values for the SKT were 17 for the treatment group and 15 in the placebo group. After three months, the SKT mean value dropped to 12 in the treatment group, whereas it increased to 17 in the placebo group. The difference between the groups was highly significant after one, two, and three months ($p = 0.00017$, $p = 0.00017$, and $p = 0.00043$, respectively). A superiority of the active substance was found in all five subscales of the SCAG. In addition, the efficacy of the preparation could be clarified in two further neurophysiological examinations (saccade test and EEG). The change in behavior of the patient documented by the subjective final assessment of the examining physician, which is also visible in various items and groups of factors of the SCAG, confirms the other positive results.

Side effects
No side effects recorded during trial.

Author's comments
The proof of efficacy of a preparation aimed at improving cerebral performance may be considered as established if, in each of the target variables, significant changes can be demonstrated by comparison with the control group in two out of three independent examination levels. In this clinical trial, EGb 761 meets this requirement.

Reviewer's comments
This small sample of dementia (Alzheimer's-type) patients responded very clearly to EGb 761 on SKT—a valid and important test of cognitive function, supported by rating scales and EEG. The study was flawed by the inappropriate randomization and the lack of description of withdrawals and dropouts. (2, 6)

Clinical Study: Rökan®

Extract name	EGb 761
Manufacturer	Intersan GmbH, Germany (Dr. Willmar Schwabe GmbH & Co., Germany)
Indication	**Cerebrovascular insufficiency**

Level of evidence   I
Therapeutic benefit   **Yes**

Bibliographic reference
Grassel E (1992). The effect of *Ginkgo biloba* extract on mental performance: Double-blind study conducted under computerized measurement
conditions in patients with cerebral insufficiency. *Fortschritte der Medizin*
110 (5): 73-76.

Trial design
Parallel. Four-week washout period before the study.

Study duration	6 months
Dose	2 (80 mg extract) tablets daily
Route of administration	Oral
Randomized	Yes
Randomization adequate	Yes
Blinding	Double-blind
Blinding adequate	Yes
Placebo	Yes
Drug comparison	No
Site description	3 trial centers
No. of subjects enrolled	72
No. of subjects completed	53
Sex	Male and female
Age	Mean: 63.8 years

Inclusion criteria
Outpatients under 80 years of age with cerebral insufficiency diagnosed on
the basis of case histories, with short-term memory capacity IQ lower than
Mehrfachwahl Wortschatz Intelligence Test (MWT) IQ (multiple choice vocabulary intelligence test). Patients also had to be able to read text on a
computer monitor and had to have an MWT IQ greater than 80.

Exclusion criteria
Patients with neurological diseases of a different origin, those with recent
myocardial infarction or severe cardiac arrhythmias, severe hepatic insufficiency, severe renal insufficiency, or pregnancy.

End points
Psychometric performance tests, computerized recordings of short-term
memory capacity and basic learning rate, were administered. Testing was
done at baseline and at 6, 12, and 24 weeks.

Results

For the ginkgo group, there was a statistically significant improvement in short-term memory capacity after six weeks ($p < 0.005$) and of learning rate after 24 weeks ($p < 0.0001$), compared to baseline. The placebo group showed no significant change compared to baseline. Comparison between the groups showed a statistically significant difference in the short-term memory capacity and learning rate at the end of the 24-week treatment phase (both $p < 0.01$).

Side effects

Four patients in the ginkgo group reported the following adverse events: alopecia, bloating, nausea with gastric pain, or facial flush.

Author's comments

Treatment with *Ginkgo biloba* extract EGb 761 results in improvement of the basic mental performance (especially "capacity for conscious information processing").

Reviewer's comments

Good study showing significant improvement in memory and learning in elderly cerebral insufficiency patients using computerized tests. More information on the tasks would have been welcomed. The only flaw was that the raw data used to evaluate the actual "effect size" were not given. (Translation reviewed) (5, 6)

Clinical Study: Tebonin® forte

Extract name	EGb 761
Manufacturer	Dr. Willmar Schwabe GmbH & Co., Germany
Indication	**Cerebrovascular insufficiency**
Level of evidence	I
Therapeutic benefit	**Yes**

Bibliographic reference

Halama P, Bartsch G, Meng G (1988). Randomized, double-blind study on the efficacy of *Ginkgo biloba* extract. *Fortschritte der Medizin* 106 (19): 408-412.

Trial design

Parallel.

Study duration	3 months
Dose	3 (40 mg extract) tablets daily
Route of administration	Oral
Randomized	Yes
Randomization adequate	Yes
Blinding	Double-blind
Blinding adequate	Yes
Placebo	Yes
Drug comparison	No
Site description	1 neurology practice
No. of subjects enrolled	40
No. of subjects completed	40
Sex	Male and female
Age	55-85 years

Inclusion criteria
Outpatients aged above 55 years and diagnosed with mild to medium cerebrovascular insufficiency (Hachinski score > 7, Crichton degree 1 to 3).

Exclusion criteria
Patients with the following diseases or symptoms were excluded: psychosis or neurosis; primary degenerative dementia; secondary insufficiency of cerebral performance (due to intoxication, metabolic disorder, alcoholism, etc.); epilepsy or other severe diseases (e.g., myocardial infarction in the past six months, severe renal insufficiency, severe, life-threatening arrhythmias, malignoma); as well as patients who were not sufficiently cooperative.

End points
The primary outcome measure was the Sandoz Clinical Assessment-Geriatric score evaluating cognitive disturbances, social behavior, lack of initiative, affective disturbances, and somatic disturbances. Additional tests included the Crichton Geriatric Behavioral Rating Scale (CRBRS), the background-interference method (Hintergrund-Interferenz-Verfahren [HIV]), the Syndrom-Kurztest (SKT), and craniocorpography (CCG). Dizziness, tinnitus, headache, and hearing deficit were investigated by questioning the patients. Assessment was completed at baseline and at weeks 4, 8, and 12.

Results
After 12 weeks, the ginkgo group values for total SCAG score dropped on average by 9 points, whereas they remained unchanged in the placebo group. The difference between the groups was highly significant ($p = 0.00005$). In addition, short-term memory and mental awareness improved, tinnitus improved compared to the placebo group (twelfth week: $p = 0.035$),

hearing deficits remained unchanged in both groups, headache improved compared to placebo, and dizziness significantly improved in the ginkgo group (twelfth week: $p < 0.001$).

Side effects
Mild to moderate headaches in one patient in the ginkgo group.

Authors' comments
On the basis of the results of the present study, *Ginkgo biloba* is very well suited for the treatment of disturbances of cerebral performance of vascular origin.

Reviewer's comments
Well-designed and well-conducted study with clear and marked improvements in SCAG, particularly items for cognitive and somatic disturbances, plus improvements to SKT for cognitive function plus reduction in dizziness. (Translation reviewed) (5, 6)

Clinical Study: Rökan®

Extract name	EGb 761
Manufacturer	Intersan GmbH, Germany (Dr. Willmar Schwabe GmbH & Co., Germany)

Indication	**Cerebrovascular insufficiency**
Level of evidence	**II**
Therapeutic benefit	**Yes**

Bibliographic reference
Hofferberth B (1991). Simultaneous determination of electrophysiological, psychometric, and rheological parameters in patients with cerebro-organic psychosyndrome and increased vascular risk—A placebo-controlled double-blind study with *Ginkgo biloba* extract EGb 761. In *Mikrozirkulation in Gehirn und Sinnesorganen*. Eds. R Stodtmeister, LE Pillunat. Stuttgart: Ferdinand Enke Verlag, pp. 64-74.

Trial design
Parallel. Treatment preceded by a two-week placebo washout phase.

Study duration	3 months
Dose	3 (40 mg extract) tablets daily
Route of administration	Oral
Randomized	Yes

Randomization adequate	No
Blinding	Double-blind
Blinding adequate	Yes

| Placebo | Yes |
| Drug comparison | No |

| Site description | Not described |

No. of subjects enrolled	24
No. of subjects completed	24
Sex	Male and female
Age	62-74 years

Inclusion criteria
Hospitalized patients with the diagnosis "cerebrovascular risk" on the basis of measurements of the venous microembolism index, the theta proportion in the quantified EEG, and clinical history.

Exclusion criteria
Unclear cardiovascular conditions, such as recent myocardial infarction; congestive heart failure; refractory hypertension; hypotension; uncontrollable diabetes; severe liver, kidney, or gastrointestinal disorders; progressive neurological diseases or brain tumors; and patients with stenoses in the carotid or the cerebral circulation or transient ischaemic attack (TIA).

End points
Patients were examined prior to the placebo phase, at baseline, and after 4 and 12 weeks of therapy. Patients were assessed according to quantified EEG, the saccade test, Vienna Determination Unit (VDU), and venous microembolism index (VMI) (a laboratory indicator of platelet aggregation).

Results
After four weeks of treatment, there was an improvement in the ginkgo group compared with the placebo for all measured parameters. The theta-wave component of the theta/alpha ratio fell significantly ($p < 0.01$, between group comparison). Latency time for saccadic eye movements fell at both four weeks ($p < 0.01$) and 12 weeks ($p < 0.001$). The number of correct answers in the VDU reaction test was increased (statistically significant after four weeks). The VMI decreased continuously in the ginkgo group, whereas in the placebo group there was no change ($p < 0.001$ at four weeks, between-group comparison).

Side effects
Two patients in the ginkgo group complained of stomachache.

Author's comments
The standardized *Ginkgo biloba* extract EGb 761 used in this study proved to be highly significantly more effective than placebo and thus fulfills the frequently stipulated criterion of a large difference in efficacy from the control.

Reviewer's comments
Another well-conducted study from this investigator showing marked and widespread improvements despite a small parallel group design. However, the randomization process and statistical methods were not adequately described. (Translation reviewed) (3, 5)

Clinical Study: Rökan®

Extract name	EGb 761
Manufacturer	Intersan GmbH, Germany (Dr. Willmar Schwabe GmbH & Co., Germany)
Indication	**Cerebrovascular insufficiency**
Level of evidence	**III**
Therapeutic benefit	**Yes**

Bibliographic reference
Hofferberth B (1989). Effect of *Ginkgo biloba* extract on neurophysiological and psychometric findings in patients with cerebro-organic syndrome. *Arzneimittel-Forschung/Drug Research* 39 (8): 918-922.

Trial design
Parallel. Treatment preceded by a two-week washout period.

Study duration	2 months
Dose	3 (40 mg extract) tablets daily
Route of administration	Oral
Randomized	Yes
Randomization adequate	No
Blinding	Double-blind
Blinding adequate	No
Placebo	Yes
Drug comparison	No
Site description	Not described
No. of subjects enrolled	36
No. of subjects completed	36

Sex	Male and female
Age	53-69 years (mean: 63)

Inclusion criteria
Hospitalized patients with cerebrovascular syndrome, pathological results in two of the four tests (EEG, saccade test, Vienna Determination Test, or Trail Making Test).

Exclusion criteria
Patients were excluded if they were taking supplementary prohibited medication, such as vasoactive drugs, CNS stimulants, tranquilizers, antihistamines, calcium antagonists, thrombocyte aggregation inhibitors, and anticoagulants. Also excluded were patients with acute heart disease, uncontrolled hypertension, hypotension, unstable diabetes, severe liver and renal disease, and gastrointestinal disease.

End points
Objective assessment by quantified EEG and saccadic eye movements, and by two psychometric tests (Vienna Determination Unit Test; number connection test). Tests were conducted at baseline and after four and eight weeks, except EEG which was conducted at commencement and at the end of treatment.

Results
After both four weeks and eight weeks of therapy, there was a highly significant improvement in the saccadic test in comparison to the placebo group ($p < 0.0001$). Similar improvements were observed in the psychometric tests. The number of correct responses in the Vienna Determination Test increased very significantly at all speed levels in the ginkgo group after four weeks, by which time it had normalized. In the placebo group, no change was documented. Similarly, the time taken in the Trail Making Test decreased dramatically in the ginkgo group after four weeks, while in the placebo group there was only a slight tendency to shorter times. Quantitative EEG analysis before the study and after eight weeks showed a significant decrease in the theta component of patients in the ginkgo group only. After four weeks of therapy, the patients' subjective evaluation of their condition and the doctor's assessment were clearly positive in the active treatment group.

Side effects
Two reports of nausea and one of ankle edema in the ginkgo group.

Author's comments
The results show *Ginkgo biloba* extract to be a therapeutic option in mild and moderate cerebro-organic syndrome.

Reviewer's comments
Well-conducted trial, with modest sample ($n = 36$), showing large benefits on saccadic eye movements, theta-band reduction in EEG, and improved cognitive function on Vienna test plus Trails A. No placebo improvement was seen, although a similar trial (Bruchert, Heinrich, and Ruf-Kohler, 1991) showed ten seconds improvement in placebo in a similar population in a trail-making test. Neither the randomization nor the blinding were adequately described. (Translation reviewed) (1, 6)

Clinical Study: Tebonin® forte

Extract name	EGb 761
Manufacturer	Dr. Willmar Schwabe GmbH & Co., Germany
Indication	**Cerebrovascular insufficiency**
Level of evidence	**III**
Therapeutic benefit	**Yes**

Bibliographic reference
Arrigo A (1986). Treatment of chronic cerebrovascular insufficiency with *Ginkgo biloba* extract. *Therapiewoche* 36: 5208-5218.

Trial design
Crossover. Washout periods of 15 days before treatment and between 45-day treatment periods.

Study duration	45 days
Dose	3 doses of 20 drops (40 mg extract) daily
Route of administration	Oral
Randomized	No
Randomization adequate	No
Blinding	Double-blind
Blinding adequate	No
Placebo	Yes
Drug comparison	No
Site description	Not described
No. of subjects enrolled	90
No. of subjects completed	80
Sex	Male and female
Age	36-88 years

Inclusion criteria

Patients with cerebral insufficiency of vascular origin (diffuse or localized tissue ischemia, localized stenoses) diagnosed predominantly on an arteriosclerotic basis. Symptoms included transient ischemic attacks, hemipareses, tinnitus, dizziness, headache, and anxiety.

Exclusion criteria

Patients with severe neurological deficits (e.g., agnosia, apraxia) and/or mental deficiency (e.g., atrophy); psychiatric pathology (e.g., hypochondriacal and depressive psychoses); chronic disease processes altering absorption, metabolism, and catabolism of drugs (e.g., gastric resection, hepatic and renal disease, severe insulin-dependent diabetes); and pathological processes that are possibly terminal (e.g., recent myocardial infarction, severe cardiac arrhythmia).

End points

Patients completed a questionnaire regarding their symptoms (e.g., asthenia, insomnia, headache, dizziness, tinnitus, vision, and stress) at baseline and every 15 days thereafter until the end of treatment. The Wechsler Adult Intelligence Scale (WAIS), which monitors general knowledge, vocabulary, language comprehension, social relationships, ability to concentrate, memory, and learning ability, was conducted before treatment and at the end of treatment periods. Other tests administered were Complex Figures According to Rey; Retentive Capacity (Memory Table); Word Recognition; and the Questionnaire for Determining State of Anxiety and Habitually Anxious Behavior (STAI).

Results

Marked improvement in the patients' self-assessment of symptoms was seen for most symptoms by day 30, and for asthenia after 45 days of treatment with ginkgo. According to the objective psychological tests, ginkgo extract improves memory, logical thinking, and vigilance. The WAIS data show that ginkgo acts upon the progressive diminution of intellectual and cognitive facilities. Concentration, retentive capacity, and ability to make logical associations were significantly improved. In the Word Recognition test, the group treated with ginkgo in each phase of the trial showed significantly greater improvement over the group treated with placebo ($p < 0.0001$). Ginkgo had a significant effect on performance compared to placebo in the Memory test ($p < 0.0001$). Treatment with ginkgo also decreased the state of anxiety ($p < 0.0001$) and anxious behavior ($p < 0.01$).

Side effects

None mentioned in paper.

Author's comments

The subjectively experienced improvement in the target symptoms of chronic cerebrovascular insufficiency (CCVI) was clearly evident after patients had been treated with *Ginkgo biloba* extract for about two weeks. According to objective psychological tests, *Ginkgo biloba* also brings about an appreciable improvement in memory, logical thinking, and vigilance.

Reviewer's comments
Well-conducted crossover study in CCVI patients. Improvement was seen in symptoms including tinnitus, anxiety, attention, higher functions, and memory. The study was not randomized, and the blinding was not adequately described. (Translation reviewed) (1, 6)

Clinical Study: Tebonin® forte

Extract name	EGb 761
Manufacturer	Dr. Willmar Schwabe GmbH & Co., Germany
Indication	**Cerebrovascular insufficiency and depressive symptoms**
Level of evidence	**III**
Therapeutic benefit	**Trend**

Bibliographic reference
Halama P (1990). Treatment with *Ginkgo biloba* in patients with cerebrovascular insufficiency and refractory depressive symptoms: Results of a placebo-controlled, randomized double-blind pilot study. *Therapiewoche* 40 (51/52): 3760-3765.

Trial design
Parallel. Patients continued their existing antidepressant medication.

Study duration	2 months
Dose	3 (80 mg extract) tablets daily
Route of administration	Oral
Randomized	Yes
Randomization adequate	No
Blinding	Double-blind
Blinding adequate	No
Placebo	Yes
Drug comparison	No
Site description	Not described

No. of subjects enrolled   20
No. of subjects completed   20
Sex   Male and female
Age   55-85 years

Inclusion criteria
Diagnosis of depression in mild to moderate cerebro-organic disturbances, with at least three months' unsuccessful treatment with antidepressants.

Exclusion criteria
Alcoholism or other addictions; concomitant treatment not dose-stable; concomitant diseases which must be expected to get worse during the period of the study; and pregnancy.

End points
Treatment was monitored using the Zung Self-Rating Depression Scale (SRDS), late auditory-evoked potentials (LAEP), and several psychometric tests, including short screening test for cerebral insufficiency (CI test); self-assessment method for the objective measurement of mild cerebral insufficiency (CI scale); the short test of general intelligence (Kurztest für Allgemeine Intelligenz [KAI]); subjective assessment of depression; and subjective assessment of the ability to concentrate. Patients were assessed at baseline and at four and eight weeks.

Results
The Zung SRDS index decreased by 5.3 points in the active medication group in the eight-week period, whereas there was an increase of 5.2 points in the placebo group. Mean latency time of P300 in the active group was reduced significantly in the eight-week period ($p = 0.048$) and increased in the placebo group. Psychometric findings showed clear differences in favor of the ginkgo group. Severity of depression improved in three patients in the ginkgo group, remained unchanged in four, and got worse in three patients. In the placebo group, no patients improved their depression, five remained the same, and five got worse. The ability to concentrate, assessed subjectively, also improved after eight weeks of treatment with ginkgo.

Side effects
No adverse drug effects occurred during treatment.

Author's comments
Because of the small number of cases and the differing baseline situations of the groups, this must be regarded as a pilot study and used as a basis for investigations in a larger group of patients.

Reviewer's comments
In this small study in depressed cerebrovascular insufficiency patients,

there are patterns of improvement in latency of evoked potential reaction times and symptoms of depression. Neither the randomization nor the blinding processes were adequately described. (Translation reviewed) (1, 5)

Clinical Study: Tebonin® forte

Extract name   EGb 761
Manufacturer   Dr. Willmar Schwabe GmbH & Co.,
                      Germany

Indication   **Peripheral vascular disease**
Level of evidence   I
Therapeutic benefit   **Yes**

Bibliographic reference
Blume J, Kieser M, Holscher U (1996). Placebo-controlled double-blind study on the efficacy of *Ginkgo biloba* special extract EGb 761 in the maximum-level trained patients with intermittent claudication. *Zeitschrift fur Gefasskrankheiten/Journal for Vascular Diseases* 25 (3): 265-274.

Trial design
Parallel. Pretrial two-week run-in phase with placebo.

Study duration   6 months
Dose   1(40 mg) tablet 3 times daily
Route of administration Oral

Randomized   Yes
Randomization adequate Yes
Blinding   Double-blind
Blinding adequate   Yes

Placebo   Yes
Drug comparison   No

Site description   Single center

No. of subjects enrolled   60
No. of subjects completed 54
Sex   Male and female
Age   47-82 years

Inclusion criteria
Patients with peripheral arterial occlusive disease of the lower extremities, Fontaine stage IIb, intermittent claudication for over six months, no improve-

ment in walking performance in spite of consistent walking three to four times per week. Pain-free walking distance had to be below 150 meters and within 30 percent of initial value at the end of the placebo run-in phase.

Exclusion criteria
Patients less than 18 years of age; cardiac infarction during the preceding six months; New York Heart Association stage III or IV cardiac insufficiency; severe circulatory hypertension; severe renal insufficiency; severe functional hepatic disorders; respiratory insufficiency as a limiting factor of the walking distance; restricted walking due to an orthopedic disorder; venous insufficiency from stage II (Basel classification); badly manageable diabetes mellitus; malabsorption; anemia; hematocrit above 48 percent; fibrinogen over 500 mg/dl; regular intake of platelet aggregation inhibitors, anti-inflammatory agents, or analgesics; pregnancy; or expected insufficient compliance.

End points
The main outcome measure was the difference in walking distance from the start of therapy and after 8, 16, and 24 weeks. Secondary parameters were the corresponding differences for the maximum walking distance, the relative increase in pain-free walking distance, the Doppler index, and the subjective evaluation of the patients.

Results
At the start of the therapy, the treatment group had a pain-free walking distance of 96 m and a maximum walking distance of 126 m. In the ginkgo group, there was a continuous improvement in pain-free walking distance compared to placebo at 8, 16, and 24 weeks ($p < 0.0001$, $p < 0.0003$, $p < 0.0001$, respectively). There was a 20 percent clinically relevant difference between the two groups. Maximum total walking distance values also increased significantly in the treatment group at 8, 16, and 24 weeks (22 m, 32 m, 50.5 m, respectively) compared to the placebo group (0 m, 7.5 m, 15.5 m, respectively) ($p < 0.005$ for between group comparison). The Doppler index remained unchanged in both groups. The results of the subjective assessment survey indicated that the treatment group felt that they had improved significantly, while the placebo group did not.

Side effects
Two ginkgo patients had gastric pains and nausea which disappeared spontaneously during continued administration of the extract.

Authors' comments
The present study confirmed the clinical efficacy of *Ginkgo biloba* special extract EGb 761 previously documented in other clinical trials involving patients with intermittent claudication and also demonstrated the additive use-

fulness of such a therapy in patients who had already reached their maximum physical capacity through previous exercise.

Reviewer's comments
This is an excellent study with clear, unequivocal results. (Translation reviewed) (5, 6)

Clinical Study: Rökan®

Extract name	EGb 761
Manufacturer	Intersan GmbH, Germany (Dr. Willmar Schwabe GmbH & Co., Germany)

Indication	**Peripheral vascular disease**
Level of evidence	**II**
Therapeutic benefit	**Yes**

Bibliographic reference
Bauer U (1984). 6-month double-blind randomized clinical trial of *Ginkgo biloba* extract versus placebo in two parallel groups in patients suffering from peripheral arterial insufficiency. *Arzneimittel-Forschung/Drug Research* 34 (6): 716-720.

Trial design
Parallel. Pretrial washout period of six weeks with placebo.

Study duration	6 months
Dose	1 (40 mg) tablet 3 times daily
Route of administration	Oral
Randomized	Yes
Randomization adequate	No
Blinding	Double-blind
Blinding adequate	Yes
Placebo	Yes
Drug comparison	No
Site description	Not described
No. of subjects enrolled	80
No. of subjects completed	79
Sex	Male and female
Age	Mean: 60.9 years

Inclusion criteria
Outpatients suffering from obliterative arterial disease of the lower limbs, Fontaine's stage IIb, with accompanying stenosis of the superficial femoral artery, with or without stenosis of other arteries, predominantly on one side, and lasting for more than a year; pain-free walking distance below 150 meters and within 30 percent of initial value at the end of the placebo run-in phase.

Exclusion criteria
Uncooperative patients; patients taking disallowed medication; other stages of Fontaine's classification; concomitant diseases such as pathology of the veins, anemia, noncompensated cardiac insufficiency, recent myocardial infarction, uncontrolled hypertension, other causes of walking impairment, poorly controlled diabetes, significant kidney or hepatic insufficiency, and treatment with anticoagulant drugs during the past six months.

End points
Examinations were performed at the beginning of the washout phase, before treatment, and after 6, 12, and 24 weeks. Efficacy was evaluated according to the following parameters: subjective assessment of pain using a visual analog scale; assessment of walking distance before onset of pain and total walking distance; Doppler pulse volume recording and ankle pressure measurements; trophicity; venous occlusion plethysmography values at rest and after application of a cuff for three minutes; blood pressure; and heart rate.

Results
After 24 weeks, decreases in subjective estimates of pain were almost four times as great for the ginkgo group compared to placebo ($p < 0.001$). There was a statistically significant improvement in the distance the ginkgo group was able to walk without pain ($p < 0.05$) as well as for total distance the patients were able to walk ($p < 0.001$) compared with placebo. Blood flow in the affected side increased significantly in the ginkgo group ($p < 0.01$) and only slightly in the placebo group. Doppler measurements showed no change in the ratio of ankle to arm pressure in either group.

Side effects
Nausea and blood in urine occurred in one patient in the ginkgo group who also had bladder cancer.

Author's comments
This trial demonstrates the beneficial effect of ginkgo extract on walking tolerance, together with an improvement of the limb perfusion. At the end of this six-month trial, this improvement is not only statistically significant, but also clinically relevant.

Reviewer's comments
This is an excellent early study showing ginkgo improving walking distance in this condition. However, the randomization process was not adequately described. (3, 6)

Clinical Study: Tanakan®

Extract name	EGb 761
Manufacturer	Ipsen, France (Dr. Willmar Schwabe Gmbh & Co., Germany)

Indication	**Peripheral vascular disease**
Level of evidence	**III**
Therapeutic benefit	**Yes**

Bibliographic reference
Thomson GJL, Vohra RK, Carr MH, Walker MG (1990). A clinical trial of *Ginkgo biloba* extract in patients with intermittent claudication. *International Angiology* 9 (2): 75-78.

Trial design
Parallel. Pretrial washout period of six weeks with placebo.

Study duration	6 months
Dose	3 tablets daily
Route of administration	Oral
Randomized	Yes
Randomization adequate	No
Blinding	Double-blind
Blinding adequate	No
Placebo	Yes
Drug comparison	No
Site description	Not described
No. of subjects enrolled	49
No. of subjects completed	37
Sex	Not given
Age	Not given

Inclusion criteria
Patients with Fontaine stage II peripheral vascular disease affecting the iliac or femoral arteries and involving predominantly one leg.

Exclusion criteria

Claudication distance of greater than 300 meters, alternating side of pain, poorly controlled diabetes, and significant concomitant illness. Improvement by 30 percent or more during pretrial washout. Smoking more than five cigarettes per day.

End points

Doppler pressures at the ankles were measured at the beginning of the washout phase, before treatment, and at weeks 6, 12, and 25. Ankle/brachial (A/B) pressure ratio, walking distance to claudication, changes in pressures in response to exercise, and recovery time were measured using a treadmill. Patients assessed pain using a 10 cm analog scale.

Results

Pain scores were significantly improved after 24 weeks in patients receiving ginkgo ($p < 0.05$), but not in those receiving placebo. Claudication distance (distance before onset of painful walking) increased for both groups but was significant only for the ginkgo group. Comparison of the actual distance walked at 24 weeks showed no significant difference between the two groups. There was no difference in A/B ratio, resting ankle pressure, ankle pressure immediately after exercise, or recovery times.

Side effects

No major side effects in either group.

Authors' comments

Ginkgo biloba extract is a safe and effective method of improving walking distance and reducing pain severity in patients with intermittent claudication, although Doppler studies have failed to suggest any gross improvement in the perfusion of the ischemic leg. A six-month course of EGb 761 results in symptomatic improvement in Fontaine stage II peripheral vascular disease.

Reviewer's comments

This is a positive trial with clear findings, but neither the randomization nor the blinding were adequately described. (1, 6)

Clinical Study: Tebonin® forte

Extract name	EGb 761
Manufacturer	Dr. Willmar Schwabe GmbH & Co., Germany
Indication	**Peripheral vascular disease**

Level of evidence   **III**
Therapeutic benefit   **Yes**

Bibliographic reference
Peters H, Kieser M, Holscher U (1998). Demonstration of the efficacy of *Ginkgo biloba* special extract EGb 761 on the intermittent claudication: A placebo-controlled, double-blind multicenter trial. *Zeitschrift fur Gefasskrankheiten/Journal for Vascular Diseases* 27 (2): 106-110.

Trial design
Parallel. Pretrial washout period of two weeks with placebo.

Study duration	6 months
Dose	1(40 mg) tablet 3 times daily
Route of administration	Oral
Randomized	Yes
Randomization adequate	No
Blinding	Double-blind
Blinding adequate	No
Placebo	Yes
Drug comparison	No
Site description	Multicenter
No. of subjects enrolled	111
No. of subjects completed	109
Sex	Male and female
Age	60-67 years (mean: 63)

Inclusion criteria
Patients with peripheral arterial occlusive disease of the lower extremities, Fontaine stage IIb, intermittent claudication for over six months, no improvement in walking performance in spite of consistent walking three to four times per week. Pain-free walking distance had to be below 150 meters and within 30 percent of initial value at the end of the placebo run-in phase.

Exclusion criteria
Patients with neuropathies; Raynaud's disease; severe restrictions in cardiac, liver, and kidney functions; restrictions in walking ability due to respiratory insufficiency or orthopedic condition; poorly managed diabetes mellitus; pathologically changed hemorheology; and regular intake of platelet aggregation inhibitors, anti-inflammatory agents, or analgesics.

End points
Main outcome was the difference in pain-free walking distance between the

start of therapy and after 8, 16, and 24 weeks. The absolute walking distance was determined and the subjective assessment of the patients was documented using a visual analog scale. Doppler pressure measurements were performed bilaterally over the posterior tibial arteries and the brachial arteries prior to inclusion, at baseline, and at 24 weeks.

Results
Pain-free walking increased continuously with treatment from 108 to 153 m after 24 weeks. Pain-free walking distance in the EGb 761 group was significantly greater than placebo at 8, 16, and 24 weeks ($p = 0.014$, $p = 0.006$, and $p = 0.012$, respectively). Total walking distance also improved under therapy with ginkgo extract compared to placebo ($p = 0.021$ after 16 weeks, and $p = 0.030$ after 24 weeks). Subjective assessment of therapy by patients showed an improvement in both groups. The Doppler quotients remained the same in both groups.

Side effects
No adverse reactions were recorded for EGb 761.

Authors' comments
This study confirms the clinical efficacy of EGb 761 in patients with peripheral arterial occlusive disease Fontaine stage IIb, with very good tolerance.

Reviewer's comments
This is a sound replication of previous trial from this group (Blume, Kieser, and Holscher, 1996). The placebo effect was larger in this study, but it did not affect the positive outcome. However, neither the randomization nor the blinding were adequately described. (1, 6)

Clinical Study: Rökan®

Extract name	EGb761
Manufacturer	Intersan GmbH, Germany (Dr. Willmar Schwabe GmbH & Co., Germany)
Indication	**Peripheral vascular disease**
Level of evidence	**III**
Therapeutic benefit	**Yes**

Bibliographic reference
Schweizer J, Hautmann C (1999). Comparison of two dosages of *Ginkgo biloba* extract Egb 761 in patients with peripheral arterial occlusive disease

Fontaine's stage IIb. *Arzneimittel-Forschung/Drug Research* 49 (11): 900-904.

Trial design

Parallel. Dose comparison with pretrial washout period of two to four weeks.

Study duration	6 months
Dose	120 mg or 240 mg daily (both in split doses)
Route of administration	Oral
Randomized	Yes
Randomization adequate	No
Blinding	Double-blind
Blinding adequate	No
Placebo	No
Drug comparison	No
Site description	Multicenter
No. of subjects enrolled	77
No. of subjects completed	74
Sex	Male and female
Age	55-71 years

Inclusion criteria

Patients with peripheral arterial occlusive disease (pAOD) Fontaine's stage IIb with occlusion of the superficial femoral artery on one leg and without occlusion of the deep femoral artery, for which there were no other therapeutic options. The pain-free walking distance, evaluated on a treadmill, had to be <200 meters and the maximum walking distance between 100 and 300 meters. The difference between the walking distances at the end of the wash-out period and at week 0 (start of treatment) had to be <25 percent. Pain associated with pAOD had to be unilateral, had to occur regularly, and the patients had to be able to describe pain precisely.

Exclusion criteria

Patients with severe kidney of hepatic insufficiency (creatinine > 140 µmol/l; serum glutamic pyruvic transaminase [SGPT] > 40U/l), gastrointestinal disturbances, malabsorption, diabetes, noncompensated cardiac insufficiency, myocardial infarction within the preceding six months, poorly controlled hypertension, hypertension below 100 mmHg systolic blood pressure, or other causes of walking impairment. Patients with coronary heart disease could be included if the disease was not a limiting factor for the walking distance.

End points
Patients were assessed at inclusion, at the beginning of treatment, and at week 6, 12, 18, and 24 for pain-free walking distances and the maximum walking distance on a treadmill. Bilateral Doppler pressure measurements were carried out above the posterior artery, the dorsal foot artery, and the brachial artery, and comparisons were made with the arm. Pain was rated subjectively by the patients.

Results
The pain-free walking distance improved in both groups. There was a mean increase of 61 meters in the group of patients who received 120 mg *Ginkgo biloba* extract daily and a statistically significant higher ($p = 0.0253$) mean increase of 107 meters in the group of patients who were treated with the higher dose of 240 mg. The maximum walking distance also increased in both groups, with the higher dose significantly superior at weeks 8 and 24 (both $p = 0.01$). There were no significant differences in Doppler pressure measurements between the two groups.

Side effects
One patient developed a rash and the association to the drug was rated as possible by an investigator.

Authors' comments
The clear-cut positive and statistically significant effects of the daily administration of 240 mg *Ginkgo biloba* extract compared 120 mg on the pain-free walking distance and the maximum walking distance in patients with pAOD demonstrated the substantial therapeutic benefit of the higher dose.

Reviewer's comments
This is another positive trial complementing previous trials. However, neither the randomization nor the blinding were adequately described. (1, 6)

Clinical Study: Tebonin® forte

Extract name	EGb 761
Manufacturer	Dr. Willmar Schwabe GmbH & Co., Germany
Indication	**Tinnitus** (ringing in the ears)
Level of evidence	**I**
Therapeutic benefit	**Yes**

Bibliographic reference
Morgenstern C (1997). *Ginkgo biloba* extract EGb 761 in the treatment of tinnitus aurium. *Fortschritte der Medizin* 115: 7-11.

Trial design
Parallel. Two-week pretrial run-in phase with placebo.

Study duration	3 months
Dose	3 × 1 tablet (each tablet contains 40 mg extract) daily
Route of administration	Oral
Randomized	Yes
Randomization adequate	Yes
Blinding	Double-blind
Blinding adequate	Yes
Placebo	Yes
Drug comparison	No
Site description	Single center
No. of subjects enrolled	99
No. of subjects completed	78
Sex	Male and female
Age	Mean: 45.5 years

Inclusion criteria
Patients with normal hearing capacity, at least three adjacent frequencies in the audiogram, experiencing a tonally defined and maskable tinnitus for at least two months previously, able to reliably reproduce and describe noises in the ears, and over 18 years of age.

Exclusion criteria
Patients hearing objectively audible noises; diseases of the middle ear; non-releasable stapedial reflex; reproducibility of otoacoustic emissions <85 percent at the initial medical examination; absolute latency period <0.5 ms in waves I through V in recordings of brainstem potential; severe organic diseases; alcohol or drug abuse; and pregnancy. Patients whose tinnitus decreased between the time of the first examination and the start of therapy two weeks later were excluded from the trial.

End points
Target parameter was a change in tinnitus sound volume in the more severely affected ear at the start of the study. As secondary parameters, the reproducibility of the click-evoked otoacoustic emissions as well as their response, the intensity of tinnitus, loss in hearing, and the subjective impression of the patient in the context of improvement or aggravation were recorded. Measurements were taken before the pretrial phase, at the beginning of treatment, and on weeks 4, 8, and 12.

Results

From the eighth week of treatment on, a clear drop in sound volume was recorded in the ginkgo group which was statistically significant after ten weeks ($p = 0.015$). The values in the placebo group did not change significantly. Recording of the otoacoustic emissions showed no changes in either group. In both groups, patients were of the opinion that their tinnitus had improved. No changes were found in either group in the measurement of hearing loss.

Side effects

No adverse drug reactions were reported by patients in either group.

Author's comments

For the long-term therapy to be expected in the case of tinnitus, the *Ginkgo biloba* extract EGb 761 is a suitable substance due to a positive influence on tinnitus sound volume and also due to its high tolerance level.

Reviewer's comments

This is a model study in conduct and reporting with clear and important clinical benefit in this unpleasant condition. (5, 6)

Clinical Study: EGb 761®

Extract name	EGb 761
Manufacturer	Intersan GmbH, Germany (Dr. Willmar Schwabe GmbH & Co., Germany)

Indication	**Sudden hearing loss**
Level of evidence	**II**
Therapeutic benefit	**Trend**

Bibliographic reference

Burschka MA, Hassan HAH, Reineke T, van Bebber L, Caird DM, Mösges R (2001). Effect of treatment with *Ginkgo biloba* extract EGb 761 (oral) on unilateral idiopathic sudden hearing loss in a prospective randomized double-blind study of 106 outpatients. *European Archives of Oto-Rhino-Laryngology* 258 (5): 213-219.

Trial design

Parallel. Dose comparison. Patients were given either 12 mg EGb 761 (L) or 120 mg EGb 761 (H) twice daily (24 or 240 mg daily).

Study duration	2 months
Dose	2 (12 or 120 mg) tablets daily

Route of administration   Oral

Randomized   Yes
Randomization adequate   Yes
Blinding   Double-blind
Blinding adequate   Yes

Placebo   No
Drug comparison   No

Site description   Multicenter

No. of subjects enrolled   106
No. of subjects completed   78
Sex   Male and female
Age   Mean: 44 years

Inclusion criteria
Patients with acute unilateral idopathic sudden sensorineural hearing loss (ISSHL) of at least 15 dB at one frequency (250, 500, 1000, 2000, or 3000 Hz). The hearing loss had to have happened within ten days of the initial hospital visit.

Exclusion criteria
Patients were excluded if in the affected ear they experienced conductive deafness; signs of inflammation; injury; suspected retrocochlear dysacousis, Ménière's disease; hearing loss greater than 75 dB. Patients with the following conditions were also excluded: severe hepatic or renal insufficiency or cardiovascular diseases; severe gastrointestinal disturbances or malabsorption syndrome; noncontrollable diabetes; breast-feeding women; women of childbearing age taking no contraception; suspected alcoholics; or patients taking disallowed concomitant medication (diuretics, aminoglycoside antibiotics, vasoactive medication, tranquilizers, CNS-stimulating drugs, antihistamines, calcium antagonists, nitrates, beta-blockers, anticoagulants, and platelet aggregation inhibitors).

End points
Patients were examined by their ear-nose-throat (ENT) specialist and given routine blood tests at baseline and on days 3, 4, 14, 28, 42, and 56. The main end point was the recovery (in dB) of the auditory threshold, averaged over the individual affected frequencies, from the baseline measurement to the final measurement at the end of treatment.

Results
A large majority of patients in both treatment groups recovered fully by the end of the trial. Overall there were no statistically or medically significant differences between the two groups. After reanalyzing the data, 13 subjects

were found to be in violation of the inclusion criteria. With these 13 subjects excluded from the analysis, risk of failing to improve measurably was lower in the high-dose group, and patients in that group had a greater chance of becoming "healed." This advantage surfaced after one week of treatment, and the high-dose group showed faster recovery in the low-tone area. This high-dose advantage in recovery occurred almost exclusively in those patients without tinnitus.

Side effects
Nine adverse effects occurred in eight patients: nausea and gastrointestinal discomfort (H: 2, L: 1), headache (H: 1), tinnitus (L: 2), and two patients in the L group reported severe effects (myocardial inflammation and severe vertigo, neither associated with the treatment).

Authors' comments
EGb 761 (oral) appears to speed up and improve the recovery of those patients with uncomplicated ISSHL who have a good chance of recovering completely. The results of this study are exploratory rather than conclusive, however, largely because the recovery rate under the low-dosage treatment had been underestimated in planning the study.

Reviewer's comments
The results need to be verified with a placebo-controlled trial. (5, 6)

Clinical Study: Tebonin® forte

Extract name	EGb 761
Manufacturer	Dr. Willmar Schwabe GmbH & Co., Germany
Indication	**Protection against hypoxia**
Level of evidence	**III**
Therapeutic benefit	**Yes**

Bibliographic reference
Schaffler K, Reeh PW (1985). Double-blind study on the protective effect against hypoxia of a standardized *Ginkgo-biloba* preparation following repeated administration to normal subjects. *Arzneimittel-Forschung/Drug Research* 35 (2): 1283-1286.

Trial design
Crossover. Two 14-day study phases were separated by a one-week washout period.

Study duration	2 weeks
Dose	2 ml extract twice daily (equivalent to 40 drops twice daily, or 160 mg extract daily)
Route of administration	Oral
Randomized	Yes
Randomization adequate	No
Blinding	Double-blind
Blinding adequate	No
Placebo	Yes
Drug comparison	No
Site description	Not described
No. of subjects enrolled	8
No. of subjects completed	8
Sex	Male
Age	Mean: 27.3 years

Inclusion criteria
Healthy young male subjects.

Exclusion criteria
None mentioned.

End points
After 14 days of administration, subjects' performance in terms of oculomotor (and complex choice reactions were evaluated with the aid of a computer-assisted oculodynamic test during three exposures to hypoxia (10.5 percent oxygen, balanced nitrogen). Concomitantly, simple cardiorespiratory parameters were recorded.

Results
The main oculomotor parameters showed an insignificant trend toward improved performance after administration of ginkgo compared to placebo. After repeated exposure to hypoxia (in the third session), the ocular adaptation time was shortened following administration of the drug ($p < 0.01$). The number of correct answers on the operational tests tended to be increased with medication, and the complex choice reaction time was slightly reduced. However, upon repeated exposure to hypoxia (second and third tests), the choice reaction time was significantly ($p < 0.05$ and $p < 0.01$, respectively) shorter with the ginkgo than with placebo.

Side effects
None mentioned in paper.

Authors' comments
The overall conclusion to be drawn is that ginkgo enhances the resistance of healthy subjects to certain consequences of repeated respiratory hypoxia. These findings are interpreted as indicative of a protective action against hypoxia relevant to the treatment of cerebrovascular insufficiency.

Reviewer's comments
This is an interesting study showing the ability of ginkgo to protect against hypoxia-induced slowing of choice reaction time and saccadic eye movements. However, the randomization and blinding were not adequately described, and the data were not described sufficiently to allow for alternative analyses or replication. (1, 5)

Clinical Study: Tanakan®

Extract name	EGb 761
Manufacturer	Ipsen, France (Dr. Willmar Schwabe GmbH & Co., Germany)
Indication	**Antioxidant effects; postoperative oxidative stress**
Level of evidence	**III**
Therapeutic benefit	**Yes**

Bibliographic reference
Pietri S, Seguin J, d'Argigny P, Drieu K, Culcasi M (1997). *Ginkgo biloba* extract (EGb 761) pretreatment limits free radical-induced oxidative stress in-patients undergoing coronary bypass surgery. *Cardiovascular Drugs and Therapy* 11 (2): 121-131.

Trial design
Parallel. Patients were treated for five days preceding aortic valve replacement surgery.

Study duration	5 days
Dose	160 mg twice daily
Route of administration	Oral
Randomized	Yes
Randomization adequate	No
Blinding	Double-blind
Blinding adequate	No
Placebo	Yes

Drug comparison	No
Site description	Single center
No. of subjects enrolled	20
No. of subjects completed	15
Sex	Male and female
Age	43-79 years (mean: 63)

Inclusion criteria
Patients undergoing aortic value replacement in nonurgent open-heart surgery.

Exclusion criteria
Patients could have no recent (<one month) myocardial infarction, no severe cardiac or renal failure, no severe hypertension, and no anti-ischemic, anti-inflammatory, vasoactive, or antioxidant medications for at least five days before surgery.

End points
Plasma samples were obtained from the peripheral circulation and the coronary sinus at crucial stages of the operation: before incision, during ischemia, and within the first 30 minutes after unclamping.

Results
Upon aortic unclamping, EGb 761 inhibited the transcardiac release of thiobarbituric acid reactive species ($p < 0.05$) and attenuated the early (five to ten minute) decrease in dimethylsulfoxide/ascorbyl free radical levels ($p < 0.05$). EGb 761 also significantly reduced the more delayed leakage of myoglobin ($p = 0.007$) and had an almost significant effect on ventricular myosin leakage ($p = 0.053$, six days postoperatively). The clinical outcome of recovery of treated patients was improved, but not significantly, compared with untreated patients.

Side effects
None mentioned by authors.

Authors' comments
The results demonstrate the usefulness of adjuvant Egb 761 therapy in limiting oxidative stress in cardiovascular surgery.

Reviewer's comments
This is an important, well-conducted study showing the utility of ginkgo in coronary artery bypass-elective patients. Ginkgo significantly limited oxidative stress and improved recovery of patients, though the sample size was too small for this to reach significance. Also, the randomization and blinding were not described adequately. (1, 5)

Clinical Study: Ginkgold®

Extract name	EGb 761
Manufacturer	Dr. Willmar Schwabe GmbH & Co., Germany
Indication	**Electrophysiological effects** in healthy volunteers
Level of evidence	**III**
Therapeutic benefit	**MOA**

Bibliographic reference
Itil T, Martorano D (1995). Natural substances in psychiatry (*Ginkgo biloba* in dementia). *Psychopharmacology Bulletin* 31 (1): 147-158.

Trial design
Crossover.

Study duration	3 hours
Dose	40 mg, 120 mg, or 240 mg extract
Route of administration	Oral
Randomized	No
Randomization adequate	No
Blinding	Double-blind
Blinding adequate	No
Placebo	No
Drug comparison	Yes
Drug name	Ginkgo Power™, Super Ginkgo™
Site description	Single center
No. of subjects enrolled	12
No. of subjects completed	12
Sex	Male
Age	18-65 years (mean: 32.2)

Inclusion criteria
Healthy.

Exclusion criteria
None mentioned.

End points
Computer electroencephalographic (CEEG: Pharmaco-EEG/dynamic brain

mapping) data were collected before, as well as one and three hours after, administration of ginkgo.

Results
After one hour, a statistical difference in CEEG effects occurred in the Ginkgold groups versus the Ginkgo Power group. Ginkgold increased alpha activity in all brain areas. Super Ginkgo had only a mild increase in alpha activity at one hour but showed greater activity than Ginkgold at three hours. Ginkgo Power showed a minimal increase in alpha activity limited to the anterior brain region.

Side effects
No major side effects.

Authors' comments
Data suggest that the only ginkgo extract which has potent alpha-enhancing effects and could be classified as a cognitive activator was Ginkgold (EGb 761). The central nervous system (CNS) effects of Ginkgold were similar to other psychoactive compounds classified as cognitive activators. In further CEEG studies, the CNS effects of three doses of Ginkgold could be differentiated from placebo, and the effects of the higher doses (120 and 240 mg) could be discriminated from the lowest dose (40 mg).

Reviewer's comments
This is a well-conducted pilot study suggesting differing EEG effects of three gingko preparations, with EGb 761 appearing best. The description of the methodology was sparse, and the blinding process was not described at all. The study was not randomized. (1, 6)

Clinical Study: Tanakan®

Extract name	EGb 761
Manufacturer	Ipsen, France (Dr. Willmar Schwabe GmbH & Co., Germany)
Indication	**Electrophysiological effects** in healthy volunteers
Level of evidence	**III**
Therapeutic benefit	**MOA**

Bibliographic reference
Luthringer R, d'Arbigny P, Macher JP (1995). *Ginkgo biloba* extract (EGb 761), EEG and event-related potentials mapping profile. In *Advances in*

Ginkgo biloba *Extract Research,* Volume 4: *Effects of* Ginkgo biloba *Extract (EGb 761) on Aging and Age-Related Disorders.* Eds. Y Christen, Y Courtois, M-T Droy-Lefaix. Paris: Elsevier, pp. 107-118.

Trial design
Two-part study. Part I compared the effects of single doses of 80 and 160 mg of ginkgo extract versus placebo in a double-blinded design. Part II investigated the effects of five days of treatment with 160 mg extract per day in a single-blinded design. A one-day washout period separated the treatment days in part 1 and preceded treatment in part 2.

Study duration	2 × 1-day treatments (part I), and 1 × 5-day period (part II)
Dose	Part I: 80 mg and 160 mg ginkgo extract; Part II: 160 mg ginkgo extract daily
Route of administration	Oral
Randomized	No
Randomization adequate	No
Blinding	Double/single-blind
Blinding adequate	No
Placebo	Yes
Drug comparison	No
Site description	Not described
No. of subjects enrolled	15
No. of subjects completed	15
Sex	Not given
Age	Mean: 30 years

Inclusion criteria
Healthy young volunteers were included in this trial.

Exclusion criteria
Psychotropic drug intake was not allowed for two weeks prior to the study. Subjects were not allowed to smoke or to drink coffee, tea, or alcohol in the hours preceding the measurements.

End points
Electroencephalography (EEG) and event-related potentials (ERP) mapping data were collected prior to drug administration and 0.5, 1, 1.5, 2, 3, 4, 5, and 6 hours after drug administration. Auditory P300 was recorded, as was contingent negative variation (CNV).

Results
After single doses of either 80 or 160 mg ginkgo extract, the alpha-1 band was significantly increased compared to placebo in terms of both absolute and relative power. For the alpha-2 band the increase was significant at the beginning and end of the recordings. After five days of treatment with ginkgo extract, the alpha increase was still present. A marked beta increase also occurred. Theta values were decreased significantly at 1.5 and 2 hours. ERP were only slightly modified in amplitude. However, there was a significant decrease in P300 latency after both single-dose and five-day administration ($p < 0.05$).

Side effects
None mentioned in the paper.

Authors' comments
These EEG data confirm that EGb 761 extract has a nootropic profile with obvious improvements of the vigilance level, concomitant with beneficial effects on some cognitive skills, such as memory. Furthermore, the fact that additional effects, such as the beta increase, occurred after five days of treatment may suggest other therapeutic indications of EGb 761, for example antistress effects after long-term treatment.

Reviewer's comments
This is a well-conducted trial indicating that ginkgo has nootropic or cognition-enhancing action on EEG and evoked potentials. The study participants did not appear to be randomized, and the blinding process was not described. (1, 6)

Clinical Study: Tebonin®

Extract name	EGb 761
Manufacturer	Dr. Willmar Schwabe GmbH & Co., Germany
Indication	**Electrophysiological effects** in healthy volunteers
Level of evidence	**II**
Therapeutic benefit	**MOA**

Bibliographic reference
Kunkel H (1993). EEG profile of three different extractions of *Ginkgo biloba*. *Neuropsychobiology* 27 (1): 40-45.

Trial design
Crossover. Two-part study. Part I: three doses (40, 80, and 160 mg) of EGb 761. Part II: 80 mg each of EGb 761 and two fractions (fraction 1: flavonoid concentrate and ginkgolides; fraction 2: flavonoid concentrate). Subjects for the two parts of the study were different; 12 subjects participated in each study part. Medication was administered for three days prior to recording sessions.

Study duration	6 tests; 3 days of treatment preceded each test
Dose	Part I: 40, 80, and 160 mg EGb 761 extract; Part II: EGb 761, subfraction 1 and 2 (all 80 mg)
Route of administration	Oral
Randomized	Yes
Randomization adequate	No
Blinding	Double-blind
Blinding adequate	Yes
Placebo	Yes
Drug comparison	No
Site description	Not described
No. of subjects enrolled	12
No. of subjects completed	12
Sex	Male
Age	Part I: 24-29 years (median: 26) Part II: 25-29 years (median: 27)

Inclusion criteria
Normal, healthy males with a typical high-alpha EEG (defined as alpha activity during 70 percent of recording period and a frequency between 9 and 11 Hz).

Exclusion criteria
None mentioned.

End points
Five 15-minute electroencephalography measurements (EEG) were obtained at hourly intervals on test days. Vigilance was examined using the critical-flicker fusion frequency (CFF) and a speeded arithmetic test (Pauli test). In addition, emotional changes were assessed with a mood-adjective checklist.

Results

Both experiments revealed a number of effects on various EEG parameters. However, the topographical distribution of effects was completely different in the two experiments. Part I: there was no clear dose-response relationship for any of the parameters. Part II: statistically marked EEG effects were observed for the extract and its two subfractions; however, there was no predictable relationship. In both studies, no drug effects were found for the CFF or speeded arithmetic test. The mood-adjective checklist did not show any consistent mood changes under any of the dosages.

Side effects

None of the subjects reported any side effects.

Author's comments

No clear EEG profile of an extract of *Ginkgo biloba* and its subfractions could be delineated through the two experiments of the present study.

Reviewer's comments

This is a carefully conducted trial showing the effect of ginkgo on EEG and differential effects for different preparations. No profile emerged, though; thus, there are central effects but they are not easily clarified by EEG. The randomization process was not described. (3, 5)

Product Profile: Ginkai™

Manufacturer	**Lichtwer Pharma AG, Germany (Indena S.p.A., Italy)**
U.S. distributor	**Lichtwer Pharma U.S., Inc.**
Botanical ingredient	**Ginkgo leaf extract**
Extract name	**LI 1370 (GinkgoSelect™)**
Quantity	50 mg
Processing	Plant to extract ratio 50:1
Standardization	25% (12.5 mg) flavone glycosides, 6% (3 mg) terpenoids (ginkgolides, bilobalide)
Formulation	Tablet

Recommended dose: Take one tablet, three times daily with cool liquid. Results observed after six weeks of usage.

DSHEA structure/function: Clinically proven to improve memory and concentration.

Cautions: If pregnant, nursing a baby, or administering to children, seek the advice of a health professional before using this product.

Other ingredients: Lactose, microcrystalline cellulose, citric acid, magnesium silicate, hydroxy propylmethyl cellulose, magnesium stearate, silicum dioxide, castor oil, stearic acid.

Comments: Sold as Ginkyo® and Kaveri® in Europe.

Source(s) of information: Product package; product information on Internet (<www.lichtwer.com/ginkai/ginkai_prod_info.html>, accessed on 1/25/02; information is currently available at <www.lichtwer.com/product_ginkai.html>); Ginkyo® product information (Lichtwer Pharma GmbH, 1996); information provided by Indena USA, Inc.

Product Profile: Ginkgo Biloba-24%

Manufacturer	**Enzymatic Therapy® (Indena S.p.A., Italy)**
U.S. distributor	**Enzymatic Therapy®**
Botanical ingredient	**Ginkgo leaf extract**
Extract name	**GinkgoSelect™**
Quantity	40 mg
Processing	Plant to extract ratio 50:1
Standardization	24% flavone glycosides, 6% terpene lactones, and 2% bilobalide
Formulation	Capsule

Recommended dose: One capsule three times daily.

DSHEA structure/function: Dietary supplement for improved short-term memory.

Other ingredients: Cellulose, gelatin, magnesium stearate, titanium dioxide.

Source(s) of information: Product label; information provided by Indena USA, Inc.

Product Profile: GB24™

Manufacturer	**Thorne Research (Indena S.p.A., Italy)**
U.S. distributor	**Thorne Research**
Botanical ingredient	**Ginkgo leaf extract**
Extract name	**GinkgoSelect™**

Quantity	40 mg
Processing	Plant to extract ratio 50:1
Standardization	24% ginkgo heterosides
Formulation	Capsule

Recommended dose: None given.

Cautions: If pregnant, consult a health care practitioner before using this or any other product.

Other ingredients: Cellulose capsule. May contain one or more of the following hypoallergenic ingredients to fill space: magnesium citrate, silicon dioxide.

Comments: This product is available only through pharmacies and health care practitioners.

Source(s) of information: Product label; information provided by Indena USA, Inc.

Product Profile: Ginkgo Biloba

Manufacturer	**Swanson Health Products (Indena S.p.A., Italy)**
U.S. distributor	**Swanson Health Products**
Botanical ingredient	**Ginkgo leaf extract**
Extract name	**GinkgoSelect®**
Quantity	60 mg
Processing	Plant to extract ratio 50:1
Standardization	24% flavone glycosides and 6% terpene lactones
Formulation	Capsule

Recommended dose: Take one capsule with water during the morning and evening meals.

Cautions: Consult a health care provider before use if taking a blood-thinning medication.

Other ingredients: Microcrystalline cellulose (plant fiber), gelatin.

Comments: Also distributed by Doctor's A-Z™.

Source(s) of information: Product label; information provided by Indena USA, Inc.

Clinical Study: LI 1370

Extract name	LI 1370
Manufacturer	Lichtwer Pharma AG, Germany
Indication	**Age-related cognitive impairment**
Level of evidence	**III**
Therapeutic benefit	**Yes**

Bibliographic reference
Bruchert E, Heinrich SE, Ruf-Kohler P (1991). Wirksamkeit von LI 1370 bei alteren patienten mit hirnleistungsschwache. *Munchener Medizinische Wochenschrift* 133 (Suppl 1): S9-S14.

Trial design
Parallel. Pretrial washout period of 14 days.

Study duration	3 months
Dose	1 (50 mg) tablet 3 times daily
Route of administration	Oral
Randomized	No
Randomization adequate	No
Blinding	Double-blind
Blinding adequate	No
Placebo	Yes
Drug comparison	No
Site description	33 general practices
No. of subjects enrolled	303
No. of subjects completed	209
Sex	Male and female
Age	45-80 years (mean: 69)

Inclusion criteria
Elderly outpatients with cerebral insufficiency or impaired cerebral function, with at least one symptom from each of four typical symptom groups.

Exclusion criteria
Patients with pronounced stenoses of the supraaortal vessels; severe internal diseases such as advanced heart or kidney failure, cirrhosis of the liver, or poorly controlled mellitus or hypertension; suspect abuse of alcohol, narcotics, or prescription drugs; and treatment with nootropic, psychotropic, or vasoactive drugs during, or in the 14 days prior to, the trial.

End points
Patients were tested for symptoms of cerebral insufficiency and asked to perform a connect-the-numbers test at admission and after 6 and 12 weeks of therapy. Both physicians and patients judged effectiveness.

Results
Statistically significant improvements were demonstrated after six weeks of therapy on 3 out of 11 typical symptoms, and after 12 weeks of therapy on 8 out of 11. Forgetfulness, depression, and headache were improved after six weeks. In addition, memory gaps, concentration, fatigue, lack of drive, and tinnitus were improved after 12 weeks. In the treatment group the time period for the figure connection test was improved by 25 percent in the ginkgo group and 14 percent in the placebo group ($p < 0.01$). Both the doctors' and the patients' judgment concerning the efficacy showed highly significant differences between the two groups, with over 50 percent giving positive assessment to ginkgo.

Side effects
Minor adverse events (the principal one being stomachache), most mentioned twice as often in the placebo group.

Authors' comments
In this trial, the parameter with the greatest statistical significance in the comparison of ginkgo and placebo was the overall integrative assessment by physician and patient. Psychometric methods are highly valued today due to their objectivity in follow-up observations of patients with impaired cerebral function. They are less significant in general practice, however, and should be viewed on the scale of the results reported here.

Reviewer's comments
Excellent, very large trial showing clear and highly believable improvements in cognitive functions, symptoms, and clinician ratings. However, the study groups were not randomized and the blinding was not adequately described. (Translation reviewed) (1, 5)

Clinical Study: Kaveri®

Extract name	LI 1370
Manufacturer	Lichtwer Pharma AG, Germany
Indication	**Age-related cognitive impairment**
Level of evidence	**I**
Therapeutic benefit	**Yes**

Bibliographic reference
Vesper J, Hansgen KD (1994). Efficacy of *Ginkgo biloba* in 90 outpatients with cerebral insufficiency caused by old age. *Phytomedicine* 1: 9-16.

Trial design
Parallel.

Study duration	3 months
Dose	1 (50 mg) tablet 3 times daily
Route of administration	Oral
Randomized	Yes
Randomization adequate	Yes
Blinding	Double-blind
Blinding adequate	Yes
Placebo	Yes
Drug comparison	No
Site description	11 practices
No. of subjects enrolled	90
No. of subjects completed	86
Sex	Male and female
Age	55-80 years (mean: 62.7)

Inclusion criteria
Elderly outpatients with cerebral insufficiency according to ICD-290.x., premorbid IQ of at least 80 (Mehrfachwahl-Worschatz-Intelligenztest [MWT-B]), affected by distinct subjective troubles (>19 points on the cerebral insufficiency [CI]-scale), and did not exhibit any pseudodementias (dementia-pseudodementia differentiation [DPD] value > 2). The use of nootropic agents, psychopharmaceuticals, vasoactive, or psychotropic substances was prohibited three weeks before and during the trial.

Exclusion criteria
Patients with cerebral/myocardial infarction in the previous six months, serious cardiac or renal insufficiency, other serious internal diseases requiring medical treatment, cardiac arrhythmia, stenoses of the supraaortic vessels, psychoses, epilepsy, cerebral tumors, abuse of alcohol, drugs, and medical remedies, and other diseases generally accepted as exclusion criteria.

End points
Medical checks were performed at the beginning of the study and after 6 and 12 weeks of treatment. The test parameters were long-term and short-term memory, concentration power, maximum stress, mental flexibility, family problems, and general satisfaction with life. Psychometric tests were: Mini

Mental Status according to Folstein; multiple verbal comprehension test version B (the MWT-B); dementia/pseudodementia differentiation sheet; and the brief form of Hachinski's ischaemia scale (K-HIS).

Results

Significant improvement in performance was seen with LI 1370 compared to placebo, particularly between the sixth and twelfth week of treatment. Particular improvement was seen in short-term memory and concentration. Improvement was observed in the patients' attention in tasks requiring quick orientation and readaptation, and consistent attentiveness level maintained over a longer period of time (long-term stress). The length of time with optimum attention was increased. There were also positive changes of the patients' subjective performance (reduction of troubles, reduction of behavioral abnormalities, and assessment of behavior by others).

Side effects

No side effects were observed.

Authors' comments

This study was the first to prove the clinical efficacy of *Ginkgo biloba* special extract in the treatment of cerebral insufficiency in a larger group of patients with the help of computer diagnostics. Due to the established favorable benefit/risk profile of LI 1370, it is among the remedies which are particularly recommended in the treatment of cerebral insufficiency.

Reviewer's comments

This is a well-conducted and written up trial with a medium sample size ($n = 90$) that shows clear benefits of ginkgo on computerized cognitive tests and symptoms. (5, 5)

Clinical Study: LI 1370

Extract name	LI 1370
Manufacturer	Lichtwer Pharma AG, Germany
Indication	**Age-related cognitive impairment**
Level of evidence	**III**
Therapeutic benefit	**Yes**

Bibliographic reference

Hofferberth B (1991). *Ginkgo biloba* special extract in patients with organic brain syndrome. *Munchener Medizinische Wochenschrift* 133 (Suppl. 1): S30-S33.

Trial design
Parallel. Pretrial washout period of 14 days.

Study duration	6 weeks
Dose	1 (50 mg) tablet 3 times daily
Route of administration	Oral
Randomized	No
Randomization adequate	No
Blinding	Double-blind
Blinding adequate	No
Placebo	Yes
Drug comparison	No
Site description	1 neurological ward
No. of subjects enrolled	50
No. of subjects completed	50
Sex	Male and female
Age	57-76 years (mean: 65)

Inclusion criteria
Inpatients with organic brain syndrome.

Exclusion criteria
None mentioned.

End points
Measurements were made before the trial and after three and six weeks of therapy. The Vienna determination instrument and the digit connection test were used as psychometric methods. Saccadic eye movements, EEG analysis, and measurement of evoked potentials served as neurophysiologic methods.

Results
For all five target criteria there was improvement in the ginkgo group compared to placebo, which was evident at three weeks ($p < 0.001$). Eleven typical symptoms assessed by the physician showed good improvement in 19 of 25 in the ginkgo group and 11 of 25 in the placebo group.

Side effects
None discussed.

Author's comments
The results show that therapy with the *Ginkgo biloba* special extract LI 1370

in patients with cerebro-organic syndrome contributes to an increased cerebral capacity.

Reviewer's comments
This is the fourth study on ginkgo from these researchers showing dramatic, widespread, and large benefits in a small sample. Dramatic improvements were seen in all measures, from tests of performance to P300 evoked potentials and saccadic eye movements. It is hard to understand, however, why such widespread, highly consistent effects should occur in a relatively small sample. The study was not randomized, the blinding was inadequately described, and the data were not described in sufficient detail to permit alternative analysis. (Translation reviewed) (1, 5)

Clinical Study: LI 1370

Extract name	LI 1370
Manufacturer	Lichtwer Pharma AG, Germany
Indication	**Age-related cognitive impairment**
Level of evidence	**III**
Therapeutic benefit	**Undetermined**

Bibliographic reference
Schulz H, Jobert M, Breuel HP (1991). Wirkung von spezialextrakt LI 1370 auf das EEG alterer patienten im schlafentzugsmodell. *Munchener Medizinische Wochenschrift* 133 (Suppl. 1): S26-S29.

Trial design
Parallel.

Study duration	2 months
Dose	1 (50 mg) tablet 3 times daily
Route of administration	Oral
Randomized	Yes
Randomization adequate	No
Blinding	Double-blind
Blinding adequate	No
Placebo	Yes
Drug comparison	No
Site description	Single center
No. of subjects enrolled	16

No. of subjects completed 15
Sex Male and female
Age Mean: 64.9 years

Inclusion criteria
Subjects age 55 to 75 years with age-dependent symptoms of forgetfulness; decreasing alertness and insufficient concentration; impairment of brain function based on assertion by subjects and according to the MWT (multiple choice vocabulary), and ZVT-G (number association) tests; and physically healthy (with allowance for age).

Exclusion criteria
Subjects with alcohol and/or drug abuse; intake of other medications which were not allowed in the study; known hypersensitivity to ginkgo extracts; participation in other clinical trials within the past 30 days; and incapacity to cooperate in the trial.

End points
EEG recordings (15 minutes duration) were taken twice: between 7:30 and 8 p.m. and between 4 and 4:30 a.m. after a sleepless night. The tests were conducted on the first and last day of the study. Sleepiness symptoms were documented hourly with a questionnaire.

Results
Ginkgo biloba extract LI 1370 did not cause changes in EEG activity in the evening but did cause changes in the early morning after a sleepless night. The output of the theta band decreased, whereas the alpha slow-wave index on average increased in the treatment group compared to the placebo group. There was no difference in the degree of tiredness.

Side effects
Not discussed.

Authors' comments
Ginkgo biloba extract LI 1370 does not cause a general change in EEG activity but does cause changes that are situation and stimulus dependent. This is corroborated by the selective influence on the EEG under sleep deprivation conditions compared to control measurements of the previous evening.

Reviewer's comments
This is an interesting pilot study suggesting ginkgo may help pharmaco-EEG in impaired elderly in sleep deprivation model. The study was flawed by the lack of details on randomization and blinding, the small sample size, the lack of description of withdrawal/dropouts, and inadequately applied/described statistical methods. (Translation reviewed) (0, 4)

Clinical Study: LI 1370

Extract name	LI 1370
Manufacturer	Lichtwer Pharma AG, Germany
Indication	**Cognitive functioning** after brain aneurysm operation
Level of evidence	**II**
Therapeutic benefit	**Yes**

Bibliographic reference
Maier-Hauff K (1991). LI 1370 after cerebral aneurysm operation; efficacy in outpatients with disorders of cerebral functional capacity. *Munchener Medizinische Wochenschrift* 133 (Suppl. 1): S34-S37.

Trial design
Parallel.

Study duration	3 months
Dose	1 (50 mg) tablet 3 times daily
Route of administration	Oral
Randomized	Yes
Randomization adequate	Yes
Blinding	Double-blind
Blinding adequate	Yes
Placebo	Yes
Drug comparison	No
Site description	Single center
No. of subjects enrolled	50
No. of subjects completed	42
Sex	Male and female
Age	21-63 years (mean: 48)

Inclusion criteria
Patients who had subarachnoidal hemorrhage and subsequent aneurysm operation in the previous 7 to 42 months.

Exclusion criteria
No psychoactive drugs or nootropics were allowed for two weeks before, as well as during, the study.

End points
Neuropsychological tests were carried out before the study as well as at the

end of the sixth and twelfth weeks. Tests included the Zimmermann test battery for attentiveness and assessment of short-term memory on verbal and nonverbal levels.

Results

After 12 weeks of treatment there was a statistically significant improvement in reaction time to stimuli in comparison to baseline as well as placebo (both $p < 0.01$). The number of errors was reduced compared to baseline ($p < 0.001$) and placebo ($p < 0.01$). Short-term verbal memory also improved compared to baseline ($p < 0.001$) and placebo ($p < 0.05$). There was no significant change to nonverbal memory which was already in the normal range.

Side effects

One report of nausea and stomach pains.

Author's comments

In summary the trial showed that cognitive disorders in patients with subarachnoidal hemorrhage and subsequent aneurysm operation can be favorably influenced with *Ginkgo biloba* extract LI 1370. Significant improvements were shown in the field of attention and verbal short-term memory. These results argue in favor of early initiation of therapy in order to improve cognitive deficits in performance after aneurysm operation.

Reviewer's comments

Well-conducted study showing cognitive improvements in patients recovering from cerebral aneurysms. Study received a Level II due to the statistical methods being inadequately described/applied and an inadequate description of data, thus preventing replication or alternative analysis. (Translation reviewed) (5, 4)

Clinical Study: LI 1370

Extract name	LI 1370
Manufacturer	Lichtwer Pharma AG, Germany
Indication	**Cognitive functioning** in normal volunteers
Level of evidence	**II**
Therapeutic benefit	**Yes**

Bibliographic reference

Rigney U, Kimber S, Hindmarch I (1999). The effects of acute doses of standardized *Ginkgo biloba* extract on memory and psychomotor performance in volunteers. *Phytotherapy Research* 13 (5): 408-415.

Trial design
Dose comparison in five-way crossover design: 150 mg (50 mg three times daily); 300 mg (100 mg three times daily); 120 mg (1 dose); 240 mg (1 dose); or placebo. Each treatment was taken for two days and separated by a minimum five-day washout period.

Study duration	2 days
Dose	(3 × 50 mg) or (3 × 100 mg) or (1 × 120 mg) or (1 × 240 mg) extract per day
Route of administration	Oral
Randomized	Yes
Randomization adequate	Yes
Blinding	Double-blind
Blinding adequate	No
Placebo	Yes
Drug comparison	No
Site description	Single center
No. of subjects enrolled	36
No. of subjects completed	31
Sex	Male and female
Age	30-59 years (mean: 43.6)

Inclusion criteria
Good physical condition and mental health and free from concomitant medication.

Exclusion criteria
None mentioned.

End points
A psychometric test battery was administered predose and at regular intervals until 11 hours postdose. Working memory was assessed using immediate word recall and Sternberg's short-term memory scanning task (STM). Long-term memory was assessed using delayed word recall. Other measures included Stroop color task (SCT), critical flicker fusion, choice reaction time, digit symbol substitution task (DSST), line analog rating scales for subjective sedation (LARS), Leeds sleep evaluation questionnaire (LSEQ), and continuous activity monitoring using an actigraphy during the two-day treatment period.

Results
Reaction times in the Sternberg STM were significantly faster under the influence of LI 1370 for all doses except 150 mg on day 2 of treatment, while reaction times with 120 mg and 300 mg were faster on both days of treatment. This effect was most evident for the group receiving 120 mg and older in age (50 to 59 years). An insignificant trend toward increased immediate word recall was seen only with the 120 mg dose. Other treatment effects were not significantly different from placebo.

Side effects
None mentioned.

Authors' comments
The results show that the effects of LI 1370 extract on aspects of cognition in normal healthy volunteers are more pronounced for memory, particularly working memory, than for arousal or selective attention. These effects may be dose dependent, though not in a linear dose-related manner. The once per day dose of 120 mg produced the most evident effect of the doses examined. The cognitive-enhancing effects are more likely to be apparent in individuals aged 50 to 59 than those aged 30 to 49 years.

Reviewer's comments
This is a well-controlled and well-powered trial with five-way crossover design and frequent assessments with a wide range of tests. Authors did not state method to blind five differing dosing regimens, however. The dose relationship of response on Sternberg test is also hard to understand. In addition, the authors should have explained their rationale between different dosing conditions and regimen and addressed the difference between 120 mg in one dose and 50 mg three times a day. (2, 6)

Clinical Study: LI 1370

Extract name	LI 1370
Manufacturer	Lichtwer Pharma AG, Germany
Indication	**Tinnitus** (ringing in the ears)
Level of evidence	**I**
Therapeutic benefit	**No**

Bibliographic reference
Drew S, Davies E (2001). Effectiveness of *Ginkgo biloba* in treating tinnitus: Double blind, placebo controlled trial. *British Medical Journal* 322 (7278): 1-6.

Trial design

Parallel. Of the participants, 956 were matched for sex, age (less than ten years difference), and tinnitus duration (489 pairs). Each pair was then given one random number corresponding to placebo treatment and one number corresponding to active treatment.

Study duration	3 months
Dose	1 (50 mg) tablet 3 times daily
Route of administration	Oral
Randomized	Yes
Randomization adequate	Yes
Blinding	Double-blind
Blinding adequate	Yes
Placebo	Yes
Drug comparison	No
Site description	Remote: via questionnaire
No. of subjects enrolled	1121
No. of subjects completed	909
Sex	Male and female
Age	Mean: 53 years

Inclusion criteria

Healthy volunteers between 18 and 70 years old with tinnitus.

Exclusion criteria

Patients who were pregnant or trying to become pregnant, had previously taken *Ginkgo biloba* extract, had tinnitus for less than 12 months, reported that their tinnitus had varied greatly in the six months before the screening questionnaire, had tried any treatment for tinnitus in the six months before the screening questionnaire (e.g., homeopathy, acupuncture, hypnotherapy, etc.), were not in generally good health, were taking antidepressants or anticoagulant drugs, or had abnormal blood pressure.

End points

The main outcome measure was the participants' assessment of tinnitus before, during, and after treatment with ginkgo (change in tinnitus). Measurement of tinnitus severity was the secondary outcome measure. In addition, subjects were asked questions about other symptoms of cerebral insufficiency besides tinnitus. These end points were measured by questionnaires completed four times: at the beginning of the study, four weeks after treatment start, at the end of the 12 weeks of treatment, and two weeks after treatment had ended.

Results

Only data from the matched pairs were reported, as the authors believed that the unmatched analysis did not provide any additional information. There were no significant differences in any of the end points for either group. After 12 weeks of treatment, 34 subjects out of 360 in the ginkgo group reported that their tinnitus was less troublesome, versus 35 out of 360 placebo subjects. However, 4.9 percent of the ginkgo group (n = 489) reported beneficial side effects (e.g., in general well-being, hearing better, improved circulation, etc.) versus only 2.2 percent of the placebo group (n = 489).

Side effects

Side effects were analyzed for the 489 matched pairs. The incidence of side effects was similar between the two groups (ginkgo: 10.4 percent, placebo: 11 percent), with the most common being gastrointestinal upset.

Authors' comments

Ginkgo biloba extract LI 1370 had no greater therapeutic effect than placebo in treating tinnitus. In addition, other symptoms of cerebral insufficiency were not significantly affected by the treatment.

Reviewer's comments

Clear and unequivocal negative results. (5, 6)

Clinical Study: LI 1370

Extract name	LI 1370
Manufacturer	Lichtwer Pharma AG, Germany
Indication	**Microcirculation; retinal blood flow** in patients with fundus hypertonicus
Level of evidence	**III**
Therapeutic benefit	**Yes**

Bibliographic reference

Koza KD, Ernst FD, Sporl E (1991). Retinal blood flow after *Ginkgo biloba* therapy in fundus hypertonicus. *Munchener Medizinische Wochenschrift* 133 (Suppl. 1): S47-S50.

Trial design

Parallel.

Study duration	6 weeks
Dose	1 (100 mg) tablet 3 times daily

Route of administration	Oral
Randomized	Yes
Randomization adequate	No
Blinding	Double-blind
Blinding adequate	No
Placebo	Yes
Drug comparison	No
Site description	Single center
No. of subjects enrolled	24
No. of subjects completed	24
Sex	Male and female
Age	28-64 years (mean: 50)

Inclusion criteria
Hypertensive patients with fundus hypertonicus phase I according to Thiel.

Exclusion criteria
None mentioned.

End points
Measurements were taken one day before beginning medication and on the fourteenth and forty-second days of treatment. The following aspects of retinal microcirculation were determined: quadrant artery diameter, blood velocity and blood flow in that artery, arteriovenous transit time, diameter of all arteries, and blood flow through these arteries. Other hemorheologic parameters measured were hematocrit values, plasma viscosity, erythrocyte aggregation, and erythrocyte filtration time.

Results
After treatment with ginkgo, blood flow in the quadrant artery and the total blood flow improved significantly in comparison to placebo (both $p < 0.05$ on day 14 and $p < 0.01$ on day 42). The arteriovenous circulation time decreased significantly. Erythrocyte aggregation and erythrocyte filtration time showed a tendency to decrease, and plasma viscosity demonstrated a significant drop in comparison to placebo.

Side effects
None reported.

Authors' comments
In summary, after administration of *Ginkgo biloba* extract LI 1370 there is a substantial increase of the retinal circulation in phase I fundus hypertonicus. (according to Thiel) in comparison with placebo. Because in advanced dia-

betic retinopathy, and in a large portion of venous occlusive diseases of the retina, arterial constriction and reduced fluidity of the blood can be of pathogenetic importance, it seems permissible to include LI 1370 in the treatment of these retinal diseases.

Reviewer's comments
Important study showing ginkgo improves retinal circulation—confirming one potential mechanism of action. The study shows that vascular effects of *Ginkgo biloba* extract may be important in its cognitive effects. The findings support the results of Jung and colleagues (1990). However, neither the randomization nor the blinding were adequately described. (Translation reviewed) (1, 5)

Clinical Study: Kaveri®

Extract name	LI 1370
Manufacturer	Lichtwer Pharma AG, Germany
Indication	**Microcirculation and blood fluidity** in healthy volunteers
Level of evidence	**III**
Therapeutic benefit	**Yes**

Bibliographic reference
Jung F, Mrowietz C, Kiesewetter H, Wenzel E (1990). Effect of *Ginkgo biloba* on fluidity of blood and peripheral microcirculation in volunteers. *Arzneimittel-Forschung/Drug Research* 40 (1) 5: 589-593.

Trial design
Crossover. One-week washout period between each one-day study period.

Study duration	1 day
Dose	45 ml (0.25 g extract/100 g solution)
Route of administration	Oral
Randomized	Yes
Randomization adequate	No
Blinding	Single-blind
Blinding adequate	No
Placebo	Yes
Drug comparison	No
Site description	Single center

No. of subjects enrolled   10
No. of subjects completed   10
Sex   Male and female
Age   21-30 years

Inclusion criteria
Healthy volunteers with limited fluidity of blood (plasma viscosity > 1.29, erythrocyte (red blood cell) aggregation > 17.3, erythrocyte rigidity > 1.14, thrombocyte (platelet) aggregation > 40).

Exclusion criteria
Subjects with hypertension, diabetes mellitus, hyperuricemia, hyperlipoproteinemia, or adiposity.

End points
Before as well as one, two, and four hours after administration, the following blood parameters were examined: hematocrit, plasma viscosity, erythrocyte aggregation, erythrocyte rigidity, spontaneous thrombocyte aggregation, number of circulating thrombocyte aggregates, thrombocyte count, and leukocyte count. Peripheral microcirculation (mean erythrocyte velocity and erythrocyte column diameter in the nail fold) was measured before and every 30 minutes for four hours after administration.

Results
A significant decrease (15.6 percent, $p < 0.0001$) in erythrocyte aggregation was observed two hours after administration of ginkgo compared to baseline. Blood flow in nail fold capillaries increased significantly by about 57 percent ($p < 0.004$) one hour after administration of ginkgo. All other parameters, blood pressure, heart rate, hemocrit, plasma viscosity, erythrocyte rigidity, thrombocyte count, and leukocyte count, as well as thrombocyte aggregation and the number of circulating thrombocyte aggregates, remained unchanged.

Side effects
None reported.

Authors' comments
In conclusion, it can be said that after administration of 45 ml *Ginkgo biloba* solution, compared to placebo, an improvement in blood viscosity, as well as an increase in the erythrocyte flow in skin capillaries, was observed.

Reviewer's comments
This is an important study with clear findings illustrating one mechanism of action of ginkgo—decrease in erythrocyte aggregation plus 57 percent increase in blood flow in nail capillaries—clear and important findings for the

actions of ginkgo on blood motility. However, the study was only single-blind and the randomization process was not adequately described. (1, 6)

Clinical Study: LI 1370

Extract name	LI 1370
Manufacturer	Lichtwer Pharma AG, Germany
Indication	**Sleep quality** in healthy volunteers
Level of evidence	I
Therapeutic benefit	**MOA**

Bibliographic reference
Murray BJ, Cowen PJ, Sharpley AL (2001). The effect of Li 1370, extract of *Ginkgo biloba,* on REM sleep in humans. *Pharmacopsychiatry* 34 (4): 155-157.

Trial design
Crossover. Subjects were given either placebo or ginkgo two hours before going to bed. After a one-week washout period, subjects were given the opposite treatment. Normal sleeping and waking schedule was maintained throughout the study. Subjects were allowed to continue their normal caffeine intake, but they were asked to refrain from alcohol on the preceeding and study nights.

Study duration	1 night
Dose	240 mg
Route of administration	Oral
Randomized	Yes
Randomization adequate	Yes
Blinding	Double-blind
Blinding adequate	Yes
Placebo	Yes
Drug comparison	No
Site description	Subjects' homes
No. of subjects enrolled	10
No. of subjects completed	10
Sex	Male and female
Age	18-48 years (mean: 35.9)

Inclusion criteria
Healthy volunteers with no current or past history of psychiatric or sleep disorder (determined by clinical interview).

Exclusion criteria
Subjects taking medication.

End points
On both study nights, sleep polysomnograms were recorded by the patients at home. REM sleep latency was calculated from these measurements. Also, after each study night, subjects were asked to rate how well they had slept.

Results
There were no significant differences between the two treatments for any sleep parameter. *Ginkgo biloba* extract did not have any shortening effect on REM sleep latency. Objective and subjective measures of sleep efficiency were also unaffected by ginkgo.

Side effects
None mentioned.

Authors' comments
The purpose of this study was to test the hypothesis that LI 1370 increases cholinergic activity as measured by its effect on latency to rapid eye movement sleep. As cholinergic effects on REM sleep can be affected by other factors such as noradrenaline or serotonin function, the results do not prove conclusively that LI 1370 does not promote cholinergic activity. The main findings are that even a reasonably high dose of *Ginkgo biloba* extract is well tolerated in healthy subjects and does not affect sleep more than placebo.

Reviewer's comments
Well-conducted trial but the statistical power was marginal. Although the power was adequate to detect a 30-minute reduction in REM latency, there is no basis to expect LI 1370 to have this magnitude of effect. (5, 5)

Product Profile: GK501™

Manufacturer	**Pharmaton S.A., Switzerland**
U.S. distributor	None
Botanical ingredient	**Ginkgo leaf extract**
Extract name	**GK501™**
Quantity	60 mg

Processing	No information
Standardization	24% flavone glycosides and 6% terpene lactones
Formulation	Capsule

Source(s) of information: Kennedy, Scholey, and Wesnes, 2000.

Clinical Study: GK501™

Extract name	GK501
Manufacturer	Pharmaton S.A., Switzerland
Indication	**Cognitive functioning** in normal volunteers
Level of evidence	**I**
Therapeutic benefit	**Yes**

Bibliographic reference
Kennedy DO, Scholey AB, Wesnes KA (2000). The dose-dependent cognitive effects of acute administration of *Ginkgo biloba* to healthy young volunteers. *Psychopharmacology* 151 (4): 416-423.

Trial design
Multidose, balanced, crossover (Latin-square design) trial comparing 120 mg, 240 mg, and 360 mg of GK501 extract to placebo. Study took place on five separate testing days, each separated by a seven-day washout period. No placebo or active medication was administered on the first study day, which was used to familiarize subjects with procedures.

Study duration	1 day
Dose	2, 4, or 6 (60 mg extract) capsules per day
Route of administration	Oral
Randomized	Yes
Randomization adequate	Yes
Blinding	Double-blind
Blinding adequate	Yes
Placebo	Yes
Drug comparison	No
Site description	Single center
No. of subjects enrolled	20

No. of subjects completed 20
Sex Male and female
Age 19-24 years (mean: 20)

Inclusion criteria
Healthy young volunteers who were taking no medication with the exception of oral contraception for female volunteers. Participants abstained from caffeine-containing products and alcohol on each study day.

Exclusion criteria
Volunteers who were heavy smokers (more than ten cigarettes per day).

End points
Cognitive performance was assessed using the Cognitive Drug Research (CDR) computerized test battery immediately prior to dosing, and at 1, 2.5, 4, and 6 hours after. Primary outcome measures were speed of attention, accuracy of attention, speed of memory, and quality of memory. Patients also completed the Bond-Lader visual analog scales (VAS) to analyze three mood factors: alertness, calmness, and contentedness.

Results
Compared with placebo, there was a dose-dependent improvement of the speed of attention factor following both 240 mg and 360 mg extract; this was evident after 2.5 hours ($p = 0.036$ and $p = 0.0001$, respectively), and still present after six hours ($p = 0.026$ and $p = 0.0004$, respectively). There was a trend toward improvement of speed of attention for the lowest dose of 120 mg. The other factor that showed a convincing pattern was quality of memory. Performance was significantly enhanced with 120 mg at one and four hours ($p = 0.033$ and $p = 0.02$, respectively), with trends toward significant enhancement for the 240 mg dose at the same time points. Changes in speed of memory and accuracy of attention did not follow a pattern. None of the three factors on the Bond-Lader VAS for mood showed a significant difference.

Side effects
None mentioned in paper.

Authors' comments
Acute administration of *Ginkgo biloba* is capable of producing a sustained improvement in attention in healthy young adults.

Reviewer's comments
This study shows clear, accurate, dose-dependent improvements to index combining speed scores on three tests of attention in healthy volunteers. (4, 6)

Clinical Study: GK501™, G115®, Ginkoba M/E™

Extract name	GK501, G115
Manufacturer	Pharmaton S.A., Switzerland
Indication	**Cognitive functioning** in normal volunteers
Level of evidence	**I**
Therapeutic benefit	**Yes**

Bibliographic reference

Scholey AB, Kennedy DO (2002). Acute, dose-dependent cognitive effects of *Ginkgo biloba, Panax ginseng* and their combination in healthy young volunteers: Differential interactions with cognitive demand. *Human Psychopharmacology* 17 (1): 35-44.

Trial design

Crossover. Three studies are reported here testing ginkgo, ginseng, and a combination of the two. All studies had a total of five test days. The first day was a training day in which subjects performed all tests but were not given any treatment. The following four test days, in which subjects were given one of four treatments, were separated by one-week washout periods. The dosing was as follows: Study I: 120, 240, or 360 mg ginkgo (GK501), or placebo; Study II: 200, 400, or 600 mg ginseng (G115), or placebo; Study III: 320, 640, or 960 mg ginkgo-ginseng combination (Ginkoba M/E), or placebo.

Study duration	1 day
Dose	120, 240, or 360 mg ginkgo; 200, 400, or 600 mg ginseng; or 320, 640, or 960 mg ginkgo plus ginseng
Route of administration	Oral
Randomized	Yes
Randomization adequate	Yes
Blinding	Double-blind
Blinding adequate	Yes
Placebo	Yes
Drug comparison	No
Site description	Single center
No. of subjects enrolled	20, each
No. of subjects completed	Not given
Sex	Male and female
Age	Mean: approximately 20 years

Inclusion criteria
Healthy volunteers taking no medication, except for some females taking the contraceptive pill.

Exclusion criteria
Heavy smokers (more than 10 cigarettes per day).

End points
Five testing sessions took place on each day: predose (to establish baseline for that day), and 1, 2.5, 4, and 6 hours after taking that day's treatment. Cognitive ability was tested using serial arithmetic tasks, consisting of a modified computerized version of the serial sevens test and the serial threes task.

Results
Study I: Ginkgo significantly improved speed of responding on the serial threes task in a dose-dependent manner. Although ginkgo did not affect the speed of responding on the serial sevens task, the accuracy was significantly increased by all doses after 2.5 hours. Study II: Ginseng had no effect compared to placebo on the serial threes task. However, various doses of ginseng significantly slowed the speed of reaction, while some increased the accuracy, on the serial sevens task. Study III: Several significant and sustained improvements in performance occurred after taking the ginkgo-ginseng combination. On the serial threes task, the speed of responding was significantly increased with 320 mg dose at four hours, compared to placebo ($p < 0.05$). Accuracy was also significantly increased for 640 mg at 2.5 hours ($p < 0.05$) and for 960 mg at all test times (all $p < 0.05$). On the serial sevens test, speed of responding significantly increased for the 320 mg dose at all test times (all $p < 0.01$). Speed of responding also increased for the 640 mg dose after four hours ($p < 0.01$). Accuracy was significantly improved for all doses after 2.5 and 6 hours, and the 640 mg dose also made fewer errors at the four-hour test session.

Side effects
None mentioned.

Authors' comments
Each of the three treatments under investigation significantly affected performance on computerized serial subtractions in a dose-, time-, and task-specific manner. The effects of single doses of ginkgo and ginseng were reasonably consistent with previous findings. The most striking (and unexpected) result, however, was a marked and sustained improvement in serial sevens performance following the ginkgo-ginseng combination. It would appear that the comprehensive improvements in performance associated with the ginkgo-ginseng combination represents a synergistic behavioral effect of the two extracts interacting with cognitive demand.

Reviewer's comments
Clear evidence of acute beneficial effects of GK501 on cognitive function. (4, 6)

Product Profile: Ginkgoforce

Manufacturer	**Bioforce AG, Switzerland**
U.S. distributor	**Bioforce USA**
Botanical ingredient	**Ginkgo leaf extract**
Extract name	None given
Quantity	50 g fresh plant (16.4 g dried plant) per 100 g tincture
Processing	Plant to extract ratio 1:9, 63% alcohol
Standardization	No information
Formulation	Liquid

Recommended dose: Take 15 to 20 drops in a small amount of water three times daily.

DSHEA structure/function: Benefits memory, mental clarity, and alertness.

Comments: Sold as Geriaforce in Europe.

Source(s) of information: Information provided by distributor.

Clinical Study: Geriaforce

Extract name	None given
Manufacturer	Bioforce AG, Switzerland
Indication	**Age-related memory impairment**
Level of evidence	**II**
Therapeutic benefit	**Trend**

Bibliographic reference
Degenring FH, Brautigam MRH (1999). Geriaforce for the treatment of age-induced memory disorders—A placebo-controlled double-blind study with two dosages. Schweizerische *Zeitschrift fur GanzheitsMedizin* 11 (5): 252-257.

Trial design
Parallel. Two different doses compared to placebo. Trial preceded by a four-week washout period.

Study duration	6 months
Dose	3 (20 or 40 drops) doses daily

Route of administration	Oral
Randomized	Yes
Randomization adequate	No
Blinding	Double-blind
Blinding adequate	Yes
Placebo	Yes
Drug comparison	No
Site description	22 general practices
No. of subjects enrolled	241
No. of subjects completed	197
Sex	Male and female
Age	55-85 years (mean: 69)

Inclusion criteria
Patients with age-induced memory disorders determined by their score on the Mini-Mental State Examination.

Exclusion criteria
Exclusion criteria were dementia, depression, loss of memory for a known cause that needed other treatment, psychoses and secondary cerebral insufficiency as the result of intoxication or metabolic disorders (including liver and renal failure, diabetes mellitus, diseases of the gastrointestinal tract, heart failure, malignant diseases, as well as abuse of alcohol and medicaments), concomitant anticholinergic medication, and prior treatment with *Ginkgo biloba* in the past 3 months.

End points
Assessment was based on objective psychometric tests: the extended mental control test (EMCT) measuring attention and concentration; the Rey test parts I and II, for measuring short- and long-term memory and learning ability; and the Benton test for measuring visual short-term memory. In addition, subjective impressions of memory and concentration were recorded by the patients. Tests were administered at baseline and after 12 and 24 weeks of treatment.

Results
A marked improvement was noted in all three groups on all psychometric tests after six months due to a learning effect. Only the Benton test for visual short-term memory showed significant improvement compared to placebo ($p = 0.0076$) for the lower dose of Geriaforce. There was a 14.2 percent improvement over baseline. The higher dose of Geriaforce also caused more improvement compared to baseline (10 percent) than the placebo compared to baseline (6.1 percent). In the EMCT and Rey tests I and II, there

were no statistically significant differences between groups. There was also no significant difference in the improvement of memory and concentration according to the subjective assessment of the patients.

Side effects
Tolerance was good in all three treatment groups. Mild symptoms included gastric symptoms, dizziness and stupor, headache, and tiredness.

Authors' comments
From the present results, it can be deduced that in patients with age-related disorders of memory and concentration the dosage corresponding to the commercial preparation (20 drops three times a day) is superior not only to the placebo but also to the double dose.

Reviewer's comments
Very large trial, but results were partially spoiled by not training subjects on tests prior to study, with the result that training effects appeared on all assessments. Nonetheless, on one of the tests (Benton Visual Retention Test), improvements were greater with ginkgo. The randomization of subjects was inadequately described. (3, 5)

Product Profile: Ginkoba M/E™

Manufacturer	**Pharmaton S.A., Switzerland**
U.S. distributor	**Pharmaton Natural Health Products**
Botanical ingredient	**Ginkgo leaf extract**
Extract name	**GK501™**
Quantity	60 mg
Processing	No information
Standardization	24% flavone glycosides and 6% terpene lactones
Formulation	Capsule
Botanical ingredient	**Ginseng root extract**
Extract name	**G115®**
Quantity	100 mg
Processing	No information
Standardization	4% ginsenosides

Recommended dose: One capsule with water twice daily. Optimal results have been shown after four weeks of continuous daily use. Ginkoba M/E works gradually over time and should be taken as part of an ongoing healthy regimen.

DSHEA structure/function: Promotes fast and accurate thinking, reduces mental fatigue, safely promoting blood circulation and oxygen supply to the brain.

Cautions: If taking a prescription medicine, such as an anticoagulant agent, are pregnant, or are lactating, please contact a doctor before taking this product. In case of accidental ingestion/overdose, seek the advice of a professional immediately.

Other ingredients: Mannitol, gelatin, silicon dioxide, magnesium stearate, titanium dioxide, synthetic iron oxides.

Comments: Sold as Gincosan® in Europe.

Source(s) of information: Product package (© Boehringer Ingelheim Pharmaceuticals, Inc. 2000); Wesnes et al., 1997.

Clinical Study: Gincosan®

Extract name	GK501 and G115
Manufacturer	Pharmaton S.A., Switzerland
Indication	**Cognitive functioning** in healthy volunteers with neurasthenic complaints
Level of evidence	**III**
Therapeutic benefit	**Yes**

Bibliographic reference
Wesnes KA, Faleni RA, Hefting NR, Hoogsteen G, Houben JJG, Jenkins E, Jonkman JHG, Leonard J, Petrini O, van Lier JJ (1997). The cognitive, subjective and physical effects of a *Ginkgo biloba/Panax ginseng* combination in healthy volunteers with neurasthenic complaints. *Psychopharmacology Bulletin* 33 (4): 677-683.

Trial design
Parallel. Compared three different doses of Ginkoba M/E to placebo.

Study duration	3 months
Dose	80 mg, 160 mg, or 320 mg Ginkoba M/E twice daily
Route of administration	Oral
Randomized	Yes
Randomization adequate	No
Blinding	Double-blind

Blinding adequate	No
Placebo	Yes
Drug comparison	No
Site description	Single center
No. of subjects enrolled	64
No. of subjects completed	64
Sex	Male and female
Age	42-65 years (mean: 55)

Inclusion criteria
Subjects with neurasthenic complaints (fatigue, lack of motivation, feeling of inadequacy) identified using the SCL-90-R questionnaire and ICD-10 F48.0 diagnosing guidelines.

Exclusion criteria
Pregnancy or lactation; mental handicap; heavy smoking (more than15 cigarettes daily); alcohol abuse or drug addiction; participation in a drug study within 90 days; insulin-dependent diabetes or epilepsy; organic psychiatric disorders; regular use of neuroleptics, antidepressants, calcium antagonists, cinnarizine, or hydergine that could not be stopped seven days before the study; the use of ginseng preparations within six weeks of the start of the study and/or the use of *Ginkgo biloba* preparations within four weeks of the study; and the inability to perform the study pharmacodynamic tests adequately.

End points
Assessments were performed at baseline and on days 1, 30, and 90 one hour after the morning dose, one hour after the afternoon dose, and again five hours later. Assessments included the Cognitive Drug Research computerized assessment system, the Vienna determination unit, cycle ergometry, and various questionnaires.

Results
Significant improvements were seen one hour after the morning dosing with all doses on day 1 (80 mg, $p = 0.003$; 160 mg, $p = 0.033$; 320 mg, $p = 0.004$). Also, one hour after the morning dosing on day 90, the 320 mg dose significantly improved the quality of memory index compared to placebo ($p = 0.003$); however, the placebo group had improved so much that there was no significant difference between it and the two lowest doses. The opposite pattern appeared on the tests one hour after afternoon dosing. The 320 mg dose impaired the global index of memory on day 1 and day 90 ($p < 0.004$ and $p < 0.001$, respectively). Afternoon memory impairments appeared to be dose dependent. After morning exercise on day 90, all doses of Ginkoba M/E showed a greater reduction in heart rate from the prestudy level com-

pared to placebo; however, the effect was not clearly dose dependent and only the 80 mg dose was significantly different from placebo ($p = 0.03$). The mean score on neurasthenic-related questions (SCL-90-R symptom checklist) showed a decrease on days 30 and 90 compared with the pre-study score for all groups, with no significant differences between groups.

Side effects
The nine adverse events considered to be possibly related to the treatment were of mild intensity. Of those, four were considered to be probably related to the treatment and were either nausea or abdominal pain.

Authors' comments
This study found that a combination of ginkgo and ginseng has beneficial effects on cognitive function and other measures. The reversal of some of the cognitive effects hours later after an additional dose suggests that a longer in-between dosing interval may be appropriate.

Reviewer's comments
This trial showed significant benefit to quality of memory. Benefits began at day 30, but they appeared to reverse later on day 90. Neither randomization nor blinding were adequately described. (0, 6)

Clinical Study: Ginkoba M/E™

Extract name	GK501 and G115
Manufacturer	Pharmaton S.A., Switzerland
Indication	**Cognitive functioning** in normal volunteers
Level of evidence	**II**
Therapeutic benefit	**Yes**

Bibliographic reference
Wesnes K, Ward T, McGinty A, Petrini O (2000). The memory enhancing effects of a *Ginkgo biloba/Panax ginseng* combination in healthy middle-aged volunteers. *Psychopharmacology* 152 (4): 353-361.

Trial design
Parallel. Comparison of two dosing regimens: 160 mg twice daily or 320 mg once daily. Twelve-week study preceded by a two-week placebo washout phase, and followed by two weeks of no treatment.

Study duration	14 weeks
Dose	2 (160 mg) capsules daily, either together or 5 hours apart

Route of administration	Oral
Randomized	Yes
Randomization adequate	No
Blinding	Double-blind
Blinding adequate	Yes
Placebo	Yes
Drug comparison	No
Site description	7 health centers
No. of subjects enrolled	279
No. of subjects completed	256
Sex	Male and female
Age	38-66 years (mean: 56)

Inclusion criteria
Healthy middle-aged volunteers.

Exclusion criteria
Volunteers with signs or history of depression, evidence of dementia, clinically relevant abnormalities in medical history or examination, history of alcohol or drug abuse, heavy smokers (more than 10 cigarettes per day), history of food or drug allergies relevant to the study compound, clinically relevant deviation from normal of any finding during prestudy medical screening, unable to perform the cognitive tests, and taking a cognition-enhancing substance or medication which may have been stopped at some time during the active dosing phase.

End points
Assessment was conducted before pretrial washout, at baseline, and after 4, 8, 12, and 14 weeks. Volunteers performed a selection of tests of attention and memory from the Cognitive Drug Research computerized cognitive assessment system prior to morning dosing, and again at one, three, and six hours later. The volunteers also completed questionnaires about mood states, quality of life, and sleep quality.

Results
The ginkgo/ginseng combination significantly improved the quality of memory index by 7.5 percent. There was no difference between the two dosing regimens, nor in the successive weeks of testing. Memory enhancement was seen throughout the 12-week treatment and after the two-week final washout. There were no significant effects of Ginkoba M/E on the secondary vari-

ables: power of attention, continuity of attention, and the speed of memory process.

Side effects
Five volunteers suffered mild adverse events leading them to withdraw from the study.

Authors' comments
This study represents the first substantial demonstration of improvements to the memory of healthy middle-aged volunteers produced by a phytopharmaceutical.

Reviewer's comments
This is the largest properly controlled study of a phytopharmaceutical in normals ever conducted. No evidence of biphasic effect seen in previous study (Wesnes et al., 1997). The selective improvement of quality of memory confirmed in this study is a new phytopharmaceutical benchmark. The only deficit to the trial was an inadequate description of the randomization process. (3, 6)

Clinical Study: Ginkoba M/E™

Extract name	GK501 and G115
Manufacturer	Pharmaton
Indication	**Cognitive functioning** in normal volunteers
Level of evidence	I
Therapeutic benefit	**Yes**

Bibliographic reference
Kennedy DO, Scholey AB, Wesnes KA (2001). Differential, dose dependent changes in cognitive performance following acute administration of a *Ginkgo biloba/Panax ginseng* combination to healthy young volunteers. *Nutritional Neuroscience* 4 (5): 399-412.

Trial design
Crossover. Subjects received 320, 640, and 960 mg Ginkoba M/E and matching placebo in order dictated by a Latin square. There was a washout period of seven days between each treatment.

Study duration	1 day
Dose	2, 4, or 6 (60 mg GK501 and 100 mg G115) capsules per day
Route of administration	Oral
Randomized	Yes
Randomization adequate	Yes
Blinding	Double-blind
Blinding adequate	Yes
Placebo	Yes
Drug comparison	No
Site description	Not described
No. of subjects enrolled	20
No. of subjects completed	20
Sex	Male and female
Age	Mean: 20.6 years

Inclusion criteria
Healthy young volunteers who were taking no medication with the exception of oral contraception for female volunteers. Participants abstained from caffeine-containing products and alcohol on each study day.

Exclusion criteria
Volunteers who were heavy smokers (more than 10 cigarettes per day) or were taking herbal supplements.

End points
Cognitive performance was assessed using a computerized test battery immediately prior to dosing and at 1, 2.5, 4, and 6 hours after treatment. Primary outcome measures were quality of memory; working memory (subfactor) and secondary memory (subfactor) (derived from quality of memory); speed of memory; speed of attention; and accuracy of attention. Patients also completed the Bond-Lader visual analog scales to analyze three mood factors: alertness, calmness, and contentedness.

Results
Compared to placebo, quality of memory was significantly improved following treatment with 960 mg both one hour and six hours postdose ($p = 0.0009$ and $p = 0.002$, respectively). Further analysis revealed that this effect was differentially targeted at the secondary memory, which improved one, four, and six hours after dosing, rather than the working memory component, which was not different from placebo. There was no improvement in quality of memory following the 320 mg dose and only a trend toward improvement six hours after the 640 mg dose. Both 320 mg and 640 mg treatments produced trend improvements in secondary memory after six hours. No dose

produced significant differences in general speed of performance. Speed of attention, however, was significantly slowed for both the 320 mg and 640 mg doses four hours after treatment ($p = 0.01$ and $p = 0.05$, respectively), and again for 320 mg at six hours ($p = 0.0006$). The 960 mg dose saw no significant drop in performance for this factor. No dose produced a significant difference in performance on the accuracy of attention factor. There were also no significant differences on the Bond-Lader VAS.

Side effects
None mentioned.

Authors' comments
The results show improvements of mnemonic performance in healthy young participants within one hour of ingestion, and this offers support to the possibility that the ginkgo-ginseng combination may have some utility in combating cognitive deficits.

Reviewer's comments
Important replication of selective enhancement of quality of memory index with ginkgo-ginseng combination, this time in a third laboratory and in young, healthy volunteers. Trial dropouts were not described, but the authors assured that there were none (4, 6).

Ginseng

Other common names: **Asian ginseng; Chinese ginseng; Korean ginseng,** *ren shen*
Latin name: ***Panax ginseng*** C.A. Meyer [Araliaceae]
Latin synonyms: ***Panax schinseng*** T. Nees
Plant part: **Root**

American Ginseng

Other common name: *xi yang shen*
Latin name: ***Panax quinquefolius*** L. [Araliaceae]
Plant part: **Root**

PREPARATIONS USED
IN REVIEWED CLINICAL STUDIES

Ginseng, or in Chinese, *ren shen,* has been translated roughly as "man-root," referring to the shape of the root. Only products of *Panax* species are properly labeled ginseng. However, the name has been used more loosely, and incorrectly, to include members of other genera, such as *Eleutherococcus senticosus* (Rupr. et Maxim) Maxim., given the nickname "Siberian ginseng." The genus *Panax* includes 11 species—the most commonly used is *Panax ginseng* C.A. Meyer, also known as Asian ginseng (Awang, 2003; Wen, 2001).

The root of Asian ginseng has been used in traditional Asian medicine for more than 2,000 years. Commercially supplied roots are graded according to their source, age, part of the root, and method of preparation (Bahrke and Morgan, 1994). The root can be used fresh, or prepared as "white" ginseng (peeled and dried) or "red" ginseng (steamed and dried). The fresh root is often sliced thinly and taken with or without honey, or it can be boiled in soup. White or red ginseng can be powdered, extracted, or made into a tea (Yun and Choi, 1998). The main active components of ginseng roots are glycosidal

GINSENG SUMMARY TABLE

Product Name	Manufacturer/ U.S. Distributor	Product Characteristics	Dose in Trials	Indication	No. of Trials	Benefit (Evidence Level-Trial No.)
Asian Ginseng Products						
Ginsana®*	Pharmaton S.A., Switzerland/ Pharmaton Natural Health Products	Extract standard- ized to 4% ginsenosides (G115®)	2-6 (100 mg) capsules; 200- 600 mg daily	Physical perfor- mance	7	Yes (I-1, II-2, III-1) Undetermined (III-1) No (II-2)
				Cognitive functioning	2	Yes (I-1, II-1)
				Vaccination potentiation	1	Yes (II-1)
				Bronchitis	2	Yes (II-1, III-1)
				Menopausal symptoms	1	Trend (II-1)
				General well-being	2	Yes (I-1) Undetermined (II-1)
Ginsana® Gold Blend	Pharmaton S.A., Switzerland/ Pharmaton Natural Health Products	Extract standard- ized to 4% ginsenosides (G115®) plus vitamins and minerals	1-2 (40 mg) capsules daily	General well-being	3	Yes (I-2, II-1)
				Physical perfor- mance	1	Yes (III-1)
				Age-related memory impairment	1	Yes (II-1)
				Geriatric re- habilitation	1	No (II-1)

Gerimax	Dansk Droge, Denmark/None	Extract standardized to 4% ginsenosides	100-400 mg daily	Cognitive functioning	1	Yes (II-1)
				Diabetes (NIDDM)	1	Yes (III-1)

American Ginseng Products

American ginseng root	Chai-Na-Ta Corp., Canada/None	Ontario grown powdered root	1-9 g	Diabetes (NIDDM)	2	Trend (II-1, III-1)
				Postprandial glycemia	3	Undetermined (III-2) No (II-1)

*See the ginkgo profile for information on the combination product Ginkoba M/E™, which contains extracts of ginseng root (G115®) and ginkgo leaves (GK501™).

saponins known as ginsenosides. There are eight commonly measured ginsenosides, in addition to three malonylginsenosides. The heating process in the production of red ginseng converts the malonylginsenosides to their ginsenoside counterparts (Chuang et al., 1995) and also results in other chemical transformations.

American ginseng, *Panax quinquefolius* L., is native to eastern North America and cultivated both in North America and in Asia. American ginseng root can be distinguished from Asian ginseng by profiling the constituent ginsenosides (Dou, Hou, and Chen, 1998; Chuang et al., 1995).

Ginsana® is manufactured by Pharmaton S.A. in Switzerland, and is sold by Pharmaton Natural Health Products in the United States. Ginsana contains the ginseng root extract G115®, which is characterized as containing 4 percent ginsenosides. This standardized extract is also sold in combination with vitamins and minerals as Ginsana® Gold Blend in the United States and Gericomplex in Europe. Three similar products also produced by Pharmaton (Geriatric Pharmaton®, Gegorvit®, Pharmaton® Capsules) contained an additional ingredient, deanol (dimethylaminoethanol bitartrate), and were used in three of the reviewed clinical trials (Le Gal, Cathebras, and Struby, 1996; Neri et al., 1995; Pieralisi, Ripari, and Vecchiet, 1991).

Gerimax Ginseng Extract is manufactured by Dansk Droge in Denmark and is characterized as containing 4 percent ginsenosides. This product is not sold in the United States.

Powdered American ginseng root is manufactured by Chai-Na-Ta Corporation in British Columbia, Canada. However, this product has not been developed commercially and is not available on the market.

SUMMARY OF REVIEWED CLINICAL STUDIES

Ginseng has been described as an "adaptogen," a substance that corrects dysfunction in sick individuals and protects healthy individuals from stresses without producing unwanted side effects. The adaptogen concept originated from Soviet scientists in the late 1950s. The concept was translated recently into Western conventional medicine as a medicinal agent with a pharmacological profile of antioxidant and/or anticancer activity, immunomodulatory, and cholesterol-lowering properties, as well as having hypoglycemic and choleretic actions (Davydov and Krikorian, 2000). Adaptogens have also been described as increasing nonspecific resistance to stress due to adverse physical, chemical, and/or biological factors (Bahrke and Morgan, 1994).

The trials reviewed in the book test ginseng for its effects on physical performance, well-being, cognitive performance, the immune system, and diabetes. Case reports indicate that the use of ginseng may reduce the risk of cancer.

Ginsana (G115)

Physical Performance

The five reviewed trials with Ginsana (G115) focus on physical fitness using the standard dose of 200 mg per day over a period of two to three months. Three studies reported positive results and two studies reported no benefit to fitness. The positive studies, including 28 to 30 male athletes each, reported an increase in fitness following nine weeks of treatment compared to placebo. The studies reported an increase in oxygen capacity during exercise, a decrease in maximum exercise heart rate, and a decrease in lactate levels following exercise. The most recent study was a good-quality placebo-controlled trial (Forgo and Schimert, 1985). Our reviewer, Keith Wesnes, observed that the results of this study showed great improvements in fitness and faster reaction times. The second study, of poor quality, compared the G115 extract (with 4 percent ginsenosides) to G115S (a special extract containing 7 percent ginsenosides) and found no difference in the effectiveness of the two products. The authors concluded that no advantage existed in increasing the ginsenoside concentration to greater than 4 percent (Forgo and Kirchdorfer, 1982). This study was rated as having poor quality because it lacked a placebo control and the study subjects were not randomized. The third study, a good-quality trial, contained three treatment groups: 200 mg G115S with 7 percent ginsenosides; 200 mg of the standard G115 plus 400 mg vitamin E; and placebo. Compared with placebo, similar increases in fitness were observed in both treatment groups (Forgo, 1983).

Two well-conducted trials on exercise capacity, conducted by a different research group, failed to find any benefit to exercise capacity with G115 after eight weeks of treatment. These trials used 19 healthy females and 31 healthy males, respectively, and a dose of 200 mg, or 200 or 400 mg extract per day, respectively (Engels, Said, and Wirth, 1996; Engels and Wirth, 1997). The contradictory data reported by these two research groups leave open the question of whether ginseng can enhance exercise capacity. It may be that larger sample sizes are needed to evaluate efficacy or that a difference exists between the effect of G115 on athletes, subjects in the positive studies, and normal healthy persons, included in the negative studies.

Two other studies reported an increase in the speed of reactions to light and sound following a dose of 200 mg G115 extract for three months. A placebo-controlled study with 120 members of a sports club reported increases in reaction times and pulmonary function, particularly in those above 40 years of age (Forgo, Kayasseh, and Staub, 1981). A smaller, poorly described study with 60 subjects reported faster responses, improved two-handed coordination, and increased recovery after exercise (Dörling, Kirchdorfer, and Ruckert, 1980).

Cognitive Functioning

Cognitive function was assessed in two trials. One placebo-controlled study with 32 healthy male students found improved mental arithmetic compared to placebo after three months of treatment with 200 mg extract per day (D'Angelo et al., 1986). A crossover trial with 20 young volunteers (mean age: 21 years) showed that single doses of 200, 400, or 600 mg improved the ability to retain information in short- and long-term memory, with the greatest benefit in quality of memory following a single dose of 400 mg. The study also reported a decrement in reaction times on attention tasks following a single dose of 200 or 600 mg but not 400 mg. The significance of the latter result is not fully understood by the researchers, who recommended further investigation (Kennedy, Scholey, and Wesnes, 2001).

Vaccination Potentiation

The clinical data suggest that G115 can protect against influenza and improve immune responses, including those in smokers with chronic bronchitis. In a large, placebo-controlled study investigating vaccination potentiation, 219 healthy subjects were vaccinated with a flu vaccine four weeks into a three-month treatment period with either G115 (200 mg per day) or placebo. As a result, G115 reduced the incidence of influenza or common cold by about two-thirds compared to placebo. In addition to the reduction in colds, the treatment group also had increased antibody titers and increased natural killer cell activity compared to the placebo group (Scaglione et al., 1996).

Bronchitis

Two trials that studied the effect of G115 on subjects with bronchitis indicated an increase in immune response following a dose of 200 mg per day. A single-blind study of 40 smokers with chronic bronchitis reported increases in immune parameters, including alveolar macrophage phagocytosis and intracellular killing, after two months of treatment (Scaglione et al., 1994). An open study, with 44 subjects with symptoms of an acute attack of chronic bronchitis reported increased bacterial clearance in the group receiving G115 plus antibiotics for nine days compared to the group receiving only antibiotics (Scaglione, Weiser, and Alessandria, 2001).

Menopausal Symptoms

A well-conducted study examined the quality of life in 379 healthy, postmenopausal women. There was a trend toward symptomatic relief of menopausal symptoms, with the strongest evidence for reduction in depression. There was no change in physiological parameters or hot flashes (Wiklund et al., 1999).

General Well-Being

Ginseng had no effect on psychological outlook or mood in a placebo-controlled study with 83 young, healthy adults (average age: 26 years). Treatment groups were given either 200 or 400 mg of G115 per day for two months, and mood was assessed using a questionnaire regarding emotional states (Cardinal and Engels, 2001). A small pilot study assessing general quality of life via a questionnaire found improvements in social functioning and mental health in young adults following four weeks of treatment with 200 mg of G115 per day compared with placebo. However, these differences did not appear at the end of the eight-week trial (Ellis and Reddy, 2002).

Ginsana Gold Blend (G115 with Vitamins and Minerals)

We reviewed six trials on a mixture of G115 with vitamins and minerals. Three studies indicated benefits in quality of life indexes, particularly when they were poor to begin with. One study reported improvement in exercise capacity. Another indicated improvements in age-associated memory impairment. The final study did not indicate a benefit in geriatric rehabilitation.

General Well-Being

Three large, good-quality trials indicated a general improvement in quality of life. Quality of life was assessed from a questionnaire scoring general well-being, satisfaction with life, activity and energy levels, sexual activity, and ability to sleep. The largest trial, well-conducted and well-described, with 501 adults subject to increased physical and mental stress, compared one capsule of the ginseng mixture to vitamins and minerals alone. After three months, quality of life was improved in the ginseng group when compared to the baseline and to the control group (Marasco et al., 1996). Another excellent study with 390 healthy adults showed no overall increase in general well-being, according to a questionnaire, following ingestion of two capsules daily for three months. However, a subset of the subjects, with the lowest well-being scores at baseline, improved in vitality and mood compared with placebo. There were, however, general improvements in behavioral aspects, such as alertness, appetite, and relaxation, for the entire treatment group (Wiklund, Karlberg, and Lund, 1994). The third large trial with 219 subjects showed improved quality of life in people who had been suffering from functional fatigue for more than 15 years. Both treatment and placebo groups improved greatly, but even so a statistically significant improvement was observed with a dose of two capsules per day compared to placebo at the end of six weeks (Le Gal, Cathebras, and Struby, 1996).

Physical Performance

A placebo-controlled study with 47 healthy male sports teachers noted an increase in exercise capacity after six weeks of administration of two capsules of the G115 formula compared with placebo (Pieralisi, Ripari, and Vecchiet, 1991).

Age-Related Memory Impairment

Improvements in memory and life satisfaction were noted in a placebo-controlled trial of 60 elderly volunteers (mean age 60 years) with age-associated memory impairment. The subjects were assessed after nine months of treatment with two capsules daily (Neri et al., 1995).

Geriatric Rehabilitation

Another well-conducted trial studied 40 nondemented geriatric patients (mean age 78 years) admitted to the hospital for treatment of cardiovascular, pulmonary, or musculoskeletal diseases. Compared with placebo, there was no difference in quality of life, cognitive function, or length of hospital stay following treatment with two capsules daily for two months (Thommessen and Laake, 1996).

Gerimax

Cognitive Functioning

In a trial including 112 healthy subjects, ages 40 to 70 years old, reaction times and ability for abstract thinking increased after receiving 400 mg Gerimax Ginseng Extract for eight to nine weeks compared to no controls. However, no difference developed between the two groups in assessments of concentration or memory (Sorensen and Sonne, 1996).

Diabetes

A trial including 36 newly diagnosed patients with non-insulin-dependent diabetes mellitus (NIDDM) recorded increased psychomotor performance, mood, and vigor after two months of treatment compared to the baseline. A dose of 200 mg for two months reduced fasting blood glucose and glycosylated hemoglobin (HbA_{1c}) levels compared to placebo (Sotaniemi, Haapakoski, and Rautio, 1995). Neither the blinding nor the randomization were adequately described in this trial, which diminished its quality.

American Ginseng Root

Diabetes

Four pilot trials focused on the ability of American ginseng root powder to reduce the rise in blood sugar following administration of oral glucose. Vuksan, Sivenpiper, and colleagues (2000) reported in a small study including ten healthy subjects and nine type II diabetics that 3 g ginseng root powder administered 40 minutes before the glucose challenge caused significant reductions (approximately 20 percent of the area under the curve) in the resulting rise in blood sugar in both groups compared to placebo. For diabetics, the reduction in blood sugar also occurred when ginseng and glucose were taken at the same time.

Other studies by the same group reported that there was no significantly different response in healthy subjects when higher doses of 6 or 9 g were administered or when lower doses of 1 or 3 g were administered. In addition, similar reductions in blood glucose were recorded whether ginseng was taken 40, 80, or 120 minutes before challenge, but not later (Vuksan, Stavro, Sievenpiper, Koo et al., 2000; Vuksan et al., 2001). Further studies with a small group of 12 type II diabetics also reported no change with response regardless of whether doses of 3, 6, or 9 g were administered. In contrast to healthy subjects, glucose levels were reduced when ginseng was administered concurrently with the challenge, as well as 40, 80, or 120 minutes before challenge (Vuksan, Stavro, Sievenpiper, Beljan-Zdravkovic et al., 2000). A weakness of these studies is the small number of participants. The size of the groups in all studies ranged from 10 to 12.

Sievenpiper and colleagues (2003) recently reported a fifth study using 12 normal healthy subjects. A different batch of powdered American ginseng was used for this study. In contrast to previous studies, this study reported no reduction in plasma glucose when 6 g ginseng was given 40 minutes before the 75 g oral glucose test. The batch of powdered American ginseng used in this study contained approximately half the amount of the previous batch. The authors suggested that the quantity of total ginsenosides or differences in the profiles of the individual ginsenosides may account for the lack of activity.

SYSTEMATIC REVIEWS

A systematic review of double-blind, randomized, placebo-controlled clinical studies was conducted on all "ginsengs." The review included 16 trials: ten of which were conducted on *Panax ginseng;* one on *Panax quinguefolius* (American ginseng); three on *Eleutherococcus senticosus* (commonly referred to as "Siberian ginseng"); and two on materials simply described as "ginseng." The indications for the trials were physical performance, psychomotor performance and cognitive function, immunomodulation, diabetes mellitus, and herpes simplex type II infections. The authors found that the evidence for these conditions was not convincing (Vogler, Pittler, and Ernst, 1999). However, with multiple species and different preparations all lumped together, it would be difficult to reach any meaningful conclusions.

EPIDEMIOLOGICAL STUDIES

A cohort study that included 4,634 adults over 40 years old in a province in Korea reported evidence that *Panax ginseng* has a non-organ-specific preventive effect against cancer. Ginseng consumers had less than half the risk of cancer compared with nonconsumers (relative risk 0.40, 95 percent confidence interval). The risk decreased with an increase in the frequency of ginseng consumption when those who consumed ginseng less than three times per year were compared with those taking ginseng more than once a month (Yun and Choi, 1998). Two case-controlled studies, wherein newly diagnosed cancer patients admitted to the hospital were paired with patients admitted to the hospital for other reasons (905 pairs and 1,987 pairs, respectively), questioned subjects regarding their use of ginseng. Fewer of the cancer patients reported taking ginseng when compared to the controls. The authors thus reported a reduction in risk of cancer of about half (relative risk 0.56 and 0.50, respectively) (Yun and Choi, 1990, 1995). These three studies were reanalyzed in a recent publication. Taking into account results from the studies, there was a significant decrease in the proportion of cancer cases with increasing frequency of intake of ginseng. Red ginseng was profiled as having the strongest anticancer activity in comparison with other ginseng preparations (Yun, Choi, and Yun, 2001).

ADVERSE REACTIONS OR SIDE EFFECTS

Ginseng was well tolerated in the reviewed studies. A systematic review of adverse effects and drug interactions was published for *Panax ginseng* (Coon and Ernst, 2002). The authors found that data from clinical trials suggest that the incidence of adverse events with ginseng (single ingredient) preparations is similar to that of placebo. The most commonly experienced events were headaches, sleep disorders, and gastrointestinal disorders. The review cited two case reports involving potential herb-drug interactions. One was a 64-year-old woman who was taking phenelzine along with triazolam and lorazepam and developed a headache and tremulousness upon adding ginseng to her regime. The second was a 47-year-old man with a mechanical heart valve taking warfarin, whose bleeding time decreased after supplementation with ginseng. The latter report was surprising since ginseng has been reported to have some platelet-inhibiting effects, and the opposite effect might be expected. The review also reported an open, nonrandomized clinical trial with 14 healthy volunteers that suggested that ginseng enhances the clearance rate of blood alcohol (Coon and Ernst, 2002).

The *British Herbal Compendium (BHC)* warns that extensive use of ginseng can lead to hypertension (Bradley, 1992). However, a placebo-controlled study including 26 subjects with mild or moderate hypertension (systolic blood pressure over 140 mmHg and diastolic blood pressure between 90 and 110 mmHg) reported opposite results. The participants were placed on a 24-hour blood pressure monitoring system. Administration of 4.5 g powdered red ginseng root (obtained from Korea) per day for eight weeks resulted in significant decreases in systolic blood pressure with only a tendency for diastolic blood pressure to decrease. The authors concluded that red ginseng might be a relatively safe medication to add to standard hypertensive therapy (Han et al., 1998).

INFORMATION FROM PHARMACOPOEIAL MONOGRAPHS

Sources of Published Therapeutic Monographs

British Herbal Compendium
German Commission E
World Health Organization

Indications

The German Commission E, the *British Herbal Compendium (BHC)*, and the World Health Organization (WHO) specify that the dried main and lateral root and root hairs of ginseng are indicated as a tonic, prophylactic, or restorative agent for invigoration and fortification in times of fatigue and debility, physical or mental exhaustion, stress, and for declining capacity for work and concentration (Blumenthal et al., 1998; Bradley, 1992; WHO, 1999). The Commission E and the WHO suggest that ginseng can be used during convalescence as well (Blumenthal et al., 1998; WHO, 1999). The *BHC* also states that ginseng can be used for inadequate resistance to infections and lists the following actions: adaptogenic, stimulant, and tonic (Bradley, 1992).

Doses

Dried root: 1 to 2 g daily (Blumenthal et al., 1998); 0.6 to 2 g daily, taken in the morning (Bradley, 1992); 0.5 to 2 g daily, taken in the morning (WHO, 1999); or equivalent preparations
Decoction: equivalent amounts to above (Bradley, 1992; WHO, 1999)

Treatment Period

Both the Commission E and the *BHC* suggest that ginseng be used for up to three months and that a repeated course is feasible (Blumenthal et al., 1998; Bradley, 1992). However, the *BHC* also states that occasional use or courses of one month followed by a two-month interval are recommended (Bradley, 1992).

Contraindications

The Commission E and the WHO list no known contraindications (Blumenthal et al., 1998; WHO, 1999). The *BHC*, however, lists the following: pregnancy, acute illness, hypertension, and use of other stimulants (including significant consumption of caffeine-containing beverages) (Bradley, 1992).

Adverse Reactions

The Commission E states no known adverse reactions, and the WHO adds that there are none if ginseng is taken at the recommended dose (Blumenthal et al., 1998; WHO, 1999). The *BHC* warns that extensive use can lead to sleeplessness, hypertension, or other side effects (Bradley, 1992).

Precautions

The WHO advises that diabetic patients should consult a physician prior to taking ginseng root, since it may slightly reduce blood glucose levels (WHO, 1999).

Drug Interactions

The Commission E lists no known drug interactions, whereas the WHO states that two reports exist of an interaction between ginseng and phenelzine, a monoamine inhibitor (Blumenthal et al., 1998; WHO, 1999).

REFERENCES

Awang DVC (2003). What in the name of *Panax* are those other "ginsengs"? *HerbalGram* 57: 30-35.

Bahrke MS, Morgan WP (1994). Evaluation of the ergogenic properties of ginseng. *Sports Medicine* 18 (4): 229-248.

Blumenthal M, Busse W, Hall T, Goldberg A, Grünwald J, Riggins C, Rister S, eds. (1998). *The Complete German Commission E Monographs: Therapeutic Guide to Herbal Medicines.* Trans. S Klein. Austin: American Botanical Council.

Bradley PR, ed. (1992.) *British Herbal Compendium: A Handbook of Scientific Information on Widely Used Plant Drugs,* Volume 1. Dorset: British Herbal Medicine Association.

Cardinal BJ, Engels H-J (2001). Ginseng does not enhance psychological well-being in healthy young adults: Results of a double-blind, placebo-controlled, randomized clinical trial. *Journal of the American Dietetic Association* 101 (6): 655-660.

Chuang WC, Wu HK, Sheu SJ, Chiou SH, Chang HC, Chen YP (1995). A comparative study on commercial samples of ginseng radix. *Planta Medica* 61: 459-465.

Coon JT, Ernst E (2002). *Panax ginseng:* A systematic review of adverse effects and drug interactions. *Drug Safety* 25 (5): 323-344.

D'Angelo L, Grimaldi R, Caravaggi M, Marcoli M, Perucca E, Lecchini S, Frigo GM, Crema A (1986). A double-blind, placebo-controlled clinical study on the effect of a standardized ginseng extract on psychomotor performance in healthy volunteers. *Journal of Ethnopharmacology* 16 (1): 15-22.

Davydov M, Krikorian AD (2000). *Eleutherococcus senticosus* (Rupr. and Maxim.) Maxim. (Araliaceae) as an adaptogen: A closer look. *Journal of Ethnopharmacology* 72 (3): 345-393.

Dörling E, Kirchdorfer AM, Rückert KH (1980). Do ginsenosides influence the performance? Results of a double-blind study. *Notabene Medici* 10 (5): 241-246.

Dou DQ, Hou WB, Chen YJ (1998). Studies on the characteristic constituents of Chinese ginseng and American ginseng. *Planta Medica* 64: 585-586.

Ellis JM, Reddy P (2002). Effects of *Panax ginseng* on quality of life. *The Annals of Pharmacotherapy* 36 (3): 375-379.

Engels HJ, Said JM, Wirth JC (1996). Failure of chronic ginseng supplementation to affect work performance and energy metabolism in healthy adult females. *Nutrition Research* 16 (8): 1295-1305.

Engels HJ, Wirth JC (1997). No ergogenic effects of ginseng (*Panax ginseng* C.A. Meyer) during graded maximal aerobic exercise. *Journal of the American Dietetic Association* 97 (10): 1110-1115.

Forgo I (1983). Effect of drugs on physical performance and hormone system of sportsmen. *Münchener Medizinische Wochenschrift* 125 (38): 822-824.

Forgo I, Kayasseh L, Staub JJ (1981). Effects of a standardized ginseng extract on general health, reaction capacity, pulmonary function, and hormones. *Medizinische Welt* 32 (19): 751-756.

Forgo I, Kirchdorfer AM (1982). The effect of different ginsenoside concentrations on physical work capacity. *Notabene Medici* 12 (9): 721-727.

Forgo I, Schimert G (1985). The duration of effect of the standardized ginseng extract G115 in healthy competitive athletes. *Notabene Medici* 15 (9): 636-640.

Han KH, Choe SC, Kim HS, Sohn DW, Nam KY, Oh BH, Lee MM, Park YB, Choi YS, Seo JD, Lee YW (1998). Effect of red ginseng on blood pressure in patients with essential hypertension and white coat hypertension. *American Journal of Chinese Medicine* 26 (2): 199-209.

Kennedy DO, Scholey AB, Wesnes KA (2001). Dose dependent changes in cognitive performance and mood following acute administration of ginseng to healthy young volunteers. *Nutritional Neuroscience* 4: 295-310.

Le Gal M, Cathebras P, Struby K (1996). Pharmaton capsules in the treatment of functional fatigue: A double-blind study versus placebo evaluated by a new methodology. *Phytotherapy Research* 10 (1): 49-53.

Marasco CA, Vargas RR, Villagomez SA, Infante BC (1996). Double-blind study of a multivitamin complex supplemented with ginseng extract. *Drugs Under Experimental and Clinical Research* 22 (6): 323-329.

Neri M, Andermarcher E, Pradelli JM, Salvioli G (1995). Influence of a double blind pharmacological trial on two domains of well-being in subjects with age associated memory impairment. *Archives of Gerontology and Geriatrics* 21 (3): 241-252.

Pieralisi G, Ripari P, Vecchiet L (1991). Effect of a standardized ginseng extract combined with dimethylaminoethanol bitartrate, vitamins, minerals, and trace elements on physical performance during exercise. *Clinical Therapeutics* 13 (3): 373-382.

Scaglione F, Cattaneo G, Alessandria M, Cogo R (1996). Efficacy and safety of the standardized ginseng extract G115 for potentiating vaccination against common cold and/or influenza syndrome. *Drugs Under Experimental and Clinical Research* 22 (2): 65-72.

Scaglione F, Cogo R, Cocuzza C, Arcidiancono M, Beretta A (1994). Immunomodulatory effect of *Panax ginseng* C.A. Meyer (G115) on alveolar macrophages from patients suffering with chronic bronchitis. *International Journal of Immunotherapy* 10 (1): 21-24.

Scaglione F, Weiser K, Alessandria M (2001). Effects of the standardized ginseng extract G115 in patients with chronic bronchitis: A non-blinded, randomized, comparative pilot study. *Clinical Drug Investigation* 21 (1): 41-45.

Sievenpiper JL, Arnason JT, Leiter LA, Vukson V (2003). Variable effects of American ginseng: A batch of American ginseng (*Panax quiquefolius* L.) with a depressed ginseng profile does not affect postprandial glycemia. *European Journal of Clinical Nutrition* 57 (2): 243-248.

Sorensen H, Sonne J (1996). A double-masked study of the effects of ginseng on cognitive functions. *Current Therapeutic Research* 57: 959-968.

Sotaniemi EA, Haapakoski E, Rautio A (1995). Ginseng therapy in non-insulin-dependent diabetic patients. *Diabetics Care* 18 (10): 1373-1375.

Thommessen B, Laake K (1996). No identifiable effect of ginseng (Geri-complex) as an adjuvant in the treatment of geriatric patients. *Aging* (Milan, Italy) 8 (6): 417-420.

Vogler BK, Pittler MH, Ernst E (1999). The efficacy of ginseng. A systematic review of randomized clinical trials. *European Journal of Clinical Pharmacology* 55 (8): 567-575.

Vuksan V, Sievenpiper JL, Koo VYY, Francis T, Beljan-Zdravkovic U, Xu Z, Vidgen E (2000). American ginseng (*Panax quinquefolius* L) reduces postprandial glycemia in nondiabetic subjects and subjects with type 2 diabetes mellitus. *Archives of Internal Medicine* 160 (7): 1009-1013.

Vuksan V, Sievenpiper JL, Wong J, Xu Z, Beljan-Zdravkovic U, Arnason JT, Assinewe V, Starvro MP, Jenkins AL, Leiter LA, et al. (2001). American ginseng (*Panax quinquefolius* L.) attenuates postprandial glycemia in a time-dependent but not dose-dependent manner in healthy individuals. *American Journal of Clinical Nutrition* 73 (4): 753-758.

Vuksan V, Stavro MP, Sievenpiper JL, Beljan-Zdravkovic U, Leiter LA, Josse RG, Xu Z (2000). Similar postprandial glycemic reductions with escalation of dose and administration time of American ginseng in type 2 diabetes. *Diabetes Care* 23 (9): 1221-1226.

Vuksan V, Stavro MP, Sievenpiper JL, Koo VYY, Wong E, Beljan-Zdravkovic U, Francis T, Jenkins AL, Leiter LA, Josse AB, et al. (2000). American ginseng improves glycemia in individuals with normal glucose tolerance: Effect of dose and time escalation. *Journal of the American College of Nutrition* 19 (6): 738-744.

Wen J (2001). Species diversity, nomenclature, phylogeny, biogeography and classification of the ginseng genus (*Panax* L., Araliaceae). In ZK Punja (ed.) *Utilization of Biotechnological, Genetic and Cultural Approaches for North American and Asian Ginseng Improvement. Proceedings of the International Ginseng Workshop* (pp. 67-88). Vancouver, Canada: Simon Fraser University Press.

Wiklund I, Karlberg J, Lund B (1994). A double-blind comparison of the effect on quality of life of a combination of vital substances including standardized ginseng G115 and placebo. *Current Therapeutic Research* 55 (1): 32-42.

Wiklund IK, Mattsson LA, Lindgran R, Limoni C (1999). Effects of a standardized ginseng extract on quality of life and physiological parameters in symptomatic postmenopausal women: A double-blind, placebo-controlled trial. *International Journal of Clinical Pharmacology Research* 19 (3): 89-99.

World Health Organization (WHO) (1999). *WHO Monographs on Selected Medicinal Plants.* Volume 1. Geneva: World Health Organization.

Yun TK, Choi SY (1990). A case-control study of ginseng intake and cancer. *International Journal of Epidemiology* 19 (4): 871-876.

Yun TK, Choi SY (1995). Preventive effect of ginseng intake against various human cancers: A case-control study on 1,987 pairs. *Cancer Epidemiology, Biomarkers, and Prevention* 4 (4): 401-408.

Yun TK, Choi SY (1998). Non-organ specific cancer prevention of ginseng: A prospective study in Korea. *International Journal of Epidemiology* 27 (3): 359-364.

Yun TK, Choi SY, Yun HY (2001). Epidemiological study on cancer prevention by ginseng: Are all kinds of cancers preventable by ginseng? *Journal Korean Medical Science* 16 (Suppl.): S19-S27.

DETAILS ON GINSENG PRODUCTS
AND CLINICAL STUDIES

Product and clinical study information is grouped in the same order as in the Summary Table. A profile on an individual product is followed by details of the clinical studies associated with that product. In some instances a clinical study, or studies, supports several products that contain the same principal ingredient(s). In these instances, those products are grouped together.

Clinical studies that follow each product, or group of products, are grouped by therapeutic indication in accordance with the order in the Summary Table.

Index to Ginseng Products

Product Profile: Ginsana®

Manufacturer	**Pharmaton S.A., Switzerland**
U.S. distributor	**Pharmaton Natural Health Products**
Botanical ingredient	**Ginseng root extract**
Extract name	**G115®**
Quantity	100 mg extract (equivalent to 500 mg root)
Processing	No information
Standardization	4% ginsenosides
Formulation	Capsule

Recommended dose: Two capsules with water in the morning, or one capsule in the morning and one in the afternoon. Optimal results have been shown with four weeks continuous use, when taken as directed.

DSHEA structure/function: Enhances physical endurance; improves oxygen utilization; helps maintain natural energy and an overall feeling of healthy well-being.

Cautions: Consult a health care professional if taking a prescription medicine, pregnant, or nursing a baby. There have been rare reports of mild allergic skin reactions with the use of the extract in this product. In case of accidental ingestion/overdose, seek the advice or a health care professional immediately.

Other ingredients: Sunflower oil, gelatin, glycerin, lecithin, beeswax, chlorophyll.

Source(s) of information: Product package (© Boehringer Ingelheim Pharmaceuticals, Inc. 2000); Engels, Said, and Wirth, 1996; Forgo, Kayasseh, and Staub, 1981.

Clinical Study: Ginsana®

Extract name	G115®
Manufacturer	GPL Ginsana Products Ltd., Switzerland (Pharmaton S.A., Switzerland)
Indication	**Physical performance** in healthy athletes
Level of evidence	**II**
Therapeutic benefit	**Yes**

Bibliographic reference
Forgo I, Schimert G (1985). The duration of effect of the standardized ginseng extract G115 in healthy competitive athletes. *Notabene Medici* 15 (9): 636-640.

Trial design
Parallel.

Study duration	9 weeks
Dose	2 (100 mg G115) capsules daily
Route of administration	Oral
Randomized	Yes
Randomization adequate	No
Blinding	Double-blind
Blinding adequate	Yes
Placebo	Yes
Drug comparison	No
Site description	Not described
No. of subjects enrolled	28

No. of subjects completed 28
Sex Male
Age Mean: 24.5 years

Inclusion criteria
Healthy male athletes whose training program consisted of at least ten hours per week with their trainer.

Exclusion criteria
None mentioned.

End points
Performance capacity was measured before treatment, at the end of 9 weeks, and 1, 3, 7, and 11 weeks following the treatment. Oxygen uptake was measured at rest and during exercise with a cyclic ergometer. Pulmonary functions and heart rate were monitored, as well as reaction times to visual signals.

Results
Following nine weeks, the Ginsana group had an increase in maximum oxygen uptake (VO2 max.) of 17 percent and a lowering of the maximum exercise heart rate by 10 percent. The oxygen pulse, oxygen uptake divided by heart rate, increased by 26 percent. Serum lactate levels decreased by 40 percent. There was an increase in parameters of pulmonary function, i.e., forced expiratory one-second volume (FEV1) and forced vital capacity (FVC), as well as a shortening of reaction time to visual stimuli. These changes persisted for three weeks following treatment.

Side effects
None mentioned.

Authors' comments
It is concluded that the increased performance is based on far-reaching metabolic effects that are of importance from the clinical point of view. Particularly significant is the approximately 26 percent increase in oxygen transport capacity of the heart, which has a positive influence on the coronary reserve.

Reviewer's comments
This is a well-conducted study. The results showed very large improvements in fitness plus faster reaction times. However, the trial lacked an adequate description of randomization, and no mention was made of withdrawals or dropouts (translation reviewed). (2, 6)

Clinical Study: Ginsana®

Extract name	G115®
Manufacturer	GPL Ginsana Products Ltd., Switzerland
	(Pharmaton S.A., Switzerland)

Indication	**Physical performance** in athletes
Level of evidence	**III**
Therapeutic benefit	**Undetermined**

Bibliographic reference

Forgo I, Kirchdorfer AM (1982). The effect of different ginsenoside concentrations on physical work capacity. *Notabene Medici* 12 (9): 721-727.

Trial design

Comparison of two standardized ginseng preparations: G115 containing 4 percent ginsenosides, and G115S containing 7 percent ginsenosides (200 mg daily). Subjects were instructed not to take any other pharmaceutical preparations during the trial period. Twenty subjects received G115 extract one summer, and ten received G115S the following summer.

Study duration	9 weeks
Dose	2 (100 mg) capsules daily
Route of administration	Oral
Randomized	No
Randomization adequate	No
Blinding	Double-blind
Blinding adequate	Yes
Placebo	No
Drug comparison	Yes
Drug name	G115S
Site description	Not described
No. of subjects enrolled	30
No. of subjects completed	30
Sex	Male
Age	18-31 years (mean: 23.5)

Inclusion criteria

Top-class male athletes engaged in karate, wrestling, or boxing.

Exclusion criteria

None mentioned.

End points
Criteria measured were the maximum oxygen absorption capacity, lactate concentration in blood, and the heart rate during effort in an ergometry test.

Results
After nine weeks of treatment, oxygen capacity (VO2) increased 17 percent in subjects treated with G115 and by 20 percent in subjects treated with G115S. No statistical difference was found between the two groups. Lactic acid levels after ergometer effort were significantly lower in both groups at the end of the nine-week period. The differences between the groups were not statistically significant. Heart rate during effort improved significantly in both groups after nine weeks of treatment with no discernible differences between the two groups.

Side effects
No discernible side effects or intolerance reactions.

Authors' comments
Our clinical experimental results validate the view that there is no advantage in using ginseng extracts with a concentration of total ginsenosides greater than 4 percent.

Reviewer's comments
There was no placebo control and no difference between two very similar treatments. The results are consistent with other work from same lab (Forgo, Kayasseh, and Staub, 1981; Forgo, 1983; Forgo and Schimert, 1985) that fitness increases in athletes with ginseng, but these results are not scientific evidence on their own. The study subjects were not randomized (translation reviewed). (2, 5)

Clinical Study: Ginsana®

Extract name	G115®
Manufacturer	GPL Ginseng Products Ltd., Switzerland (Pharmaton S.A., Switzerland)
Indication	**Physical performance** in athletes
Level of evidence	I
Therapeutic benefit	**Yes**

Bibliographic reference
Forgo I (1983). Effect of drugs on physical performance and hormone sys-

tem of sportsmen. *Münchener Medizinische Wochenschrift* 125 (38): 822-824.

Trial design

Parallel. Comparison of G115S (200 mg of 7 percent ginsenoside extract), Ginsana G115 plus vitamin E (200 mg 4 percent ginsenosides plus 400 mg vitamin E), and placebo in a three-arm study. Subjects were instructed to abstain from eating or drinking alcohol for two hours before tests and not to participate in heavy work/exercise for the preceding 24 hours.

Study duration	9 weeks
Dose	2 (100 mg G115 + 200 mg vitamin E) capsules daily
Route of administration	Oral
Randomized	Yes
Randomization adequate	Yes
Blinding	Double-blind
Blinding adequate	Yes
Placebo	Yes
Drug comparison	Yes
Drug name	G115S
Site description	Not described
No. of subjects enrolled	30
No. of subjects completed	30
Sex	Male
Age	18-31 years (mean: 24.2)

Inclusion criteria

Top-class male athletes engaged in karate, wrestling, or boxing.

Exclusion criteria

Subjects were not allowed to take other pharmaceutical preparations during the trial.

End points

Aerobic capacity was measured using a cyclic ergometer. Heart rates were monitored. Serum lactate levels and hormone levels (testosterone and luteinizing hormone in plasma and cortisol in urine) were determined.

Results

Following nine weeks of treatment, oxygen capacity (VO2) increased from 4.0 to 4.3 liters/minute to 5.2 and 4.9 for the G115S and G115 + vitamin E groups, respectively. There was no change for the placebo group, with a significant difference, $p < 0.01$. Lactate levels two minutes following exercise were significantly lower for both Ginsana groups. Heart rates were also lower for the Ginsana groups compared to placebo. There was no change in hormone levels.

Side effects
None mentioned.

Author's comments
The significantly increased oxygen absorption capacity and significantly reduced lactate levels in both Ginsana groups are indicative of greater fitness and a shorter recovery time. In addition, the decrease in heart rate attests to the improvement in physical work capacity.

Reviewer's comments
This is a well-reported study. The sample size is small (< 40) but adequate for this purpose (translation reviewed). (4, 6)

Clinical Study: G115®

Extract name	G115
Manufacturer	Pharmaton S.A., Switzerland
Indication	**Physical performance** in healthy volunteers
Level of evidence	**II**
Therapeutic benefit	**No**

Bibliographic reference
Engels HJ, Said JM, Wirth JC (1996). Failure of chronic ginseng supplementation to affect work performance and energy metabolism in healthy adult females. *Nutrition Research* 16 (8): 1295-1305.

Trial design
Parallel.

Study duration	2 months
Dose	2 (100 mg) capsules daily
Route of administration	Oral
Randomized	Yes
Randomization adequate	No
Blinding	Double-blind
Blinding adequate	Yes

Placebo	Yes
Drug comparison	No
Site description	Single center
No. of subjects enrolled	19
No. of subjects completed	19
Sex	Female
Age	21-35 years

Inclusion criteria
Healthy females maintaining normal diet and nonconsumption of other dietary supplements at least three to four weeks prior to initial pretest and throughout test period, maintaining regular physical activity habits throughout the study, and abstaining from food and caffeine products for at least three hours and from strenuous exertion for 24 hours prior to each laboratory testing session.

Exclusion criteria
Not mentioned.

End points
Test sessions were conducted before treatment and after eight weeks. Physical work capacity was measured while seated on a cycle ergometer. Volunteers cycled until voluntary exhaustion. Recovery oxygen uptake (VO2), respiratory exchange ratio (RER), minute ventilation (VE), heart rate, and blood lactic acid levels were measured at baseline rest, submaximal exercise, maximal exercise, and during postexercise recovery.

Results
Chronic ginseng supplementation had no effect on maximal work performance, resting, exercise, and recovery oxygen uptake, respiratory exchange ratio, minute ventilation, heart rate, and blood lactic acid levels. Habitual physical activity scores of study participants were found to be similar between the placebo and ginseng treatment groups at the beginning and end of the eight-week trial period.

Side effects
None reported.

Authors' comments
The present data in healthy adult females indicate that chronic dietary supplementation with a standardized extract of *Panax ginseng* C.A. Meyer does not result in an enhancement of work performance or a change in energy metabolism and improvement of the recovery response from maximal physical work.

Reviewer's comments
This well-conducted and well-reported study found no benefits in fitness of 19 normal, young, healthy females. The sample size may be inappropriate, but Forgo and Schimert (1985) found large effects among 28 athletes. In conclusion, either nonathletes will not benefit from ginseng, a larger sample is required, or there are problems with the following trials: Forgo, 1983; Forgo and Kirchdorfer, 1982; and Forgo and Schimert, 1985. (2, 5)

Clinical Study: G115®

Extract name	G115
Manufacturer	Pharmaton S.A., Switzerland
Indication	**Physical performance** in healthy volunteers
Level of evidence	**II**
Therapeutic benefit	**No**

Bibliographic reference
Engels HJ, Wirth JC (1997). No ergogenic effects of ginseng (*Panax ginseng* C.A. Meyer) during graded maximal aerobic exercise. *Journal of the American Dietetic Association* 97 (10): 1110-1115.

Trial design
Parallel.

Study duration	2 months
Dose	200 or 400 mg G115 daily
Route of administration	Oral
Randomized	Yes
Randomization adequate	No
Blinding	Double-blind
Blinding adequate	Yes
Placebo	Yes
Drug Comparison	No
Site description	Single center
No. of subjects enrolled	36
No. of subjects completed	31
Sex	Male
Age	Mean (range for 3 groups): 23-27 years

Inclusion criteria

Healthy males maintaining a normal diet and nonconsumption of other dietary supplements at least three to four weeks prior to initial pretest and throughout test period, maintaining regular physical activity habits throughout the study, and abstaining from food and caffeine products for at least three hours, and from strenuous exertion for 24 hours, prior to each laboratory testing session.

Exclusion criteria

None mentioned.

End points

Participants were evaluated before and after eight weeks of treatment. Assessment of submaximal and maximal exercise responses were performed using a standard, graded maximal exercise protocol on a mechanically-braked cycle ergometer. Recovery oxygen uptake (VO2), respiratory exchange ratio (RER), minute ventilation (VE), heart rate, and blood lactic acid levels were measured, and the subjects rated perceived exertion.

Results

Supplementation with ginseng had no effect on the following physiologic and psychological parameters: oxygen consumption, respiratory exchange ratio, minute ventilation, blood lactic acid concentration, heart rate, and perceived exertion ($p > 0.05$).

Side effects

None mentioned.

Authors' comments

Our data in healthy men do not offer support for claims that *Panax ginseng* C.A. Meyer is an ergogenic aid to improve submaximal and maximal aerobic exercise performance.

Reviewer's comments

This well-conducted and reported trial showed no effects of ginseng on fitness in normal males. The data were not inconsistent with Forgo, Kayasseh, and Staub (1981) in which males (30 to 39 years) showed no benefits on fitness from ginseng. The randomization was not adequately described. (3, 5)

Clinical Study: Ginsana®

Extract name	G115®
Manufacturer	GPL Ginseng Products Ltd., Switzerland (Pharmaton S.A., Switzerland)
Indication	**Physical performance**
Level of evidence	**II**
Therapeutic benefit	**Yes**

Bibliographic reference
Forgo I, Kayasseh L, Staub JJ (1981). Effects of a standardized ginseng extract on general health, reaction capacity, pulmonary function and hormones. *Medizinische Welt* 32 (19): 751-756.

Trial design
Parallel. Each test group was divided into two age groups: 30 to 39 and 40 to 60 years old.

Study duration	3 months
Dose	2 (100 mg extract) capsules daily
Route of administration	Oral
Randomized	No
Randomization adequate	No
Blinding	Double-blind
Blinding adequate	Yes
Placebo	Yes
Drug comparison	No
Site description	Single center
No. of subjects enrolled	120
No. of subjects completed	120
Sex	Male and female
Age	30-60 years

Inclusion criteria
Members of sports clubs.

Exclusion criteria
None mentioned.

End points
Visual and acoustic reactions were tested using the Vienna reaction unit. Subjects were tested before the study and after 3, 6, 9, and 12 weeks. Pul-

monary function was measured by a Sandoz analyzer before the trial and after 6 and 12 weeks. Luteinizing hormone, follicle stimulating hormone, estradiol (women), and testosterone (men) levels were determined before the study and after 12 weeks. Subjective variables were determined using a self-assessment questionnaire before the study as well as after 6 and 12 weeks.

Results

Reaction time and pulmonary function showed significant improvement in the Ginsana group, compared with the placebo group, in the 40- to 60-year-old men and women. Men and women ages 30 to 39 showed no significant change in reaction time, and men ages 30 to 39 showed no change in pulmonary function. In the self-evaluation (performance, mood, concentration) a clear improvement was evident in the subjects treated with Ginsana (men and women 40 to 60, $p = 0.001$, women 30 to 39, $p = 0.01$), with the exception of the men ages 30 to 39. No significant changes in hormone levels were observed.

Side effects

Not mentioned.

Authors' comments

The results obtained, particularly with regard to reaction, pulmonary function, self-assessment and compatibility have shown that Ginsana, a standardized ginseng extract, has a positive influence on the mental and physical functions investigated.

Reviewer's comments

Large well-conducted trial with clearly defined outcome measures and appropriately applied statistical methods. Older men and women showed improved reaction times with ginseng. All except males (30 to 39 years) showed enhanced pulmonary function. The study subjects were not randomized (translation reviewed). (2, 6)

Clinical Study: Ginsana®

Extract name	G115®
Manufacturer	GPL Ginseng Products Ltd., Switzerland (Pharmaton S.A., Switzerland)
Indication	**Physical performance**
Level of evidence	**III**
Therapeutic benefit	**Yes**

Bibliographic reference
Dörling E, Kirchdorfer AM, Ruckert KH (1980). Do ginsenosides influence the performance? Results of a double-blind study. *Notabene Medici* 10 (5): 241-246.

Trial design
Parallel.

Study duration	3 months
Dose	2 (100 mg extract) capsules daily
Route of administration	Oral
Randomized	No
Randomization adequate	No
Blinding	Double-blind
Blinding adequate	Yes
Placebo	Yes
Drug comparison	No
Site description	Not described
No. of subjects enrolled	60
No. of subjects completed	60
Sex	Male and female
Age	22-80 years

Inclusion criteria
None mentioned.

Exclusion criteria
None mentioned.

End points
Subjects' response time to light and sound, assessment of the critical flicker fusion threshold, two-hand coordination, and the recovery quotient were measured. Each subject was questioned before commencement of the trial and after 2, 4, 6, 8, 10, and 12 weeks concerning general subjective physical condition, physical fitness, mental alertness, attitude to life/mood, concentration/memory, and sleep behavior.

Results
Reaction times to light and auditory stimuli improved in 81.6 percent of subjects in the Ginsana group, compared to 33.3 percent of subjects in the placebo group—a statistically significant difference. Improvement in critical flicker fusion thresholds was seen in 59.4 percent of Ginsana patients and 29.7 percent of placebo patients. Hand coordination in the Ginsana group

improved steadily from weeks 4 to 12, reaching 74.4 percent improvement at week 12. This was significantly different from the placebo group, in which improvement of coordination measured 16.6 percent. Recovery quotient for climbing exercise improved in 29 patients in the Ginsana group, and in 9 patients in the placebo group. After three months, recovery periods after exercise decreased in 97 percent of Ginsana patients and 33.3 percent of placebo patients. Results of self-assessments indicated that many Ginsana patients felt more fit after the trial, compared to only a few placebo patients.

Side effects
None mentioned.

Authors' comments
The test results indicate beneficial effects of several weeks of Ginsana treatment, especially on reaction time, two-hand coordination, recovery period, and recovery quotient. Questioning showed the results in the Ginsana group to be markedly superior to those of the placebo group, especially in the parameters of subjective physical condition, physical fitness, and sleep behavior.

Reviewer's comments
The trial was not well-reported, but it was run on a good sized sample. It was also placebo-controlled and double-blind. The data were favorable for reaction time, critical flicker fusion frequency and exercise capacity (translation reviewed). (2, 3)

Clinical Study: Ginsana®

Extract name	G115®
Manufacturer	GPL Ginsana Products Ltd., Switzerland (Pharmaton S.A., Switzerland)
Indication	**Cognitive functioning** in healthy volunteers
Level of evidence	**II**
Therapeutic benefit	**Yes**

Bibliographic reference
D'Angelo L, Grimaldi R, Caravaggi M, Marcoli M, Perucca E, Lecchini S, Frigo GM, Crema A (1986). A double-blind, placebo-controlled clinical study on the effect of a standardized ginseng extract on psychomotor performance in healthy volunteers. *Journal of Ethnopharmacology* 16 (1): 15-22.

Trial design
Parallel.

Study duration	3 months
Dose	2 (100 mg G115) capsules daily
Route of administration	Oral
Randomized	Yes
Randomization adequate	No
Blinding	Double-blind
Blinding adequate	Yes
Placebo	Yes
Drug comparison	No
Site description	Single center
No. of subjects enrolled	32
No. of subjects completed	32
Sex	Male
Age	20-24 years

Inclusion criteria
Students in good physical condition.

Exclusion criteria
None mentioned.

End points
Patients were assessed before the trial and during the last week of treatment. Psychomotor assessments included a tapping test, simple and choice reaction time, cancellation test, digit symbol substitution test, mental arithmetic, and logical deduction. Blood tests were also preformed before the trial and in the last week. Subjects were asked to refrain from drinking caffeine or alcoholic beverages on assessment days.

Results
End performance of the G115 group was statistically superior to the placebo group only in mental arithmetic. Four other assessments showed an improvement over baseline for the G115 group compared to one assessment for the placebo group. However, no significant differences between G115 and placebo were found in other psychomotor tests.

Side effects
None reported.

Authors' comments
It is generally recognized in experimental and clinical studies that an improvement in psychomotor performance by pharmacological agents can be induced more easily when brain function is disturbed or impaired; therefore, the significant effect of G115 in these young, intellectually active volunteers appears remarkable.

Reviewer's comments
This study provides the first evidence of improved cognitive function in normal subjects with ginseng: one of eight tests showed significant improvement in the 12-week trial (mental arithmetic). However, no tests of memory were used. The randomization was inadequately described in this otherwise well-conducted trial. (3, 6)

Clinical Study: G115®

Extract name	G115
Manufacturer	Pharmaton S.A., Switzerland
Indication	**Cognitive functioning** in healthy volunteers
Level of evidence	I
Therapeutic benefit	**Yes**

Bibliographic reference
Kennedy DO, Scholey AB, Wesnes KA (2001). Dose dependent changes in cognitive performance and mood following acute administration of ginseng to healthy young volunteers. *Nutritional Neuroscience* 4: 295-310.

Trial design
Crossover. Subjects received 200, 400, and 600 mg of G115, as well as a matching placebo, in counterbalanced order, with a seven-day washout period between treatments.

Study duration	1 day
Dose	2, 4, or 6 (100 mg extract) capsules per day
Route of administration	Oral
Randomized	Yes
Randomization adequate	Yes
Blinding	Double-blind
Blinding adequate	Yes

| Placebo | Yes |
| Drug comparison | No |

| Site description | Single center |

No. of subjects enrolled	20
No. of subjects completed	Not given
Sex	Male and female
Age	20-27 years (mean: 21.3)

Inclusion criteria
Healthy young volunteers taking no medication with the exception of oral contraception for female volunteers. Participants abstained from caffeine-containing products and alcohol on each study day.

Exclusion criteria
Heavy smokers (more than ten cigarettes per day).

End points
Cognitive performance was assessed using a computerized test battery immediately prior to dosing, and at 1, 2.5, 4, and 6 hours after. Primary outcome measures were quality of memory, speed of memory, speed of attention, and accuracy of attention. Secondary outcome measures of working memory (subfactor) and secondary memory (subfactor) were derived from quality of memory. Patients also completed the Bond-Lader Visual Analogue Scales (VAS) to analyze three mood factors: alertness, calmness and contentedness.

Results
For the "quality-of-memory" factor, 400 mg of ginseng saw improvements in the accuracy-of-memory task at 1, 2.5, 4, and 6 hours after dose ($p = 0.0043$, $p = 0.026$, $p = 0.035$, $p = 0.002$, respectively) in comparison with placebo. The 600 mg dose saw improvement at 2.5 hours after dosing ($p = 0.02$), but 200 mg saw no improvement. Only the 200 mg saw any difference in "speed of memory," which decreased four hours after dosing ($p = 0.0045$). Speed of performance on the attention tasks was reduced at four hours post dose for both 200 mg and 600 mg ($p = 0.0001$, $p = 0.0019$, respectively), as well as six hours post dose ($p = 0.0006$, $p = 0.0003$, respectively); 400 mg was not affected. For the secondary outcome measures, only the "secondary memory" subfactor reflected any differences from placebo: the 600 mg dose enhanced performance at 1, 2.5, and 4 hours after dosing ($p = 0.046$, $p = 0.0034$, $p = 0.034$, respectively); the 400 mg dose produced improvements at all time points (1, 2.5, 4, and 6 hours after dosing; $p = 0.0022$, $p = 0.0027$, $p = 0.013$, $p = 0.0036$, respectively); and the 200 mg dose caused a difference at four hours after dosing ($p = 0.039$). The 200 and 400 mg groups

also saw reductions on the "alert" factor of the Bond-Lader VAS six hours after dosing ($p = 0.001$, $p = 0.01$, respectively).

Side effects
None mentioned.

Authors' comments
The results of the current study show that ingestion of ginseng can affect cognitive performance in a time and dose-dependent manner. Moreover, these modulatory effects were caused by single doses of ginseng. Although this modulation was overwhelmingly beneficial for the middle dose (400 mg), there was evidence of cognitive and subjective mood costs associated with the other doses.

Reviewer's comments
This is a clear demonstration of acute cognitive effects of ginseng on young volunteers. Quality of memory is enhanced, but attention is disrupted. (4, 6)

Clinical Study: Ginsana®

Extract name	G115®
Manufacturer	Pharmaton S.A., Switzerland
Indication	**Vaccination potentiation**
Level of evidence	**II**
Therapeutic benefit	**Yes**

Bibliographic reference
Scaglione F, Cattaneo G, Alessandria M, Cogo R (1996). Efficacy and safety of the standardized ginseng extract G115 for potentiating vaccination against common cold and/or influenza syndrome. *Drugs Under Experimental and Clinical Research* 22 (2): 65-72.

Trial design
Parallel. Vaccination with Agrippal® influenza polyvalent vaccine (0.5 ml) took place four weeks after the start of administration of G115 or placebo.

Study duration	3 months
Dose	2 (100 mg G115) capsules daily
Route of administration	Oral
Randomized	Yes
Randomization adequate	No
Blinding	Double-blind

Blinding adequate	Yes
Placebo	Yes
Drug comparison	No
Site description	3 private practices
No. of subjects enrolled	227
No. of subjects completed	219
Sex	Male and female
Age	31-65 years (mean: 48)

Inclusion criteria
Over 18 years of age, recommended for influenza vaccination.

Exclusion criteria
Already vaccinated for influenza; already taking ginseng; with granulocytes <1,000 mm; hypersensitivity to ginseng; receiving any investigational agent or antineoplastic chemotherapy; with underlying terminal diseases (e.g., AIDS) or liver disease; pregnant or nursing women; and subjects with severe gastritis.

End points
Incidences of influenza/common cold were recorded at 2, 4, 8, 10, and 12 weeks. Natural killer activity (peripheral blood mononuclear cells) and antibody titers were measured before the trial and after 4, 8, and 12 weeks. Laboratory safety parameters were measured before the trial and after 12 weeks. Adverse events were recorded every two weeks after the trial.

Results
The frequency of influenza or common cold between weeks 4 and 12 was 42 cases in the placebo group and 15 cases in the G115 group, the difference being statistically highly significant ($p < 0.001$). Whereas antibody titers by week 8 rose to an average of 171 units in the placebo group, they rose to an average of 272 units in the G115 group ($p < 0.0001$). Natural killer activity levels at weeks 8 and 12 were nearly twice as high in the G115 group as compared to the placebo group ($p < 0.0001$).

Side effects
Of the eight adverse events reported for G115, four were insomnia, three were gastrointestinal, and one was anxiety.

Authors' comments
The results obtained from this study show that the standardized ginseng extract G115 Ginsana is able to improve the immune response in vivo in humans and can protect against influenza and the common cold.

Reviewer's comments
Well-conducted study showing that ginseng protects against influenza and improves immune response. The randomization was inadequately described. (3, 6)

Clinical Study: G115®

Extract name	G115
Manufacturer	Pharmaton S.A., Switzerland
Indication	**Bronchitis**
Level of evidence	**III**
Therapeutic benefit	**Yes**

Bibliographic reference
Scaglione F, Cogo R, Cocuzza C, Arcidiancono M, Beretta A (1994). Immunomodulatory effect of *Panax ginseng* C.A. Meyer (G115) on alveolar macrophages from patients suffering with chronic bronchitis. *International Journal of Immunotherapy* 10 (1): 21-24.

Trial design
Parallel.

Study duration	2 months
Dose	1 (100 mg G115) capsule every 12 hours
Route of administration	Oral
Randomized	Yes
Randomization adequate	No
Blinding	Single-blind
Blinding adequate	No
Placebo	Yes
Drug comparison	No
Site description	Single center
No. of subjects enrolled	40
No. of subjects completed	Not given
Sex	Male and female
Age	Not given

Inclusion criteria
Smokers (less than 20 cigarettes per day) who suffered from chronic bronchitis.

Exclusion criteria
Subjects who underwent vaccination within 20 days prior to the study, and those with suspected or known hypersensitivity toward the tested drug and/or its excipients. No treatment with corticosteroids or immunomodulatory agents was allowed during the study.

End points
Alveolar macrophages were collected by bronchoalveolar lavage before and after four and eight weeks of treatment. Macrophages were immediately assayed for phagocytic activity and killing power toward *Candida albicans.*

Results
The phagocytosis index and the phagocytosis fraction show an increase in the G115 group that was statistically significant at the end of the eighth week. Intracellular killing also showed a significant increase in the G115 group detectable at the end of the eighth week. No modification of these parameters was seen in the placebo group.

Side effects
The treatment was well-tolerated in all patients enrolled in the study.

Authors' comments
These results show that G115 extract is able to improve the immune response of alveolar macrophages in chronically compromised subjects. These findings suggest that substances such as G115 may play an important role in the prevention and therapy of respiratory disorders.

Reviewer's comments
This is an important pilot study showing that ginseng may protect by increasing immune response in smokers with chronic bronchitis. The study showed improvements under placebo that were not statistically evaluated, but may have been significant. Such findings stress the need for placebo-controlled trials in this field. However, the placebo effects do not affect the outcome of this study since the effect of G115 was far greater. This study needs replication: the randomization process was not described and blinding was only single. (0, 5)

Clinical Study: G115®

Extract name	G115
Manufacturer	Pharmaton S.A., Switzerland
Indication	**Bronchitis**
Level of evidence	**II**
Therapeutic benefit	**Yes**

Bibliographic reference

Scaglione F, Weiser K, Alessandria M (2001). Effects of the standardized ginseng extract G115 in patients with chronic bronchitis: A non-blinded, randomized, comparative pilot study. *Clinical Drug Investigation* 21 (1): 41-45.

Trial design

Parallel. Patients received 875 mg amoxicillin and 125 mg clavulanic acid twice daily for nine days. They were then divided into two groups. Both groups continued with the antibacterial treatment, and one group also received G115, for an additional nine days.

Study duration	9 days
Dose	2 (100 mg G115) capsules daily
Route of administration	Oral
Randomized	Yes
Randomization adequate	Yes
Blinding	Open
Blinding adequate	No
Placebo	No
Drug comparison	No
Site description	Single center
No. of subjects enrolled	75
No. of subjects completed	44
Sex	Male and female
Age	Not given

Inclusion criteria

More than 18 years old with symptoms of acute bacterial attack of chronic bronchitis (ACB). Chronic bronchitis was defined as a productive cough present on most days of a minimum of three consecutive months over two or more successive years. ACB was defined as a rapid onset of cough with production of purulent sputum. In addition, the patients had to have one or more of the following: dyspnea, tachypnea, wheezing, fever (> 38°C), and be suitable for therapeutic treatment with amoxicillin and clavulanic acid.

Exclusion criteria

Concurrent pneumonia, systemic use of an anti-infective drug seven days prior to enrollment, systemic corticosteroid therapy (excluding inhaled or intranasal aerosolized corticosteroids), hypersensitivity to penicillins, a history of significant renal or hepatic impairment, or treatment with a drug within the last 30 days that had not received regulatory approval at the time of study entry. Immediate family of investigators and site personnel were also excluded.

End points
Each morning of the trial period, a sample of bronchial secretion was taken by protected expectoration. The sample was plated out and the bacterial count (colony forming units) was determined. Patients were considered cured and antibacterial therapy was stopped upon elimination of symptoms of infection.

Results
In the group receiving G115, bacterial clearance was significantly faster than those receiving antibacterials alone. Significant improvement in the G115 group was observed on days 4, 5, 6, and 7 ($p < 0.01$), whereas a borderline trend was observed on day 8 ($p = 0.055$). A significant decrease in time for clearance of infection was also observed.

Side effects
None mentioned.

Authors' comments
These results indicate a beneficial effect of G115 ginseng extract on the reduction of bacterial counts in the bronchial systems of patients with acute attacks of chronic bronchitis. Patients in whom the elimination of bacteria from the bronchial system is particularly difficult may benefit from the use of ginseng.

Reviewer's comments
An interesting, nonblinded pilot study showing ability of ginseng to speed recovery of patients treated with antibacterials. Lack of placebo control may present a problem, however, as an improvement in the placebo group was seen in a similar study (Scaglione et al., 1994). (3, 6)

Clinical Study: Ginsana®

Extract name	G115®
Manufacturer	Pharmaton S.A., Switzerland
Indication	**Menopausal symptoms**
Level of evidence	**II**
Therapeutic benefit	**Trend**

Bibliographic reference
Wiklund IK, Mattsson LA, Lindgran R, Limoni C (1999). Effects of a standardized ginseng extract on quality of life and physiological parameters in symptomatic postmenopausal women: A double-blind, placebo-controlled trial. *International Journal of Clinical Pharmacology Research* 19 (3): 89-99.

Trial design
Parallel. Two-week run-in period before allocation to treatment groups.

Study duration	4 months
Dose	2 (100 mg G115) capsules daily
Route of administration	Oral
Randomized	Yes
Randomization adequate	No
Blinding	Double-blind
Blinding adequate	Yes
Placebo	Yes
Drug comparison	No
Site description	Multicenter
No. of subjects enrolled	384
No. of subjects completed	379
Sex	Female
Age	45-65 years (mean: 53)

Inclusion criteria
Healthy postmenopausal women, ages 45 to 65 years, without hormone replacement therapy for the previous two months and with no bleeding during the previous six months, reporting at least six episodes of hot flashes during at least three days over the past seven days.

Exclusion criteria
Previous or concomitant serious or chronic medical conditions, uncontrolled hypertension (>160/95), psychiatric illness, taking concomitant medication such as tranquilizers, and those who were unable to understand and complete the questionnaires.

End points
Patients completed the following validated questionnaires at baseline and after 16 weeks of treatment to assess the effects of the extract on quality of life: Psychological General Well-Being (PGWB) index, Women's Health Questionnaire (WHQ), and Visual Analogue Scales (VAS).

Results
Ginseng treatment when compared with placebo showed only a tendency for a slightly better overall symptomatic relief according to the total score of the PGWB ($p < 0.1$). Analysis of PGWB subsets reported p values <0.05 for depression, well-being, and health subscales. No statistically significant effects were seen for the WHQ and the VAS of the physiological parameters, including vasomotor symptoms (hot flashes).

Side effects
Tolerability was rated as good or very good by more than 90 percent of subjects. Similar numbers of adverse events were seen in both the active and placebo groups. One patient on ginseng withdrew from the study due to a treatment-related adverse event (nausea).

Authors' comments
The data of the present study suggest that ginseng extract may offer effective relief in quality-of-life-related aspects in healthy postmenopausal women. The positive effects of ginseng on depression, well-being, and health deserve further attention.

Reviewer's comments
Well-conducted and well-presented study. The large sample validated instruments, yet results, while consistent and close to significant, were not robust. The effect on depression is interesting. The randomization was not adequately described. (3, 6)

Clinical Study: G115®

Extract name	G115
Manufacturer	Pharmaton, S.A., Switzerland
Indication	**Psychological well-being** in healthy volunteers
Level of evidence	**II**
Therapeutic benefit	**Undetermined**

Bibliographic reference
Cardinal BJ, Engels H-J (2001). Ginseng does not enhance psychological well-being in healthy young adults: Results of a double-blind, placebo-controlled, randomized clinical trial. *Journal of the American Dietetic Association* 101 (6): 655-660.

Trial design
Parallel. Patients received either 200 or 400 mg G115 per day, or placebo.

Study duration	2 months
Dose	200 or 400 mg daily
Route of administration	Oral
Randomized	Yes
Randomization adequate	Yes
Blinding	Double-blind

Blinding adequate	Yes
Placebo	Yes
Drug comparison	No
Site description	Lab
No. of subjects enrolled	96
No. of subjects completed	83
Sex	Male and female
Age	21-31 (mean: 25.7)

Inclusion criteria
Healthy volunteers (determined by a medical history/health status question-naire) who agreed to not change their physical activity level substantially, to maintain their usual diets, and to not take other dietary supplements during the study period.

Exclusion criteria
None mentioned.

End points
Subjects were assessed before the trial start (baseline) and at the end of the trial (between 56 to 60 days after starting supplementation). Three psycho-logical variables were assessed: positive affect, negative aspect (both deter-mined by the Positive Affect-Negative Affect Scale [PANAS]), and total mood disturbance (determined by the Profile of Mood States inventory [POMS]).

Results
No changes were observed in the assessed psychological variables for any of the treatments. Compared with published norms, subjects had normal psychological profiles both pre- and postintervention for positive affect, neg-ative affect, and total mood disturbance.

Side effects
None mentioned.

Authors' comments
The present study offers no support for commercial manufacturers', distribu-tors', and suppliers' claims that *Panax ginseng* C.A. Meyer enhances healthy, young adults' psychological well-being beyond "normal" levels. In our experiment, chronic ginseng supplementation—at both its clinically rec-ommended level and twice that level—was no more effective in enhancing healthy, young adults' mental health than was a sugar pill.

Reviewer's comments
Although well conducted, this study is severely compromised by relying on

end points for which no previous history of sensitivity is presented. Further, having established that the study had adequate statistical power for one outcome, they raised the required significance level, but did not report final *p* values. Good trial methodology, but poor science. (5, 5)

Clinical Study: Ginsana®

Extract name	G115®
Manufacturer	Pharmaton S.A., Switzerland
Indication	**General well-being; quality of life**
Level of evidence	I
Therapeutic benefit	**Yes**

Bibliographic reference
Ellis JM, Reddy P (2002). Effects of *Panax ginseng* on quality of life. *The Annals of Pharmacotherapy* 36 (3): 375-379.

Trial design
Parallel. Subjects consumed no ginseng-containing products one week prior to the study. Treatment (ginseng or placebo) was taken with a full glass of water before 10 a.m.

Study duration	2 months
Dose	200 mg daily
Route of administration	Oral
Randomized	Yes
Randomization adequate	Yes
Blinding	Double-blind
Blinding adequate	Yes
Placebo	Yes
Drug comparison	No
Site description	Not described
No. of subjects enrolled	30
No. of subjects completed	23
Sex	Male and female
Age	18-25 years (mean: 21.6)

Inclusion criteria
Volunteers at least 18 years old.

Exclusion criteria

Subjects taking anticoagulants; with previous adverse reaction to any ginseng extract (*Panax,* American, or Siberian) or lactose; with history of alcohol abuse; who were pregnant or planning on becoming pregnant; with a history of auto-immune, hepatic, or renal dysfunction; with a history of supraventricular or ventricular arrhythmias; or who did not provide informed consent.

End points

In order to assess health-related quality of life (HRQOL), subjects were given the Short Form-36 Health Survey version 2 (SF-36v2) at baseline and at weeks 4 and 8. This questionnaire assesses eight domains: mental health, physical functioning, social functioning, role limitation due to physical health, role limitations due to emotional problems, vitality, and general health perceptions.

Results

After four weeks of treatment, the ginseng group had significantly higher scores than the placebo group in social functioning ($p = 0.014$) and the mental component summary ($p = 0.019$). A trend toward a higher score in mental health ($p = 0.075$) was observed. These differences did not persist through the end of the eight-week trial. No significant differences in the other scored domains were found between groups at either 4 or 8 weeks after beginning treatment. Compared to the placebo group, the ginseng group was more likely to state that they thought they received ginseng and that they felt differently during the study ($p < 0.05$, $p = 0.03$, respectively).

Side effects

The incidence of side effects for ginkgo and placebo were similar (33 percent and 17 percent, respectively, $p < 0.40$). One report of each of the following adverse effects occurred in the ginseng group: nausea/vomiting, rebound irritability, insomnia, and headache.

Authors' comments

We found that *P. ginseng* 200 mg/day improved social functioning and mental component summary scores after four weeks of therapy, but these differences did not persist with continued use. Caution should be taken in interpretation because of the small sample size and the young population studied. Future studies should examine the effect of *P. ginseng* on HRQOL using a larger sample size, measure the effects at earlier time points, and investigate the effects of ginseng withdrawal.

Reviewer's comments

Sound study, even though the statistical power was marginal. The major flaw of the analysis was the substitution of data for dropouts. (5, 5)

Product Profile: Ginsana® Gold Blend

Manufacturer	**Pharmaton S.A., Switzerland**
U.S. distributor	**Pharmaton Natural Health Products**
Botanical ingredient	**Ginseng root extract**
Extract name	**G115®**
Quantity	40 mg
Processing	No information
Standardization	4% ginsenosides
Formulation	Gelcap

Recommended dose: Take two gelcaps with water in the morning or one gelcap in the morning and one in the afternoon. Effectiveness as early as four weeks of continuous uninterrupted use.

DSHEA structure/function: Clinically proven to increase vitality and reduce fatigue. Nourishes, fortifies, and revitalizes.

Cautions: Accidental overdose of iron-containing products is a leading cause of fatal poisoning in children under 6. Keep this product out of reach of children. In case of accidental overdose, call a doctor or poison control center immediately.

Other ingredients: Vitamin A (beta carotene) 2,000 IU, vitamin C (ascorbic acid) 60 mg, vitamin D (cholecalciferol) 200 IU, vitamin E (dl-alpha tocopherol) 15 IU, thiamine (Vitamin B1) 1.2 mg, riboflavin (vitamin B2) 1.7 mg, niacin (vitamin B3) 15 mg, vitamin B6 (pyridoxine HCl) 2 mg, folic acid 200 mcg, vitamin B12 (cobalamin conc.) 1 mcg, calcium (calcium phosphate) 100 mg, iron (ferus sulfate) 9 mg, phosphorus 80 mg, magnesium 10 mg, zinc (zinc sulfate) 1 mg, copper (copper sulfate) 1 mg, manganese (manganese sulfate) 1 mg; microcrystalline cellulose, gelatin, hydrogenated corn syrup, providone, glycerin, croscarmellose sodium, magnesium stearate, colloidal silica, hydroxypropyl methylcellulose, ethylcellulose, titanium dioxide, dibutyl sebecate, stearic acid powder, polysorbate 80, FD&C yellow lake #6, FD&C red lake #40, vanillin powder, polyethylene glycol 8000, caramel color, FD&C blue lake #1.

Comments: Previously sold as Vitasana™. Sold as Gericomplex® and Pharmaton® Capsules in Europe.

Source(s) of information: Product package (© Boehringer Ingelheim Pharmaceuticals, Inc. 2001); Vitasana™ Supplement Facts (© Boehringer Ingelheim Pharmaceuticals, Inc. 1998); Engels, Said, and Wirth, 1996.

Clinical Study: Pharmaton® Capsules

Extract name	G115®
Manufacturer	Pharmaton S.A., Switzerland
Indication	**General well-being; physical or mental stress**
Level of evidence	I
Therapeutic benefit	**Yes**

Bibliographic reference

Marasco CA, Vargas RR, Villagomez SA, Infante BC (1996). Double-blind study of a multivitamin complex supplemented with ginseng extract. *Drugs Under Experimental and Clinical Research* 22 (6): 323-329.

Trial design

Parallel. Comparison of ginseng combined with multivitamins to multivitamins alone.

Study duration	3 months
Dose	One capsule (G115 + vitamins, minerals, trace elements, and lipotropic substances: inositol, choline, linoleic, and linolenic acid) daily
Route of administration	Oral
Randomized	Yes
Randomization adequate	Yes
Blinding	Double-blind
Blinding adequate	Yes
Placebo	No
Drug comparison	Yes
Drug name	Multivitamin capsules
Site description	Single center
No. of subjects enrolled	625
No. of subjects completed	501
Sex	Male and female
Age	18-65 years (mean: 37-39)

Inclusion criteria

Adults known to be subject to increased physical and mental stress and/or to present fatigue symptoms not related to any of the exclusion criteria.

Exclusion criteria
Pregnancy, interaction with other medication not normally allowed, or protocol violation.

End points
At each of the four monthly visits, quality of life (physical and sexual activity,
well-being) was assessed by a standardized 11-item questionnaire validated by the Medical School of the National Autonomous University of Mexico. Pulse rate, arterial pressure and general clinical history were also assessed.

Results
Administration of either the Pharmaton complex or the multivitamins alone
induced a significant increase in the quality-of-life index. However, improvement of 11.9 points for the Pharmaton Capsules was significantly superior to
the 6.4 average increase with the multivitamin capsules. When indices at
visit 4 were compared with visit 1, the Pharmaton group showed significant
improvement in every one of the 11 questionnaire items ($p < 0.0001$),
whereas the multivitamin group did not show significant improvement in any
of these items. No differences were observed between the two groups' systolic blood pressure and heart rate, but the diastolic pressure at visit 4 was
significantly lower for the Pharmaton group ($p < 0.01$). Significant increases
in body weight were recorded in the multivitamin group.

Side effects
Adverse effects were minimal in both groups.

Authors' comments
This study demonstrated that Pharmaton Capsules were more effective
than multivitamins alone in improving the quality of life in a population subjected to high levels of physical and mental stress.

Reviewer's comments
This is a well-conducted and well-designed large trial showing ginseng plus
vitamins is better than vitamins alone in quality-of-life index. (4, 6)

Clinical Study: Gericomplex®

Extract name	G115®
Manufacturer	Pharmaton SA, Switzerland
Indication	**General well-being; quality of life** in healthy volunteers

Level of evidence   I
Therapeutic benefit   **Yes**

Bibliographic reference

Wiklund I, Karlberg J, Lund B (1994). A double-blind comparison of the effect on quality of life of a combination of vital substances including standardized ginseng G115 and placebo. *Current Therapeutic Research* 55 (1): 32-42.

Trial design

Parallel.

Study duration	3 months
Dose	2 (40 mg G115 + vitamins, minerals, and trace elements) capsules daily
Route of administration	Oral
Randomized	Yes
Randomization adequate	Yes
Blinding	Double-blind
Blinding adequate	Yes
Placebo	Yes
Drug comparison	No
Site description	Single center
No. of subjects enrolled	417
No. of subjects completed	390
Sex	Male and female
Age	33-51 years (mean: 42.7)

Inclusion criteria

Healthy volunteers older than 25 years.

Exclusion criteria

Subjects with a systolic blood pressure greater than or equal to 200 mmHg or diastolic blood pressure greater than or equal to 100 mmHg were excluded. Other exclusion criteria were sensitivity to ginseng extracts, a history of alcohol or drug abuse, pregnancy or breastfeeding, inability or unwillingness to cooperate, and the use of concomitant medication (except short-term medication, for example, for headache or gastrointestinal discomfort).

End points

Quality of life was evaluated in two standard, self-administered questionnaires, the Psychological General Well-Being (PGWB) index and the Sleep Dysfunction scale. In addition, bipolar adjectives in Visual Analogue Scales

(VAS) were used to quantify changes in other behavioral aspects. Assessment was carried out at baseline and after 12 weeks of treatment.

Results
General well-being (PGWB index) improved significantly in both groups during the 12-week trial. No significant difference was observed between the two groups, either in the total score or in the dimensions. In terms of sleep, there was a similar slight improvement during the course of active treatment, but no statistical difference between the groups. On the VAS, subjects receiving ginseng showed significant improvement in alertness ($p = 0.05$), appetite ($p = 0.04$), relaxation ($p = 0.02$), and the overall score ($p = 0.03$). Among a subgroup of subjects with the 20 percent lowest scores at baseline, ginseng improved both vitality ($p = 0.03$) and depressed mood ($p = 0.05$). Benefits of ginseng therapy were more pronounced for the 20 percent of subjects who had the lowest quality-of-life rating for each measure.

Side effects
Nine subjects in the ginseng group and six subjects in the placebo group withdrew prematurely because of adverse effects that could be related to the medication.

Authors' comments
It was concluded that in healthy subjects the combination of vital substances including G115 offers significant advantages over placebo treatment in terms of improvement in self-assessed feelings of vitality, alertness, less time urgency (feeling more relaxed), and appetite. The beneficial effects appear to be more pronounced in those subjects who were at a disadvantage and worse off before the study started.

Reviewer's comments
Well-conducted, large, and well-reported study. (5, 6)

Clinical Study: Pharmaton® Capsules

Extract name	G115®
Manufacturer	Pharmaton S.A., Switzerland
Indication	**General well-being; functional fatigue**
Level of evidence	**II**
Therapeutic benefit	**Yes**

Bibliographic reference
Le Gal M, Cathebras P, Struby K (1996). Pharmaton Capsules in the treat-

ment of functional fatigue: A double-blind study versus placebo evaluated by a new methodology. *Phytotherapy Research* 10 (1): 49-53.

Trial design
Parallel.

Study duration	6 weeks
Dose	2 (40 mg G115 + vitamins, minerals, and deanol [dimethylaminoethanol bitartrate, 26 mg])
Route of administration	Oral
Randomized	Yes
Randomization adequate	Yes
Blinding	Double-blind
Blinding adequate	No
Placebo	Yes
Drug comparison	No
Site description	Multicenter
No. of subjects enrolled	232
No. of subjects completed	219
Sex	Male and female
Age	25-60 years

Inclusion criteria
Patients included in the study were suffering from functional fatigue for at least 15 years.

Exclusion criteria
Excluded from the study were patients suffering from an acute or chronic disease (endocrine, neurological, infectious, malignant) that could have been responsible for the fatigue, liver disease, calcium lithiasis, or psychiatric illness, especially depression. Also excluded from the study were alcoholic patients and alcoholics undergoing detoxification therapy, patients being treated with psychotropic drugs, antibiotics, or antiasthenic preparations, including vitamins, trace elements and homeopathy, pregnant women or those likely to become pregnant, and women who had given birth less than three months before or who were still breast-feeding.

End points
Each patient was allowed to choose, from a preestablished list of 20 suggestions, the five items that best described his or her complaints. An individual fatigue score was calculated for each patient on the basis of the sum of the scores given by the patient for each of the five items selected (each item was

evaluated on a four-point scale). Assessment was carried out at baseline and on days 21 and 42.

Results

At the beginning of the study, 28 patients in the Pharmaton group and 29 patients taking placebo had signs or symptoms related to fatigue (the numbers of related signs/symptoms in each group were 46 and 52, respectively). Both groups had improved after 21 days, with 16 patients taking the active substance and 22 taking placebo having signs or symptoms associated with fatigue (number of associated symptoms in each group: 10 and 20, respectively). At the end of the study, both groups had improved even more. Only six patients in the Pharmaton group and 16 in the placebo group reported signs or symptoms associated with fatigue (the number of associated signs/symptoms in each group were 4 and 14, respectively). The difference between the groups was statistically significant ($p = 0.023$). The efficacy of Pharmaton Capsules was assessed as better than placebo by both the patients and the doctors.

Side effects

The most common unwanted effects were nausea and/or vomiting in six patients of the Pharmaton group and in one patient of the placebo group; sleep disorders in three patients of each group; abdominal pain in three patients of each group; bowel disorder in two Pharmaton patients; and headache in two placebo patients.

Authors' comments

The efficacy of Pharmaton Capsules on the complaints caused by a state of functional fatigue, after six weeks of treatment, has been proven by the results of this study.

Reviewer's comments

It is hard to judge the importance of active versus placebo after 42 days due to the large placebo effect. However, the final difference between groups was statistically significant. The blinding was not adequately described. (3, 5)

Clinical Study: Geriatric Pharmaton®

Extract name	G115®
Manufacturer	Pharmaton S.A., Switzerland
Indication	**Physical performance** in healthy volunteers
Level of evidence	**III**
Therapeutic benefit	**Yes**

Bibliographic reference

Pieralisi G, Ripari P, Vecchiet L (1991). Effect of a standardized ginseng extract combined with dimethylaminoethanol bitartrate, vitamins, minerals, and trace elements on physical performance during exercise. *Clinical Therapeutics* 13 (3): 373-382.

Trial design

Three phase trial. First two phases were crossover trials of six weeks each. Third phase was a single-blind placebo washout period of one week.

Study duration	6 weeks
Dose	2 (G115 + dimethylaminoethanol bitartrate, vitamins, minerals, and trace elements)
Route of administration	Oral
Randomized	Yes
Randomization adequate	No
Blinding	Double-blind
Blinding adequate	No
Placebo	Yes
Drug comparison	No
Site description	Single center
No. of subjects enrolled	50
No. of subjects completed	47
Sex	Male
Age	21-47 years (mean: 33)

Inclusion criteria

Healthy male sports teachers.

Exclusion criteria

None mentioned.

End points

Blood samples were taken for lab tests at the beginning of the study and at the end of each phase. An exercise test up to maximal load was performed on a treadmill with a seven-step protocol. Before and after each step, and three, six, and nine minutes after exercise, heart rate, oxygen consumption, ventilation, carbon dioxide production, the respiratory quotient, systolic and diastolic blood pressure, and plasma lactic acid levels were measured. At the end of each exercise test the total maximal work load and the maximal oxygen consumption were determined.

Results

The total work load and maximal exercise were significantly greater after ginseng consumption than after placebo. At the same work load, oxygen consumption, plasma lactate levels, ventilation, carbon dioxide production, and heart rate during exercise were significantly lower after the ginseng preparation than after placebo. The effects of ginseng were more pronounced in the subjects with maximal oxygen consumption less than 60 ml/kg per minute during exercise than in the subjects with levels of 60 ml/kg per minute or greater. The results indicate that the ginseng preparation increased the subjects' work capacity by improving muscular oxygenation.

Side effects

None reported.

Authors' comments

The results of this study showed that the administration of two capsules of a ginseng preparation per day for six weeks increased the subjects' work capacity, probably by improving muscular oxygen utilization.

Reviewer's comments

This is a good trial with interesting results. However, it did not adequately describe randomization and blinding, nor important aspects of the analysis of study results. (1, 5)

Clinical Study: Gegorvit® Pharmaton

Extract name	G115®
Manufacturer	Pharmaton S.A., Switzerland
Indication	**Age-related memory impairment**
Level of evidence	**II**
Therapeutic benefit	**Yes**

Bibliographic reference

Neri M, Andermarcher E, Pradelli JM, Salvioli G (1995). Influence of a double blind pharmacological trial on two domains of well-being in subjects with age associated memory impairment. *Archives of Gerontology and Geriatrics* 21 (3): 241-252.

Trial design

Parallel. Fifteen-day run-in period before baseline evaluation and treatment phase.

Study duration	9 months
Dose	2 (G115 + dimethylaminoethanol bitartrate [deanol], minerals and vitamins) capsules daily
Route of administration	Oral
Randomized	Yes
Randomization adequate	No
Blinding	Double-blind
Blinding adequate	Yes
Placebo	Yes
Drug comparison	No
Site description	Single center
No. of subjects enrolled	60
No. of subjects completed	Not given
Sex	Male and female
Age	51-65 years (mean: 60.7)

Inclusion criteria

Subjects with age-associated memory impairment (AAMI). Specifically, subjects older than 50 years with subjective memory disturbances exceeding the threshold value of a metamemory scale (De Vreese, forgetfulness scale threshold: 20) and memory deficit revealed by a paragraph recall test adjusted for age and education level (Babcock tale). Global cognitive deficit was ruled out by a score of at least 24 on the Mini Mental State Examination. A monotonic psychopathology rating scale (Scala di Valutazione del Benessere Affettiro [SVEBA]) graded and validated for the Italian population was applied to screen for clinically significant affective disorders.

Exclusion criteria

Medical or neurological disorders producing cognitive deterioration and current psychiatric diagnosis according to the *Diagnostic and Statistical Manual of Mental Disorders,* Third Edition, Revised (DSM-III-R). Subjects on long-term medication.

End points

Testing performed before and after 15-day run-in period as well as at three-month intervals over nine months. Subjects were evaluated by the following tests: the Life Satisfaction in the Elderly Scale (LSES) evaluating eight categories of well-being; the Symptom Rating Scale (SRT), a checklist evaluating the frequency and intensity of depression, anxiety, somatisation, and inadequacy; and the Randt Memory Test, a battery of seven subtest scores to evaluate Acquisition-Recall (AR), Delayed Memory (DM), and the sum, indexed to age, yields the Memory Index (MI).

Results

At final evaluation, the SRT did not differ in the drug and placebo groups, whereas MI and LSES were significantly higher in the drug-treated group. Moreover, the negative correlation between the affective SRT and cognitive MI component of psychological well-being waned in the drug-treated group, but not in the placebo group. In the drug-treated group, a positive correlation emerged between the cognitive index and social contacts, mood, and self-concept factors of the LSES. Drug-treated subjects differed from controls in part by improved scores on objective cognitive tests, but even more so by modification of the correlations among indexes of psychological well-being and quality of life.

Side effects

None requiring withdrawal from study were reported.

Authors' comments

The effect of aging on cerebral function appears to be multidimensional in nature. Therefore a medication that is presumed to act on some of the mechanisms underlying AAMI meets the prerequisites as a candidate for drug therapy.

Reviewer's comments

Interesting, well-conducted study showing improved memory with treatment and a suggestion of enhanced quality of life. The trial lacked an adequate description of randomization and withdrawals or dropouts. (2, 6)

Clinical Study: Gericomplex®

Extract name	G115®
Manufacturer	Pharmaton S.A., Switzerland
Indication	**Geriatric rehabilitation**
Level of evidence	**II**
Therapeutic benefit	**No**

Bibliographic reference

Thommessen B, Laake K (1996). No identifiable effect of ginseng (Gericomplex) as an adjuvant in the treatment of geriatric patients. *Aging* (Milan, Italy) 8 (6): 417-420.

Trial design

Parallel.

Study duration	2 months
Dose	2 (40 mg G115 + vitamins, minerals, and trace elements) capsules daily
Route of administration	Oral
Randomized	Yes
Randomization adequate	No
Blinding	Double-blind
Blinding adequate	Yes
Placebo	Yes
Drug comparison	No
Site description	Single center
No. of subjects enrolled	60
No. of subjects completed	49
Sex	Male and female
Age	65-87 years (mean: 77.9)

Inclusion criteria
Patients admitted to a department of geriatric medicine for treatment and rehabilitation. Main diagnoses were cardiovascular, pulmonary, or musculoskeletal diseases, and depression/anxiety.

Exclusion criteria
Cognitive impairment Mini Mental State Examination (MMSE) score < 20, cancer, difficulties in swallowing, or in a terminal state of disease.

End points
Patients were assessed at baseline in the hospital and after eight weeks of treatment at home by the same physician. Activities of daily living (ADL) score was determined according to the Barthel ADL index. Cognitive function was assessed at baseline and after eight weeks using the MMSE, the Kendrick Object Learning test and the Trail-Making test. Somatic symptoms and symptoms of depression and anxiety were scored on a 23-question version of the Hopkins Symptom Checklist.

Results
Length of stay in hospital did not differ in the two groups. The groups also improved to the same degree on the various functional outcome measures, except for the Kendrick Object Learning test, on which the placebo group improved more markedly.

Side effects
None reported.

Authors' comments
We conclude that Gericomplex has no significant effect as an adjuvant in the rehabilitation of geriatric patients ages 65 years and older.

Reviewer's comments
A well-conducted and well-written study that failed to mention the randomization technique but nonetheless has a clear negative finding. (3, 6)

Product Profile: Gerimax Ginseng Extract

Manufacturer	**Dansk Droge, Denmark**
U.S. distributor	None
Botanical ingredient	**Ginseng root extract**
Extract name	None given
Quantity	100 mg
Processing	No information
Standardization	No information
Formulation	Tablet

Recommended dose: One tablet per day.

Comments: According to personal correspondence, Gerimax is a copy of the G115® extract (Pharmaton S.A.).

Source(s) of information: Sotaniemi, Haapakoshi, and Rautio, 1995; <www.nycomed. at/allgemein/detail_allgemein.php?produkt_id=21>.

Clinical Study: Gerimax Ginseng Extract

Extract name	None given
Manufacturer	Dansk Droge, Denmark
Indication	**Cognitive functioning** in healthy volunteers
Level of evidence	**II**
Therapeutic benefit	**Yes**

Bibliographic reference
Sorensen H, Sonne J (1996). A double-masked study of the effects of ginseng on cognitive functions. *Current Therapeutic Research* 57: 959-968.

Trial design
Parallel.

Study duration	8 to 9 weeks
Dose	400 mg ginseng extract
Route of administration	Oral
Randomized	Yes
Randomization adequate	No
Blinding	Double-blind
Blinding adequate	Yes
Placebo	Yes
Drug comparison	No
Site description	Not described
No. of subjects enrolled	127
No. of subjects completed	112
Sex	Male and female
Age	42-61 years (mean: 51)

Inclusion criteria
Healthy subjects ages 40 to 70.

Exclusion criteria
Serious illness, diseases of the central nervous system, and abuse of alcohol or drugs. Patients taking psychoactive medication that might interact with ginseng were also excluded.

End points
Patients received a battery of cognitive tests at baseline and again at the end of the study. The battery consisted of psychomotor tests (Simple Auditive Reaction Times Test, Simple Visual Reaction Times Test, and Finger-Tapping Test), attention and concentration tests (D2 Test and Fluency Test), learning and memory tests (Selective Reminding Test, Logical Memory and Reproduction Test, and Rey-Oestrich Complex Figure Test), and abstraction tests (Wisconsin Card Sorting Test). A questionnaire was also provided at the end of the trial for the subjects to discusses changes during the treatment period in their general well-being, energy, memory, concentration, and speed.

Results
The ginseng group showed a tendency toward faster simple reactions (Simple Auditive Reaction Times Tests; especially the most rapid auditive reaction time) and significantly better abstract thinking (Wisconsin Card Sorting Test) than the controls. No other differences in test scores reached signifi-

cance. With regards to the questionnaire, both groups reported a small improvement in general well-being and energy, but this did not reach significance.

Side effects
No side effects were identified.

Authors' comments
The group that received ginseng for eight to nine weeks showed slightly faster reaction times than the placebo group. Similarly, the subjects who received ginseng performed significantly better on an abstraction test. These findings conform to the assumption that ginseng causes increased alertness and arousal.

Reviewer's comments
This is a well-conducted trial showing some benefit of ginseng on reaction times and executive function. The results are also suggestive of enhancement on the Selective Reminding Test, which is relevant to a similar finding in Kennedy, Scholey, and Wesnes (2001). (3, 5)

Clinical Study: Gerimax Ginseng Extract

Extract name	None given
Manufacturer	Dansk Droge, Denmark
Indication	**Diabetes (NIDDM)**
Level of evidence	**III**
Therapeutic benefit	**Yes**

Bibliographic reference
Sotaniemi EA, Haapakoski E, Rautio A (1995). Ginseng therapy in non-insulin-dependent diabetic patients. *Diabetics Care* 18 (10): 1373-1375.

Trial design
Parallel. Pretrial run-in period of eight weeks. Patients were instructed to follow a diet consisting of 20 percent protein, 50 percent carbohydrates, and 30 percent fat.

Study duration	2 months
Dose	100 or 200 mg ginseng daily
Route of administration	Oral
Randomized	Yes
Randomization adequate	No

Blinding	Double-blind
Blinding adequate	No
Placebo	Yes
Drug comparison	No
Site description	Not described
No. of subjects enrolled	36
No. of subjects completed	36
Sex	Male and female
Age	48-61 years (mean: 58.7)

Inclusion criteria
Newly diagnosed non-insulin-dependent diabetes mellitus (NIDDM) patients.

Exclusion criteria
None mentioned.

End points
Patients kept diaries to monitor their physical activity, and the change was compared to the pretrial period. Patients self-rated subjective tests of mood, well-being, and vigor. Psychoperformance and memory (Digit Span test) were also tested. Patients were interviewed with a questionnaire about their sleep, degree of fatigue, and lifestyle. The following were also measured to evaluate efficacy: blood glucose and insulin levels; serum lipids; glycated hemoglobin (HbA1c); serum aminoterminalpropeptide (PIIINP); and body weight.

Results
Both doses of ginseng improved psychomotor performance, mood, and vigor significantly, and the 200 mg dose also improved well-being and physical activity significantly, all compared to baseline. Sleep and memory did not change significantly. Body weight was reduced significantly by all three groups. Fasting blood glucose was improved by both the 100 mg and 200 mg dose compared to placebo. The 200 mg dose also reduced serum HbA_{1c} and PIIINP values. Ginseng did not change serum lipid values.

Side effects
No side effects associated with the treatment.

Authors' comments
Our study demonstrates that drugs that activate mood and psychophysical performance may improve glucose balance.

Reviewer's comments
This is an important study showing improved cognition and mood in non-

insulin-dependent diabetics plus a lowering of fasting blood glucose. Neither the blinding nor the randomization were adequately described. (1, 6)

Product Profile: American Ginseng

Manufacturer	**Chai-Na-Ta Corporation, Canada**
U.S. distributor	None
Botanical ingredient	**Ginseng, American root**
Extract name	N/A
Quantity	500 mg
Processing	3-year-old Ontario dried and ground ginseng root
Standardization	No information
Formulation	Capsule

Comments: Product is not yet available on the market.

Source(s) of information: Vuksan et al., 2001; information provided by manufacturer.

Clinical Study: American Ginseng

Extract name	N/A
Manufacturer	Chai-Na-Ta Corporation, Canada
Indication	**Diabetes (NIDDM)**
Level of evidence	**III**
Therapeutic benefit	**Trend**

Bibliographic reference
Vuksan V, Sievenpiper JL, Koo VYY, Francis T, Beljan-Zdravkovic U, Xu Z, Vidgen E (2000). American ginseng (*Panax quinquefolius* L) reduces postprandial glycemia in nondiabetic subjects and subjects with type 2 diabetes mellitus. *Archives of Internal Medicine* 160 (7): 1009-1013.

Trial design
Crossover. Ten nondiabetic (ND) and nine diabetic (D) subjects participated in the study. Participants received one of two treatments (placebo or 3 g ginseng) at 0 or 40 minutes before an oral glucose challenge. Subjects were required to fast overnight (10 to 12 hours) before testing. A minimum of one week separated each of the four test days.

Study duration	1 day
Dose	3 g powdered root
Route of administration	Oral
Randomized	Yes
Randomization adequate	No
Blinding	Single-blind
Blinding adequate	No
Placebo	Yes
Drug comparison	No
Site description	One hospital
No. of subjects enrolled	ND:10; D: 9
No. of subjects completed	ND:10; D: 9
Sex	Male and female
Age	Means: ND: 34 ± 7 years; D: 62 ± 7 years

Inclusion criteria
Nondiabetic subjects and subjects with reasonably well-controlled type 2 diabetes mellitus (current treatments included diet, sulfonylurea, and a combination of sulfonylurea and metformin; these treatments were maintained constant during the study).

Exclusion criteria
None mentioned.

End points
Thirty minutes before the beginning of each test, the subjects with type 2 diabetes mellitus took their regular medication. Capillary blood was then collected for both sets of subjects before the administration of treatment, and at 0, 15, 30, 45, 60, and 90 minutes after the start of a 25 g oral glucose challenge. The diabetic subjects were also tested again at 120 minutes after the glucose challenge. Blood glucose levels of samples were later calculated.

Results
In nondiabetic subjects, ginseng did not significantly lower incremental glycemia after the glucose challenge when the administration was at the time of the challenge. Incremental glycemia was significantly lowered compared with placebo at 45 and 60 minutes after the challenge when ginseng was administered 40 minutes before the challenge (both $p < 0.05$). In addition, when ginseng was administered before, the area under the blood glucose curve was significantly lower than with placebo ($p < 0.05$), with a reduction of 18 percent. In subjects with diabetes, incremental glycemia was significantly lowered compared with placebo at 45 and 60 minutes when ginseng was given with the challenge (both $p < 0.05$) and at 30 and 45 minutes

when ginseng was given 40 minutes before the challenge (both $p < 0.05$). The areas under the curve were also significantly lower for ginseng than placebo for both administration times (both $p < 0.05$), with reductions of 22 percent (with challenge) and 19 percent (40 minutes before).

Side effects
Mild insomnia was reported by one subject with diabetes after taking ginseng.

Authors' comments
To our knowledge, we are the first to demonstrate an effect of American ginseng on postprandial glycemia in humans. We noticed significant blood glucose-lowering action both in nondiabetic subjects and subjects with type 2 diabetes mellitus when ginseng was given 40 minutes prior to the test meal.

Reviewer's comments
Despite the limitations of sample size and scope, this study offers valuable information regarding the acute effects of American ginseng in both normoglycemic individuals and those with type 2 diabetes. The results suggest a possible effect in individuals with impaired glucose tolerance; however, the duration of the experiments (less than two hours) makes it impossible to comment on long-term clinical significance in the treatment of diabetes. (1, 5)

Clinical Study: American Ginseng

Extract name	N/A
Manufacturer	Chai-Na-Ta Corporation, Canada

Indication	**Diabetes (NIDDM)**
Level of evidence	**II**
Therapeutic benefit	**Trend**

Bibliographic reference
Vuksan V, Stavro MP, Sievenpiper JL, Beljan-Zdravkovic U, Leiter LA, Josse RG, Xu Z (2000). Similar postprandial glycemic reductions with escalation of dose and administration time of American ginseng in type 2 diabetes. *Diabetes Care* 23 (9): 1221-1226.

Trial design
Crossover. Participants received one of four treatments (placebo, 3 g, 6 g, or 9 g powdered ginseng) at 0, 40, 80, or 120 minutes before an oral glucose challenge. Subjects were required to fast overnight (10 to 12 hours) before testing. A minimum of three days separated each of the 16 test days.

Study duration	1 day
Dose	3, 6, or 9 g powdered root
Route of administration	Oral
Randomized	Yes
Randomization adequate	Yes
Blinding	Single-blind
Blinding adequate	No
Placebo	Yes
Drug comparison	No
Site description	One hospital
No. of subjects enrolled	10
No. of subjects completed	10
Sex	Male and female
Age	Mean: 63 ± 2 years.

Inclusion criteria
Subjects with type 2 diabetes mellitus (current treatments included diet, sulfonylurea, and a combination of sulfonylurea and metformin).

Exclusion criteria
None mentioned.

End points
Capillary blood was collected before the administration of treatment and at 0, 15, 30, 45, 60, 90, and 120 minutes after the start of a 25 g oral glucose challenge. Blood glucose levels of samples were later calculated.

Results
For all doses of American ginseng, a significant effect was observed on incremental glycemia at 30, 45, 60, 90, and 120 minutes ($p < 0.05$). Reductions in the areas under the blood glucose curve occurred for all doses (3 g: 19.7 percent; 6 g: 15.3 percent; 9 g: 15.9 percent) and were significant ($p < 0.05$). No differences were observed between the doses. The time of administration did not affect either incremental glycemia or the area under the blood glucose curve. However, for the area under the curve, there was a significant interaction between dose and time of administration ($p = 0.037$).

Side effects
None reported.

Authors' comments
Consistent with our previous study, the present findings demonstrated the efficacy of American ginseng in reducing postprandial glycemia in type 2 di-

abetes. The reductions, however, occurred independent of the dose used or the time of administration. Taken together, these data indicate that 3 g administered within two hours of the test may be sufficient to achieve reductions in postprandial glycemia in type 2 diabetic individuals.

Reviewer's comments
Despite the preliminary nature of the study, these results suggest a possible therapeutic benefit in patients with type 2 diabetes. Further investigations are needed in larger, longer-term trials with end points such as hemoglobin A_{1C}. (3, 5)

Clinical Study: American Ginseng

Extract name	N/A
Manufacturer	Chai-Na-Ta Corporation, Canada
Indication	**Postprandial glycemia** in healthy volunteers
Level of evidence	**III**
Therapeutic benefit	**Undetermined**

Bibliographic reference
Vuksan V, Stavro MP, Sievenpiper JL, Koo VYY, Wong E, Beljan-Zdravkovic U, Francis T, Jenkins AL, Leiter LA, Josse AB, et al. (2000). American ginseng improves glycemia in individuals with normal glucose tolerance: Effect of dose and time escalation. *Journal of the American College of Nutrition* 19 (6): 738-744.

Trial design
Crossover. Participants received one of four treatments (placebo, 3 g, 6 g, or 9 g powdered ginseng) at 40, 80, or 120 minutes before an oral glucose challenge. Subjects were required to fast overnight (10 to 12 hours) before testing. A minimum of three days separated each of the 12 test days.

Study duration	1 day
Dose	3, 6, or 9 g powdered root
Route of administration	Oral
Randomized	Yes
Randomization adequate	No
Blinding	Single-blind
Blinding adequate	No
Placebo	Yes

Drug comparison	No
Site description	One hospital
No. of subjects enrolled	10
No. of subjects completed	10
Sex	Male and female
Age	Mean: 41 ± 2 years

Inclusion criteria
Nondiabetic individuals.

Exclusion criteria
None mentioned.

End points
Capillary blood was collected before the administration of treatment and at 0, 15, 30, 45, 60, and 90 minutes after the start of a 25 g oral glucose challenge. Blood glucose levels of samples were later calculated.

Results
Independent of administration time, incremental glucose values for all doses of ginseng were significantly lower than placebo ($p < 0.05$) at 30, 45, and 60 minutes after the glucose challenge. Both 3 and 9 g of ginseng were significantly lower than placebo at 90 minutes ($p < 0.05$). At 45 minutes post-challenge, the incremental glucose concentration for 9 g was significantly lower than 3 g ginseng ($p < 0.05$). Reductions in the areas under the blood glucose curve for 3, 6, or 9 g ginseng were 26.6 percent, 29.3 percent, and 38.5 percent, respectively. No significant differences were found between the ginseng administration times.

Side effects
None reported.

Authors' comments
The results of this study coincided with our previous finding that 3 g of American ginseng (AG) consumed 40 minutes before a 25 g glucose challenge improves glucose tolerance in normoglycemic individuals. However, the current results contraindicated our study hypothesis, such that no further enhancement of glucose tolerance occurred with escalating AG doses above 3 g, and/or administering them earlier than 40 minutes before the glucose challenge.

Reviewer's comments
The study is limited by its small sample size, single-blinding, short duration of the experiments, and limited description of the inclusion and exclusion criteria. Although the results provide information on acute postprandial effects on individuals with normal glucose tolerance, conclusions cannot be made

regarding longer-term therapeutic effects on subjects with impaired glucose tolerance or diabetes. (1, 3)

Clinical Study: American Ginseng

Extract name	N/A
Manufacturer	Chai-Na-Ta Corporation, Canada
Indication	**Postprandial glycemia** in healthy volunteers
Level of evidence	**III**
Therapeutic benefit	**Undetermined**

Bibliographic reference
Vuksan V, Sievenpiper JL, Wong J, Xu Z, Beljan-Zdravkovic U, Arnason JT, Assinewe V, Starvro MP, Jenkins AL, Leiter LA, et al. (2001). American ginseng (*Panax quinquefolius* L.) attenuates postprandial glycemia in a time-dependent but not dose-dependent manner in healthy individuals. *American Journal of Clinical Nutrition* 73 (4): 753-758.

Trial design
Crossover. Participants received one of four treatments (placebo, 1 g, 2 g, or 3 g powdered ginseng) at 40, 20, 10, or 0 minutes before an oral glucose challenge. Subjects were required to fast overnight (10 to 12 hours) before testing. A minimum of three days separated each of the 16 test days.

Study duration	1 day
Dose	1, 2, or 3 g powdered root
Route of administration	Oral
Randomized	Yes
Randomization adequate	No
Blinding	Single-blind
Blinding adequate	No
Placebo	Yes
Drug comparison	No
Site description	One hospital
No. of subjects enrolled	12
No. of subjects completed	12
Sex	Male and female
Age	Mean: 42 years

Inclusion criteria
Healthy subjects without diabetes.

Exclusion criteria
None mentioned.

End points
Capillary blood was collected before the administration of treatment and at 0, 15, 30, 45, 60, and 90 minutes after the start of a 25 g oral glucose challenge. Blood glucose levels of samples were later calculated.

Results
The main effects of treatment and administration time were significant ($p < 0.05$) by way of two-way analysis of variance. Over the last 45 minutes of the test, glycemia was lower than placebo with all doses of ginseng ($p < 0.05$), but no significant differences were observed between doses. Reductions in the areas under the blood glucose curve for 1, 2, or 3 g ginseng were 14.4 percent, 10.6 percent, and 9.1 percent, respectively. In the last hour of the test, glycemia was significantly lower when ginseng was given 40 minutes before the glucose challenge than when it was given 20, 10, or 0 minutes before the challenge ($p < 0.05$).

Side effects
No adverse effects were reported.

Authors' comments
The American ginseng used in the present study reduced postprandial glycemia in healthy subjects without diabetes in a manner that was dependent on the time of administration but not the dose. An effect was seen only when administration was 40 minutes before the challenge, and doses within the range of 1 to 3 g were equally effective. This lack of a dose response suggests that the next step should be to study lower doses.

Reviewer's comments
This study suggests that lower doses (1 g) can still affect glucose tolerance, as compared to higher doses used in the investigators' previous studies. However, the conclusions that can be drawn from the study are limited, and no statements can be made regarding longer-term therapeutic effects. The study was limited by the small sample size, the short-term nature of the experiments, and the limited description of the inclusion and exclusion criteria. (1, 4)

Clinical Study: American Ginseng

Extract name	N/A
Manufacturer	Chai-Na-Ta Corporation, Canada
Indication	**Postpriandial glycemia** in healthy volunteers
Level of evidence	**II**
Therapeutic benefit	**No**

Bibliographic reference

Sievenpiper JL, Arnason JT, Leiter LA, Vuksan V (2003). Variable effects of American ginseng: A batch of American ginseng (*Panax quinquefolius* L.) with a depressed ginsenoside profile does not affect postprandial glycemia. *European Journal of Clinical Nutrition* 57 (2): 243-248.

Trial design

Crossover. Volunteers were given either ginseng or placebo on two test days, separated by at least three days. Treatment was given 40 minutes prior to the start of a 75 g oral glucose tolerance test. Subjects were asked to maintain the same exercise and dietary patterns the evening before each test and to consume at least 150 g of carbohydrates each day in the three days preceding the test.

Study duration	1 day
Dose	6 g powdered root
Route of administration	Oral
Randomized	Yes
Randomization adequate	No
Blinding	Single-blind
Blinding adequate	No
Placebo	Yes
Drug comparison	No
Site description	1 hospital
No. of subjects enrolled	12
No. of subjects completed	12
Sex	Male and female
Age	Mean: 31 ± 3 years

Inclusion criteria

Healthy volunteers.

Exclusion criteria

Younger than 18 years or older than 75 years; previous diagnosis of dysglycemia, kidney or liver disease, morbid obesity, or a major surgery in the last six months.

End points

A fasting blood sample was collected before the administration of treatment, and blood was again collected at 0, 15, 30, 45, 60, 90, and 120 minutes after the start of the 75 g oral glucose tolerance test. Blood glucose levels of samples were later calculated.

Results

American ginseng had no significant effects on incremental plasma glucose, incremental plasma insulin, or their areas under the curve (indices of insulin sensitivity) compared to placebo.

Side effects

No difference in side effects reported by the ginseng and placebo groups, which included: nausea, belching, bloating, headache, dizziness, light-headedness, diarrhea, flatulence, polyuria, numbness, anxiety, insomnia, cramping, or thirst.

Authors' comments

The present study demonstrated a favorable safety profile for the present batch of American ginseng but a lack of effect in postprandial indices of glycemia and insulinemia. This lack of efficacy is in direct contrast to previous studies (Vuksan, Sievenpiper, et al., 2000; Vuksan, Stavro, Sievenpiper, Beljan-Zdravkovic, et al., 2000; Vuksan, Stavro, Sievenpiper, Koo., et al., 2000; Vuksan et al., 2001). The reasons for this difference are unknown but might be due to differences in composition between the batch of ginseng used in this study compared to the batch used in previous studies. Although the ginsenoside profile confirmed that the present batch was also *Panax quinquefolius* L., marked differences in ginsenosides were observed compared to the original batch.

Reviewer's comments

This study demonstrates the complex nature of herbs and the inherent difficulties in studying them in clinical trials. Differences in ginsenoside profiles between ginseng batches used in the different trials may have been the cause of the different results. It seems that we must further understand these active components before a specific preparation is studied in a larger, longer-term trial. (1, 5)